TOCOTRIENOLS
VITAMIN E BEYOND TOCOPHEROLS
Second Edition

AOCS MISSION STATEMENT

To be a global forum to promote the exchange of ideas, information, and experience; to enhance personal excellence; and to provide high standards of quality among those with a professional interest in the science and technology of fats, oils, surfactants, and related materials.

AOCS BOOKS AND SPECIAL PUBLICATIONS COMMITTEE

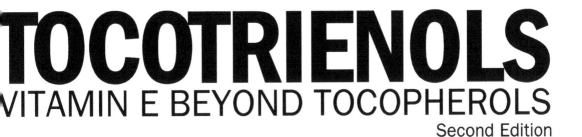

TOCOTRIENOLS
VITAMIN E BEYOND TOCOPHEROLS
Second Edition

Edited by

Barrie Tan

Ronald Ross Watson

Victor R. Preedy

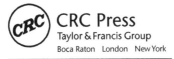

CRC Press
Taylor & Francis Group
Boca Raton   London   New York

CRC Press is an imprint of the
Taylor & Francis Group, an **informa** business

Cover: Design & photography by Thong Vo of annatto seed pod with thanks to Harrison Tan for his assistance. Annatto (*Bixa orellana*) is a plant from which tocopherol-free tocotrienol is obtained.

CRC Press
Taylor & Francis Group
6000 Broken Sound Parkway NW, Suite 300
Boca Raton, FL 33487-2742

First issued in paperback 2016

© 2013 by American Oil Chemists Society
CRC Press is an imprint of Taylor & Francis Group, an Informa business

No claim to original U.S. Government works

Version Date: 20120719

ISBN 13: 978-1-138-19972-9 (pbk)
ISBN 13: 978-1-4398-8441-6 (hbk)

Library of Congress Cataloging-in-Publication Data

Tocotrienols : vitamin E beyond tocopherols / editors, Barrie Tan, Ronald Ross Watson, Victor R. Preedy.
-- 2nd ed.
  p. ; cm.
Includes bibliographical references and index.
ISBN 978-1-4398-8441-6 (hardcover : alk. paper)
I. Tan, Barrie. II. Watson, Ronald R. (Ronald Ross) III. Preedy, Victor R.
[DNLM: 1. Tocotrienols. QU 179]

612.3'99--dc23   2012027080

Visit the Taylor & Francis Web site at
http://www.taylorandfrancis.com

and the CRC Press Web site at
http://www.crcpress.com

Contents

Preface

For 90 years, vitamin E research has produced prolific and notable discoveries, including isolation from plants, chemical identifications, and total syntheses. Until the last few decades, however, attention has been given mostly to the biological activities and underlying mechanisms of alpha-tocopherol, which we now know is only one of more than eight vitamin E isomers. Beginning in 1922 with the announcement by Herbert Evans and Katherine Bishop that "the mysterious substance X" would henceforth be known as vitamin E, "a hitherto unrecognized dietary factor essential for reproduction" [1], there have been many good days for the science of this "birth vitamin." Following the discovery of vitamin E's antioxidant function [2], the preponderant research in subsequent decades (1965–1985) focused on food protection, an activity offered particularly by, once again, alpha-tocopherol [3].

Tocotrienol discovery came much later, in 1965 [4,5], but existed for almost 20 years as an obscure vitamin E [6]. Vitamin E was erroneously named tocopherol, an error that remained uncorrected [7] for 30 years—appearing as such in the Merck Index as recently as 1996—until eventually changed in 2001 [8]. Recognition for tocotrienol began to emerge in the early 1980s at the University of Wisconsin, Madison, through the efforts of Asaf Qureshi and Charles Elson. They were the first to delineate the function of tocotrienol to lower cholesterol [9,10]. The mechanism, initially shown by a group at Bristol-Myers Squibb (1992) [11], was validated nearly 15 years later at the University of Texas, Dallas (2006) [12], by studies on the regulation of HMG CoA reductase by delta-tocotrienol and gamma-tocotrienol, but not alpha-tocopherol. This 2006 study was endorsed by Joseph Goldstein and Michael Brown, the 1985 Nobel Prize recipients for the discovery of the LDL receptor [13]. Another noteworthy development took place in 1985 when the ability of tocotrienol, but not alpha-tocopherol, to inhibit tumors was first shown [14,15] by the research group with Kanki Komiyama of Kitasato Institute, Tokyo, Japan.

I personally became very excited about tocotrienols back in 1982. I remember meeting A. Kato who was working on vitamin E and cancer inhibition when almost everyone was talking about "rich vitamin E" in palm oil. I became curious to figure out more about this vitamin E. In 1983, I met Asaf Qureshi and Charles Elson at an annual Palm Oil Research Institute of Malaysia grant update meeting, and even then they had a hunch that alpha-tocotrienol may not be the strongest tocotrienol for cholesterol reduction. Subsequently, I continued to follow the flow of research and clinical trials while developing patents for extracting tocotrienols from natural sources—initially palm, and then rice and annatto.

Tocotrienols have now stepped into the limelight of vitamin E research and have proven to contain some exceptional benefits that are not shared by their "older" tocopherol siblings. Today, the brightest spot for tocotrienol research is in cancer and CVD (Figure F.1). Tocopherols and tocotrienols are powerful antioxidants—known as early as 1937 [2]—for improving food protection and are shown today [16] to potentially protect from cognitive decline. This antioxidant vitamin E function never gets old! Emergent fields of tocotrienol research are promising—with many covered in this volume—including angiogenesis, bioavailability, bone health, gastric injury, inflammation, life extension, obesity, radiation protection, skin health, tocopherol interference, and, recently, cognitive impairment.

The availability of tocotrienol samples and standards has helped to catalyze the research forward. The three major sources of tocotrienols are rice, palm, and annatto. The ratio of tocopherol-to-tocotrienol in each is 50:50, 25:75, and 0.1:99.9, respectively [17]. Tocotrienol's natural abundance is important as alpha-tocopherol has repeatedly been shown to be ineffective, or worse, to interfere with the function of tocotrienols.

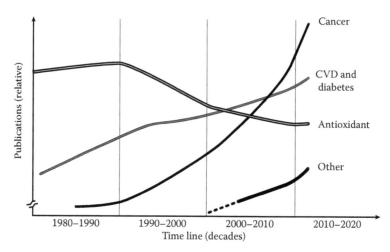

FIGURE F.1   Progress in tocotrienol research.

Research published in the last decade warranted the publication of the first-ever tocotrienol book, forwarded by Chandan Sen, indicating a wealth of vitamin E literature (greater than 95%) focused on alpha-tocopherol. Currently, tocotrienols have reached a new measure of research height: more than one-third of all vitamin E tocotrienol research of the last 30 years was published in the last 3 years (2009–2011). The thriving field of tocotrienol research gives ground for this second edition, launched in conjunction with the *103rd Annual AOCS Meeting* (April 29, 2012, Long Beach, California). It is an excellent time to continue the vitamin E research with a new focus on tocotrienols, the late arrival in the vitamin E family.

Barrie Tan
American River Nutrition
Hadley, Massachusetts

REFERENCES

1. Evans HM, Bishop KS. On the existence of a hitherto unrecognized dietary factor essential for reproduction. *Science* 1922 (December 8); LVI: 650–651.
2. Olcott HS, Emerson OH. Antioxidants and autoxidation of fats: The antioxidant properties of tocopherols. *J Am Chem Soc* 1937; 59: 1008–1009.
3. Eitenmillar R, Lee J. *Vitamin E: Food Chemistry, Composition and Analysis*, Marcel Dekker, New York, 2004.
4. Pennock JF et al., Reassessment of tocopherol chemistry. *BBRC* 1964; 17: 542–548.
5. Whittle KJ et al., The isolation and properties of delta-tocotrienol from Hevea latex. *Biochem J* 1966; 100: 138–145.
6. Tan B, Appropriate spectrum vitamin E and new perspectives on desmethyl tocopherols and tocotrienols. *J Am Nutr Assoc* 2005; 8: 35–42.
7. Merck Index, *Tocols: 9631 through 9638*, 12th edn. Merck Publishing Group, Rahway, NJ, 1996, pp. 1620–1621.
8. Merck Index, *Tocols: 9570 through 9577*, 13th edn. Merck Publishing Group, Rahway, NJ, 2001, pp. 1693–1694.
9. Burger WC et al., Effects of different fractions of the barley kernel on the hepatic lipid metabolism of chickens. *Lipids* 1982; 17: 956–963.
10. Qureshi AA et al., The structure of an inhibitor of cholesterol biosynthesis isolated from barley. *J Biol Chem* 1986; 261: 10544–10550.
11. Pearce BC et al., Hypercholesterolemic activity of synthetic and natural tocotrienols. *J Med Chem* 1992; 35: 3595–3606.

12. Song BL, DeBose-Boyd RA. Insig-dependent ubiquitination and degradation of 3-hydroxy-3-methylgl-utaryl coenzyme A reductase (HMGR) stimulated by delta- and gamma-tocotrienols. *J Biol Chem* 2006; 281: 25054–25061.
13. Nobel Prize.org, http://nobelprize.org/nobel_prizes/medicine/laureates/1985/
14. Kato A et al., Physiological effect of alpha-tocotrienol. *J Jpn Oil Chem Soc* 1985; 34: 375–376.
15. Komiyama K et al., Studies on the biological activity of tocotrienols. *Chem Pharm Bull* 1989; 37: 1369–1371.
16. Mangialasche F et al., Tocopherols and tocotrienols plasma levels are associated with cognitive impairment. *Neurobiol Aging* (2012). doi: 10.1016/j. neurobiolaging.2011.11.019.
17. Tan B, Mueller A. Tocotrienols in cardiometabolic diseases. In Tocotrienols: *Vitamin E Beyond Tocopherols* (Eds. Watson RS, Preedy VR), CRC & AOCS Press, Boca Raton, FL, 2009, Chapter 19, pp. 257–273.

Acknowledgments

It is a pleasure to take a moment and acknowledge the work of some very dedicated individuals and organizations who greatly contributed to this book.

The second edition of *Tocotrienols: Vitamin E Beyond Tocopherols* inspired the decision to hold a *Second International Tocotrienol Symposium*, which took place in conjunction with the *103rd Annual Meeting of the AOCS* in Long Beach, California (April 29, 2012). The symposium allowed many of the authors to take to the podium and present their latest groundbreaking discoveries, including how tocotrienols work, novel product formulations and combinations, as well as the latest animal studies and clinical outcomes. American River Nutrition, Inc.—a company committed for more than 15 years to support research in lipid-soluble nutrients (especially vitamin E tocotrienols)—and the Natural Health Research Institute (Elwood Richards) cosponsored the symposium in an effort to educate the public on vitamin E tocotrienols.

For this book, the editorial work landed squarely on the desk of Anne Trias who, besides being an excellent tocotrienol researcher in antibacterial functions of tocotrienols, handled the bulk of correspondence with manuscripts. Anne received expert assistance from AOCS and staff members of Taylor & Francis Group. Along the way, editorial assistance was gratefully received from Dr. Elizabeth Bachrach, Dr. Huanbiao Mo, and Bethany Stevens.

Editors

Barrie Tan received his PhD in analytical chemistry from the University of Otago, New Zealand, and later became a professor at the University of Massachusetts Amherst (chemistry and food science/nutrition). He has almost 30 years of research experience in lipid soluble vitamins, with particular focus in tocotrienols, tocopherols, carotenoids, cholesterol, CoQ10, and omega 3s.

Dr. Tan has commercialized natural carotenoids (e.g., lutein and zeaxanthin, alpha- and beta-carotene, lycopene) and was the first to introduce tocotrienol from current sources (palm, rice, and annatto) to the nutrition industry. He is the inventor of numerous tocotrienol extractions from natural sources and their application in product formulation. The continuous string of discoveries includes tocotrienols from palm (1992), then rice (1998), and finally annatto (2002).

Dr. Tan founded American River Nutrition, Inc. (www.AmericanRiverNutrition.com) in 1998 and developed the first ever tocopherol-free tocotrienol product derived from annatto beans. The annatto plant originates from the Amazon rainforest and has been used since ancient times. In addition to gaining expert status on developing tocotrienol as a condition-specific product, Dr. Tan has been involved in numerous studies on tocotrienols for cancer, prediabetes/diabetes, antioxidant potential, and lipidemia. His research in phytonutrients resulted in the development of many products, largely of natural origin, that impact chronic and degenerative conditions.

Ronald Ross Watson, PhD, attended the University of Idaho but graduated from Brigham Young University in Provo, Utah, with a degree in chemistry in 1966. He received his PhD in biochemistry from Michigan State University in 1971. His postdoctoral schooling in nutrition and microbiology was completed at the Harvard School of Public Health, where he gained two years of postdoctoral research experience in immunology and nutrition.

From 1973 to 1974, Dr. Watson was assistant professor of immunology and performed research at the University of Mississippi Medical Center in Jackson. He was assistant professor of microbiology and immunology at the Indiana University Medical School from 1974 to 1978 and associate professor at Purdue University in the Department of Food and Nutrition from 1978 to 1982. In 1982, Dr. Watson joined the faculty at the University of Arizona Health Sciences Center in the Department of Family and Community Medicine of the School of Medicine. He is currently professor of health promotion sciences in the Mel and Enid Zuckerman Arizona College of Public Health.

Dr. Watson is a member of several national and international nutrition, immunology, cancer, and alcoholism research societies. Among his patents is on a dietary supplement-passion fruit peel extract-with more pending. He has been researching melatonin effects on mouse AIDS and immune function for 20 years, and has edited a book on melatonin (Watson RR. *Melatonin in the Promotion of Health*, CRC Press, 1998, 224 pp). For 30 years, Dr. Watson has been funded by Wallace Research Foundation to study dietary supplements in health promotion. He has edited more than 35 books on nutrition, dietary supplements, and over-the-counter agents, and 53 other scientific books. He has also published more than 500 research and review articles.

Professor Victor R. Preedy, BSc, DSc, FIBiol, FRCPath, FRSPH, currently serves as professor of nutritional biochemistry in the Department of Nutrition and Dietetics, King's College London, and honorary professor of clinical biochemistry in the Department of Clinical Biochemistry, King's College London. He is also the director of the Genomics Centre, King's College London. Professor Preedy received his PhD in 1981, and in 1992 he received his membership of the Royal College of Pathologists, based on his published works. He was elected a fellow of the Royal College of Pathologists in 2000. In 1993, he received his DSc for outstanding contribution to protein metabolism. Professor Preedy was elected as a fellow of the Royal Society for the Promotion of Health (2004) and the Royal Institute of Public Health (2004). In 2009, he was elected as a fellow of the Royal Society for Public Health (RSPH). The RSPH is governed by Royal Charter, and Her Majesty The Queen is its patron. Professor Preedy has written or edited over 550 articles, which include over 160 peer-reviewed manuscripts based on original research, 85 reviews, and 30 books. His interests pertain to matters concerning nutrition and health at the individual and societal levels.

Contributors

Chisato Abe
Department of Life and
   Environmental Science
Tsu City College
Tsu, Japan

Bharat B. Aggarwal
Cytokine Research Laboratory
Department of Experimental Therapeutics
MD Anderson Cancer Center
The University of Texas
Houston, Texas

María A. Asensi-Fabado
Faculty of Biology
Department of Plant Biology
University of Barcelona
Barcelona, Spain

Philip J. Breen
Department of Pharmaceutical Sciences
University of Arkansas for Medical Sciences
Little Rock, Arkansas

Lindsay Brown
Department of Biological and Physical
   Sciences
University of Southern Queensland
Toowoomba, Queensland, Australia

Sharon E. Campbell
Department of Biochemistry
James H. Quillen College of Medicine
East Tennessee State University
Johnson City, Tennessee

Jana Cela
Faculty of Biology
Department of Plant Biology
University of Barcelona
Barcelona, Spain

A. Chatterjee
Faculty of Medicine
MARA University of Technology
Shah Alam, Malaysia

Silvia Ciffolilli
Department of Internal Medicine
University of Perugia
Perugia, Italy

Amy Clewell
AIBMR Life Sciences
Bloomington, Indiana

Cesar M. Compadre
Department of Pharmaceutical Sciences
University of Arkansas for Medical Sciences
Little Rock, Arkansas

Peter A. Crooks
Department of Pharmaceutical Sciences
University of Arkansas for Medical Sciences
Little Rock, Arkansas

Takahiro Eitsuka
Faculty of Applied Life Sciences
Niigata University of Pharmacy and Applied
   Life Sciences
Niigata, Japan

Manal Elfakhani
Department of Nutrition and Food Sciences
Texas Woman's University
Denton, Texas

John R. Endres
AIBMR Life Sciences, Inc.
Puyallup, Washington

Yukiko Fujikura
Department of Food and Human Health Sciences
Graduate School of Human Life Science
Osaka City University
Osaka, Japan

Francesco Galli
Department of Internal Medicine
University of Perugia
Perugia, Italy

Sanchita Ghosh
Armed Forces Radiobiology
    Research Institute
Uniformed Services University of the Health
    Sciences
Bethesda, Maryland

Arvind Goja
Department of Nutrition and Food Science
Wayne State University
Detroit, Michigan

Smiti V. Gupta
Department of Nutrition and Food Science
Wayne State University
Detroit, Michigan

Subash C. Gupta
Cytokine Research Laboratory
Department of Experimental Therapeutics
MD Anderson Cancer Center
The University of Texas
Houston, Texas

Martin Hauer-Jensen
Department of Pharmaceutical Sciences
University of Arkansas for Medical Sciences
Little Rock, Arkansas

Mark Houston
School of Medicine
Vanderbilt University
and
Hypertension Institute
Saint Thomas Hospital
Nashville, Tennessee

Kazim Husain
Department of Gastrointestinal Oncology
Moffitt Cancer Center
Tampa, Florida

Ibrahim Abdel Aziz Ibrahim
Faculty of Medicine
MARA University of Technology
Shah Alam, Malaysia

Saiko Ikeda
Department of Nutritional Sciences
Nagoya University of Arts and Sciences
Nisshin, Japan

Nafeeza Mohd Ismail
Faculty of Medicine
MARA University of Technology
Shah Alam, Malaysia

Xiangming Ji
Department of Nutrition and Food Science
Wayne State University
Detroit, Michigan

Mary Kaileh
Laboratory of Molecular Biology
    and Immunology
National Institute on Aging
Baltimore, Maryland

Y.S. Kamsani
Faculty of Medicine
MARA University of Technology
Shah Alam, Malaysia

Noriko Kashima
Department of Food and Human Health
    Sciences
Graduate School of Human Life Science
Osaka City University
Osaka, Japan

Tomomi Komura
Department of Food and Human Health
    Sciences
Graduate School of Human Life Science
Osaka City University
Osaka, Japan

Koymangalath Krishnan
Division of Hematology-Oncology
Department of Internal Medicine
James H. Quillen College of Medicine
East Tennessee State University
Johnson City, Tennessee

K. Sree Kumar
Armed Forces Radiobiology
    Research Institute
Bethesda, Maryland

Mao-Jung Lee
Susan Lehman Cullman Laboratory
    for Cancer Research
Department of Chemical Biology
and
Center for Cancer Prevention Research
Ernest Mario School of Pharmacy
Rutgers, The State University
    of New Jersey
Piscataway, New Jersey

Mokenge P. Malafa
Department of Gastrointestinal Oncology
Moffitt Cancer Center
Tampa, Florida

Teruo Miyazawa
Food and Biodynamic Chemistry Laboratory
Graduate School of Agricultural Science
Tohoku University
Sendai, Japan

Huanbiao Mo
Department of Nutrition and Food
    Sciences
Texas Woman's University
Denton, Texas

Norazlina Mohamed
Faculty of Medicine
Department of Pharmacology
National University of Malaysia
Kuala Lumpur, Malaysia

N. Mokhtar
Department of Physiology
National University of Malaysia
Kuala Lumpur, Malaysia

Norliza Muhammad
Faculty of Medicine
Department of Pharmacology
National University of Malaysia
Kuala Lumpur, Malaysia

Maren Müller
Faculty of Biology
Department of Plant Biology
University of Barcelona
Barcelona, Spain

Sergi Munné-Bosch
Faculty of Biology
Department of Plant Biology
University of Barcelona
Barcelona, Spain

Yuji Naito
Department of Molecular Gastroenterology
    and Hepatology
Kyoto Prefectural University of Medicine
Kyoto, Japan

Kiyotaka Nakagawa
Food and Biodynamic Chemistry Laboratory
Graduate School of Agricultural Science
Tohoku University
Sendai, Japan

Hapizah Mohd Nawawi
Faculty of Medicine
Centre for Pathology Diagnostics
    and Research Laboratories
MARA University of Technology
Buloh, Malaysia

Etsuo Niki
Health Research Institute
National Institute of Advanced Industrial
    Science and Technology
Osaka, Japan

Yoshikazu Nishikawa
Department of Food and Human Health
    Sciences
Graduate School of Human Life Science
Osaka City University
Osaka, Japan

Sridevi Patchva
Cytokine Research Laboratory
Department of Experimental Therapeutics
MD Anderson Cancer Center
The University of Texas
Houston, Texas

Elisa Pierpaoli
Advanced Technology Center for Aging Research
Scientific Technological Area
INRCA-IRCCS, Ancona, Italy
Istituto Nazionale di Ricovero e Cura per Anziani
Istituto di Ricovero e Cura a Carattere Scientifico
Ancona, Italy

Francesca Pilolli
Department of Internal Medicine
University of Perugia
Perugia, Italy

Marta Piroddi
Department of Internal Medicine
University of Perugia
Perugia, Italy

Sahdeo Prasad
Cytokine Research Laboratory
Department of Experimental Therapeutics
MD Anderson Cancer Center
The University of Texas
Houston, Texas

Mauro Provinciali
Advanced Technology Center for Aging
   Research
Scientific Technological Area
INRCA-IRCCS, Ancona, Italy
Istituto Nazionale di Ricovero e Cura per
   Anziani
Istituto di Ricovero e Cura a Carattere Scientifico
Ancona, Italy

M.H. Rajikin
Faculty of Medicine
MARA University of Technology
Shah Alam, Malaysia

Victoria P. Ramsauer
Department of Pharmaceutical Sciences
Bill Gatton College of Pharmacy
East Tennessee State University
Johnson City, Tennessee

Aida Hanum Ghulam Rasool
Pharmacology Vascular Laboratory
School of Medical Sciences
Universiti Sains, Malaysia
Kota Bharu, Malaysia

Shengmin Sang
Susan Lehman Cullman Laboratory
   for Cancer Research
Department of Chemical Biology
and
Center for Cancer Prevention Research
Ernest Mario School of Pharmacy
Rutgers, The State University of New Jersey
Piscataway, New Jersey

Alexander G. Schauss
AIBMR Life Sciences, Inc.
Puyallup, Washington

Ranjan Sen
Laboratory of Molecular Biology
   and Immunology
National Institute on Aging
Baltimore, Maryland

Anureet Shah
Department of Nutrition and Food
   Sciences
Texas Woman's University
Denton, Texas

Ahmad Nazrun Shuid
Faculty of Medicine
Department of Pharmacology
National University of Malaysia
Kuala Lumpur, Malaysia

Awantika Singh
Department of Pharmaceutical Sciences
College of Pharmacy
University of Arkansas for Medical Sciences
Little Rock, Arkansas

Ima Nirwana Soelaiman
Faculty of Medicine
Department of Pharmacology
National University of Malaysia
Kuala Lumpur, Malaysia

William L. Stone
Department of Pediatrics
James H. Quillen College of Medicine
Tennessee State University
Johnson City, Tennessee

Bokyung Sung
Cytokine Research Laboratory
Department of Experimental Therapeutics
MD Anderson Cancer Center
The University of Texas
Houston, Texas

Barrie Tan
American River Nutrition, Inc.
Hadley, Massachusetts

Keiji Terao
CycloChem Co., Ltd
Kobe, Japan

Anne M. Trias
American River Nutrition, Inc.
Hadley, Massachusetts

Tomono Uchida
Department of Nutritional Sciences
Nagoya University of Arts and Sciences
Nisshin, Japan

Kottayil I. Varughese
Department of Physiology and Biophysics
University of Arkansas for Medical Sciences
Little Rock, Arkansas

Sayori Wada
Division of Applied Life Sciences
Laboratory of Health Science
Graduate School of Life and Environmental
    Sciences
Kyoto Prefectural University
Kyoto, Japan

Wong Weng-Yew
School of Biomedical Sciences
The University of Queensland
Brisbane, Queensland, Australia

Chi-Wai Wong
NeuMed Pharmaceuticals Limited
New Territories, Hong Kong

Chung S. Yang
Susan Lehman Cullman Laboratory
    for Cancer Research
Department of Chemical Biology
and
Center for Cancer Prevention Research
Ernest Mario School of Pharmacy
Rutgers, The State University of New Jersey
Piscataway, New Jersey

Zhihong Yang
Susan Lehman Cullman Laboratory
    for Cancer Research
Department of Chemical Biology
and
Center for Cancer Prevention Research
Ernest Mario School of Pharmacy
Rutgers, The State University of New Jersey
Piscataway, New Jersey

Daniel Yee Leng Yap
BASF South East Asia Pte. Ltd
Nutrition and Health Division
Singapore, Singapore

Hoda Yeganehjoo
Department of Nutrition and Food Sciences
Texas Woman's University
Denton, Texas

1 Tocotrienols in Plants
Occurrence, Biosynthesis, and Function

Maren Müller, Jana Cela, María A. Asensi-Fabado, and Sergi Munné-Bosch

CONTENTS

1.1 INTRODUCTION

Tocopherols and tocotrienols, which are collectively known as tocochromanols, belong to the group of vitamin E compounds and play a pivotal role as essential, fat-soluble nutrients that function as antioxidants in the human body. Humans, as well as other animals and nonphotosynthetic organisms, however, cannot synthesize their own vitamin E, and this must be obtained from food. The roles of vitamin E have been extensively studied and at present more than 32,000 papers on vitamin E are listed in databases such as PubMed. However, just over 700 from this list are related to tocotrienols. As a consequence of their importance for human health, the role of tocotrienols in plants is often overlooked. Obviously plants do not synthesize tocotrienols for the benefit of humans and animals, but rather they may play a role in plant metabolism. However, the biological significance of tocotrienols in plants is rather complex, at least more than that of tocopherols. While tocopherols are synthesized in all photosynthetic organisms and are found in chloroplasts playing a role in the protection of photosynthesis-derived reactive oxygen species (ROS), tocotrienols are not universally found within the plant kingdom. Hence, they can be considered secondary metabolites, not in the sense of performing a "secondary" nonessential function, but because they are present in some specific plant families and species only, and usually in seeds or other nonphotosynthetic tissues playing an important role. In this chapter, we will present a current overview about the occurrence, biosynthesis, and function of tocotrienols in plants.

1.2 OCCURRENCE OF TOCOTRIENOLS IN PLANTS

The IUCN (International Union for Conservation of Nature) estimated that about 320,000 plant species are identified in the plant kingdom (published March 11, 2010). While tocopherols are present in all plant species examined (algae, fungi, and photosynthetic bacteria), tocotrienols have only been found in seed plants (Munné-Bosch and Alegre 2002). To date, the presence of tocotrienols has been reported in 176 plant species belonging to 56 unrelated families; thereof 53 families are angiosperm plants and 3 families are gymnosperm plants (Table 1.1) (Bagci and Karaagaçli 2004, Horvath et al. 2006, Falk and Munné-Bosch 2010, Cela et al. 2011). Within angiosperms, most of the species known to have tocotrienols belong to 147 plants of the eudicot group, of which 20 belong to the family Orobancheaceae (*Orobanche* genus), 19 species to the Fabaceae family, 10 species to the Clusiaceae family, 9 species to the Lamiaceae (mainly the *Salvia* genus), 7 species to the Rosaceae family (mainly the *Prunus* genus), and 6 species to the Solanaceae family. Nevertheless, it is remarkable that within the monocots the Poaceae family also concentrates a relatively high number of six species containing tocotrienols (Table 1.1).

Tocotrienols are generally located in seeds and fruits (Asensi-Fabado and Munné-Bosch 2010) (Table 1.2); however, there is a high variation in the relative abundance of each tocotrienol homologue (α-, β-, γ- or δ-) depending on the species. δ-Tocotrienol tends to be the predominant form found in seeds, followed by α- and γ-forms, whereas γ-tocotrienol is the predominant form in fruits. It is unusual that all four tocotrienol forms are present together. Tocopherols are always found accompanying tocotrienols in these organs, mainly in the α form. Although tocopherols are generally more abundant than tocotrienols (e.g., more than twofold or threefold higher in *Elaeis guineensis* and *Rosmarinus officinalis*, respectively) (Firestone 1999, Horvath et al. 2006), there are a number of exceptions such as *Litchi chinensis, Calophyllum inophyllum, Garcinia mangostana, Passiflora edulis* var. *flavicarpa, Passiflora ligularis, Ananas sativus,* and *Diospyros kaki*, in which tocotrienol levels are higher than those of tocopherols (Crane et al. 2005, Horvath et al. 2006, Cela et al. 2011).

Although the most usual location of tocotrienol accumulation are seeds and fruits, with yields up to 1.53, 1.42, or 1.33 mg/g DW in seeds of *Bixa orellana* (lipstick tree), *Zea mays* (maize), and fruits of *Garcinia mangostana* (purple mangosteen), respectively, or 1.08 mg/g oil from fruits of *Elaeis guineensis* (palm tree), to our knowledge the highest tocotrienol concentrations in plants have been found thus far in the latex of the rubber tree *Hevea brasiliensis*, which contains 2.59 mg/g DW (Franzen and Haass 1991, Firestone 1999, Horvath et al. 2006, Cela et al. 2011). In the latex of this tree, δ-tocotrienol constitutes the 72% of total tocotrienols, which are nearly twofold higher than total tocopherols (Table 1.2). So far, this seems to be a characteristic of this particular species, since no tocotrienols have been detected in the latex of other latex producing species such as *Ficus elastica, Ficus carica*, and *Euphorbia helioscopa* (Horvath et al. 2006).

In many occasions a specific type of tocotrienol has higher levels than its tocopherol homologous in the same seed or fruit, particularly regarding δ-tocotrienol. Examples of this are seeds of *Bixa orellana*, with 5.6-fold higher δ-tocotrienol than δ-tocopherol levels (977.9 vs. 174.7 μg/g DW, respectively) or fruits of *Garcinia mangostana*, with 2015-fold higher δ-tocotrienol than δ-tocopherol levels (1243.2 vs. 0.6 μg/g DW, respectively). δ-Tocotrienol has also been found in the bark of *Garcinia virgata*, from the Clusiaceae family (Merza et al. 2004), and in the bark of four medicinal species belonging to the Canellaceae family, that is, *Cinnamosma madagascariensis, Cinnamosma fragrans, Cinnamosma macrocarpa*, and *Pleodendron costaricense* (Amiguet et al. 2006, Harinantenaina and Takaoka 2006, Harinantenaina et al. 2007, 2008).

In contrast to tocopherols, which are widespread in photosynthetic tissues (although at 10–20 times lower levels compared to seeds or fruits), there are only two reports about the presence of tocotrienols in leaves. The aforementioned work by Amiguet et al. (2006) described the presence of δ-tocotrienol not only in the bark, but also in the leaves of *Pleodendron costaricense*. Besides, Franzen et al. (1991) reported low amounts of tocotrienols in needles of *Picea* sp.; however, subsequent analysis by Horvath et al. (2006) could not confirm this, leading these authors to suggest that tocotrienols in these species might be located in resin ducts rather than in photosynthetic tissues. Furthermore, Horvath et al. (2006) found transient accumulation of α-tocotrienol in the coleoptiles of four Poaceae seedlings a few days after seed imbibition; it was hypothesized that tocotrienol had been translocated from the seeds. Other plant

TABLE 1.1
Distribution of Tocotrienols within Seed Plants

Clade		Family	No. Species	References
Gymnosperms		Gnetaceae	*Gnetum* sp.	Matthäus et al. (2003)
		Cupressaceae	*Juniperus communis*	Ivanov and Aitzetmüller (1998)
		Pinaceae[a]	*Pinus nigra* ssp. *pallasiana*	Bagci and Karaagaçli (2004)
			Pinus nigra ssp. *pallasiana* var. *pyramidata*	Bagci and Karaagaçli (2004)
			Pinus halepensis	Bagci and Karaagaçli (2004)
			Pinus sylvestris	Bagci and Karaagaçli (2004)
			Pinus pinea	Bagci and Karaagaçli (2004)
			Pinus brutia	Bagci and Karaagaçli (2004)
			Pinus radiata	Bagci and Karaagaçli (2004)
			Pinus pinaster	Bagci and Karaagaçli (2004)
Angiosperms	Monocots	Arecaceae	*Attalea speciosa*	SOFA[b]
			Elaeis guineensis	Ong (1993), Choo et al. (2004)
			Cocos nucifera	Sheppard et al. (1993), Chun et al. (2006)
			Maximiliana maripa	Bereau et al. (2001)
		Bromeliaceae	*Ananas comosus*	Kato et al. (1983)
			Ananas sativus var. *Queen Victoria*	Cela et al. (2011)
		Poaceae	*Avena sativa*	Horvath et al. (2006)
			Triticum sp.	Horvath et al. (2006)
			Secale cereale	Horvath et al. (2006)
			Hordeum vulgare	Horvath et al. (2006)
			Oryza sativa	Horvath et al. (2006)
			Zea mays	Horvath et al. (2006), Franzen and Haass (1991)
	Magnoliids	Canellaceae	*Cinnamosma fragrans*	Harinantenaina and Takaoka (2006)
			Cinnamosma macrocarpa	Harinantenaina et al. (2007)
			Cinnamosma madagascariensis	Harinantenaina et al. (2008)
			Pleodendron costaricense	Amiguet et al. (2006)
		Lauraceae	*Persea americana*	Beringer and Nothdurft (1979), Chun et al. (2006)
		Myristicaceae	*Iryanthus grandis*	Silva et al. (2001)
	Eudicots	Actinidaceae	*Actinidi chinensis*	Chun et al. (2006)
		Amaranthaceae	*Amaranthus* sp.	Lehmann et al. (1994), Qureshi et al. (1996)
		Anacardiaceae	*Anacardia occidentale*	Sheppard et al. (1993)
			Mangifera indica	Matthäus et al. (2003)
			Pistacia terebinthus	Lehmann et al. (1994), Matthäus and Özcan (2006)
		Apiaceae	*Anethum graveolens*	Matthäus et al. (2003)
			Carum carvi	Ivanov and Aitzetmüller (1995)
			Coriandrum sativum	Ivanov and Aitzetmüller (1995)
			Foenuculum vulgare	Ivanov and Aitzetmüller (1995)
			Bifora sp.	SOFA[b]
		Asteraceae	*Carthamus tinctorius*	Firestone (1999)
			Chrysanthemum coronarium	Matthäus et al. (2003)

(*continued*)

TABLE 1.1 (continued)
Distribution of Tocotrienols within Seed Plants

Clade	Family	No. Species	References
	Betulaceae	*Corylus avellana*	Crews et al. (2005)
	Bixaceae	*Bixa orellana*	Frega et al. (1998)
	Bombacaceae	*Adansonia* sp.	Firestone (1999)
	Boraginaceae	*Onosma armeniacum*	Bagci et al. (2004a)
		Onosma polioxanthum	Bagci et al. (2004a)
		Anchusa leptophylla	Bagci et al. (2004a)
		Anchusa froedini	Bagci et al. (2004a)
	Brassicaceae	*Brassica napus*	Sheppard et al. (1993)
		Camelina sativa	Budin et al. (1995)
		Raphanus sativus	Matthäus et al. (2003)
	Cactaceae	*Opuntia ficus-indica*	Cela et al. (2011)
		Selenicereus megalanthus	Cela et al. (2011)
	Caesalpinioideae	*Erythrophleum fordii*	Matthäus et al. (2003)
	Cannabaceae	*Cannabis sativa*	Mölleken (1999)
	Capparaceae	*Capparis spinosa*	Matthäus and Özcan (2005)
		Capparis ovata	Matthäus and Özcan (2005)
	Caricaceae	*Carica papaya*	Cela et al. (2011)
	Celastraceae	*Euonymus europaea*	Ivanov and Aitzetmüller (1998)
	Clusiaceae	*Garcinia brasiliensis*	Bertoli et al. (1998)
		Cartoxylum sumatranum	Seo et al. (2002)
		Calophyllum inophyllum	Matthäus et al. (2003)
		Calophyllum calaba	Crane et al. (2005)
		Garcinia virgata	Merza et al. (2004)
		Garcinia mangostana	Cela et al. (2011)
	Convolvulaceae	*Ipomoea aquatica*	Matthäus et al. (2003)
		Cuscuta sp.	van der Kooij et al. (2005)
	Cucurbitaceae	*Cucumis sativus*	Matthäus et al. (2003)
		Cucurbita pepo	Murkovic et al. (1996)
		Momordica charantia	Matthäus et al. (2003)
		Cucumis melo var. lymphothelialisis	Cela et al. (2011)
		Cucumis metuliferus	Cela et al. (2011)
	Dipterocarpaceae	*Shorea* sp.	Soulier et al. (1989)
	Ebenaceae	*Diospyros kaki*	Cela et al. (2011)
	Elaeagnaceae	*Hippophae rhamnoides*	Kallio et al. (2002)
	Ericaceae	*Vaccinium myrtillus*	Chun et al. (2006)
		Vaccinium macrocarpon	Chun et al. (2006)
		Vaccinium corymbosum	Cela et al. (2011)
	Euphorbiaceae	*Aleurites montana*	Matthäus et al. (2003)
		Hevea brasiliensis	Ong (1993), Horvath et al. (2006), Hess (1993)
		Plukenetia volubilis	SOFA[b]
		Sapium sebiferum	Aitzetmüller et al. (1992)
	Fabaceae	*Canavalia ensiformis*	Matthäus et al. (2003)
		Cicer arietinum	Krishna et al. (1997)
		Glycine max	Sheppard et al. (1993)
		Robinia pseudoacacia	Ivanov and Aitzetmüller (1998)

TABLE 1.1 (continued)
Distribution of Tocotrienols within Seed Plants

Clade	Family	No. Species	References
		Vigna radiata	Krishna et al. (1997)
		Tamarindus indica	Cela et al. (2011)
		Colutea melanocalyx	Bagci et al. (2004b)
		Hedysarum cappadocicum	Bagci et al. (2004b)
		Lathyrus inconspicuus	Bagci et al. (2004b)
		Lathyrus laxiflorus ssp. *laxiflorus*	Bagci et al. (2004b)
		Gomocyctis dirmilensis	Bagci et al. (2004b)
		Lupinus varius	Bagci et al. (2004b)
		Trigonella cretica	Bagci et al. (2004b)
		Vicia michauxii var. *stenophylla*	Bagci et al. (2004b)
		Vicia cappadocica	Bagci et al. (2004b)
		Onobrychis major	Bagci et al. (2004b)
		Onobrychis huetiana	Bagci et al. (2004b)
		Onobrychis altissima	Bagci et al. (2004b)
		Onobrychis hypargyrea	Bagci et al. (2004b)
	Grossulariaceae	*Ribes nigrum*	Clough (2001)
		Ribes rubrum	Cela et al. (2011)
	Hippocastanaceae	*Aesculus sinensis*	Matthäus et al. (2003)
	Juglandaceae	*Juglans regia*	Amaral et al. (2005)
	Lamiaceae	*Rosmarinus officinalis*	Horvath et al. (2006)
		Salvia bracteata	Bagci et al. (2004c)
		Salvia euphratica var. *euphratica*	Bagci et al. (2004c)
		Salvia crytantha	Bagci et al. (2004c)
		Salvia limbata	Bagci et al. (2004c)
		Salvia virgata	Bagci et al. (2004c)
		Salvia syiaca	Bagci et al. (2004c)
		Salvia staminea	Bagci et al. (2004c)
		Salvia cilicica	Bagci et al. (2004c)
	Lythraceae	*Punica granatum*	Cela et al. (2011)
	Malvaceae	*Gossypium* sp.	Firestone (1999)
		Abutilon sp.	SOFA[b]
	Myrtaceae	*Psidium guajava*	Cela et al. (2011)
	Oleaceae	*Olea europea*	Hassapidou and Manoukas (1993)
		Jasminum fructicans	Ivanov and Aitzetmüller (1998)
	Onagraceae	*Oenothera biennis*	Clough (2001)
	Orobanchiaceae	*Orobanche arenaria*	Velasco et al. (2000)
		Orbranchelavendulacea	Velasco et al. (2000)
		Orobanche mutelii	Velasco et al. (2000)
		Orobanche purpurea	Velasco et al. (2000)
		Orobanche ramosa	Velasco et al. (2000)
		Orobanche schultzii	Velasco et al. (2000)
		Orobanche tunetana	Velasco et al. (2000)
		Orobanche cernua	Velasco et al. (2000)
		Orobranche cumana	Velasco et al. (2000)

(continued)

TABLE 1.1 (continued)
Distribution of Tocotrienols within Seed Plants

Clade	Family	No. Species	References
		Orobanche crenata	Velasco et al. (2000)
		Orobanche amethystea	Velasco et al. (2000)
		Orobanche densiflora	Velasco et al. (2000)
		Orobanche hederae	Velasco et al. (2000)
		Orobanche minor	Velasco et al. (2000)
		Orobanchesantolinae	Velasco et al. (2000)
		Orobanche alsatica	Velasco et al. (2000)
		Orobanche lucorum	Velasco et al. (2000)
		Orobanche rapum-genistae	Velasco et al. (2000)
		Orobanche gracilis	Velasco et al. (2000)
		Orobanche foetida	Velasco et al. (2000)
	Oxalidaceae	*Averrhoa carambola L.*	Cela et al. (2011)
	Passifloraceae	*Passiflora edulis f. edulis*	Cela et al. (2011)
		Passiflora edulis f. flavicarpa	Cela et al. (2011)
	Polygonaceae	*Fagopyrum esculentum*	Balz et al. (1992)
	Proteaceae	*Gevuina avellana*	Bertoli et al. (1998)
		Macadamia tetraphylla	Sheppard et al. (1993)
	Ranunculaceae	*Delphinium ajacis*	Matthäus et al. (2003)
		Nigella sativa	SOFA[b]
	Rosaceae	*Rosa canina*	Zlatanov (1999)
		Prunus amygdalus	Slover (1971)
		Prunus tenella (amygdalus nana)	Ivanov and Aitzetmüller (1998)
		Prunus americana	Sheppard et al. (1993)
		Prunus domestica	Chun et al. (2006)
		Prunus persica	Chun et al. (2006)
		Rosa canina	Ivanov and Aitzetmüller (1998)
	Rutaceae	*Fortunella margarita*	Cela et al. (2011)
	Sapindaceae	*Litchi chinensis*	Matthäus et al. (2003)
		Delavaya toxocarpa	Matthäus et al. (2003)
		Nephelium lappaceum	Matthäus et al. (2003)
		Sapindus mukorossi	Matthäus et al. (2003)
	Sapotaceae	*Manilkara zapota*	Cela et al. (2011)
	Solanaceae	*Nicotianna tabacum*	Falk et al. (2003)
		Nicandra physaloides	SOFA[b]
		Physalis peruviana	Cela et al. (2011)
		Solanum quitoense	Cela et al. (2011)
		Solanum lycopersicum	Cela et al. (2011)
		Solanum betaceum	Cela et al. (2011)
	Tiliaceae	*Tilia arentea*	Lehmann et al. (1994)
	Vitaceae	*Vitis vinifera*	Sheppard et al. (1993), Horvath et al. (2006)

[a] Additionally, Franzen et al. (1991) reported the presence of tocotrienols in *Picea* species; however, it was not stated clearly which of the 28 analyzed species contained tocotrienols. Therefore, they have not been included within the Pinaceae family.

[b] SOFA is the database "Seed Oil Fatty Acids," which is no longer accessible online. For a description of this database, see Matthäus et al. (2002).

TABLE 1.2
Occurrence of Tocopherols and Tocotrienols within Plant Organs and Tissues. The Approximate Relative Abundance of These Compounds in Each Organ or Tissue Is Denoted by (+), whereas (–) Indicates that these Compounds Were Not Detected or Not yet Described

Organ or Tissue	Tocopherols	Tocotrienols
Leaves	+	–[a]
Flowers	+	–
Fruits	++	+
Seeds	+++	++
Roots	+	–
Tubers	+	–
Bulbs	+	–
Latex[b]	++	+++
Bark[b]	–	++

[a] Only Amiguet et al. (2006) have reported the presence of δ-tocotrienol in the leaves of *Pleodendron costaricense*. Other contrasting results on *Picea* sp. are described in the text.

[b] Despite tocotrienol abundance in latex and bark, they have only been found in a very low number of species as reported in the text.

organs where tocopherols are found (flowers, roots, tubers, and bulbs) have not been reported to contain tocotrienols (Table 1.2).

At the subcellular level, despite the general belief that tocochromanols are exclusively present in plastids, they have also been found in cytoplasmic lipid bodies in seeds (Fisk et al. 2006). In photosynthetic tissues, tocopherols are located in chloroplasts; however, tocotrienols were found neither in chloroplasts nor in etioplasts of the coleoptiles containing tocotrienols (Horvath et al. 2006).

Curiously, the model plant *Arabidopsis thaliana* does not produce tocotrienols (Herbers 2003), although they have been found in other species of the same family (Brassicaceae), such as *Brassica napus*, *Camelina sativa*, and *Raphanus sativus* (Sheppard et al. 1993, Budin et al. 1995, Matthäus et al. 2003).

Finally, although tocotrienols have a very restricted distribution in comparison to tocopherols, the range of species containing tocotrienols is broadening with new studies. Strikingly, only 24 out of 80 species analyzed by Horvath et al. (2006) were found to contain tocotrienols, while a much higher proportion of species (26 out of 32) showed tocotrienols in the work by Cela et al. (2011). This suggests that tocotrienols are present in many plant species not yet analyzed, and future positive discoveries may depend on the particular species selected for further studies. Also, there are contradictory results about the presence of tocotrienols in several species, such as *Olea europea*, *Zea mays*, and *Nicotiana tabacum* (Franzen and Haass 1991, Hassapidou and Manoukas 1993, Falk et al. 2003, Horvath et al. 2006), and it has been shown that tocotrienol composition highly varies between different varieties of the same species. This is the case of *Triticum vulgare* (Hall and Laidman 1968), *Oryza sativa* (Horvath et al. 2006), and *Passiflora edulis* (Cela et al. 2011). These discrepancies should be taken into account when constructing the database of plant species containing tocotrienols and may be due to different methods of analyzing plant varieties or growth conditions used for studies. Further research is needed to have a wider picture of tocotrienol distribution and accumulation in seeds and fruits within the plant kingdom. It is important to improve our knowledge of the plant species that accumulate tocotrienols to get a deeper understanding of the tocotrienol levels present in our diet and to obtain new oils with commercial interest.

1.3   TOCOTRIENOL BIOSYNTHESIS

Tocotrienols are a group of four amphipathic molecules (α-, β-, γ-, and δ-tocotrienol) that differ in the number and position of the methyl groups in the polar head (Figure 1.1). Tocotrienols, like tocopherols, have a hydrophobic tail associated with membrane lipids and a polar head remaining at the membrane surface. The polar chromanol head group is derived from the shikimate pathway (Norris et al. 1998) and it is bound to a C_{20} isoprenoid-derived hydrocarbon tail with three *trans* double bonds derived from the methylerythritol phosphate (MEP) pathway (Rohmer 2003). Since tocotrienols are not present in all plants, their function and biosynthesis have remained unclear for a long time, but in the last years, some works have shed new light on these questions.

Tocotrienol biosynthesis differs little from tocopherol biosynthesis. Basically the prenylation of homogentisic acid is different because the geranylgeranyl diphosphate (GGDP) is used instead of the phytyl diphosphate (PDP). At the cellular level, the biosynthesis of tocotrienols occurs in plastids (Sun et al. 2009), and it has not been proved thus far that any isoform can be transported within the plant.

The differential step in the biosynthesis of tocotrienol compared to that of the biosynthesis of tocopherol was discovered in monocots. A new specific enzyme, the homogentisate geranylgeranyl transferase (HGGT), was characterized in wheat, barley, and rice (Cahoon et al. 2003) based on its homology with homogentisate phytyl transferase (HPT) gene, the latter implicated in tocopherol biosynthesis. A subsequent work showed that HGGT was more active (6 times more) with geranyl-geranyl diphosphate than with phytyl diphosphate but was capable to use the PDP in the presence of elevated ratios of PDP:GGDP (Yang et al. 2011) (Table 1.3). This suggested that HGGT is the only enzymatic activity that is unique to the tocotrienol biosynthetic pathway in plants. Although the presence of HGGT clarifies the particularities of the biosynthesis of tocotrienols in monocots, in other

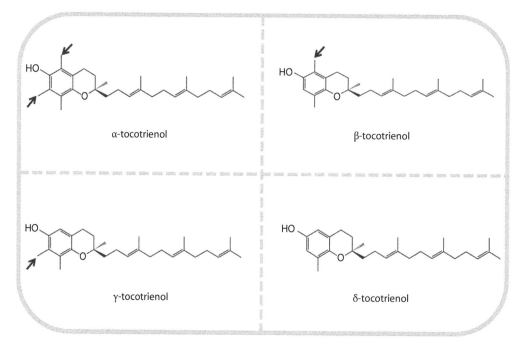

FIGURE 1.1   Chemical structures of different tocotrienol homologues. Arrows indicate the different positions of the methyl groups.

TABLE 1.3

Tocotrienol Biosynthetic Enzymes, Cellular Localization, Substrate, and Product of Each Enzyme and Locus for Each Gene in *Arabidopsis thaliana*, as a Dicot Plant Model, *Synechocystis*, as a Cyanobacterium Model, and *Oryza sativa*, as a Monocot Model Plant

Pathway Enzyme	Cellular Localization	Substrate	Product	A. thaliana Locus/Gene	Synechocystis Gene	Oryza sativa Gene
HPT	Inner chloroplast membranes	HGA+PDP HGA+GGDP(minor)	MPBQ MGGBQ	VTE2/At2g18950	slr1736	LOC_Os06g44840
HGGT	Inner chloroplast membranes	HGA+GGDP HGA+PDP(minor)	MGGBQ MPBQ	-/At3g11945.2	—	LOC_Os06g43880
MPBQ MT	Inner chloroplast membranes	MPBQ MGGBQ	DMPBQ DMGGBQ	VTE3/At3g63410	sll0418	LOC_Os07g08200 LOC_Os12g42090
TC	Plastoglobule	MPBQ MGGBQ DMPBQ DMGGBQ	δ-tocopherol δ-tocotrienol γ-tocopherol γ-tocotrienol	VTE1/At4g32770	slr1737	LOC_Os02g17650
α-TMT	Inner chloroplast membranes	δ-tocopherol δ-tocotrienol γ-tocopherol γ-tocotrienol	β-tocopherol β-tocotrienol α-tocopherol α-tocotrienol	VTE4/At1g64970	slr0089	LOC_Os02g47310

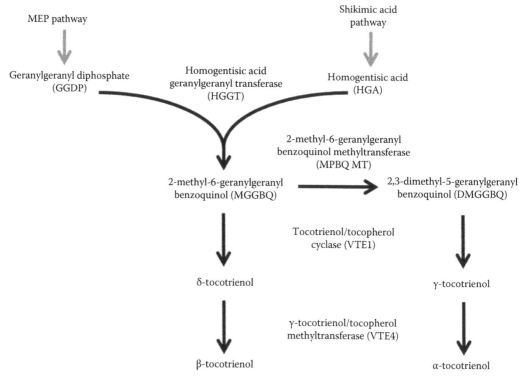

FIGURE 1.2   Biosynthesis of tocotrienols in plants and detail of enzymes involved.

plants much less is known (Figure 1.2). The *Arabidopsis thaliana* (At2g18950) and *Synechocystis PCC680* (*slr*1736) HPT that lead to tocopherol biosynthesis showed similar properties on its substrate specificities (Sadre et al. 2006). Both enzymes were more active with PDP, but were able to use GGDP too, although the specificity of the *A. thaliana* enzyme was more pronounced than that of *Synechocystis*. In a previous work, the differences between both enzymes were detected, but the low GGDP-dependent activity was not detected, presumably because of the very low activity of the plant enzyme reported (Collakova and DellaPenna 2001). A surprising HGGT-independent tocotrienol biosynthesis was accidentally found in tobacco, when a yeast (*Saccharomyces cerevisiae*) prephenate dehydrogenase (PDH), which catalyzes the production of hydroxyphenylpyruvate (HPP) (the immediate precursor of homogentisic acid (HGA)) directly from prephenate, and an *A. thaliana* hydroxyphenylpyruvate dioxygenase (HPPD) were expressed in tobacco plants (Rippert et al. 2004). The PDH-HPPD overexpressors had 10- to 11-fold more vitamin E than wild type plants, and this increase in vitamin E content was almost completely caused by tocotrienols, which are not normally synthesized in tobacco leaves. Their results suggested that these mutants were able to increase the HGA flux and altered the substrate specificity of HPT, and therefore, it was able to use GGDP as a cosubstrate (Table 1.3).

Prenylation, two methylations and one cyclation are shared steps during the biosynthesis of both tocopherol and tocotrienol and are necessary to form the different forms of tocochromanols. The two methylations and cyclation are catalyzed by 2-methyl-6-phytyl benzoquinol methyltransferase (MPBQ MT), tocopherol cyclase (TC), and γ-tocopherol methyltransferase (γ-TMT), in this order, which are able to convert the HGGT product, 2-methyl-6-geranylgeranylbenzoquinol (MGGBQ) into tocotrienols (Soll and Schultz 1979) (Table 1.3).

These two methylation steps determine the position and number of methyl substituents of the polar head. MPBQ MT adds a second methyl group to MGGBQ to form 2,3-dimethyl-5-geranylgeranyl benzoquinol (DMGGBQ), the precursor of γ-tocotrienol. Without this activity, the result will be δ-tocotrienol (Shintani and DellaPenna 1998). The tocopherol cyclase (TC) converts MGGBQ or DMGGBQ into γ- or δ-tocotrienol, depending on the methylation degree of the polar head. The TC has been localized to plastoglobules in chloroplasts (Vidi et al. 2006, Austin et al. 2006) and shows an equal preference for tocopherols and tocotrienols (Porfirova et al. 2002, Hofius et al. 2004), since—when tobacco callus are transformed with barley HGGT—it is possible to find all forms of tocotrienols (Cahoon et al. 2003). The last step in tocochromanol biosynthesis is the methylation of the C5 of the chromanol ring. Although the enzyme is called γ-tocopherol methyltransferase (VTE4), it also shows activity for the γ- and δ-form of both, tocopherols and tocotrienols, as it happens with TC (Cahoon et al. 2003).

Although all these enzymes can participate in the biosynthesis of both tocotrienols and tocopherols, it remains to be determined if the endosperm of monocot seeds have a variant form that evolved for a more efficient synthesis, as occurs with HGGT. More investigation is needed to better understand the biosynthesis of tocotrienols, especially in eudicots capable of producing tocotrienols.

1.4 FUNCTION OF TOCOTRIENOLS IN PLANTS

Tocotrienols are considered to be important vitamin E compounds in humans with functions in health and disease; however, the function of tocotrienols in plants is still largely unclear. Based on the similar structure of tocotrienols and tocopherols, it was suggested that these compounds could have comparable antioxidant functions in plants (Munné-Bosch et al. 2011). Tocochromanols are known to be lipophilic molecules with excellent antioxidant activity, which is mainly due to the capacity of their heterocyclic chromanol ring system to donate the phenolic hydrogen to lipid-free radicals (Kaman-Eldin and Appelqvist 1996). In addition, they show high activity as quenchers and scavengers of singlet oxygen (Falk and Munné-Bosch 2010). Apart from their role as radical scavengers, tocochromanols also act as important membrane structure-stabilizing agents (Wang and Quinn 2000). It has been suggested that α-tocotrienol is located closer to the membrane surface due to their threefold unsaturated polyprenyl chain and imposes more motional anisotrophy on the membrane than α-tocopherol (Suzuki et al. 1993). As a consequence of their higher recycling efficiency, more uniform distribution in the membrane bilayer, and stronger disordering effect on membrane lipids, it has been assumed that α-tocotrienol exhibits a higher antioxidant activity than α-tocopherol (Kamal-Eldin and Appelqvist 1996). An example is given when tocochromals were incorporated into phosphatidylcholine liposomes and α-tocotrienol showed significantly greater peroxyl radical scavenging activity than α-tocopherol (Suzuki et al. 1993). In contrast to tocopherols, tocotrienols are not synthesized in photosynthetically active tissues of plants and were only found in certain plant families, being preferentially found in seeds and fruits (Ong 1993, Lehmann et al. 1994, Horvath et al. 2006, Cela et al. 2011). However, after genetic manipulation plants were also capable of synthesizing and accumulating tocotrienols in leaves (Cahoon et al. 2003, Rippert et al. 2004) at even higher concentrations than tocopherols (Matringe et al. 2008). In double transgenic tobacco plants, tocotrienols accumulated as the major tocochromanol form in leaves by coexpression of the prephenate dehydrogenase (PDH) and hydroxyphenylpyruvate dioxygenase (HPPD) genes (Matringe et al. 2008). These modified tocotrienol-accumulating plants were able to protect membrane lipids in leaves from lipid peroxidation and it has been proposed that tocotrienols fulfill a similar function in plant tissues in which tocotrienols usually are accumulated, such as plant seeds.

The potential antioxidant function of tocotrienols leads to the following question: Why are tocotrienols only distributed in certain plant families and plant tissues whereas tocopherols are presented in all plants? However, to date we have no answer to this question. The exact localization of tocotrienols in tissues of seeds and fruits could be helpful to gain more insights about their possible functions in plants. Horvath et al. (2006) proposed that tocotrienols can also be translocated from seeds to coleoptiles, after the observation of α-tocotrienol molecules in the newly formed leaves of germination seedlings of *Tricticum aestivum*. In the mesocarp of *Elaeis guineensis*, tocotrienol levels are much higher compared to tocopherols, however, only during the final phase of fruit ripening (Choo et al. 2004). In cereals (barley, corn, oat, and wheat), tocochromanols are present in the pericarp, whereas in the endosperm only tocotrienols are located and in the germ tocopherols (Grams et al. 1970, Morrison et al. 1982, Balz et al. 1992, Peterson 1995, Hoa et al. 2003, Falk et al. 2003). Interestingly, in dry seeds α-tocopherol is accumulated in those parts that survive and are necessary to build up the new plant, whereas tocotrienols are located in those parts that finally die before or during germination, respectively. In nonendospermic seeds of *Gevuina avellana* and *Macadamia tetraphylla*, tocotrienols were almost exclusively found in the embryo. Curiously, these seeds have a relative short viability and are desiccation sensitive (Halloy et al. 1996).

1.5 FUTURE PERSPECTIVES

In the last years tocotrienols have been of increasing interest, although many questions mainly related to their roles in plants are still not clearly understood. Therefore, it is of importance to collect more information about their distribution in the plant kingdom as well as their exact localization in plant cells and tissues. Although tocopherols and tocotrienols seem to share the same biosynthetic pathways, in cereals the presence of the additional enzyme HGGT could be shown as responsible for specific production of tocotrienols. However, further investigations are necessary to clarify if the presence of tocotrienols, especially in eudicots, is also a result of a second prenyltransferase, as in cereals, or a less restricted or convertible substrate specificity of their HPT. Further experiments are also needed to confirm if tocotrienols can be translocated from seeds. It is still unclear which target membranes tocotrienols are supposed to protect, and whether they act as antioxidants only or have other as yet unknown functions.

REFERENCES

Aitzetmüller, K., Xin, Y., Werner, G., Grönheim, M. 1992. High performance liquid chromatographic investigations of stillingia oil. *Journal of Chromatography* 603: 165–173.

Amaral, J.S., Alves, M.R., Seabra, R.M., Oliviera, B.P. 2005. Vitamin E composition of walnuts (*Juglans regia* L.): A 3-year comparative study of different cultivars. *Journal of Agricultural and Food Chemistry* 53: 5467–5472.

Amiguet, V.T., Petit, P., Ta, C.A. et al. 2006. Phytochemistry and antifungal properties of the newly discovered tree *Pleodendron costaricense*. *Journal of Natural Products* 69: 1005–1009.

Asensi-Fabado, M.A., Munné-Bosch, S. 2010. Vitamins in plants: Occurrence, biosynthesis and antioxidant function. *Trends in Plant Science* 15: 582–592.

Austin, J.R., Frost, E., Vidi, P.A., Kessler, F., Staehelin, L.A. 2006. Plastoglobules are lipoprotein subcompartments of the chloroplast that are permanently coupled to thylakoid membranes and contain biosynthetic enzymes. *Plant Cell* 18: 1693–1703.

Bagci, E., Bruehl, L., Aitzetmüller, K., Altan, Y. 2004a. Fatty acid and tocochromanol patterns of some Turkish Boraginaceae—A chemotaxonomic approach. *Nordic Journal of Botany* 22: 719–726.

Bagci, E., Bruehl, L., Özçelik, H., Aitzetmüller, K., Vural, M., Sahim, A. 2004b. A study of the fatty acid and tocochromanol patterns of some Fabaceae (Leguminosae) plants from Turkey I. *Grasas y Aceites* 55: 378–384.

Bagci, E., Karaagaçli, Y. 2004. Fatty acid and tocochromanol patterns of Turkish pines. *Acta Biologica Cracoviensia, Series Botanica* 46: 95–100.

Bagci, E., Vural, M., Dirmenci, T., Bruehl, L., Aitzetmüller, K. 2004c. Fatty acid and tocochromanol patterns of some *Salvia* L. species. *Zeitschrift für Naturforschung* 59c: 305–309.

Balz, M., Schulte, E., Their, H.P. 1992. Trennung von Tocopherolen und Tocotrienolen durch HPLC. *Fat Science Technology* 94: 209–213.

Bereau, D., Benjelloun-Mlayah, B., Delmas, M. 2001. *Maximiliana maripa* drude mesocarp and kernel oils: Fatty acid and total tocopherol compositions. *Journal of the American Oil Chemists' Society* 78: 213–214.

Beringer, H., Nothdurft, F. 1979. Plastid development and tocochromanol accumulation in oil seeds. In *Advances in Biochemistry and Physiology of Plant Lipids*, eds. L.A. Appelqvist, and C. Liljenberg, pp. 133–137. Amsterdam, the Netherlands: Elsevier/North Holland Biomedical Press.

Bertoli, C., Fay, L.B., Stancanelli, M., Gumy, D., Lambelet, P. 1998. Characterization of Chilean hazelnut (*Gevuina avellana* Mol) seed oil. *Journal of the American Oil Chemists' Society* 75: 1037–1040.

Budin, J.T., Breene, W.M., Putnam, D.H. 1995. Some compositional properties of camelina (*Camelina sativa* L. Crantz) seeds and oils. *Journal of the American Oil Chemists' Society* 72: 309–315.

Cahoon, E.B., Hall, S.E., Ripp, K.G., Ganzke, T.S., Hitz, W.D., Coughlan, S.J. 2003. Metabolic redesign of vitamin E biosynthesis in plants for tocotrienol production and increased antioxidant content. *Nature Biotechnology* 21: 1082–1087.

Cela, J., Müller, M., Munné-Bosch, S. 2011. Tocopherol and tocotrienol (vitamin E) composition of some edible fruits. In *Vitamin E: Nutrition, Side Effects and Supplements*, ed. A. Lindberg, pp. 277–287. Hauppauge, NY: Nova Science Publishers.

Choo, Y.M., Ma, A.N., Chuah, C.H., Khor, H.T., Bong, S.C. 2004. A developmental study on the appearance of tocopherols and tocotrienols in developing palm mesocarp (*Elaeis guineensis*). *Lipids* 39: 561–564.

Chun, J., Lee, J., Ye, L., Exler, J., Eitenmiller, R.R. 2006. Tocopherol and tocotrienol contents of raw and processed fruits and vegetables in the United States diet. *Journal of Food Composition and Analysis* 19: 196–200.

Clough, P.M. 2001. Specialty vegetable oils containing γ-linolenic acid and stearidonic acid. In *Structured and Modified Lipids 4*, ed. F.D. Gunstone, pp. 75–107. New York: Dekker.

Collakova, E., DellaPenna, D. 2001. Isolation and functional analysis of homogentisate phytyltransferase from *Synechocystis* sp. PCC 6803 and *Arabidopsis*. *Plant Physiology* 127: 1113–1124.

Crane, S., Aurore, G., Joseph, H., Mouloungui, Z., Bourgeois, P. 2005. Composition of fatty acids triacylglycerols and unsaponifiable matter in *Calophyllum calaba* L. oil from Guadeloupe. *Phytochemistry* 66: 1825–1831.

Crews, C., Hough, P., Godward, J. et al. 2005. Study of the main constituent of some authentic hazelnut oils. *Journal of Agricultural and Food Chemistry* 53: 4843–4852.

Falk, J., Andersen, G., Kernebeck, B., Krupinska, K. 2003. Constitutive overexpression of barley 4-hydroxy-phenylpyruvate dioxygenase in tobacco results in elevation of the vitamin E content in seeds but not in leaves. *FEBS Letters* 540: 35–40.

Falk, J., Munné-Bosch, S. 2010. Tocochromanol functions in plants: Antioxidation and beyond. *Journal of Experimental Botany* 61: 1549–1566.

Firestone, D. 1999. Physical and chemical characteristics of oils, fats, and waxes. *Database 'Seed Oil Fatty Acids' (SOFA)*.

Fisk, I.D., White, D.A., Carvalho, A., Gray, D.A. 2006. Tocopherol—An intrinsic component of sunflower seed oil bodies. *Journal of the American Oil Chemists Society* 83: 341–344.

Franzen, J., Bausch, J., Glatzle, D., Wagner, E. 1991. Distribution of vitamin E in spruce seedlings and mature tree organs, and within the genus. *Phytochemistry* 30: 147–151.

Franzen, J., Haass, M. 1991. Vitamin E content during development of some seedlings. *Phytochemistry* 30: 2911–2913.

Frega, N., Mozzon, M., Bocci, F. 1998. Identification and estimation of tocotrienols in the annatto lipid fraction by gas chromatography–mass spectrometry. *Journal of the American Oil Chemists' Society* 75: 1723–1727.

Grams, G.W., Blessin, C.W., Inglett, G.E. 1970. Distribution of tocopherol within the corn kernel. *Journal of the American Oil Chemists' Society* 47: 337–339.

Hall, G.S., Laidman, D.L. 1968. The pattern and control of isoprenoid quinone and tocopherol metabolism in the germinating grain of wheat (*Triticum vulgare*). *Biochemical Journal* 108: 475–482.

Halloy, S., Garu, A., McKenzie, B. 1996. Gevuina nut (*Gevuina avellana*, Proteaceae), a cool climate alternative to macadamia. *Economic Botany* 50: 224–235.

Harinantenaina, L., Asakawa, Y., De Clercq, E. 2007. Cinnamacrins A-C, cinnafragrin D, and cytostatic metabolites with α-glucosidase inhibitory activity from *Cinnamosma macrocarpa*. *Journal of Natural Products* 70: 277–282.

Harinantenaina, L., Matsunami, K., Otsuka, H., Kawahata, M., Yamaguchi, K., Asakawa, Y. 2008. Secondary metabolites of *Cinnamosma madagascariensis* and their α-glucosidase inhibitory properties. *Journal of Natural Products* 71: 123–126.

Harinantenaina, L., Takaoka, S. 2006. Cinnafragrins A-C, dimeric and trimeric drimane sesquiterpenoids from *Cinnamosma fragrans*, and structure revision of capsicodendrin. *Journal of Natural Products* 69: 1193–1197.

Hassapidou, M.N., Manoukas, A.G. 1993. Tocopherol and tocotrienol compositions of raw table olive fruit. *Journal of the Science of Food and Agriculture* 61: 277–280.

Herbers, K. 2003. Vitamin production in transgenic plants. *Journal of Plant Physiology* 160: 821–829.

Hess, J.L. 1993. Vitamin E, α-tocopherol. In *Antioxidants in Higher Plant*, eds. R.G. Alscher, and J.L. Hess, pp. 111–134. Boca Raton, FL: CRC Press.

Hoa, T.T., Al-Babili, S., Schaub, P., Potrykus, I., Beyer, P. 2003. Golden indica and japonica rice lines amenable to deregulation. *Plant Physiology* 133: 161–169.

Hofius, D., Hajirezaei, M.R., Geiger, M., Tschiersch, H., Melzer, M., Sonnewald, U. 2004. RNAi-mediated tocopherol deficiency impairs photoassimilate export in transgenic potato plants. *Plant Physiology* 135: 1256–1268.

Horvath, G., Wessjohann, L., Bigirimana, J. et al. 2006. Differential distribution of tocopherols and tocotrienols in photosynthetic and non-photosynthetic tissues. *Phytochemistry* 67: 1185–1195.

Ivanov, S.A., Aitzetmüller, K. 1995. Untersuchungen über die Tocopherol-und Tocotrienolzusammensetzung der Samenöle einiger Vertreter der Familie Apiaceae. *Fat Science Technology* 97: 24–29.

Ivanov, S.A., Aitzetmüller, K. 1998. Untersuchungen über die Tocopherol-und Tocotrienolzusammensetzung der Samenlipide einiger Arten der bulgarischen Flora. *Fett/Lipid* 100: 348–352.

Kallio, H., Yang, B., Peippo, P., Tahvonen, R., Pan, R. 2002. Triacylglycerols, glycerophospholipids, tocopherols, and tocotrienols in berries and seeds of two subspecies (ssp. *sinensis* and *mongolica*) of sea buckthorn *(Hippophaë rhamnoides)*. *Journal of Agricultural and Food Chemistry* 50: 3004–3009.

Kamal-Eldin, A., Appelqvist, L. 1996. The chemistry and antioxidant properties of tocopherols and tocotrienols. *Lipids* 31: 671–701.

Kato, A., Yamaoka, M., Tanaka, A. 1983. Vitamin E extraction. UK Patent application GB 2117381 A.

van der Kooij, T.A.W., Krupinska, K., Krause, K. 2005. Tocochromanol content and composition in different species of the parasitic flowering plant genus *Cuscuta*. *Journal of Plant Physiology* 162: 777–781.

Krishna, A.G.G., Prabhakar, J.V., Aitzetmüller, K. 1997. Tocopherol and fatty acid composition of some Indian pulses. *Journal of the American Oil Chemists' Society* 74: 1603–1606.

Lehmann, J.W., Putnam, D.H., Qureshi, A.A. 1994. Vitamin E isomers in grain amaranths (*Amaranthus spp.*). *Lipids* 29: 177–181.

Matringe, M., Ksas, B., Rey, P., Havaux, M. 2008. Tocotrienols, the unsaturated forms of vitamin E, can function as antioxidants and lipid protectors in tobacco leaves. *Plant Physiology* 147: 764–778.

Matthäus, B., Aitzetmüller, K., Friedrich, H. 2002. Description of the database 'Seed Oil Fatty Acids' (SOFA). *Agro Food Industry Hi-tech* 13: 38–43.

Matthäus, B., Özcan, M. 2005. Glucosinolates and fatty acid, sterol, and tocopherol composition of seed oils from *Capparis spinosa* var. spinosa and *Capparis ovata* Desf. var. canescens (Coss.) Heywood. *Journal of Agricultural and Food Chemistry* 53: 7136–7141.

Matthäus, B., Özcan, M. 2006. Quantitation of fatty acids, sterols, and tocopherols in turpentine (*Pistacia terebinthus* Chia) growing wild in Turkey. *Journal of Agricultural and Food Chemistry* 54: 7667–7671.

Matthäus, B., Vosmann, K., Quoc Pham, L., Aitzetmüller, K. 2003. Fatty acids and tocopherol composition of Vietnamese oilseeds. *Journal of the American Oil Chemists' Society* 80: 1013–1020.

Merza, J., Aumond, M.C., Rondeau, D. et al. 2004. Prenylated xanthones and tocotrienols from *Garcinia virgata*. *Phytochemistry* 65: 2915–2920.

Mölleken, H. 1999. Hanf (*Cannabis sativa*) als novel food. *Bioforum–Forschung and Entwicklung* 22: 452–457.

Morrison, W.R., Conventry, A.M., Barnes, P.J. 1982. The distribution of acyl lipids and tocopherols in flour millstreams. *Journal of the Science of Food and Agriculture* 33: 925–933.

Munné-Bosch, S., Alegre, L. 2002. The function of tocopherols and tocotrienols in plants. *Critical Reviews in Plant Sciences* 21: 31–57.

Munné-Bosch, S., Oñate, M., Olivera, P.G., Garcia, Q.S. 2011. Changes in phytohormones and oxidative stress markers in buried seeds of *Vellozia alata*. *Flora* 206: 704–711.

Murkovic, M., Hillebrand, A., Winkler, J., Pfannhauser, W. 1996. Variability of vitamin E content in pumpkin seeds (*Cucurbita pepo* L.). *Zeitschrift für Lebensmittel-Untersuchung und-Forschung A* 202: 275–278.

Norris, S.R., Shen, X., DellaPenna, D. 1998. Complementation of the *Arabidopsis* pds1 mutation with the gene encoding *p*-hydroxyphenylpiruvate dioxygenase. *Plant Physiology* 117: 1317–1323.

Ong, A.S.H. 1993. Natural sources of tocotrienols. In *Vitamin E in Health and Disease*, eds. L. Packer, and J. Fuchs, pp. 3–8. New York: Dekker.

Qureshi, A.A., Lehmann, J.W., Peterson, D.M. 1996. Amaranth and its oil inhibit cholesterol biosynthesis in 6-week-old female chickens. *Journal of Nutrition* 126: 1972–1978.

Peterson, D.M. 1995. Oat tocols: Concentration and stability in oat products and distribution within in the kernel. *Cereal Chemistry* 72: 21–24.

Porfirova, S., Bergmüller, E., Tropf, S., Lemke, R., Dörman, P. 2002. Isolation of an *Arabidopsis* mutant lacking vitamin E and identification of a cyclase essential for all tocopherol biosynthesis. *Proceedings of the National Academy of Sciences USA* 99: 12495–12500.

Rippert, P., Scimemi, C., Dubald, M., Matringe, M. 2004. Engineering plant shikimate pathway for production of tocotrienol and improving herbicide resistance. *Plant Physiology* 134: 92–100.

Rohmer, M. 2003. Mevalonate-independent methylerythritol phosphate pathway for isoprenoid biosynthesis. *Pure and Applied Chemistry* 75: 375–387.

Sadre, R., Gruber, J., Frentzen, M. 2006. Characterization of homogentisate prenyltrasnferase involved in plastoquinone-9 and tocochromanol biosynthesis. *FEBS Letters* 580: 5357–5362.

Seo, E.K., Kim, N.C., Wani, M.C. et al. 2002. Cytotoxic prenylated xanthones and the unusual compounds anthraquinobenzophenones from *Cratoxylum sumatranum*. *Journal of Natural Products* 65: 299.

Sheppard, A.J., Weihrauch, J.L., Pennington, J.A.T. 1993. Analysis and distribution of vitamin E in vegetable oils and foods. In *Vitamin E in Health and Disease,* eds. L. Packer, and J. Fuchs, pp. 9–31. New York: Marcel Dekker.

Shintani, D., DellaPenna, D. 1998. Elevating the vitamin E content of plants through metabolic engineering. *Science* 282: 2098–2100.

Silva, D.H.S., Pereira, F.C., Zanoni, M.V.B., Yoshida, M. 2001. Lipophyllic antioxidants from *Iryanthera juruensis* fruits. *Phytochemistry* 57: 437–442.

Slover, H.T. 1971. Tocopherols in food and fats. *Lipids* 6: 291–296.

Soll, J., Schultz, G. 1979. Comparison of geranylgeranyl and phytyl substituted methylquinols in the tocopherol synthesis of spinach chloroplasts. *Biochemical Biophysical Research Communications* 91: 715–720.

Soulier, P., Lecerf, J.-C., Farines, M., Soulier, J. 1989. Composition chimique des beurres de sal et d'illipé. *Revue Francaise des Corps Gras* 36: 361–365.

Sun, Q., Zybailov, B., Majeran, W., Friso, G., Olinares, P.D.B., van Wijk, K.J. 2009. PPDB, the plant proteomics database at Cornell. *Nucleic Acids Research,* 37: 969–974.

Suzuki, Y., Tsuchiya, M., Wassall, S.R. et al. 1993. Structural and dynamic membrane properties of alpha-tocopherol and alpha-tocotrienol. Implication to the molecular mechanism of the antioxidant potency. *Biochemistry* 32: 10692–10699.

Velasco, L., Goffman, F.D., Pujadas-Salva, A.J. 2000. Fatty acids and tocochromanols in seeds of *Orobanche*. *Phytochemistry* 54: 295–300.

Vidi, P.A., Kanwischer, M., Baginsky, S. et al. 2006. Tocopherol cyclase (VTE1) localization and vitamin E accumulation on chloroplast plastoglobule lipoprotein particles. *Journal of Biological Chemistry* 281: 11225–11234.

Wang, X., Quinn, P.J. 2000. The location and function of vitamin E in membranes. *Molecular Membrane Biology* 17: 143–156.

Yang, W., Cahoon, R.E., Hunter, S.C. et al. 2011. Vitamin E biosynthesis: Functional characterization of the monocot homogentisate geranylgeranyl transferase. *Plant Journal* 65: 206–211.

Zlatanov, M.D. 1999. Lipid composition of Bulgarian chokeberry, black currant and rose hip seed oils. *Journal of Agricultural and Food Chemistry* 79: 1620–1624.

2 Safety of Unsaturated Vitamin E Tocotrienols and Their Isomers

Alexander G. Schauss, John R. Endres, and Amy Clewell

CONTENTS

2.1 INTRODUCTION

As late as 2002, major reviews on vitamin E made surprisingly little to no mention of the presence of tocotrienols (Brigelius-Flohe et al., 2002), despite the discovery of these classes of compounds by Pennock and Whittle (Pennock et al., 1964; Whittle et al., 1966) in 1964, and their biological significance delineated in the early 1980s and thereafter (Schauss, 2009). Lack of interest is partially due to the very low levels found in most plants and food sources. So it is not surprising that evidence supporting the safety of tocotrienols is somewhat sparse, as normal food sources are limited. However, with the dramatic increase in the sales of dietary supplements containing tocotrienols higher in concentration than would be found in the daily diet, the need to evaluate the safety of these compounds is imperative.

2.2 CHEMISTRY

The vitamin E natural tocochromanols (tocopherols + tocotrienols) consist of four tocopherols and four tocotrienols each of which contains a chroman ring head, and either a phytyl or a farnesyl tail (Mayer et al., 1967). The 6-hydroxychroman moiety with a lipid-soluble chain is what constitutes vitamin E.

Tocopherols and tocotrienols have α, β, γ, and δ isomers that differ in number and position of the methyl groups in the chroman ring: β- and γ-are structural isomers (5,8-dimethyltocol and 7,8-dimethyltocol), while α- and δ-(5,7,8-trimethyltocol and 8-methyltocol) differ from each other and from β- and γ-because they possess either one more or one less methyl group in the aromatic ring (Mayer et al., 1967; Colombo, 2010).

Figure 2.1 shows the schematic representation of the vitamin E isomers: D-α-tocopherol, D-β-tocopherol, D-γ-tocopherol, D-δ-tocopherol, D-α-tocotrienol, D-β-tocotrienol, D-γ-tocotrienol, and D-δ-tocotrienol. Tocotrienols have an unsaturated farnesyl isoprenoid tail with three trans double bonds in their structure, whereas tocopherols have a saturated phytyl tail (Watson and Preedy, 2009).

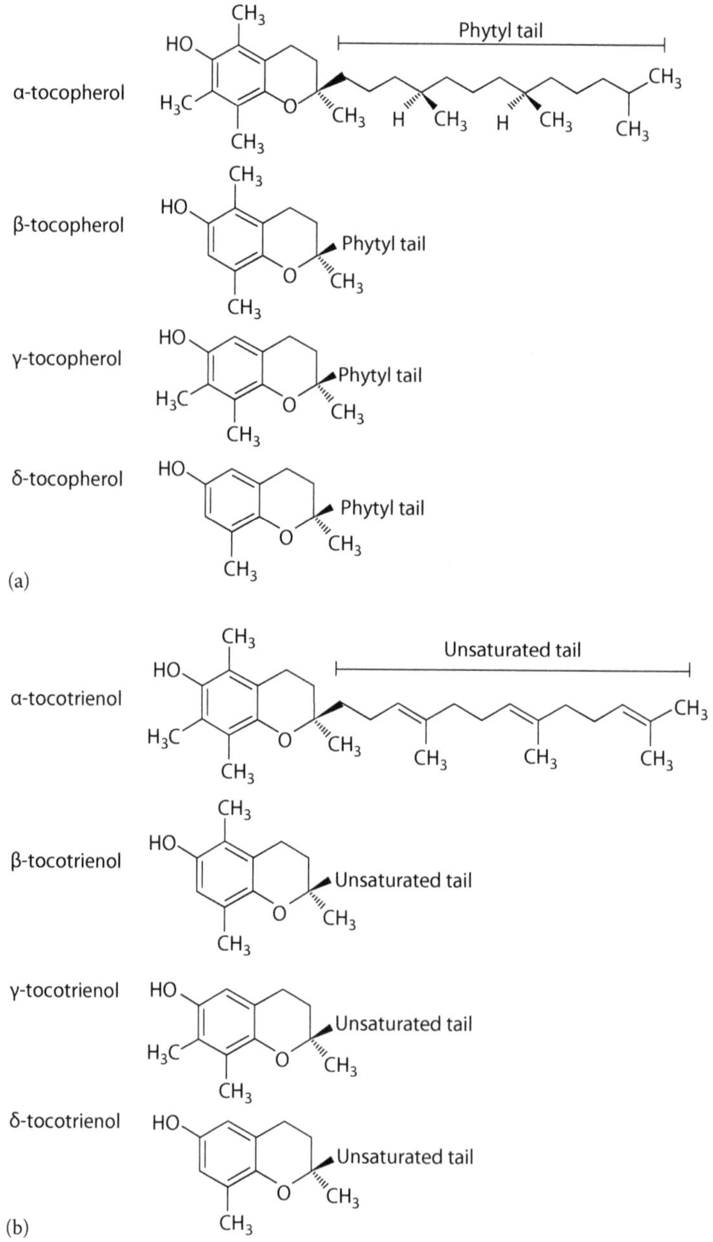

FIGURE 2.1 Schematic structures of (a) tocopherol and (b) tocotrienol isomers.

Compound	Formula	R1	R2	R3	MW
α-tocopherol	$C_{29}H_{50}O_2$	CH_3	CH_3	CH_3	430
α-tocotrienol	$C_{29}H_{44}O_2$	CH_3	H	CH_3	424
β-tocopherol	$C_{28}H_{48}O_2$	CH_3	H	CH_3	416
β-tocotrienol	$C_{29}H_{42}O_2$				410
γ-tocopherol	$C_{28}H_{48}O_2$	H	CH_3	CH_3	416
γ-tocotrienol	$C_{28}H_{42}O_2$				410
δ-tocopherol	$C_{27}H_{46}O_2$	H	H	CH_3	402
δ-tocotrienol	$C_{27}H_{40}O_2$				396

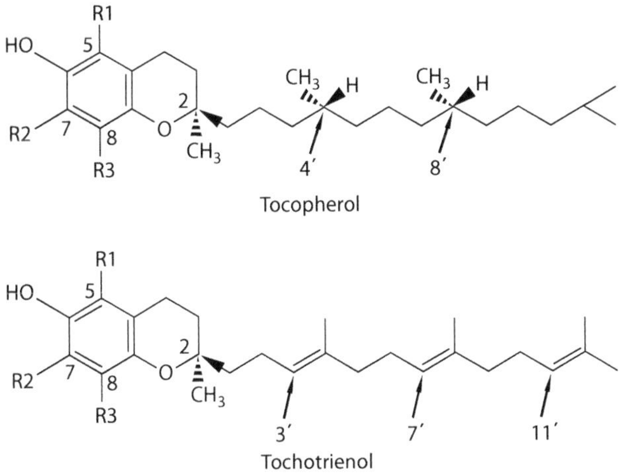

FIGURE 2.2 Structural differences of tocopherol and tocotrienol isomers.

Figure 2.2 provides the molecular formula, number and position of the methyl groups at the five, seven, and eight positions, and molecular weight of each isomer. Tocotrienols have the same basic structure as tocopherols, only with three unsaturated bonds in the side chain. This structural difference accounts for why tocopherols do not have tocotrienol's cholesterol-lowering properties, as tocotrienols down-regulate 3-hydroxy-3-methylglutaryl coenzyme A (HMG-CoA) reductase activity, the rate limiting activity in the mevalonate pathway that contributes to the synthesis of cholesterol (Brown and Goldstein, 1980; Parker et al., 1990; Pearce et al., 1992; Tan et al., 2008).

Tocotrienols are found throughout the plant kingdom, with the highest concentration found in the bright red seeds of *Bixa orellana L.*, a shrub native to tropical America. Known as the "annatto plant," its seeds have a unique composition of 90% δ-tocotrienol and 10% γ-tocotrienol, without any tocopherols. By comparison, other rich sources of tocotrienols have quite different vitamin E isomer ratios. For example, the oil-rich kernels of the palm tree, *Elaeis guineensis* L., the major source of palm oil, have a tocopherol-to-tocotrienol ratio of 25:75, while the ratio in rice is 50:50. Other foods with detectable levels of tocotrienols include rice bran oil, wheat germ, barley oil, and oats (Rao and Perkins, 1972; Ong, 1993; Souci et al., 2002; Moreau et al., 2007; Engelsen and Hansen, 2009).

The levels of tocotrienols in the diet have been studied by several investigators. Franke et al. (2007) analyzed 79 food items commonly consumed in Hawaii for tocotrienol levels, which ranged from nondetectable to 432 mg/kg. The sum of all E vitamers (tocopherols plus tocotrienols) in the foods ranged from 0.6 to 827.7 mg/kg. Mean levels of δ- and γ-tocotrienols in the foods were 37.0 and 36.4 mg/kg, respectively. Overall daily consumption of tocotrienols from foods is thought to be around several milligrams per day, which is well below levels typically studied clinically for health benefits (Sookwong et al., 2008).

The abundance of vitamin E homologues (tocopherols and tocotrienols) in a product depends on the species of the plant from which it is extracted, as well as the extraction methods used to prepare it. For example, a tocotrienol-tocopherol preparation derived from refining rice oil can be prepared by extracting the tocotrienol distillate with methanol until crystallized and then distilling it to remove residual methanol.

Oils that oxidize during processing may induce adverse effects due to the ingestion of oxidative toxicants, and thereby lose their health benefits. Tocotrienols are relatively stable in foods, but can suffer oxidation when exposed to heat, air, metal ions, or extremes of pH. Plants avoid lipid oxidation by accumulating tocochromanols in oily seeds and fruits or in young tissues undergoing active cell divisions (Colombo, 2010). This is one reason why fresh foods lack detectable levels of vitamin E oxidation products.

Only recently have tocotrienols been studied to determine the effects of food storage and processing, or the nature of oxidation products following degradation, especially that of α-tocotrienol, as this isomer is the least stable and has the highest rate of degradation. Using high-performance liquid chromatography (HPLC) with diode array detection, fluorescence detection, and a particle beam interface electron mass spectroscopy, it has been possible to separate the primary oxidation products of α-tocotrienol from eight tocochromanol isomers (Busing and Ternes, 2011). Among several previously unknown oxidation products, only 5-formyl-γ-tocotrienol has been fully characterized by Fourier transform infrared spectroscopy and 1H- and 13C-nuclear magnetic resonance (NMR) spectroscopy, suggesting that much knowledge is still to be obtained about tocotrienol oxidation products and their potential health effects.

2.3 DIFFERENTIAL BIOACTIVITIES OF VITAMIN E ISOMERS

As tocopherols may interfere with tocotrienols' cholesterol-lowering bioactivity (Qureshi et al., 1995; Tan, 2005), this has clinical implications not only in the management of dyslipidemias but also in the outcome of clinical trials that administered either single tocopherol isomers (i.e., D-α-tocopherol) or a mixture of tocopherols lacking tocotrienols.

The complement of vitamin E isomers primarily functions as a chain-breaking antioxidant that prevents the propagation of lipid peroxidation, especially in biological membranes (Watson and Preedy, 2009). During the 1990s, a clearer distinction between the properties of tocotrienols and tocopherols emerged beyond its antioxidant bioactivity, especially for γ- and δ-tocopherols and tocotrienols (Schauss, 2009). For example, tocotrienols have been found to have superior anticancer, antihypertensive, immunomodulatory, and neuroprotective properties in addition to having molecular targets such as apoptotic regulators, cytokines, adhesion molecules, enzymes, kinases, receptors, transcription factors, and growth factors (Koba et al., 1992; Newaz and Nawal, 1999; Yu, 1999; Gu, 1999; O'Byrne, 2000; Sen et al., 2006; Khanna et al., 2006; Patel et al., 2011; Nesaretnam and Meganathan, 2011; Husain et al., 2011; Das et al., 2012). Tocotrienols exhibit antiangiogenic activity, resulting in limiting tumor growth via regulation of growth factor-dependent signaling in endothelial cells (Kannappan et al., 2011; Miyazawa et al., 2011). They also exhibit cardioprotective effects including raising serum HDL-cholesterol, and inhibiting oxidation of low-density lipoproteins, plaque instability and thrombogenesis, platelet aggregation and monocyte adhesion, smooth muscle proliferation, and other cardiovascular dysfunctions (Vasanthi et al., 2011; Prasad, 2011). Tocotrienol fractions have been shown to reduce DNA damage and enhance elongation of telomere length in senescent human diploid fibroblasts, suggesting a potential life extension role (Makpol et al., 2011; Wilankar et al., 2011).

2.4 PHARMACOKINETICS OF TOCOTRIENOLS

The rates of absorption of vitamin E isomers consumed with food vary from as high as 51%–86% to as low as 21%–29% depending on the diet (EFSA Authority 2008). All isomers of vitamin E are absorbed in the lumen of the small intestine into the enterocytes by passive diffusion (Traber, 2007).

Once consumed, emulsification is facilitated by bile acids and salts secreted by the liver. Formation of micelles follows, which contain the vitamin E isomer(s) that are then absorbed at the brush border of the enterocytes in the intestinal mucosa and secreted by the enterocytes into the lymphatics in the form of chylomicrons. (Chylomicrons are among the five major groups of lipoproteins that enable fatty acids and cholesterol to move in the aqueous-based solution of the bloodstream. For this reason, the lipoprotein chylomicron particles contain exogenous lipids, such as vitamin E.) As tocotrienols are transported by the chylomicrons, they eventually disappear from plasma during chylomicron clearance (Hayes et al., 1993). Elimination of nonabsorbed tocotrienols and tocotrienols released by chylomicrons occurs via biliary recycling and fecal excretion (Machlin, 1991). Although tocotrienols are distributed throughout the body via the bloodstream, accumulation of tocotrienols has been found in adipose tissue and the skin, based on studies in different rodent species (Podda et al., 1996; Ikeda et al., 2000).

Human cytochrome P450 4F2 (CYP4F2) catalyzes the hydroxylation reaction in the metabolism of tocopherols and tocotrienols to carboxyethylhydroxychromanols (CEHC). CEHC appears to be the primary metabolite of tocotrienols (Hensley et al., 2004). By studying hydroxylation reactions, it has been determined that CYP4F2-mediated tocopherol-omega-hydroxylation is the primary mechanism that affects the biological half-life and biopotency of tocotrienols (Sontag and Parker, 2007). The influence of the number and positions of methyl groups on the chromanol ring, stereochemistry, and saturation of the side chain has been explored. This led to the determination that methylation at C5 of the chromanol ring is associated with markedly low activity, with tocotrienols exhibiting much higher V_{max} values than that of tocopherols. In the case of α-tocotrienol supplementation in humans, it has been shown that it peaks at a concentration of 3 μmol in the plasma (Khanna et al., 2006). Conjugated long-chain carboxychromanols may be novel excreted metabolites, with γ-tocotrienol more extensively metabolized than γ-tocopherol (Freiser and Jiang, 2009).

The superfamily of ATP-binding cassette transporters carry various molecules across extra- and intra-cellular membranes and thus serve an important role as efflux pumps for xenobiotic compounds with broad substrate specificity, thereby decreasing drug accumulation. Within this superfamily of proteins is the permeability glycoprotein (P-glycoprotein), also known as the multidrug resistance protein 1 (MDR1) which is expressed in humans by the ABCB1 gene in certain cells in the liver, kidney, jejunum, pancreas, and colon. The interaction of γ-tocotrienol has been investigated to determine if it can cause significant alteration of the pharmacokinetic properties of P-glycoprotein (P-gp) when taken with P-gp substrate drugs (Abznait et al., 2011). Natural products can up-regulate P-gp expression and functionality, which may induce food–drug interactions when taken with P-gp substrate medications. Treatment with γ-tocotrienol resulted in a ~2.5-fold increase in P-gp expression when concomitantly used with P-gp substrate drugs.

Ralla et al. (2011) assessed intestinal absorption of tocotrienols in dogs. 40 mg/kg bw of a tocotrienol-rich fraction containing 32% α-tocotrienol, 2% β-tocotrienol, 27% γ-tocotrienol, 14% δ-tocotrienol, and 25% α-tocopherol was given by intubation. The results showed that tocotrienols were detected in plasma with a noticeable increase in antioxidant capacity. α-tocopherol that was detected in plasma was unaffected by tocotrienols.

Tocotrienols have gained considerable attention as anticancer agents. Their antiproliferative, antiangiogenic, and apoptotic effects, and ability to induce immunologic activity suggest they may be potent antitumor agents. Tocotrienol isomers display potent apoptotic activity against a range of cancer cell types, yet have little to no effect on normal cell function or viability (Sylvester, 2007). Determining the intracellular mechanisms as to how the isomers mediate apoptic effects on different types of cancer cells has been an ongoing area of research. Certain tocotrienol isomers have been found to have a high affinity for estrogen receptor-beta (ER-β) but not ER-α signaling, based on *in silico* and *in vitro* binding analyses (Nesaretnam et al., 2011). These studies have demonstrated that specific tocotrienols increase ER-β translocation into the nucleus to activate expression of various estrogen responsive genes in breast cancer cells. Such binding of tocotrienol isomers to ER-β is associated with caspase-3 activation, DNA fragmentation, apoptosis, and changes in cell morphology. The results suggest the need for further research on tocotrienols as a potential adjunctive treatment for breast cancer.

Erlotinib and gefitinib are anticancer agents that inhibit the activation of individual human epidermal growth factor receptor subtypes, but have shown limited clinical success because of heterodimerization between different receptor family members that can rescue cancer cells from agents directed against a single receptor subtype. Known as epidermal growth factor receptors (EGFR), their excessive signaling is associated in humans with the development of numerous neurodegenerative diseases, including Alzheimer's disease, and the development of malignancies associated with a wide variety of tumors. Studies have investigated the anticancer effectiveness of low-dose treatment of statins or EGFR inhibitors alone and in combination with γ-tocotrienol on highly malignant +SA mouse mammary epithelial cells *in vitro*. In one study, combined treatment with γ-tocotrienol and chemotherapeutic agents resulted in a synergistic inhibition of +SA cell growth and viability, suggesting that combined treatment of γ-tocotrienol with anticancer agents may not only provide an enhanced therapeutic response, but also offer a means to avoid the toxicity associated with high-dose chemotherapy (Sylvester, 2011). A study determined that the meachanism of action of tocotrienol-induced apoptosis in neoplastic +SA mammary epithelial cells grown *in vitro* occurs independent of mitochondrial stress apoptic signaling (Shah and Sylvester, 2005).

Yap et al. (2001), reported on a study of healthy subjects administered a single dose of 300 mg of mixed tocotrienols under fasting or fed conditions to study their bioavailability. No significant differences were observed between the fasted and fed peak plasma concentrations (T_{max}) or area under the plasma concentration-time curve values of the three isomers. The mean apparent elimination half-life of α-, γ-, and δ-tocotrienols was estimated to be 4.4, 4.3, and 2.3 h, respectively, between 4.5-fold and 8.7-fold shorter than that reported for α-tocopherol. The authors also reported that the mean apparent volume of distribution values under the fed state were significantly smaller than those of the fasted state, which they attributed to increased absorption of tocotrienols in the fed state. No adverse effects were reported.

2.5   DRUG–NUTRIENT INTERACTIONS

The molecular mechanism by which tocotrienols affect absorption and efficacy of certain drugs has been studied. The steroid and xenobiotic receptor (SXR) (also, known as pregnane X receptor, and pregnane-activated receptor), an orphan nuclear receptor, has been of particular interest as its expression regulates xenobiotic, endobiotic, and dietary clearance in the liver and intestine. SXR also plays an important role in the regulation of the cytochrome CYP3A4 gene and multidrug resistance gene 1 (MDR1). Zhou et al. (2004) demonstrated that all four tocotrienols bind to and activate SXR, whereas tocopherols do not (Zhou et al., 2004). Tocotrienols upregulate CYP3A4, but not MDR1 or UDP-glucuronosyltransferase 1A1 (UGT1A1) in primary hepatocytes, yet induce MDR1 and UGT1A1, but not CYP3A4 in intestinal LS180 cells, suggesting tocotrienols show tissue-specific induction of SXR target genes. These investigations have also found that expression of nuclear receptor corepressors (NCoR) enhance the ability of tocotrienols to induce CYP3A4 in LS180 cells.

Since tocotrienols have a natural blood thinning effect, lower doses of the blood thinner warfarin (Coumadin®) may be needed. Individuals should consider stopping tocotrienol supplementation directly prior to and after surgery. Certain medications are known to impede Vitamin E absorption, such as: cholestyramine (Questran®, Questran Light®, Cholybar®), a bile acid sequestrant; colestipol (Colestid®), a cholesterol lowering drug; isoniazid (Tubizid®), an antibiotic to treat tuberculosis; mineral oil; or, sucralfate (Carafate®; Xactdose®), a gastro-protective drug. Also, tocotrienol supplementation could hypothetically affect liver metabolism of certain drugs.

2.6 EXPERIMENTAL STUDIES ASSESSING THE SAFETY OF TOCOTRIENOLS

2.6.1 *In Vitro* and *In Vivo* Genotoxicity Studies

Tasaki et al. (2008) mentions unpublished studies on a mixed tocotrienol sample; the sample was negative for mutagenic activity in bacteria, negative for chromosome aberration activity in mammalian cells, and negative for the induction of micronuclei when administered to mice. Polasa and Rukmini (1987) reported no mutagenic activity of a dimethylsulfoxide (DMSO)-based extract of rice bran oil in a modified Ames test using *Salmonella typhimurium* strains TA98 and TA100 with or without metabolic activation. However, although tocotrienols are found at detectable levels in rice, no information was provided on the percentage of the tocotrienol content of RBO, as pointed out by Raghuram et al. (1995).

Oliveira et al. (1994) investigated the genotoxicity of red palm oil on bone marrow cells from 8 to 10 week old Balb/C female mice. Experimental groups received five daily gavage doses of 4.5 g/kg supernatant and sediment of red palm oil. The negative control group received corn oil and the positive control group received cyclophosphamide at 20 mg/kg intraperitoneally. There were no differences in the frequency of chromosomal aberrations between mice that were treated with red palm oil and those that received corn oil. However, although tocotrienols are found at detectable levels in red palm oil, no information was provided on tocotrienol content.

2.6.2 Acute and Subchronic Animal Toxicity Studies

Oo et al. (1992) administered a palm oil extract containing 80% tocotrienols to rats and mice by intubation up to a dose of 25,000 mg/kg bw in an acute toxicology study. No mortality or adverse effects were observed in animals at any dose.

Ima-Nirwana et al. (2011) performed 14 day acute and 42 day subchronic toxicity studies in mice given a palm oil extract by intubation that contained 18.43% α-tocopherol, 14.62% α-tocotrienol, 32.45% γ-tocotrienol, and 23.93% δ-tocotrienols. Doses of the extract administered were 200, 500, and 1000 mg/kg bw; the control group received vitamin E free palm oil. No deaths were reported in the acute toxicity study. In the subchronic study, 1 death occurred in the 200 mg group, 3 deaths in the 500 mg group, and 1 death, in the fourth week of treatment in the 1000 mg group. While no differences were noted related to weight in the acute study, in the subchronic study body weight was lower in the 500 mg group from 5 weeks onward, as well as after 4 weeks in the 1000 mg group. Bleeding time was increased in the 500 mg group in the acute study, as well as in the 500 and 1000 mg/kg groups in the subchronic study. Thus, the anticoagulant effects of tocotrienols need further study. Some renal impairment was seen by an increase in serum creatinine in the 500 and 1000 mg groups in the subchronic study. This coincided with the reduction in kidney weights seen in the 200 and 500 mg groups and in the acute toxicity study in the 1000 mg group. No previous animal or human toxicology or clinical trial study has reported renal impairment, which suggests the need to confirm and further elucidate the extract that was tested.

Whereas the studies of Ima–Nirwana used an extract that contained 80% tocotrienols, Nakamura et al. (2001) studied a palm oil extract that contained 70% tocotrienols in a 13 week oral toxicity study in rats at doses of 0, 119, 474, and 2130 mg/kg bw in males, and 0, 130, 491, and 2,047 mg in females. The study established a no-observed-adverse-event-level (NOAEL) of 1.9 g/kg in the diet, which corresponded to 120 mg/kg/day for males and 130 mg/kg/day for females, as adverse events were observed and measured in the two highest dose groups, including increased liver and adrenal weight in all treated male animals, and ovary and uterus weights in the highest dose females. Serum biochemical examinations revealed an increase in albumin/globulin ratio and alkaline phophastase in all treated males, and decreased mean corpuscular hemoglobin and mean corpuscular hemoglobin concentration in females in the two highest dose groups, while also reducing hematocrit in females of the highest dose group. Histopathological examinations were unremarkable except for a reduction in vacuolation observed in the adrenal cortical region in males. This was attributed to the hypocholesterolemic bioactivity of tocotrienols, as these compounds can reduce cholesterol and steroid precursors.

2.6.3 Chronic Animal Toxicity Studies

Tasaki et al. (2008) evaluated the toxicological effects of a 52 week exposure to tocotrienol concentrate from palm oil extract (21.4% α-tocotrienol, 3.5% β-tocotrienol, 36.5% γ-tocotrienol, 8.6% δ-tocotrienol) in Wistar Hannover rats of both sexes. Four groups (10 rats/sex/group) were fed daily doses of 0%, 0.08%, 0.4%, or 2% of a preparation in powdered diet. By week 50, six male rats had died at the 2% dose. At necropsy, these rats were found to have hemorrhaging observed at the cerebral base and in the thoracic cavity, testes, prostate, and/or bladder. Because of this, for the last 2 weeks of the study, the 2% dose was decreased to 1% in both sexes.

The final body weights of male and female rats were significantly decreased in the initially 2% treated group. Relative but not absolute weights of brain, heart, lungs, and kidneys were significantly increased in male rats receiving the initial 2% dose. Absolute weights were significantly increased for heart, liver, and kidney at 0.4% and decreased for lung at 2% dose for female rats. A significant decrease in hematocrit (Ht) and white blood cells (WBC) at the 0.08% dose was noted, as well as a significant decrease in mean corpuscular volume (MCV) at the dose of 0.4% for male rats. In female rats, significant decreases of hemoglobin (Hb), Ht, and mean corpuscular hemoglobin (MCH) were observed at the 2% dose only. The changes in the serum biochemical data were not considered to have toxicological significance, as the values were within normal range.

Contrary to other studies, there was no change in the serum cholesterol levels among the groups. In males, significant increases of A/G, P, ALT, ALP, and D.Bil, and decreases of LDH and TG were observed at the dose of 2%. At necropsy, multiple cystic nodules were found with high incidence in the livers of male and female rats in the 2% dose group. Upon histopathological examination of these rats, nodular hepatocellular hyperplasia was evident with distortion of hepatic cords and compression of the surrounding tissue, resulting in a diagnosis of spongiosis hepatis, the precise pathogenesis of which is unknown. However, since Ito cells produce a number of growth factors, the simultaneous incidence of spongiosis hepatis may have contributed to the proliferative activity of hepatocytes in the nodules.

The authors stated that there was no toxicological change in any of the parameters examined with a tocotrienol dose of 0.4% or less given to male or female rats, although a significant increase in the absolute weight of heart, liver, and kidney organs of female rats were reported without histopathological findings. Based on the results demonstrating nodular hepatocellular hyperplasia only at the high dose for both sexes, the authors concluded that the NOAEL is 0.4%, which corresponds to 303 mg/kg/day for males, and 472 mg/kg/day for females (Tasaki et al., 2008). Two of the authors from the aforementioned Nakamura study were coauthors for this study, which is of a similar design and used an identical test article with respect to the tocotrienol composition.

Rahmat et al. (1993) investigated the effects of long-term (9 month) administration of tocotrienol on hepatocarcinogenesis (induced by diethylnitrosamine (DEN) and 2-acetylaminofluorene (AAF)) in rats. Twenty-eight male 7–8 week old *Rattus norvegicus* rats, weighing 120–160 g were divided into four treatment groups: a control group on a basal diet, a group fed a basal diet supplemented with tocotrienol (30 mg/kg food), a group treated with DEN/AAF, and a group treated with DEN/AAF and fed a diet supplemented with tocotrienol (30 mg/kg food). The tocotrienol was composed of 80% γ-tocotrienol, and 20% α- and β-tocotrienol. The rats were sacrificed after 9 months and the livers were examined morphologically. Grayish white nodules (2/liver) were found in all the DEN/AAF-treated rats ($n = 10$), but only one of the rats treated with DEN/AAF and supplemented with tocotrienol ($n = 6$) had liver nodules. The authors concluded that tocotrienol supplementation attenuated the impact of carcinogenesis in the rats.

2.6.4 Reproductive and Developmental Animal Toxicity Studies

Rukmini (1988) investigated the toxicological effects of consumption of rice bran oil by rats over three generations. Thirty (15 females, 15 males) weanling albino rats of NIN/Wistar strain were fed a diet containing 20% protein and 10% rice bran oil or 10% groundnut oil (control). The rice bran oil did not affect the balance of nitrogen, phosphorus, and calcium in rats (calculated based on dietary and fecal levels of these nutrients) or percentages of conception, birth weight, litter size, weaning weight, and pre-weaning mortality. In addition, no differences in mutagenicity and teratogenicity were observed. No specific information about tocotrienol content was provided.

2.7 HUMAN STUDIES

2.7.1 Human Requirements and Recommended Intake Levels of Vitamin E

In the United States, the panel on Dietary Antioxidants and Related Compounds, Subcommittee on Upper Reference Levels of Nutrients and Interpretation and Uses or Dietary Reference Intakes (DRIs), Standing Committee on the Scientific Evaluation of Dietary Reference Intakes, and Food and Nutrition Board of the Institute of Medicine, have concluded that Vitamin E is safe for chronic use in the general population at levels up to 1000 mg/day (1000 IU synthetic Vitamin E, 1500 IU natural Vitamin E) (Institute of Medicine 2000a). The panel concluded that the Recommended Dietary Allowance (RDA) for vitamin E is the same for men and women regardless of age, and α-tocopherol alone is used for estimating vitamin E requirements and recommending daily vitamin E intake, since the other naturally occurring forms of vitamin E (β-, γ-, δ-tocopherols, and the tocotrienols) are not converted to α-tocopherol transfer protein in the liver. (In referring to α-tocopherol, the panel includes RRR-α-tocopherol, the only form of α-tocopherol that occurs naturally in foods, and the 2R-stereoisomeric forms of α-tocopherol (RRR-, RSR-, RRS-, and RSS-α tocopherol) that occur in fortified foods and supplements. They also concluded that the 2R-stereoisomeric forms of α-tocopherol are the only forms of vitamin E that have been shown to meet human requirements.)

To estimate the requirement for vitamin E, the panel examined data on induced vitamin E deficiency in humans and the intake that correlated with *in vitro* hydrogen peroxide-induced hemolysis and plasma α-tocopherol concentrations (Institute of Medicine 2000b). They also recognized that vitamin E acts as an *in vivo* antioxidant, supporting normal physiological function related to endogenous antioxidant defense systems.

As has been the case in review papers on vitamin E, the panel gave scant attention to the role of tocotrienols in their recommendations. The panel determined that the Tolerable Upper Intake Levels (UL) by life stage for α-tocopherol ranged from 200 mg to 1000 mg/day, as it is their opinion that intakes above the UL from food, water, and supplements increases the risk of adverse effects, particularly impaired bleeding and clotting time as seen in rat studies (Traber, 2008). But this pertains only to α-tocopherol, not tocotrienols. These recommendations disregard the compelling body of biological evidence—when setting the UL for vitamin E and other antioxidants—that at high enough levels such as that occurring during oxidative stress, reactive oxygen and nitrogen species can cause considerable damage to cells and cell membranes, leading to cellular dysfunction and disease. The recommended UL for vitamin E also neglects to take into consideration the etiology of excessive oxidation and nitrogen species *in vivo* to carcinogenesis, cardiovascular and neurodegenerative diseases, and the whole spectrum of metabolic diseases, such as diabetes and obesity.

What is of significance in reading the panel's conclusions is their statement that

> Because the various forms of vitamin E are not intraconvertible and because plasma concentrations of α-tocopherol are dependent upon the affinity of the hepatic α-tocopherol transfer protein for the various forms, it is recommended that relative biological potencies of the various forms of vitamin E be reevaluated. Until this is done, the actual concentrations of each of the various vitamin E forms in food and biological samples should be reported separately, whenever possible (Institute of Medicine, 2000b, p. 19).

In Europe, the RDA for vitamin E is set at 10 mg/day (European Council Directive 90/496/EEC [1990]). The lack of attention by the U.S. panel to the tocotrienol content of vitamin E, contrasts significantly with that of the European Food Safety Authority (EFSA). In 2008, the EFSA reported on their panel of expert's "opinion on mixed tocopherols, tocotrienol, tocopherol, and tocotrienols as sources for vitamin E added as a nutritional substance in food supplements" (EFSA Authority 2008).

2.7.2 CLINICAL STUDIES

Clinical trials of vitamin E have reported few side effects. The exception has been two studies that found an association between increased deaths due to hemorrhagic stroke and all-cause mortality. The former was a study of long-term Finnish smokers given alpha-tocopherol or beta-carotene treatment for 5–8 years, known as the Alpha-Tocopherol, Beta-Carotene Cancer Prevention study (ABTC 1994). The latter study is known as the Cambridge Heart Anti-oxidant Study (CHAOS) (Stephens et al., 1996). The explanation for these findings remains controversial, but in neither study were tocotrienols given to participants.

Major clinical studies conducted on tocotrienols are summarized in Table 2.1 and are individually discussed in the following.

Qureshi et al. (1991) investigated the effect of a mix of vitamin E compounds on serum lipids of hypercholesterolemic adults who had cholesterol levels ranging from 6.21 to 8.02 mmol/L. All subjects were first observed for a 2 week baseline period. In this double-blind crossover study, subjects were randomly assigned to receive four 50 mg capsules of a tocotrienol-enriched fraction of palm oil, containing 15%–20% α-tocopherol, 12%–15% α-tocotrienol, 35%–40% γ-tocotrienol, and 25%–30% δ-tocotrienol, mixed with 250 mg of palm superolein (palmvitee), or 300 mg of corn oil (control), for 4–6 weeks. The authors reported significant decreases in serum total cholesterol, LDL-C, apo B, thromboxane, platelet factor 4, and glucose concentration in the treatment group. The LDL-cholesterol lowering effect was only significant after exclusion of three poor responders among those in the 15-subject tocotrienol group. No adverse events were reported.

Tomeo et al. (1995) conducted a randomized, placebo-controlled study to investigate the antioxidant effects of daily ingestion of 300 mg capsules that each contained 16 mg α-tocopherol, 40 mg γ- and α-tocotrienols, 240 mg palm superolein, or 300 mg palm superolein (placebo) for 18 months in 50 patients with carotid artery atherosclerosis. During the first 3 months of the study, subjects received four capsules daily. The daily dosage increased to five capsules for months 4–6, and then to six capsules for the remainder of the study. The authors reported no improvement in blood lipids with tocotrienol supplementation, but observed regression of carotid stenosis as evidenced by improved blood flow in the carotid arteries in 24% of the subjects supplemented for 12 months. No adverse events were reported.

Qureshi et al. (1995) conducted a follow up study with 36 hypercholesterolemic (cholesterol levels above 5.7 mmol/L) individuals. Subjects were maintained on the American Heart Association (AHA) Step I diet throughout the study and received 4 weeks of palmvitee, a tocotrienol-rich fraction of palm oil containing 48 mg α-tocotrienol, 112 mg γ-tocotrienol, 60 mg δ-tocotrienol, and 40 mg α-tocopherol, or 200 mg of γ-tocopherol, a tocopherol-free preparation. The authors reported significant decreases in serum total cholesterol, apo B, and thromboxane in subjects taking tocotrienols. No adverse events were reported.

Qureshi et al. (1997) obtained similar results in a later study with a similar design, in which 20 subjects consumed a 4 week diet put forth by the National Cholesterol Education Program instead of the AHA Step I diet followed by a 4 week daily supplementation with a processed oil extracted from rice bran that contained 12.5% α-tocopherol, 21% γ-tocotrienol, 10% δ-tocotrienol, 4.5% d-tocotrienol, 17% P_{25}-tocotrienol, 6% α-tocopherol, and 18% unidentified tocotrienols. No adverse events were reported.

Mensink et al. (1999) reported on a 6 week study of 20 subjects men with mild hypercholesterolemia given 240 mg/day of palm olein, 20 mg α-tocopherol, and 40 mg tocotrienols, or control capsules containing 280 mg palm olein and 20 mg DL-α-tocopherol. The tocotrienol-containing capsules did not have beneficial effects on serum lipoproteins, lipid peroxide concentrations, or hemostatic measures. No adverse effects were reported.

TABLE 2.1
Summary of Notable Clinical Studies on Tocotrienol

Study	Number of Subjects in Study	Duration	Total T3 Dose (mg/day)	Source	Adverse Events
Qureshi et al. (1991)	25	4 weeks	160	Palm	The authors reported no adverse events
Tomeo et al. (1995)	50	18 months	Approx 240	Palm	The authors reported no adverse events
Qureshi et al. (1995)	36	4–8 weeks	220 and 200	Palm	The authors reported no adverse events
Qureshi et al. (1997)	41	4 weeks	166	Rice bran	The authors reported no adverse events
Mensink et al. (1999)	20	6 weeks	140	Palm	The authors reported no adverse events
Kooyenga et al. (2001)	50	3 years 1 year	52	Palm Rice bran	Authors state there were "no reports of side effects such as headache, intestinal upset, muscle weakness, or persistent liver function abnormalities"
Qureshi et al. (2001)	14 14	35 days 70 days	50	Rice bran	The authors reported no adverse events
Qureshi et al. (2002)	90	35 days	22%–174%	Rice bran	The authors reported no adverse events
O'Byrne et al. (2003)	51	8 weeks	250	Palm	Authors report that subjects tolerated tocotrienol acetates, except four subjects who received γ-tocotrienols acetate and had transient abdominal distention, gastric upset, and pain during the first week. Two subjects reported persistent flatulence. One subject, who had a hiatal hernia and gastric reflux, reported nausea and vomiting 1 h after taking α-tocotrienol acetate with their evening meal—symptoms stopped when taken with their afternoon meal
Baliar-singh et al. (2005)	19	8 weeks	390	Rice bran	The authors reported no adverse events
Tan (2005)	10 (5 × 2)	2 months	75	Annatto	The authors reported no adverse events
Rasool et al. (2006)	36	8 weeks	59–237	Palm	The authors reported no adverse events; treatment was well tolerated
Ajuluchukwu et al. (2007)	28	4 weeks	50	Palm	The authors reported no adverse events
Rasool et al. (2008)	36	8 weeks	39–154	Palm	The authors reported no adverse events; treatment was well tolerated
Radhakrishnan et al. (2008)	53	56 days	140	Palm	The authors reported no adverse events
Mahalingam et al. (2010)	108	56 days	400	Palm	No vaccine-related serious adverse events were reported. The authors reported no adverse events

Kooyenga et al. (2001) conducted a 4 year clinical study to investigate the effect of supplementation with an extract from palm oil for 3 years and rice bran for 1 year on carotid atherosclerosis. Each rice bran oil capsule provided 52 mg of tocotrienol, 60 mg of α-tocopherol, and 76 mg of non-saponifiables. No information about the percentage of different tocotrienols was provided. Placebo capsules contained 300 mg oil (oil is not further specified; however, "vehicle is described as 17.5% palmitic and stearic acids, 42.5% oleic acid, and 40% linoleic acid by weight). The authors stated that there were no reports of side effects "such as headache, intestinal upset, muscle weakness, or persistent liver function abnormalities" in the 50 subjects studied. No improvement in blood lipids was observed during the first 36 months, although blood flow appeared to improve for 10 of 25 patients. Decreases in serum cholesterol, LDL, and triglyceride levels and an increase in HDL occurred from month 36–48 during the period of consumption of rice bran oil. Eight of the subjects who consumed the supplement moved to a lower category of stenosis, two subjects moved two categories lower, three subjects increased in progression of disease, and the remaining subjects showed no difference in disease progression.

Qureshi et al. (2001) investigated the efficacy of tocotrienol-rich fraction of rice bran (TRF_{25}), both alone and in combination with the cholesterol-lowering drug, lovastatin. TRF_{25} consisted of 8.7% α-tocopherol, 15.5% α-tocotrienol, 1.6% β-tocotrienol, 39.4% γ-tocotrienol, 4.4% δ-tocopherol, 5.2% δ-tocotrienol, and 25.2% other tocotrienol-like compounds. In this five-phase study, with each phase lasting 35 days, 28 hypercholesterolemic subjects were placed on the AHA Step I diet (during phase II of the study) and divided into two groups (14 subjects per group). Group A subjects were given 10 mg lovastatin per day in the third phase, 10 mg lovastatin plus 50 mg TRF_{25} per day in the fourth phase, and 10 mg lovastatin plus 50 mg alpha-tocopherol per day, in the fifth phase of the study. Group B subjects were given 50 mg TRF_{25} per day instead of lovastatin in the third phase, but were otherwise treated according to the same protocol. TRF_{25} or lovastatin plus AHA Step I diet lowered serum total cholesterol (14%, 13%) and LDL-cholesterol (18%, 15% $p < 0.001$), respectively. The combination of TRF_{25} and lovastatin plus AHA Step I diet significantly reduced lipid parameters by 20% and 25% ($p < 0.001$) in these subjects. However, replacement of TRF_{25} with alpha-tocopherol produced insignificant changes when given with lovastatin. No side effects were reported during the 25 week study.

Qureshi et al. (2002) investigated the effect of four doses (25, 50, 100, and 200 mg/day) of a tocotrienol-rich fraction (8.7% α-tocopherol, 15.5% α-tocotrienol, 1.6% β-tocotrienol, 39.4% γ-tocotrienol, 5.2% δ-tocotrienol, and 4.4% δ-tocopherol, 20.9% D-desmethyl (D-P_{21}-tocotrienol), plus D-didesmethyl (D-P_{25}-tocotrienol) tocotrienols, 4.3% unidentified tocotrienols) from rice bran oil on the suppression of serum cholesterol in adults. Ninety hypercholesterolemic subjects were divided into five groups and the study was carried out in three phases (adaptation, AHA Step I diet, and AHA Step I diet plus tocotrienol supplementation), each of which lasted for 35 days. The placebo group received 200 mg/day of vitamin E-stripped rice bran oil plus AHA Step I diet. Maximum decreases in serum cholesterol, LDL-C, apoB, and triglycerides were achieved with a dose of 100 mg/day of the tocotrienol-rich fraction. No adverse events were reported.

O'Byrne et al. (2000) investigated whether 250 mg/day of (α-, γ-, or δ-) tocotrienyl acetates isolated from a palm oil tocotrienol mixture would alter serum cholesterol or LDL oxidative resistance in hypercholesterolemic subjects. In a double-blind study, 51 subjects were randomly assigned to a treatment or placebo group and followed a low-fat diet plus supplements for 8 weeks. Neither serum LDL cholesterol nor apo-B was significantly decreased by tocotrienyl acetate supplementation. The authors reported that subjects tolerated the tocotrienyl supplements, except for four subjects receiving γ-tocotrienyl acetate supplements who had a transient abdominal distention, gastric upset, and pain during the first week of supplementation. Two of the subjects also reported flatulence that persisted during the study. One subject who had a hiatal hernia and gastric reflux reported nausea and vomiting 1 h after taking α-tocotrienyl supplements with the evening meal. However, these symptoms stopped when supplements were taken with the afternoon meal.

Baliarsingh et al. (2005) studied the effect of consumption of a tocotrienol-tocopherol mixture on lipid profiles and glycemic parameters in subjects with Type 2 diabetes and hyperlipidemia. A total of 19 subjects participated in this study with a randomized, double-blind, placebo-controlled crossover design. Throughout the study, subjects were advised to follow a diabetic diet composed of 50%–55% carbohydrate, 15%–20% protein, 30%–35% fat, and 15–20 g of dietary fiber per day. Subjects were then randomly assigned to receive 6 mg/kg bw of a vitamin E mix composed of 14.6% α-tocotrienol, 2.2% β-tocotrienol, 38.8% γ-tocotrienol, 29.9% δ-tocotrienol, 7.5% α-tocopherol, 4.6% δ-tocopherol, and 2.4% unidentified tocotrienols, or a placebo that contained 100 mg of rice bran oil free of vitamin E for 60 days (phase I). In the second phase of the study, which lasted another 60 days, subjects who received the placebo during phase I received the treatment and subjects who received the treatment in phase I received the placebo. The combined results showed that fasting and postprandial sugar levels did not change significantly after 60 days of treatment, indicating a stable glycemic status. A significant decline in total cholesterol and LDL-C with no effect on HDL-C was observed. The authors concluded that daily supplementation by Type 2 diabetics with the mix of tocopherols/tocotrienols given in the study will be useful in the prevention and treatment of hyperlipidemia and atherogenesis. No adverse events were reported.

Tan (2008) describes two open human studies performed using annatto tocotrienols. The studies each involved five subjects who took 75 mg/day of a 90% δ-tocotrienol and 10% γ-tocotrienol annatto product for 2 months. On average, total cholesterol and LDL-cholesterol dropped 13%, triglycerides dropped 23%, and HDL-cholesterol increased by 6%. No adverse events were reported. Without a control group, it is not possible to separate time or placebo effects from treatment effects.

Rasool et al. (2006) assessed the effects of three doses (80, 160, and 320 mg/day) of a tocotrienol-rich vitamin E supplement [34.6% α-tocotrienol, 24.6% γ-tocotrienol, 15% δ-tocotrienol, and 26.2% α-tocopherol] consumed for 2 months by 36 healthy men in a randomized, blinded, placebo-controlled trial with a parallel design. Treatment significantly increased α-, γ-, and δ-tocotrienol concentrations in plasma, but did not affect arterial compliance, plasma antioxidant status, serum cholesterol or LDL-cholesterol levels. The authors concluded that the tocotrienol-rich vitamin E supplements at doses up to 320 mg daily were well tolerated with no serious adverse events recorded.

Ajuluchukwu et al. (2007) studied the effect of tocotrienols on the serum lipid profiles of 28 individuals aged 18–80 with mild hypercholesterolemia (5.18–7.77 mmol/L). Subjects were randomly assigned to receive tocotrienols (consisting of 15.38 mg D-α-tocotrienol, 28.20 mg D-γ-tocotrienol, 6.42 mg D-δ-tocotrienol, and 22.90 mg D-α tocopherol) or 500 or 1000 mg vitamin E (α-tocopherol) capsules per day or every other day (n = 16). All subjects were on the AHA Step I diet. Levels of lipids were compared prior to and after 4 weeks of receiving the treatment. The authors reported a significant decrease in the total cholesterol and LDL-cholesterol for subjects who took the tocotrienol supplement compared to subjects who took the tocopherol supplement, but no difference in HDL-cholesterol or triglycerides for either group. No adverse events were reported.

Rasool et al. (2008) studied the effect of 50, 100, and 200 mg of "self-emulsifying tocotrienol-rich vitamin E" (a soft gel able to emulsify under the gentle agitation produced in the gastrointestinal tract) in 36 healthy males in a randomized, placebo-controlled, blinded end-point clinical study of 2 months duration. The supplement was Tocovid Suprabio® (Hovid, Malaysia) and comprised of 23.54% α-tocotrienol, 43.16% γ-tocotrienol, 9.83% δ-tocotrienol, and 23.5% α-tocopherol. Treatment led to a trend toward improvement in arterial compliance. The tocotrienol-rich vitamin E was overall well tolerated, and no adverse events occurred that required withdrawal from the supplement.

Radhakrishnan et al. (2008) looked at the potential immunomodulatory effects of a tocotrienol-rich fraction (TRF) derived from palm oil in 53 healthy Asian men and women. The TRF contained 70% tocotrienols (113 mg α-tocotrienol, 91 mg γ-tocotrienol, 36 mg δ-tocotrienol, 10 mg β-tocotrienol) and 30% tocopherols. It was a randomized, double-blind placebo-controlled study with three groups. The groups were given either 200 mg TRF, 200 mg α-tocopherol or placebo for 56 days. No significant differences in the immune parameters measured were noted. No adverse events were reported.

Mahalingam et al. (2010) studied the effect of TRF derived from palm oil in 108 healthy women, aged 18–25, to measure the immune response to a challenge of a tetanus toxoid vaccine. This study was of similar design to the Radhakrishnan et al. (2008) study, with the addition of an immune challenge. The double-blind, placebo-controlled trial used a dose of 400 mg of TRF per day or placebo for 56 days. The composition of each tablet (of which two were given) was 61.52 mg D-α-tocotrienol, 112.80 mg D-γ-tocotrienol, 25.68 mg D-δ-tocotrienol, and 91.60 D-α-tocopherol. Tetanus toxoid vaccine was given on day 28. Those in the treatment group had a significant increase in total vitamin E levels (including tocotrienol levels) in the plasma as compared to the placebo. They also had a significantly enhanced production of IFN-γ and IL4, a significant decrease in IL6, and significant augmentation of anti tetanus toxoid-IgG production. No adverse events were reported.

As is evident, adverse events in human clinical trials associated with tocotrienol-containing supplements are rare, offering the strong supporting evidence that tocotrienols and tocopherol–tocotrienol mixtures are safe within the dose ranges studied.

2.8   GENERALLY RECOGNIZED AS SAFE (GRAS) STATUS

Tocotrienols as a group or as specific isomers have in recent decades been added to the food supply, either as ingredients added to foods or in dietary supplements. Under sections 201(s) and 409 of the U.S. Federal Food, Drug, and Cosmetic Act, any substance that is intentionally added to food is a food additive that is subject to premarket review and approval by the FDA, unless the substance is generally recognized, among qualified experts, as reasonably certain to be safe under the conditions of its intended use, or unless the use of the substance is otherwise excluded from the definition of a food additive. A GRAS substance is distinguished from a food additive on the basis of the common knowledge about the safety of the substance for its intended use. Thus, the difference between use of a food additive and use of a GRAS substance relates to the widespread awareness of the data and information about the substance, i.e., who has access to the data and information and who has reviewed those data and information with regard to safety.

Currently in the United States, a food ingredient can attain GRAS status if it has been in "common use in foods" prior to 1958, or if it has been affirmed as GRAS by a panel of experts qualified by training and experience to evaluate the safety of food ingredients. Ingredient suppliers or manufacturers also have the option to notify the FDA of an ingredient's GRAS status. FDA may question the reasoning behind the notifier's GRAS conclusion, or they may more favorably "file the notification without question."

In reference to vitamin E, the tocopherols are GRAS when produced in accordance with good manufacturing practices (21 CRF 182.8890 and 182.3890). On October 27, 1978, the FDA proposed a rule (*Federal Register,* docket no. 78N-0213) that recognized DL-α-tocopherol to be GRAS, along with D-α-tocopheryl acid succinate, D-α-tocopheryl acetate, and DL-α-tocopheryl acetate derivatives. On November 26, 2004, however, the agency reversed its 1978 ruling by withdrawing the proposed rule, along with numerous others, in order to reduce FDAs regulatory backlog (*Federal Register*, docket no. 2002N-0434). The agency has not mentioned tocotrienols in any of its rulings related to GRAS.

As tocotrienols have not been declared GRAS—despite claims that they are since vitamin E includes tocotrienols (Qureshi et al., 2001; Yu et al., 2006)—efforts have successfully been made in recent years to "self-affirm" tocotrienols as GRAS through scientific procedures. A determination of the safety of tocotrienol must include information about its characteristics, scientific toxicological evaluations, the estimated dietary intake under the intended conditions of use, and the population that will consume the substance (proposed 21 CFR 170.36 (c)(1)(iii)). Dietary intake of a substance depends on the food categories in which it will be used and the level of use in each of those food categories, as well as background levels that are naturally present in the food supply.

A GRAS notification for a palm oil–derived ingredient containing tocotrienols and α-tocopherol as the principle components received a favorable "no comment" decision by the U.S. FDA on April 23, 2010 (GRAS Notice No. GRN 000307) for use as an ingredient in a wide range of foods. The notification was submitted by the Malaysian Palm Oil Board in America. Other tocotrienol products, such as annatto seed-derived tocotrienols (e.g., DeltaGold®), have self-affirmed GRAS status in the United States. Hence, both may be legally sold in foods under the conditions of their stated intended use.

2.9 DIETARY SUPPLEMENTS AND COLOR ADDITIVES

In the United States, dietary supplements containing tocotrienols are regularly sold and consumed as part of the diet at much higher levels than found in food, and have been available for many years. A survey conducted by the authors found that dietary supplements containing 25–205 mg of tocotrienols, based on suggested usage, are widely available through different channels of distribution. The vast majority of such supplements suggested doses of 25–100 mg/day.

A search of the U.S. FDA MedWatch database did not reveal any significant warnings or recalls related to the use of dietary supplements containing tocotrienol (US FDA, 2011—retrieved Nov 11, 2011). The manufacturer of annatto tocotrienols (DeltaGold® American River Nutrition: Hadley, MA, USA), which is 10% gamma-tocotrienol and 90% delta-tocotrienol, verified that approximately 51.7 million doses of annatto tocotrienols were sold between 2002 and 2011. These estimates are based on dosages consisting of 100 mg active tocotrienol. To the best of their knowledge, no adverse events have been reported to them or to the FDA via MedWatch since sales began in 2002 (Personal Communications 2011).

The extract of the annatto seed is an acceptable color additive according to FDA for use in foods, drugs, and cosmetics (21 CFR 73.30, 73.1030, and 73.2030). The Joint FAO/WHO Expert Committee on Food Additives (JECFA) originally determined an acceptable daily intake (ADI) level for annatto extract, based on the available research at the time, as 0–0.065 mg/kg bw/day of annatto extract expressed as bixin.

In a more recent 2004 committee meeting, new data were evaluated. Six different preparations of annatto extract were reviewed, and new toxicological data (in the form of 28 and 90 day animal studies) were available for four of the extracts. Because a generic ADI for the various types of annatto extract preparations that were reviewed could not be established, temporary ADIs for the different preparations were determined (World Health Organization 2004; World Health Organization 2005):

Annatto B (*solvent-extracted extract containing 92% pigment; 97% was bixin and 1.7% norbixin*) (World Health Organization 2000)

> ADI = 0–7.0 mg/kg bw (based on no observed effect levels (NOELs) of 1311 mg and 1446 mg/kg bw per day in male and female mice, respectively).

Annatto C (*solvent-extracted extract containing 91.6% norbixin*)

> ADI = 0 – 0.4 mg/kg bw (based on NOELs of 69 mg and 76 mg/kg bw per day in male and female rats, respectively).

Annatto E (*aqueous-processed extract containing 26% pigment, of which 90% was bixin and 4.2% norbixin*)

> ADI = 0 – 4.0 mg/kg bw (based on NOELs of 734 mg and 801 mg/kg bw per day in male and female rats, respectively).

Annatto F (*alkali-processed norbixin*)

> ADI = 0 – 0.4 mg/kg bw (based on NOELs of 79 mg and 86 mg/kg bw per day in male and female rats, respectively).

In 2008, EFSA evaluated the safety and bioavailability of three preparations of vitamin E: tocotrienols, tocotrienol plus tocopherol, and mixed tocopherols as nutritional substances in food supplements (EFSA Authority 2008). The committee found that the tocotrienol plus tocopherol supplement, containing 13.5 mg of tocotrienols (amounting to an intake of 0.23 mg tocotrienols/kg bw/day for a 60 kg person) is at least 500 times lower than the

NOAEL for the tocotrienols in a subchronic toxicity study in rats (which was equivalent to 120 mg/kg bw/day for males, and 130 mg/kg bw/day for females). Hence, it concluded that the proposed level of use is not of safety concern.

However, the authority determined that there were insufficient safety data to conclude that the tocotrienol supplement, containing up to 1000 mg of tocotrienols per daily serving, was safe, as it would result in a daily intake of 16.7 mg tocotrienols/kg bw/day for a 60 kg person, which is only seven times below the NOAEL of the subchronic rat toxicology study, and is "higher than the 5 mg/kg bw/day frequently demonstrated to be without adverse effects in human studies."

2.10 CONCLUSION

"Vitamin E" has traditionally been associated only with "tocopherols." It is now known that the vitamin consists of eight compounds, four tocopherols, and four tocotrienols. The two groups differ in the hydrophobic tridecyl side chain that is saturated (phytyl) in the tocopherols and unsaturated in tocotrienols with three double bonds.

A lack of understanding of the differential therapeutic effects and mechanism of action of tocopherols and tocotrienols has led to unwarranted concerns that tocotrienols might contribute to an increase in all-cause mortality given the traditional viewpoint of what vitamin E is (Miller et al., 2005; Dotan et al., 2009). People may die during any long-term study; all-cause mortality refers to deaths from any cause, whether or not the cause has anything to do with the purpose of the study. Concerns that high dose "vitamin E" may be a risk have been based on meta-analyses that used questionable criteria in selecting studies for analysis, and a surprising disregard or awareness of the significant impact the ratio of tocotrienols and tocopherols can have on clinical trial outcomes or epideminological investigations.

Fortunately, a significant body of experimental evidence has emerged in recent years that can provide guidance regarding the safety of tocotrienols. The genotoxicity data, though limited, do not raise safety concerns. Toxicological studies in rats reported NOAELs of 120 mg/kg/day for males and 130 mg/kg/day for females (subchronic study) and 303 mg/kg/day for males and 473 mg/kg/day for females (chronic study). Studies in humans at levels of 50–400 mg/day (equivalent to up to 6.7 mg/kg for a 60 kg human) for periods of 2 weeks to 18 months (56 days for the 400 mg/day study) have not been reported to cause adverse effects, other than occasional transient effects. Taken together, and given the pharmacokinetics of tocotrienols including their short half-life, consumption of 3–5 mg/kg/day, and possibly higher, would not be expected to cause adverse effects, which is in agreement with conclusions reached by bodies such as the EFSA and GRAS expert panel members. Tocotrienols are initially omega-oxidized by cytochrome P450 enzymes, during which time they go through beta-oxidation and are then conjugated and excreted. As all of these mechanisms are closely regulated, the potential for adverse effects is limited.

It seems likely, given the lack of adverse effects in humans reported to date, that a twofold-to-threefold higher intake of tocotrienols than recommended by scientific bodies would be safe. In time, the dose of tocotrienols that is considered safe in humans will likely be raised, and its increased consumption encouraged due to its potential therapeutic and preventive bioactivities. However, what dose is safe is subject to continued reevaluation, as would be true for any substance of nutritive and functional value sold as dietary supplement or added to a wide range of foods.

REFERENCES

ABTC. 1994. The effect of vitamin E and beta-carotene on the incidence of lung cancer and other cancers in male smokers. The Alpha-Tocopherol, Beta-Carotene Cancer Prevention Study Group. *New Engl J Med*, 330: 1029–1035.

Abznait AH et al. 2011. Induction of expression and functional activity of P-glucoprotein efflux transporter by bioactive plant natural products. *Food Chem Toxicol*, 49: 2765–2772.

Ajuluchukwu JN et al. 2007. Comparative study of the effect of tocotrienols and -tocopherol on fasting serum lipid profiles in patients with mild hypercholesterolaemia: A preliminary report. *Niger Postgrad Med J*, 14: 30–33.

Baliarsingh S et al. 2005. The therapeutic impacts of tocotrienols in type 2 diabetic patients with hyperlipidemia. *Atherosclerosis*, 182: 367–374.

Brigelius-Flohe R et al. 2002. The European perspective on vitamin E: Current knowledge and future research. *Am J Clin Nutr*, 76: 703–716.

Brown MS and Goldstein JL. 1980. Multivalent feedback regulation of HMG CoA reductase, a control mechanism coordinating isoprenoid synthesis and cell growth. *J Lipid Res*, 21: 505–517.

Busing A and Ternes W. 2011. Separation of α-tocotrienol oxidation products and eight tocochromanols by HPLC with DAD, PBI-EIMS, FTIR, and NMR. *Anal Bioanal Chem*, 401: 2843–2854.

Colombo ML. 2010. An update on vitamin E, tocopherol and tocotrienol—Perspectives. *Molecules*, 15: 2103–2113.

Das S et al. 2012. Tocotrienols confer resistance to ischemia in hypercholesterolemic hearts: Insight with genomics. *Mol Cell Biochem*, 360: 35–45.

Dotan Y et al. 2009. No evidence supports vitamin E indiscriminate supplementation. *Biofactors*, 35: 469–473.

EFSA Authority. 2008. Opinion on mixed tocopherols, tocotrienol tocopherol and tocotrienols as sources for vitamin E added as a nutritional substance in food supplements. Scientific Opinion of the Panel on Scientific Panel on Food Additives, Flavourings, Processing Aids and Materials in Contact with Food. (Question No EFSA Q-2005-146, Q-2005-172, Q-2006-265). *EFSA J*, 604: 1–34.

Engelsen MM and Hansen A. 2009. Tocopherol and tocotrienol content in commercial wheat mill streams. *Cereal Chem*, 86: 499–502.

Franke AA et al. 2007. Tocopherol and tocotrienol levels of foods consumed in Hawaii. *J Agric Food Chem*, 55: 769–778.

Freiser H and Jiang Q. 2009. Gamma-tocotrienol and gamma-tocopherol are primarily metabolized to conjugated 2-(beta-carboxyethyl)-6-hydroxy-2,7,8-trimethylchroman and sulfated long-chain carboxychromanols in rats. *J Nutr*, 139: 884–889.

Gu JY et al. 1999. Dietary effect of tocopherols and tocotrienols on the immune function of spleen and mesenteric lymph node lymphocytes in Brown Norway rats. *Biosci Biotechnol Biochem*, 63: 1697–1702.

Hayes KC et al. 1993. Differences in the plasma transport and tissue concentrations of tocopherols and tocotrienols: Observations in humans and hamsters. *Proc Soc Exp Biol Med*, 202: 353–359.

Hensley K et al. 2004. New perspectives on vitamin E: Gamma-tocopherol and carboxyelthylhydroxychroman metabolites in biology and medicine. *Free Radic Biol Med*, 36: 1–15.

Husain K et al. 2011. Vitamin E δ-tocotrienol augments the anti-tumor activity of gemcitabine and suppresses constitutive NF-kappa-B activation in pancreatic cancer. *Mol Cancer Ther*, 10: 2363–2372.

Ikeda S et al. 2000. Selective uptake of dietary tocotrienols into rat skin. *J Nutr Sci Vitaminol*, 46: 141–143.

Ima-Nirwana S et al. 2011. Subacute and subchronic toxicity studies of palm vitamin E in mice. *J Pharmacol Toxicol*, 6: 166–173.

Institute of Medicine. 2000a. *Dietary Reference Intakes of Vitamin C, Vitamin E, Selenium, and Carotenoids*. National Academies Press: Washington, DC.

Institute of Medicine. 2000b. *Dietary Reference Intakes of Vitamin C, Vitamin E, Selenium, and Carotenoids (Free Executive Summary)*. http:www.nap.edu/catalog/9810.html (retrieved on September 5, 2011).

Kannappan R et al. 2011. Tocotrienols fight cancer by targeting multiple cell signaling pathways. *Genes Nutr*, 7: 43–52.

Khanna S et al. 2006. Characterization of the potent neuroprotective properties of the natural vitamin E α-tocotrienol. *J Neurochem*, 98: 1474–1486.

Koba K et al. 1992. Effects of alpha-tocopherol and tocotrienols on blood pressure and linolenic acid metabolism in the spontaneously hypertensive rat (SHR). *Biosci Biotechnol Biochem*, 56: 1420–1423.

Kooyenga DK et al. 2001. Antioxidants modulate the course of carotid atherosclerosis: A four-year report. In: *Micronutrients and Health: Molecular Biological Mechanisms*, Higuchi Y, Nesaretnam K, and Packer L. (Eds.). AOCS Press: Urbana, IL.

Machlin L. 1991. Vitamin E. In: *Handbook of Vitamins*, Machlin L. (Ed.). Marcel Dekker: New York, pp. 99–144.

Mahalingam D et al. 2010. Effects of supplementation with tocotrienol-rich fraction on immune response to tetanus toxoid immunization in normal healthy volunteers. *Eur J Clin Nutr*, 65: 63–69.

Makpol S et al. 2011. Tocotrienol-rich fraction prevents cell cycle arrest and elongates telomere length in senescent human diploid fibroblasts. *J Biomed Biotechnol*, 2011: 506171.

Mayer H et al. 1967. The stereochemistry of natural gamma-tocotrienol (plastochromanol-3), plastochromanol-8 and plastochromenol-8. *Helv Chim Acta*, 50: 1376–1393.

Mensink RP et al. 1999. α-tocopherol was added to the placebo oil so that the only difference between capsules was the tocotrienol content. The vitamin E capsules with tocotrienols had no effect on serum lipoproteins, platelet function in men with mildly elevated serum lipid concentrations. *Am J Clin Nutr*, 69: 213–219.

Miller ER et al. 2005. Meta-analysis: High-dose vitamin E supplementation may increase all-cause mortality. *Ann Intern Med*, 142: 37–42.

Miyazawa T et al. 2011. Health benefits of vitamin E in grains, cereals and green vegetables. *Trends Food Sci Tech*, 22: 651–654.

Moreau RA et al. 2007. Tocopherols and tocotrienols in barley oil prepared from germ and other fractions from scarification and sieving of hullness barley. *Cereal Chem*, 84: 587–592.

Nakamura H et al. 2001. Oral toxicity of a tocotrienol preparation in rats. *Food Chem Toxicol*, 39: 799–805.

Nesaretnam K et al. 2011. Tocotrienols and breast cancer: The evidence to date. *Genes Nutr*, 7: 3–9.

Nesaretnam K and Meganathan P. 2011. Tocotrienols: Inflammation and cancer. *Ann NY Acad Sci*, 1229: 18–22.

Newaz MA and Nawal NN. 1999. Effect of gamma-tocotrienol on blood pressure, lipid peroxidation and total antioxidant status in spontaneously hypertensive rats (SHR). *Clin Exp Hypertens*, 21: 1297–1313.

O'Byrne D et al. 2000. Studies of LDL oxidation following alpha-, gamma-, or delta-tocotrienyl acetate supplementation of hypercholesterolemic humans. *Free Radic Biol Med*, 29: 834–845.

Oliveira SV et al. 1994. Absence of genotoxic effects of crude and refined red palm oil on mouse bone marrow cells. *Rev Bras Genét*, 17: 409.

Ong A. 1993. Natural sources of tocotrienols. In: *Vitamin E in Health and Disease*. Packer L. (Ed.). Marcel Dekker: New York, pp. 3–8.

Oo S et al. 1992. Toxicological and pharmacological studies on palm vitee. *Nutr Res*, 12: S217–S222.

Parker RA et al. 1990. Selective inhibition of cholesterol synthesis in liver versus extrahepatic tissues by HMG-CoA reductase inhibitors. *J Lipid Res*, 37: 1271–1282.

Patel V et al. 2011. Tocotrienols: The lesser known form of natural vitamin E. *Indian J Exp Biol*, 49: 732–738.

Pearce BC et al. 1992. Hypocholesterolemic activity of synthetic and natural tocotrienols. *J Med Chem*, 35: 3595–3606.

Pennock JF et al. 1964. Reassessment of tocopherol chemistry. *Biochim Biophys Res Commun*, 17: 542.

Podda M et al. 1996. Simultaneous determination of tissue tocopherols, tocotrienols, ubiquinols, and ubiquinones. *J Lipid Res*, 37: 893–901.

Polasa K and Rukmini C. 1987. Mutagenicity tests of cashewnut shell liquid, rice-bran oil and other vegetable oils using the Salmonella typhimurium/microsome system. *Food Chem Toxicol*, 25: 763–766.

Prasad K. 2011. Tocotrienols and cardiovascular health. *Curr Pharm Des*, 17: 2147–2154.

Qureshi AA et al. 1991. Lowering of serum cholesterol in hypercholesterolemic humans by tocotrienols (palmvitee). *Am J Clin Nutr*, 53: 1021S–1026S.

Qureshi AA et al. 1995. Response of hypercholesterolemic subjects to administration of tocotrienols. *Lipids*, 30: 1171–1177.

Qureshi AA et al. 1997. Novel tocotrienols of rice bran modulate cardiovascular disease risk parameters of hypercholesterolemic humans. *J Nutr Biochem*, 8: 290–298.

Qureshi AA et al. 2001. Synergistic effect of tocotrienol-rich fraction (TRF(25)) of rice bran and lovastatin on lipid parameters in hypercholesterolemic humans. *J Nutr Biochem*, 12: 318–329.

Qureshi AA et al. 2002. Dose-dependent suppression of serum cholesterol by tocotrienol-rich fraction (TRF25) of rice bran in hypercholesterolemic humans. *Atherosclerosis*, 161: 199–207.

Radhakrishnan AK et al. 2008. Daily supplementation of tocotrienol-rich fraction or alpha-tocopherol did not induce immunomodulatory changes in healthy human volunteers. *Br J Nutr*, 101: 810–815.

Raghuram TC and Rukmini C. 1995. Nutritional significance of rice bran oil. *Indian J Med Res*, 102: 241–244.

Rahmat A et al. 1993. Long-term administration of tocotrienols and tumor-marker enzyme activities during hepatocarcinogenesis in rats. *Nutr*, 9: 229–232.

Ralla J et al. 2011. Increased antioxidant capacity in the plasma of dogs after a single oral dosage of tocotrienols. *Br J Nutr*, 106: S116–S119.

Rao MK and Perkins EG. 1972. Identification and estimation of tocopherols and tocotrienols in vegetable oils using gas chromatography-mass spectrometry. *J Agric Food Chem*, 20: 240–245.

Rasool AH et al. 2006. Dose dependent elevation of plasma tocotrienol levels and its effect on arterial compliance, plasma total antioxidant status, and lipid profile in healthy humans supplemented with tocotrienol rich vitamin E. *J Nutr Sci Vitaminol (Tokyo)*, 52: 473–478.

Rasool AH et al. 2008. Arterial compliance and vitamin E blood levels with a self emulsifying preparation of tocotrienol rich vitamin E. *Arch Pharm Res*, 31: 1212–1217.

Rukmini C. 1988. Chemical, nutritional and toxicological studies of rice bran oil. *Food Chem*, 30: 257–268.

Schauss AG. 2009. Tocotrienols: A review. In: *Tocotrienols: Vitamin E Beyond Tocopherols*. Watson RR and Preedy VR. [Eds.]. AOCS Press: Urbana, IL; Taylor & Francis/CRC Press: Boca Raton, FL, pp. 1–12.

Sen CK et al. 2006. Tocotrienols: Vitamin E beyond tocopherols. *Life Sci*, 78: 2088–2098.

Shah SJ and Sylvester PW. 2005. Tocotrienol-induced cytotoxicity is unrelated to mitochondrial stress apoptotic signaling in neoplastic mammary epithelial cells. *Biochem Cell Biol*, 83: 86–95.

Sontag TJ and Parker RS. 2007. Influence of major structural features of tocopherols and tocotrienols on their omega-oxidation by tocopherol-omega-hydroxylase. *J Lipid Res*, 48: 1090–1098.

Sookwong P et al. 2008. Tocotrienol content in hen eggs: Its fortification by supplementing the feed with rice bran scum oil. *Biosci Biotechnol Biochem*, 72: 3044–3047.

Souci SW, Fachman W, Kraut H. 2002. *Food Composition and Nutrition Tables*, 6th edn., CRC Press: Boca Raton, FL.

Stephens NG et al. 1996. Randomised controlled trial of vitamin E in patients with coronary disease: Cambridge Heart Antioxidant Study (CHAOS). *Lancet*, 347: 781–786.

Sylvester PW et al. 2005. Intracellular mechanisms mediating tocotrienol-induced apoptosis in neoplastic mammary epithelial cells. *Asia Pac J Clin Nutr*, 14: 366–373.

Sylvester PW. 2007. Vitamin E and apoptosis. *Vitam Horm*, 76: 326–356.

Sylvester PW. 2011. Synergistic anticancer effects of combined γ-tocotrienol with statin or receptor tyrosine kinase inhibitor treatment. *Genes Nutr*, 7: 63–74.

Tan B. 2005. Appropriate spectrum vitamin E and new perspectives on desmethyl tocopherols and tocotrienols. *JANA*, 8: 35–42.

Tan B and Mueller M. 2008. Tocotrienols in cardiometabolic diseases. *Tocotrienols: Vitamin E beyond Tocopherols*. Watson R and Preedy VR. [Eds.] Taylor & Francis/CRC Press: Boca Raton, FL, pp. 257–274.

Tasaki M et al. 2008. Induction of characteristic hepatocyte proliferative lesion with dietary exposure of Wistar Hannover rats to tocotrienol for 1 year. *Toxicol*, 250: 143–150.

Tomeo AC et al. 1995. Antioxidant effects of tocotrienols in patients with hyperlipidemia and carotid stenosis. *Lipids*, 30: 1179–1183.

Traber MG. 2007. Vitamin E regulatory mechanisms. *Annu Rev Nutr*, 27: 347–362.

Traber MG. 2008. Vitamin E and K interactions—A 50 year-old problem. *Nutr Rev*, 66: 624–629.

Vasanthi HR et al. 2011. Tocotrienols and its role in cardiovascular health: A lead for drug design. *Curr Pharm Des*, 17: 2170–2175.

Watson R and Preedy VR. [Eds.] 2009. *Tocotrienols: Vitamin E Beyond Tocopherols*. Taylor & Francis/CRC Press: Boca Raton, FL.

Whittle KJ et al. 1966. The isolation and properties of delta-tocotrienol from *Hevea* latex. *Biochem J*, 100: 138.

Wilankar C et al. 2011. Role of immunoregulatory transcription factors in differential immunomodulatory effects of tocotrienols. *Free Radic Biol Med*, 51: 129–143.

World Health Organization. 2000. *Evaluation of National Assessments of Intake of Annatto Extracts (Bixin)*. Geneva, Switzerland.

World Health Organization. 2004. *Annatto Extracts*. Geneva, Switzerland.

World Health Organization. 2005. *Summary of Evaluations Performed by the Joint FAO/WHO Expert Committee on Food Additives: Annatto Extracts*. Geneva, Switzerland.

Yap SP et al. 2001. Pharmacokinetics and bioavailability of α-, γ-, and δ-tocotrienols under different food status. *J Pharm Pharmacol*, 53: 67–71.

Yu SG et al. 2006. Dose-response impact of various tocotrienols on serum lipid parameters in 5-week-old female chickens. *Lipids*, 41: 453–461.

Yu W et al. 1999. Induction of apoptosis in human breast cancer cells by tocopherols and tocotrienols. *Nutr Cancer*, 33: 26–32.

Zhou C et al. 2004. Tocotrienols activate the steroid and xenobiotic receptor, SXR, and selectively regulate expression of its target genes. *Drug Metab Disp*, 32: 1075–1082.

3 Bioavailability and Metabolism of Tocotrienols

Zhihong Yang, Mao-Jung Lee,
Shengmin Sang, and Chung S. Yang

CONTENTS

3.1 INTRODUCTION

Tocotrienols (T3s), together with their tocopherol counterparts, compose the vitamin E family. The difference between T3s and tocopherols is that T3s possess an unsaturated isoprenoid side chain with 3 double bonds, whereas tocopherols contain a 16-carbon saturated phytyl side chain. Based on the number and location of the methyl groups on their chromanol rings, T3s and tocopherols exist in α-, β-, γ-, and δ-forms. Emerging evidence suggests that T3s exhibit more potent anticancer effects than tocopherols (reviewed in Aggarwal et al., 2010). In addition, T3s also display activity in stimulating immune response (Mahalingam et al., 2011; Ren et al., 2010) and reducing the risk of cardiovascular diseases (Das et al., 2005, 2008). To better evaluate the efficacy of vitamin E *in vivo*, it is essential to understand their bioavailability and metabolism. This chapter will discuss the bioavailability and metabolism of T3s and the factors that may influence these processes *in vivo*.

3.2　BIOAVAILABILITY OF TOCOTRIENOLS

3.2.1　Routes of Tocotrienol Administration

A direct and effective delivery method for T3s in animal studies is intravenous injection (i.v.), particularly when T3s are prepared in emulsion form to enhance their solubility. However, the application of this method is limited, particularly in human studies due to its complexity of operation. In human and animal studies, oral administration such as dietary and intragastric (i.g.) delivery is the most common route to deliver T3s to animals. T3s in diets are fairly stable as more than 99.5% of the T3s can still be detected in animal diets containing 0.1% δ- or γ-T3 when stored at 4°C in sealed bags for 8 months (our unpublished data). Therefore, it is convenient to deliver T3s to animals through diet consumption. T3s are lipophilic compounds and it is well established that the bioavailability of lipophilic compounds can be greatly increased when they were taken with fat-rich foods. A study conducted with healthy human volunteers demonstrated that the bioavailability of α-, δ-, and γ-T3 was increased about threefold when they were delivered together with a high-fat breakfast (Yap et al., 2001). Moreover, the bioavailability of T3s was less variable when they were taken with food than under fasting (Yap et al., 2001). As vitamin E is solubilized in mixed micelles or emulsion before intestinal uptake, T3s delivered by i.g. were usually prepared as emulsion with sodium taurocholate (or other detergent), fatty acid–free bovine serum albumin, and oil (such as safflower oil) in water (Okabe et al., 2002) or in micelles by mixing with bile salts, lipid metabolites, and lysophospholipid to increase the delivery efficiency (Tsuzuki et al., 2007). The cellular concentration of γ-T3 in Caco-2 cells incubated with medium containing micelle packed γ-T3 was significantly higher than that incubated with medium containing dispersed γ-T3. After one dose i.g. administration of 10 mg γ-T3 emulsion, the serum level of T3 in mice reached about 8 μM in 2–4 h (Tsuzuki et al., 2007). Yap et al. (2003) conducted a systematic comparison of several routes to deliver T3s, in which an emulsion containing 5 mg mixed T3 (1.50, 2.75 and 0.75 mg of α-, γ- and δ-T3, respectively) was administered to male Sprague-Dawley rats either intravenously or intragastrically. They found that all three T3s reached their peak concentration in serum at about 3 h after administration, a similar result to the mouse study in terms of the time to reach peak concentration. The absolute bioavailabilities (estimated by dividing the total area under the plasma concentration-time curve ($AUC_{0-\infty}$) obtained from i.g. administration by the $AUC_{0-\infty}$ from i.v. administration) of T3s were 27.7%, 9.1%, and 8.9% for α-, γ-, and δ-T3, respectively, suggesting that the absorption of T3s was not complete and it appears that there is bio-discrimination for the absorption of different T3 forms to the blood. The discrimination is likely to be due to the different number of methyl groups in their chromanol ring, which in turn renders different lipophilicity for different T3 forms. In contrast to i.v. and i.g., intraperitoneal delivery and intramuscular administration of T3s were negligibly absorbed, possibly due to the lack of the formation of micelles, an essential step for the absorption of lipophilic compounds. In addition, for certain tissues, some specialized methods may be used to deliver T3s. For example, α- and γ-T3 in rat eye tissues could be markedly increased after topical ophthalmic administration, whereas no significant increase was observed when the same amount of T3s was administered orally (Tanito et al., 2004). In another study, topically applied α-tocopherol (α-T), α-T3 and γ-T3 could penetrate through the entire skin to the subcutaneous fat layer within half an hour after administration (Traber et al., 1998). Although the concentrations of vitamin E forms were the highest in the uppermost layer of the skin (stratum corneum), the papillary dermis layer contained the highest percentage of all vitamin E forms absorbed. The percentage of absorbed α-T and α-T3 were different in different skin layers, indicating possible preference of α-T and α-T3 in different skin layers. Minko et al. (2002) also reported that intratracheally delivered liposomal α-T could effectively reduce hypoxic lung injury. It is reasonable to believe that this method can also be applied to deliver T3s to the lung.

3.2.2 UPTAKE AND TRANSPORT OF TOCOTRIENOLS AND TOCOPHEROLS

Vitamin E forms are mainly absorbed in the intestine and then secreted with triacylglycerol-rich chylomicron into the lymph and blood (Kayden and Traber, 1993). In addition, high-density lipoproteins (HDL) may also contribute to vitamin E absorption and transport in enterocytes (Anwar et al., 2007). The uptake of T3s is thought to be a simple diffusion mechanism (reviewed in Traber and Sies, 1996). The unsaturated side chain renders more lipophilicity to T3s and allows them to be incorporated into the cell membrane more easily than their tocopherol counterparts (Yoshida et al., 2003). For example, Serbinova et al. (1991) suggested that the inter-membrane mobility of α-T3 is larger than that of α-T and α-T3 is more readily incorporated into membranes. Therefore, the uptake of T3s is faster than tocopherols; the higher uptake of T3s may partly explain their higher biological activities (Viola et al., 2011).

After lipolysis of chylomicron triacylglycerol by lipoprotein lipase in the intestine, vitamin E forms are transported to the liver where α-T transfer protein (α-TTP) selectively transfers them to lipoproteins. Then T3s and tocopherols are released into the circulation and transported to various tissues. All vitamin E forms were detected in triacylglycerol-rich particle (TRP), containing chylomicron and very low density lipoproteins (VLDL), low density lipoproteins (LDL) and HDL (Kayden and Traber, 1993). Fairus et al. analyzed the postprandial distributions of α-T and T3s after a single dose administration of α-T (1074 mg) or palm T3-rich fraction (1011 mg) in human. The concentration of α-T gradually increased in TRP after postprandial intervals beginning at 2 h, peaked at 4 h, and then steadily decreased. However, α-T was present mainly in LDL and HDL at the time points of 0 and 24 h after α-T administration. T3 concentrations were high in TRP and HDL from 2 to 6 h after administration, peaked at 4 h. Then T3s were mainly detected in HDL from 4 to 8 h before they were cleared from plasma (Fairus et al., 2006).

α-TTP is essential in maintaining normal concentrations of α-T in the plasma and extrahepatic tissues. The loss of function of α-TTP in human caused vitamin E deficiency, leading to ataxia and retinitis pigmentosa (Ouahchi et al., 1995). α-TTP knockout mouse also showed α-T deficiency in the serum (Leonard et al., 2002). α-TTP occurs mainly in the liver (Yoshida et al., 1992), and its RNA was also detected in rat brain, spleen, lung, and kidney (Hosomi et al., 1998), and in mouse liver, adrenals, and uterus; but α-TTP level was low or undetectable in mouse cerebral cortex, lung, heart, and spleen (Gohil et al., 2004; Kaempf-Rotzoll et al., 2002). In human, α-TTP has been detected in the brain and placenta (Copp et al., 1999; Kaempf-Rotzoll et al., 2003), implying an important role of α-T in the neural and reproductive tissues. The affinities of T3s and tocopherols to hepatic α-TTP and hence their retention in the body is a key factor in the bioactivity of vitamin E. α-TTP has the highest affinity to α-T (100%) in comparison with β-T (38%), γ-T (9%), and δ-T (2%), respectively (Hosomi et al., 1997). The affinity of α-TTP to α-T3 is only 12% of that to α-T. The crystal structure of α-TTP has been solved in two different confirmations at 1.9 Å resolution, shedding lights on the molecular mechanisms of how α-TTP transfers α-T (Meier et al., 2003). The structure reveals that α-TTP has a hinge and a cover that entraps α-T on the binding pocket which is enriched in hydrophobic amino acids. The relatively low binding affinity of other tocopherol forms is due to the absence of one or more methyl groups in the chromanol ring, which reduces the surface available for hydrophobic interactions and diminishes the packing density (Meier et al., 2003). The high affinity of α-T relative to other tocopherols and T3s leads to the secretion and transfer of α-T from the liver to other tissues, whereas other forms of tocopherols and T3s are restrained in the liver for degradation. The uptake of tocopherols/T3s may also be independent of α-TTP as orally supplemented α-T and α-T3 could still be delivered to vital organs in α-TTP deficient mice (Khanna et al., 2005). In this context, multidrug resistance-associated protein 1 (MRP1) may be a protein involved in the functions of vitamin E. MRP1 knockdown attenuated the protection against glutamate-induced neurotoxicity by α-T3 *in vitro*. MRP1 level was elevated in the stroke-affected cortical tissue of α-T3-supplemented mice, suggesting MRP1 is a target in the protection against ischemic stroke by α-T3 (Park et al., 2011).

The bioavailabilities of vitamin E forms are associated with their biological activities. In a study to compare the cytoprotective effects of vitamin E against glutamate-induced cell death in immature primary cortical neuron cultures, the apparent higher capacity of α-T3 compared to α-T was suggested to be ascribed to the faster uptake of T3 (Saito et al., 2010). The uptake of γ-T3 was also higher than α-T in cerebella granule neurons in culture, suggesting a link between the higher uptake of γ-T3 and its stronger neuroprotective effect than α-T at lower dose as well as its neurotoxicity at higher dose (Then et al., 2009). The antiproliferative effects of vitamin E on murine C6 glioblastoma cells were correlated to the uptake of vitamin E; when α-T and γ-T reached similar cellular concentration, their inhibitory activity was comparable (Betti et al., 2006). However, these studies were all performed in cultured cells, which are greatly different from *in vivo* situation where all vitamin E forms except α-T are not effectively transferred to the blood and hence to the target tissues. The bioavailability of vitamin E forms in target tissues and their metabolism must be considered when studying their biological activities although the biological activities of vitamin E involve many other biological processes and signaling pathways, in addition to the uptake (reviewed in Viola et al., 2011).

Another tocopherol-binding protein is tocopherol-associated protein (TAP), later renamed as Bloch's supernatant protein factor (SPF), which was identified in the cytosol of bovine liver with radioactive-labeled α-T as a tracer. Human TAP/SPF is widely distributed in human tissues, with high levels in the liver, brain, and prostate, and binds to biotinylated tocopherol within physiological concentrations (Zimmer et al., 2000). The crystal structures of TAP/SPF with and without α-tocopherol quinone (α-TQ), the oxidative product of α-T, were achieved and the structural information provided the hints that SPF may serve as a putative carrier of α-TQ (Stocker and Baumann, 2003; Stocker et al., 2002). TAP/SPF was also found to be downregulated in breast cancer cells (Wang et al., 2009).

3.2.3 DISTRIBUTION OF TOCOTRIENOLS IN DIFFERENT ORGANISMS AND TISSUES

3.2.3.1 Studies in Rat Tissues

The bioavailability of T3s in rats has been extensively studied. The distribution of T3s varies in different organs depending on the experimental system used. In Wistar rats, after 8 weeks diet administration of T3s (containing 220 mg T3-rich fraction (TRF)/kg diet), the T3 levels were high in the skin epidermal fat and adipose tissues, but the T3 levels in the liver, spleen, and serum were negligible (Ikeda et al., 2001). In another study using the same strain of rats fed T3s (50 mg α-T3 or γ-T3 per kg diet), T3s were detected in the plasma as well as in various tissues, but the concentrations in the skin and adipose tissues (>10 nmol/g) were much higher than those in the liver, kidney, and lung (Ikeda et al., 2003b). In Sprague-Dawley rats given different doses of γ-T3-rich mixed T3s together with mixed tocopherols (4.3 mg tocopherols only, or 0.8 mg T3s + 3.5 mg tocopherols, or 3.2 mg T3s + 1.1 mg tocopherols per kg body weight per day) by oral intubation for 3 weeks, a similar pattern of T3 distribution in tissues was achieved in that γ-T3 was predominantly in adipose tissues and was also detected in the skin, kidney, lung, muscle, and heart and the levels of γ-T3 were significantly higher than those in the control groups; but little γ-T3 was found in the liver and spleen. In comparison, the levels of α-T were high in the lung, spleen, and liver, but low in the skin, muscle, and brain (Kawakami et al., 2007). When an emulsion containing 67 or 200 mg of T3 mixture was intragastrically administered to Sprague-Dawley rats, the T3 levels in adipose tissues were maintained or increased for 24 h after administration; whereas T3s were not detected in the blood clot, brain, thymus, testes, vice testes, and muscles. T3s were also detected in the serum, liver, mesenteric lymph node, spleen, and lungs, with the highest levels at 8 h after administration (Okabe et al., 2002).

3.2.3.2 Studies in Mouse Tissues

The studies of the distribution of T3s in mouse tissues were rather limited; published studies only examined limited organs. Yang et al. studied the bioavailability in mice fed diets containing γ- and δ-T3 and the corresponding forms of tocopherols. The levels of T3s in various mouse tissues were studied and compared with those of tocopherols. In an experiment to study the inhibitory effect of tocopherols and T3s on xenograft tumor growth, NCr Nu/Nu mice were supplemented with 0.1% γ-T3, 0.1% δ-T3, 0.1% γ-T, or 0.1% δ-T for 6 weeks (Yang et al., 2011). The levels of α-T in different tissues of the control diet group were 4–20 μmol/kg (the basal diet contains 400 U/g α-T). Supplementation of T3s increased the levels of corresponding T3s in the serum and all the organs examined. The levels of T3s were relatively low in the liver (about 0.5 μmol/kg), but high in the spleen, kidney, small intestine, and colon (>10 μmol/kg). The levels of T3s in the xenograft tumor and lung were in the range from 1 to 10 μmol/kg. The plasma T3 levels in the T3-treated mice (1.63 ± 0.61 μM and 0.59 ± 0.08 μM for γ-T3 and δ-T3, respectively) were lower than the tocopherol levels in the corresponding tocopherol groups (4.75 ± 1.29 μM and 1.60 ± 0.21 μM for γ-T and δ-T, respectively). In contrast, the T3s levels in the spleen, kidney, small intestine, and colon in the T3 groups were higher than the tocopherol levels in the corresponding tocopherol groups. The levels of T3s and tocopherols were similar in the lung, liver, and xenograft tumors. The level of α-T was reduced in the liver after supplementation of δ-T, γ-T, and T3s, suggesting a possible interference of α-T uptake by other forms of tocopherols and T3s. Taken together, the concentrations of T3s reached about 1–10 μmol/kg (equal to 1–10 μM in solution if 1 g of tissue is regarded as 1 mL) in most mouse tissues, which is close to the levels of T3s that can be achieved in human plasma under fed status (Yap et al., 2001).

3.3 METABOLISM OF TOCOTRIENOLS

3.3.1 Proposed Side-Chain Degradation Pathway of Tocotrienols

Similar to tocopherols, T3s are metabolized through the oxidative degradation of their side chains. The degradation involves cytochromes P450 (CYP)-catalyzed ω-hydroxylation; the two major CYPs in human that have been reported to be involved in this process are CYP3A4 and CYP4F2 (Parker et al., 2000; Sontag and Parker, 2002). CYP3A11 was reported as a human CYP3A4 counterpart in mice to catalyze the hydroxylation of tocopherols (Kluth et al., 2005). The role of CYPs in metabolizing vitamin E is supported by the observations that some CYP inhibitors greatly increase the levels of vitamin E forms and reduce the levels of vitamin E metabolites in various tissues. Ketoconazole is a general CYP inhibitor to inhibit the activity of both CYP3A and 4F (Sheets and Mason, 1984). Ketoconazole decreased urinary excretion of γ-CEHC and elevated the levels of γ-T and T3s in the serum and various tissues after their administration (Abe et al., 2007). Sesamin and sesaminol, two lignans from sesame seeds, also reduced the levels of vitamin E metabolites and increased vitamin E level *in vivo*, likely through the inhibition of CYP activity (Ikeda et al., 2003a, 2007; Parker et al., 2000). Vitamin E forms have been reported to increase the level of CYPs (Landes et al., 2003; Traber et al., 2005). This induction involves the activation of pragnane X receptor (PXR), a nuclear receptor responds to the oxidative status in cells, which binds to specific *cis*-elements in the promoter region of CYP3A and mediates its gene transcription (Landes et al., 2003). The induction was most strong by α- and γ-T3 followed by δ-, α-, and γ-T in HepG2 cells (Landes et al., 2003). However, in mice the induction of CYP only specifically responded to α-T, as γ-T or γ-T3 did not change the level of CYP3A (Kluth et al., 2005; Traber et al., 2005), possibly due to the retention of α-T and the fast degradation of γ-T and γ-T3 to γ-CEHC *in vivo*, as γ-CEHC was not able to activate PXR-mediated transcription (Landes et al., 2003). Taken together, the half-life of α-T is higher than that of T3s and other tocopherols and the existence of α-T reduces the bioavailability of other vitamin E forms.

The ω-hydroxylated tocopherols and T3s are then oxidized to carboxylic acid, followed by five cycles of β-oxidation to remove a two-carbon moiety each cycle from the side chain. Several intermediate metabolites were produced during β-oxidation with 11-, 9-, and 7-carbon side chain. The final products of the vitamin E degradation are carboxyethtyl hydroxychromans (CEHCs, with a three-carbon side chain) and their precursors, carboxymethylbutyl hydroxychromans (CMBHCs, with a five-carbon side chain). Most of CEHCs are excreted in the urine (Chiku et al., 1984; Schultz et al., 1995;

Wechter et al., 1996), whereas biliary excretion is also a route for T3 and tocopherol metabolites from the liver (Traber, 2007). The liver is the major organ of vitamin E metabolism, but it is very likely that other organs such as the lung, colon, and immune cells also contain CYPs that oxidize T3s (Abe et al., 2007). Cells from different tissue origins may produce metabolites in different manners. For example, lung adenocarcinoma A549 cells produced more long-chain metabolites (Jiang et al., 2008; You et al., 2005), whereas hepatic cancer Hep2G cells mostly produced short-chain metabolites (You et al., 2005).

3.3.2 MEDIATION OF TOCOTRIENOL SIDE-CHAIN METABOLISM

In addition to the binding affinity to hepatic α-TTP, the rate of vitamin E metabolism also contributes to the discriminated retention and elimination of vitamin E forms. The metabolism rate of vitamin E is associated with their structural features of both the chromanol ring (the extent and position of the methyl groups) and the side chain (the saturation status of the side chain). A systematic study of the catabolism of vitamin E forms by Sontag and Parker demonstrated that non-methylated and monomethylated tocopherol (δ-T) were most effectively catalyzed to their water-soluble metabolites, followed by dimethylated tocopherol (γ-T), whereas triple-methylated tocopherol (α-T) was poorly catabolized (Sontag and Parker, 2007). In all dimethylated tocopherols, microsomes containing CYPs showed more activity on γ-T (dimethylated at carbon position 7 and 8 in the chromanol ring) than ε-T (dimethylated at position 5 and 7) and β-T (dimethylated at position 5 and 8). T3s, with unsaturated side chain, underwent higher degradation than their tocopherol counterparts. Further kinetic studies demonstrated that the majority of tocopherols displayed typical Michaelis-Menten kinetics, whereas T3s, and to a lesser extent, δ-T, exhibited a concentration-dependent auto-inhibitory effect on their own metabolism at high substrate concentration. The apparent K_m values positively related to the number of methyl groups with α-T show the highest K_m value while non-methylated tocopherol and δ-T show the least K_m; and the position of methyl groups and the side-chain stereochemistry displayed no significant effect. Unsaturated phytyl side chain exerted the strongest effect on apparent K_m in that all T3s exhibited lower K_m values. It seems that the K_m value is related to the ability of vitamin to incorporate into cell membrane system, particularly the microsome membrane where the CYPs are located; less number of methyl groups, and especially, the unsaturation of the side chain resulted in low K_m value. In terms of V_{max}, the number of methyl groups on the chromanol ring did not have a significant effect, but the position of methyl group played a more significant role in that methylation at C-5 attenuated activity and methylation at C-7 may enhance the activity. Again, T3s showed higher V_{max} values as compared with tocopherols, whereas stereochemistry of the side chain had no effect (Sontag and Parker, 2007).

In addition to phase I enzymes such as CYP3A, several phase II detoxification enzymes have been reported to be induced by T3s. For example, γ-T3-induced inhibition of cell cycle regulation in MCF-7 human breast cancer cells was related to redox changes and the induction of NAD(P)H:quinone oxidoreductase 2 (NQO2), a phase II detoxification enzyme under the control of the redox-sensitive transcription factor Nrf2 (Hsieh et al., 2010). Other phase II enzymes induced by T3s include sulfotransferases and glucuronyltransferases (Freiser and Jiang, 2009). It seems that the beneficial effects and cytotoxicity of T3s are associated with the induction of detoxification enzymes, although the mechanisms of how the induction of these detoxification enzymes contributes to the biological activity and the toxicity of T3s still needs to be further clarified. Therefore, caution should be used when T3s are applied in combination with other drugs as the detoxification enzymes induced by T3 supplementation may interfere with the metabolism and hence the therapeutic efficacy of other drugs.

3.3.3 DETECTION OF TOCOTRIENOL METABOLITES

CEHCs and some other metabolites from tocopherols have been well characterized and detected in animal samples (Chiku et al., 1984; Schultz et al., 1995; Wechter et al., 1996). Methods such as GC-MS, HPLC/electrochemical detection, HPLC/fluorescent detection, and LC-MS have been applied in the detection of vitamin E metabolites. All the methods include a sample preparation procedure to extract metabolites from the biological matrix to organic solvents. Birringer et al. (2002) identified some tocopherol/T3 metabolites in HepG2 cells using HPLC and gas chromatography/mass spectrometry. They found that γ-T3 was degraded to γ- CEHC, γ-CMBHC, γ-carboxymethylhexenyl hydroxychroman (CMHenHC), γ-carboxydimethyloctenyl hydroxychroman (CDMOenHC), and γ-carboxydimethyldecadienyl hydroxychroman (CDMD(en)₂HC). Likewise, α-T3 yielded α-CEHC, α-CMBHC, α-CMHenHC and α-CDMOenHC, but α-CDMD(en)₂HC was not detected. Sontag and Parker et al. (2002) also detected a series of carboxychromanol long-chain metabolites in HepG2 cells incubated with vitamin E (Parker et al., 2004; Sontag and Parker, 2002). Both studies support the concept that T3s are essentially metabolized similarly to tocopherols. However, the detection of metabolites was not complete and some essential metabolites were missing in these studies to construct a clear T3 degradation diagram.

Zhao et al. (2010) established a sensitive HPLC/electrochemical detection (ECD) method to analyze T3s and their metabolites. This sensitive HPLC/ECD was combined with LC-MS to identify and characterize different side-chain metabolites of T3s in mouse fecal and urine samples. A representative chromatogram of tocopherols/T3s and their side-chain metabolites in mouse fecal samples and representative MS spectra of γ-T derived metabolites are shown in Figure 3.1. In fecal samples from the mice fed diets supplemented with mixed T3s and tocopherols (20.2% α-T3, 4.0% β-T3, 16.1% γ-T3, 9.9% δ-T3, 14.8% α-T and 3.1% γ-T), δ-, γ-, and α-CEHCs

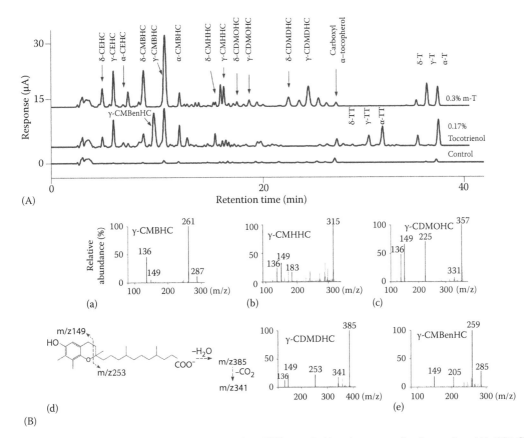

FIGURE 3.1 Identification of multiple tocopherol/T3 metabolites in mouse fecal samples. (A) HPLC chromatogram of tocopherol/T3 metabolites. The peaks eluted between 13.5 and 30 min for the T3 group were not assigned. (B) Representative MS² spectra and structural elucidation of deprotonated ions from γ-T derived metabolites. (From Zhao, Y. et al., *Agric. Food Chem.,* 58, 4844, 2010.)

and CMBHCs, as well as some new metabolites, were observed in HPLC chromatogram. A new metabolite was identified as γ-carboxymethylbutenyl hydroxychroman (CMBenHC), which was not detected by Birringer et al. (2002). More short-chain metabolites of T3s were present than long-chain metabolites. Further analysis of the fecal samples by LC-MS/MS revealed that T3 metabolites included CEHCs, CMBHCs, CMHenHCs, CDMOenHCs, and CDMD(en)₂HCs. These metabolites are similar to those reported in HepG2 cells (Birringer et al., 2002). Importantly, three additional groups of T3 metabolites were identified: one major peak of CMBenHCs with one double bond in the side chain, and two minor peaks of carboxydimethyloctadienyl hydroxychromans (CDMO(en)₂HCs) with two double bonds and carboxyl tocotrienols (Zhao et al., 2010). Based on these results, we proposed a degradation pathway of T3s as shown in Figure 3.2. In the urine samples from mice fed the diet supplemented with mixed T3s, short-chain metabolites including CEHCs, CMBHCs, and CMHenHCs were detected, whereas the parental compounds of T3s were not detected.

3.3.4 DISTRIBUTION OF TOCOTRIENOL SIDE-CHAIN METABOLITES IN DIFFERENT ORGANISMS AND TISSUES

CHECs have been reported to be excreted in human and rat urine, and several long-chain metabolites of T3s were detected in rat livers (Freiser and Jiang, 2009; Schultz et al., 1995). Yang et al. (2011) reported the distribution of T3 metabolites in mouse tissues. Athymic nude mice bearing A549 lung cancer cell xenograft tumors were fed a modified AIN76 control diet (AIN76*m*) or AIN76*m* diet supplemented with 0.05% γ-T3 for 2 weeks. γ-T3 and its short chain metabolites were detected in the serum samples as well as in several organs (lung, liver, spleen, and colon) from the mice in the γ-T3 group, but not in the control diet group. Several putative medium and long chain metabolites were also detected in the γ-T3 group, particularly in colon samples. Hydrolysis of the metabolites by glucuronidase and sulfatase in the urine samples markedly increased the levels of γ-CEHC and γ-CMBHC, suggesting that γ-CEHC and γ-CMBHC were excreted in mouse urine as glucuronidated or sulfated forms. This conclusion is similar to the detection of sulfated/glucuronidated T3 long-chain metabolites with 9- 11- and 13-carbon side-chains, and the result that most of the γ- CEHC was in conjugated forms in plasma samples, from a study of rats gavaged with a single dose of γ-T3 (10 and 50 mg γ-T3/kg body weight) (Freiser and Jiang, 2009). Consistent with previous experiments, the γ-T3 level in the liver was the lowest among the organs examined. γ-T3 metabolites were high in the colon and urine, suggesting that γ-T3 is metabolized in the liver and the metabolites are excreted from bile and urine. In the second experiment, seven groups of athymic nude mice were fed AIN76*m* diet or diets containing either tocopherol (0.2% δ-T and 0.2% γ-T) or T3 (0.05% and 0.1% δ-T3, 0.05% and 0.1% γ-T3) 1 week before the injection of H1299 lung cancer cells (1 × 10⁶), and the mice were maintained on the respective diets for 6 weeks. γ- and δ-T (0.2%) were introduced with the aim to compare the metabolism between tocopherols and T3s in mice. Both the serum and tumor levels of the two short chain metabolites, CEHCs, CMBHCs, were higher in groups treated with 0.1% δ-T3 and γ-T3 than with 0.2% δ-T and γ-T, respectively; and the levels of δ-CEHC and δ-CMBHC were higher than those of γ-CEHC and γ-CMBHC, respectively (our unpublished data). This result is consistent with the rat data reported by Freiser and Jiang that T3s are more extensively metabolized than tocopherols (Freiser and Jiang, 2009). The free long-chain metabolites were only detected in the tocopherol treated groups, but not the T3 treated groups, suggesting that the long-chain metabolites from T3s are more extensively metabolized through conjugation similarly to the situation in rats (Freiser and Jiang, 2009). Tocotrienol quinones (T3Qs) were also detected in the tumor samples. It is likely that the T3Qs are from oxidation of T3s *in vivo* rather than a direct accumulation from the diets because there were no T3Qs detected in the T3-containing diets (our unpublished data).

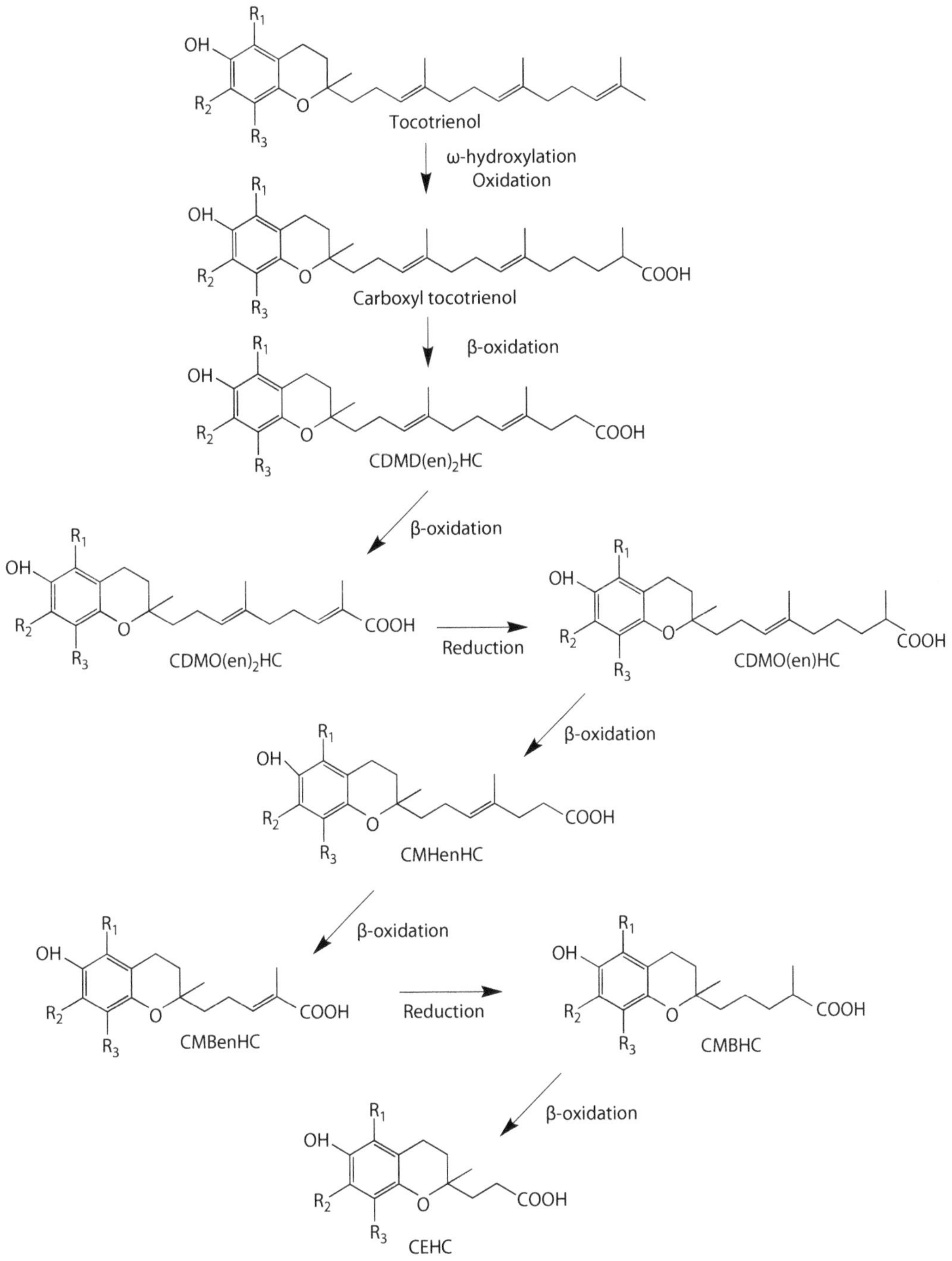

FIGURE 3.2 A proposed tocotrienol degradation pathway. (From Yang, Z. et al., *Genes Nutr.,* 7, 11, 2011.)

3.3.5 CONJUGATED TOCOTRIENOL SIDE-CHAIN METABOLITES

It has been demonstrated that CEHCs, the terminal side-chain degradation metabolite of tocopherols and T3s, are excreted in the urine in conjugated (either sulfated or glucuronidated) forms (Pope et al., 2002; Schultz et al., 1995; Swanson et al., 1999). In addition, the conjugated forms of CMBHCs, the precursor of CEHCs, were also identified in the urine and liver (Jiang et al., 2007;

Parker and Swanson, 2000). Jiang and Freiser showed that A549 cells metabolized γ-T3 to sulfated 9′-, 11′-, and 13′-carboxychromanols (9′-, 11′-, and 13′-COOH) and their unconjugated counterparts, a similar pattern as for γ-T (Freiser and Jiang, 2009; Jiang et al., 2007). In addition, γ-T3 was more rapidly metabolized, as more metabolites from γ-T3 were accumulated at 24 h than those from γ- and δ-T. Importantly, after 72 h incubation with cells, 90% of the long-chain carboxychromanols in the culture medium from γ-T3 were in sulfated forms, as compared to <45% from γ-T. In rats, γ-T3 was primarily metabolized to glucuronidated and sulfated γ-CEHC and sulfated long chain carboxychromanols, and again the plasma concentrations of most metabolites in γ-T3 supplemented rats were higher than those of rats fed γ-T. These data suggest γ-T3 is more extensively metabolized than γ-T (Freiser and Jiang, 2009).

Sang et al. detected more conjugated T3 metabolites in the fecal samples from nude mice fed γ- and δ-T3 diets using LC/ESI-MS (our unpublished data). The novel conjugated T3 metabolites were glucuronidated δ-CEHC, sulfated and glucuronidated γ- and δ-CMBHC, and sulfated γ- and δ-CMHenHC. Base on this result and the previously identified conjugated T3 metabolites, it is reasonable to state that conjugation occurs parallel to β-oxidation during the catabolism of T3s. Emerging evidences showed that some sulfated and glucuronidated drug metabolites may play a role in mediating specific biological processes (Mehta et al., 1991; Strott and Higashi, 2003; Totta et al., 2005). The potential biological functions of conjugated vitamin E metabolites are worth further elucidating.

3.3.6 Possible Biological Functions of Tocotrienol Side-Chain Metabolites

3.3.6.1 Natriuretic and Anti-Nephrotoxic Activity of γ-CEHC

γ-CEHC was shown to possess natriuretic activity by inhibiting the 70 pS potassium channel in the thick ascending limb cells of the kidney, whereas α-CEHC exhibited no corresponding activity (Wechter et al., 1996); 4.8 μg/kg γ-CEHC led to significant natriuresis, as indicated by an enhanced excretion of sodium ion, and mild diuresis with no evidence of kaliuresis in male Sprague-Dawley rats. Consistent with the effect of CEHC, supplementation of γ-T or γ-T3 resulted in an increase of γ-CEHC excretion to the urine and led to the enhancement of urinary sodium excretion in rats fed high-NaCl diet (Saito et al., 2003; Uto et al., 2004). γ-CEHC was also reported to more effectively reduce chromate nephrotoxicity induced by sodium dichromate or thallium sulfate in rats than α-T or γ-T (Appenroth et al., 2001). This protective effect of γ-CEHC seemed to be related to its stronger antioxidant activity than α-T and γ-T (as determined by iron-stimulated lipid peroxidation and lumino and lucigenin-amplified chemiluminescence) (Appenroth et al., 2001; Yoshida and Niki, 2002).

3.3.6.2 Anti-Inflammatory Activity

Several studies demonstrated that vitamin E side-chain metabolites possess anti-inflammatory activity. The main target is cyclooxygenase (COX), the enzyme for oxidation of arachidonic acid to prostaglandin H2 (PGH2), a common precursor of various prostaglandins (such as PGE2) and thromboxane, which play an essential role to regulate inflammation response. γ-T and its short chain metabolite, γ-CEHC, have been shown to inhibit the production of PGE2 in lipopolysaccharide (LPS)-activated RAW264.7 macrophages and interleukin-1β (IL-1β)-stimulated A549 human lung epithelial cells (Jiang et al., 2000). γ-T3 exhibited higher activity to inhibit COX-2 catalyzed production of PGE2 in IL-1β-stimulated A549 cells with the relative potency γ-T3 ≈ δ-T > γ-T > α-T (Jiang et al., 2008). Noticeably, this inhibition effect was partially diminished by sesamin, a CYP inhibitor to block the catabolism of vitamin E (Parker et al., 2000), suggesting that the inhibitory effect on prostaglandin production comes from vitamin E metabolites. Further investigation showed that long chain metabolites of vitamin E, including the δ-forms of 9′- and 13′-COOH, inhibited COX activity (Jiang et al., 2008). In addition, vitamin E long chain metabolites δ-13′-COOH suppressed the generation of leukotiene-B4 (LTB4) in ionophore-stimulated human blood neutrophils or differentiated

HL-60 cells and inhibited the activity of recombinant human 5-lipoxygenase (5-LOX) (Jiang et al., 2011). Therefore, the side-chain metabolites of T3s may serve as novel anti-inflammatory agents and contribute to the beneficial effects of vitamin E forms.

3.3.6.3 Anticancer Activity

Birringer et al. (2010) reported that both α- and δ-13′-COOH induced apoptosis in hepatocellular carcinoma HepG2 cells, with an IC_{50} of 13.5 and 6.5 μM, respectively. The induction of apoptosis was further supported by the activation of caspase-3 and caspase-9 as well as PARP-1 cleavage. Li et al. (2011) recently reported that δ-T was more active than other tocopherols in inhibiting the growth of H1299 lung cancer cell xenograft tumors. The blood and tissue levels of δ-T were lower than those of α-T and γ-T, whereas δ-T metabolites were greater than γ-T and far greater than α-T metabolites in the serum and tumors, suggesting a possible anticancer role of δ-T metabolites (Li et al., 2011).

3.3.7 OTHER TOCOTRIENOL METABOLITES

Tocopherols can be oxidized to form tocopheryl quinones (TQs). The 5-position methyl group of TQs seems to affect the cytotoxicity of TQs (Behan et al., 1976). Accordingly, TQs can be categorized into two classes: the nonarylating α-TQ and the arylating γ- and δ-TQs. The latter two TQs lack the 5-methyl groups and are highly cytotoxic in terms of inhibiting colony formation and inducing apoptosis in mammalian cells (Calviello et al., 2003; Cornwell et al., 2002; Jones et al., 2002, and our unpublished results). Similarly, T3s may also be oxidized to their TQ forms (T3Qs). They have been detected in the tissue samples of mice fed T3 diets (our unpublished data). However, studies on the biological functions of T3Qs are limited. α-T3Q has been reported to behave as a redox molecule with similar function as coenzyme Q_{10} to protect cells from oxidative stress and aging (Shrader et al., 2011).

α-tocopheryl phosphate (α-TP) has been reported to be present in tissues and food stuffs (Gianello et al., 2005; Mathias et al., 1981). α-TP has been reported to induce apoptosis, prevent inflammation, and provide cardioprotection (Libinaki et al., 2010; Negis et al., 2006). It has been suggested that α-TP exerted its effects by modulating the levels of Akt, VEGF, and the cell-membrane level of the scavenger receptor CD36 (Zingg et al., 2010). However, studies of other forms of TPs are rather limited. We have suggested that γ- and δ-TP may be more potent in inhibiting cancer cell growth by inducing apoptosis and inhibiting the colony formation of colon cancer cells (our unpublished data). TPs are redox-silent derivatives of tocopherols, and their anticancer activities may represent the portion that is independent of the antioxidant activities of tocopherols. The phosphorylated forms of T3s have not been studied.

3.4 CONCLUDING REMARK

Tocotrienols, a class of members in the vitamin E family, have drawn attention in recent years. They exhibit higher activities against cancers and other chronic diseases as compared to their tocopherol counterparts (reviewed in Aggarwal et al., 2010). The uptake and metabolism processes of T3s essentially follow a similar pattern to their tocopherol counterparts, but with a higher uptake, less retention, and more extensive catabolism *in vivo*. A key issue is how to interpret the different biological activities among different forms of T3s as well as between tocopherols and T3s. Our and others' data suggest a possible correlation between the high biological activities of T3s and their high metabolic rate in the production of active metabolites. In addition, other derivatives such as TPs, TQs, and T3Qs may also contribute to the biological activities of vitamin E forms. On the other hand, some studies showed that the vitamin E forms, rather than their metabolites, exert the biological effects (Conte et al., 2004; Wang et al., 2011), and this again elucidates our lack of understanding of the mechanisms of T3 actions. Further studies on the bioavailability and metabolism of T3s will contribute to the elucidation of biological actions of their group of compounds as well as to their applications in disease prevention.

REFERENCES

Abe, C., Uchida, T., Ohta, M., Ichikawa, T., Yamashita, K., and Ikeda, S. (2007). Cytochrome P450-dependent metabolism of vitamin E isoforms is a critical determinant of their tissue concentrations in rats. *Lipids 42*, 637–645.

Aggarwal, B.B., Sundaram, C., Prasad, S., and Kannappan, R. (2010). Tocotrienols, the vitamin E of the 21st century: Its potential against cancer and other chronic diseases. *Biochem Pharmacol 80*, 1613–1631.

Anwar, K., Iqbal, J., and Hussain, M.M. (2007). Mechanisms involved in vitamin E transport by primary enterocytes and in vivo absorption. *J Lipid Res 48*, 2028–2038.

Appenroth, D., Karge, E., Kiessling, G., Wechter, W.J., Winnefeld, K., and Fleck, C. (2001). LLU-alpha, an endogenous metabolite of gamma-tocopherol, is more effective against metal nephrotoxicity in rats than gamma-tocopherol. *Toxicol Lett 122*, 255–265.

Behan, J.M., Dean, F.M., and Johnstone, R.A.W. (1976). Photoelectron spectra of cyclic aromatic ethers: The question of the mills-nixon effect. *Tetrahedron 32*, 167–171.

Betti, M., Minelli, A., Canonico, B., Castaldo, P., Magi, S., Aisa, M.C., Piroddi, M., Di Tomaso, V., and Galli, F. (2006). Antiproliferative effects of tocopherols (vitamin E) on murine glioma C6 cells: Homologue-specific control of PKC/ERK and cyclin signaling. *Free Radic Biol Med 41*, 464–472.

Birringer, M., Lington, D., Vertuani, S., Manfredini, S., Scharlau, D., Glei, M., and Ristow, M. (2010). Proapoptotic effects of long-chain vitamin E metabolites in HepG2 cells are mediated by oxidative stress. *Free Radic Biol Med 49*, 1315–1322.

Birringer, M., Pfluger, P., Kluth, D., Landes, N., and Brigelius-Flohe, R. (2002). Identities and differences in the metabolism of tocotrienols and tocopherols in HepG2 cells. *J Nutr 132*, 3113–3118.

Calviello, G., Di Nicuolo, F., Piccioni, E., Marcocci, M.E., Serini, S., Maggiano, N., Jones, K.H., Cornwell, D.G., and Palozza, P. (2003). gamma-Tocopheryl quinone induces apoptosis in cancer cells via caspase-9 activation and cytochrome c release. *Carcinogenesis 24*, 427–433.

Chiku, S., Hamamura, K., and Nakamura, T. (1984). Novel urinary metabolite of D-delta-tocopherol in rats. *J Lipid Res 25*, 40–48.

Conte, C., Floridi, A., Aisa, C., Piroddi, M., and Galli, F. (2004). Gamma-tocotrienol metabolism and antiproliferative effect in prostate cancer cells. *Ann NY Acad Sci 1031*, 391–394.

Copp, R.P., Wisniewski, T., Hentati, F., Larnaout, A., Ben Hamida, M., and Kayden, H.J. (1999). Localization of alpha-tocopherol transfer protein in the brains of patients with ataxia with vitamin E deficiency and other oxidative stress related neurodegenerative disorders. *Brain Res 822*, 80–87.

Cornwell, D.G., Williams, M.V., Wani, A.A., Wani, G., Shen, E., and Jones, K.H. (2002). Mutagenicity of tocopheryl quinones: Evolutionary advantage of selective accumulation of dietary alpha-tocopherol. *Nutr Cancer 43*, 111–118.

Das, S., Lekli, I., Das, M., Szabo, G., Varadi, J., Juhasz, B., Bak, I., Nesaretam, K., Tosaki, A., Powell, S.R. et al. (2008). Cardioprotection with palm oil tocotrienols: Comparison of different isomers. *Am J Physiol Heart Circ Physiol 294*, H970–H978.

Das, S., Powell, S.R., Wang, P., Divald, A., Nesaretnam, K., Tosaki, A., Cordis, G.A., Maulik, N., and Das, D.K. (2005). Cardioprotection with palm tocotrienol: Antioxidant activity of tocotrienol is linked with its ability to stabilize proteasomes. *Am J Physiol Heart Circ Physiol 289*, H361–H367.

Fairus, S., Nor, R.M., Cheng, H.M., and Sundram, K. (2006). Postprandial metabolic fate of tocotrienol-rich vitamin E differs significantly from that of alpha-tocopherol. *Am J Clin Nutr 84*, 835–842.

Freiser, H. and Jiang, Q. (2009). Gamma-tocotrienol and gamma-tocopherol are primarily metabolized to conjugated 2-(beta-carboxyethyl)-6-hydroxy-2,7,8-trimethylchroman and sulfated long-chain carboxychromanols in rats. *J Nutr 139*, 884–889.

Gianello, R., Libinaki, R., Azzi, A., Gavin, P.D., Negis, Y., Zingg, J.M., Holt, P., Keah, H.H., Griffey, A., Smallridge, R. et al. (2005). Alpha-tocopheryl phosphate: A novel, natural form of vitamin E. *Free Radic Biol Med 39*, 970–976.

Gohil, K., Godzdanker, R., O'Roark, E., Schock, B.C., Kaini, R.R., Packer, L., Cross, C.E., and Traber, M.G. (2004). Alpha-tocopherol transfer protein deficiency in mice causes multi-organ deregulation of gene networks and behavioral deficits with age. *Ann NY Acad Sci 1031*, 109–126.

Hosomi, A., Arita, M., Sato, Y., Kiyose, C., Ueda, T., Igarashi, O., Arai, H., and Inoue, K. (1997). Affinity for alpha-tocopherol transfer protein as a determinant of the biological activities of vitamin E analogs. *FEBS Lett 409*, 105–108.

Hosomi, A., Goto, K., Kondo, H., Iwatsubo, T., Yokota, T., Ogawa, M., Arita, M., Aoki, J., Arai, H., and Inoue, K. (1998). Localization of alpha-tocopherol transfer protein in rat brain. *Neurosci Lett 256*, 159–162.

Hsieh, T.C., Elangovan, S., and Wu, J.M. (2010). gamma-Tocotrienol controls proliferation, modulates expression of cell cycle regulatory proteins and up-regulates quinone reductase NQO2 in MCF-7 breast cancer cells. *Anticancer Res 30*, 2869–2874.

Ikeda, S., Abe, C., Uchida, T., Ichikawa, T., Horio, F., and Yamashita, K. (2007). Dietary sesame seed and its lignan increase both ascorbic acid concentration in some tissues and urinary excretion by stimulating biosynthesis in rats. *J Nutr Sci Vitaminol (Tokyo) 53*, 383–392.

Ikeda, S., Kagaya, M., Kobayashi, K., Tohyama, T., Kiso, Y., Higuchi, N., and Yamashita, K. (2003a). Dietary sesame lignans decrease lipid peroxidation in rats fed docosahexaenoic acid. *J Nutr Sci Vitaminol (Tokyo) 49*, 270–276.

Ikeda, S., Tohyama, T., Yoshimura, H., Hamamura, K., Abe, K., and Yamashita, K. (2003b). Dietary alpha-tocopherol decreases alpha-tocotrienol but not gamma-tocotrienol concentration in rats. *J Nutr 133*, 428–434.

Ikeda, S., Toyoshima, K., and Yamashita, K. (2001). Dietary sesame seeds elevate alpha- and gamma-tocotrienol concentrations in skin and adipose tissue of rats fed the tocotrienol-rich fraction extracted from palm oil. *J Nutr 131*, 2892–2897.

Jiang, Q., Elson-Schwab, I., Courtemanche, C., and Ames, B.N. (2000). gamma-tocopherol and its major metabolite, in contrast to alpha-tocopherol, inhibit cyclooxygenase activity in macrophages and epithelial cells. *Proc Natl Acad Sci USA 97*, 11494–11499.

Jiang, Q., Freiser, H., Wood, K.V., and Yin, X. (2007). Identification and quantitation of novel vitamin E metabolites, sulfated long-chain carboxychromanols, in human A549 cells and in rats. *J Lipid Res 48*, 1221–1230.

Jiang, Q., Yin, X., Lill, M.A., Danielson, M.L., Freiser, H., and Huang, J. (2008). Long-chain carboxychromanols, metabolites of vitamin E, are potent inhibitors of cyclooxygenases. *Proc Natl Acad Sci USA 105*, 20464–20469.

Jiang, Z., Yin, X., and Jiang, Q. (2011). Natural forms of vitamin E and 13′-carboxychromanol, a long-chain vitamin E metabolite, inhibit leukotriene generation from stimulated neutrophils by blocking calcium influx and suppressing 5-lipoxygenase activity, respectively. *J Immunol 186*, 1173–1179.

Jones, K.H., Liu, J.J., Roehm, J.S., Eckel, J.J., Eckel, T.T., Stickrath, C.R., Triola, C.A., Jiang, Z., Bartoli, G.M., and Cornwell, D.G. (2002). Gamma-tocopheryl quinone stimulates apoptosis in drug-sensitive and multidrug-resistant cancer cells. *Lipids 37*, 173–184.

Kaempf-Rotzoll, D.E., Horiguchi, M., Hashiguchi, K., Aoki, J., Tamai, H., Linderkamp, O., and Arai, H. (2003). Human placental trophoblast cells express alpha-tocopherol transfer protein. *Placenta 24*, 439–444.

Kaempf-Rotzoll, D.E., Igarashi, K., Aoki, J., Jishage, K., Suzuki, H., Tamai, H., Linderkamp, O., and Arai, H. (2002). Alpha-tocopherol transfer protein is specifically localized at the implantation site of pregnant mouse uterus. *Biol Reprod 67*, 599–604.

Kawakami, Y., Tsuzuki, T., Nakagawa, K., and Miyazawa, T. (2007). Distribution of tocotrienols in rats fed a rice bran tocotrienol concentrate. *Biosci Biotechnol Biochem 71*, 464–471.

Kayden, H.J. and Traber, M.G. (1993). Absorption, lipoprotein transport, and regulation of plasma concentrations of vitamin E in humans. *J Lipid Res 34*, 343–358.

Khanna, S., Patel, V., Rink, C., Roy, S., and Sen, C.K. (2005). Delivery of orally supplemented alpha-tocotrienol to vital organs of rats and tocopherol-transport protein deficient mice. *Free Radic Biol Med 39*, 1310–1319.

Kluth, D., Landes, N., Pfluger, P., Muller-Schmehl, K., Weiss, K., Bumke-Vogt, C., Ristow, M., and Brigelius-Flohe, R. (2005). Modulation of Cyp3a11 mRNA expression by alpha-tocopherol but not gamma-tocotrienol in mice. *Free Radic Biol Med 38*, 507–514.

Landes, N., Pfluger, P., Kluth, D., Birringer, M., Ruhl, R., Bol, G.F., Glatt, H., and Brigelius-Flohe, R. (2003). Vitamin E activates gene expression via the pregnane X receptor. *Biochem Pharmacol 65*, 269–273.

Leonard, S.W., Terasawa, Y., Farese, R.V., Jr., and Traber, M.G. (2002). Incorporation of deuterated RRR- or all-rac-alpha-tocopherol in plasma and tissues of alpha-tocopherol transfer protein–null mice. *Am J Clin Nutr 75*, 555–560.

Li, G.X., Lee, M.J., Liu, A.B., Yang, Z., Lin, Y., Shih, W.J., and Yang, C.S. (2011). delta-tocopherol is more active than alpha- or gamma-tocopherol in inhibiting lung tumorigenesis in vivo. *Cancer Prev Res (Phila) 4*, 404–413.

Libinaki, R., Tesanovic, S., Heal, A., Nikolovski, B., Vinh, A., Widdop, R.E., Gaspari, T.A., Devaraj, S., and Ogru, E. (2010). Effect of tocopheryl phosphate on key biomarkers of inflammation: Implication in the reduction of atherosclerosis progression in a hypercholesterolaemic rabbit model. *Clin Exp Pharmacol Physiol 37*, 587–592.

Mahalingam, D., Radhakrishnan, A.K., Amom, Z., Ibrahim, N., and Nesaretnam, K. (2011). Effects of supplementation with tocotrienol-rich fraction on immune response to tetanus toxoid immunization in normal healthy volunteers. *Eur J Clin Nutr 65*, 63–69.

Mathias, P.M., Harries, J.T., Peters, T.J., and Muller, D.P. (1981). Studies on the in vivo absorption of micellar solutions of tocopherol and tocopheryl acetate in the rat: Demonstration and partial characterization of a mucosal esterase localized to the endoplasmic reticulum of the enterocyte. *J Lipid Res 22*, 829–837.

Mehta, R.G., Barua, A.B., Olson, J.A., and Moon, R.C. (1991). Effects of retinoid glucuronides on mammary gland development in organ culture. *Oncology 48*, 505–509.

Meier, R., Tomizaki, T., Schulze-Briese, C., Baumann, U., and Stocker, A. (2003). The molecular basis of vitamin E retention: Structure of human alpha-tocopherol transfer protein. *J Mol Biol 331*, 725–734.

Minko, T., Stefanov, A., and Pozharov, V. (2002). Selected contribution: Lung hypoxia: Antioxidant and antiapoptotic effects of liposomal alpha-tocopherol. *J Appl Physiol 93*, 1550–1560; discussion 1549.

Negis, Y., Aytan, N., Ozer, N., Ogru, E., Libinaki, R., Gianello, R., Azzi, A., and Zingg, J.M. (2006). The effect of tocopheryl phosphates on atherosclerosis progression in rabbits fed with a high cholesterol diet. *Arch Biochem Biophys 450*, 63–66.

Okabe, M., Oji, M., Ikeda, I., Tachibana, H., and Yamada, K. (2002). Tocotrienol levels in various tissues of Sprague-Dawley rats after intragastric administration of tocotrienols. *Biosci Biotechnol Biochem 66*, 1768–1771.

Ouahchi, K., Arita, M., Kayden, H., Hentati, F., Ben Hamida, M., Sokol, R., Arai, H., Inoue, K., Mandel, J.L., and Koenig, M. (1995). Ataxia with isolated vitamin E deficiency is caused by mutations in the alpha-tocopherol transfer protein. *Nat Genet 9*, 141–145.

Park, H.A., Kubicki, N., Gnyawali, S., Chan, Y.C., Roy, S., Khanna, S., and Sen, C.K. (2011). Natural vitamin E {alpha}-tocotrienol protects against ischemic stroke by induction of multidrug resistance-associated protein 1. *Stroke 42*, 2308–2314.

Parker, R.S., Sontag, T.J., and Swanson, J.E. (2000). Cytochrome P4503A-dependent metabolism of tocopherols and inhibition by sesamin. *Biochem Biophys Res Commun 277*, 531–534.

Parker, R.S., Sontag, T.J., Swanson, J.E., and McCormick, C.C. (2004). Discovery, characterization, and significance of the cytochrome P450 omega-hydroxylase pathway of vitamin E catabolism. *Ann NY Acad Sci 1031*, 13–21.

Parker, R.S. and Swanson, J.E. (2000). A novel 5'-carboxychroman metabolite of gamma-tocopherol secreted by HepG2 cells and excreted in human urine. *Biochem Biophys Res Commun 269*, 580–583.

Pope, S.A., Burtin, G.E., Clayton, P.T., Madge, D.J., and Muller, D.P. (2002). Synthesis and analysis of conjugates of the major vitamin E metabolite, alpha-CEHC. *Free Radic Biol Med 33*, 807–817.

Ren, Z., Pae, M., Dao, M.C., Smith, D., Meydani, S.N., and Wu, D. (2010). Dietary supplementation with tocotrienols enhances immune function in C57BL/6 mice. *J Nutr 140*, 1335–1341.

Saito, H., Kiyose, C., Yoshimura, H., Ueda, T., Kondo, K., and Igarashi, O. (2003). Gamma-tocotrienol, a vitamin E homolog, is a natriuretic hormone precursor. *J Lipid Res 44*, 1530–1535.

Saito, Y., Nishio, K., Akazawa, Y.O., Yamanaka, K., Miyama, A., Yoshida, Y., Noguchi, N., and Niki, E. (2010). Cytoprotective effects of vitamin E homologues against glutamate-induced cell death in immature primary cortical neuron cultures: Tocopherols and tocotrienols exert similar effects by antioxidant function. *Free Radic Biol Med 49*, 1542–1549.

Schultz, M., Leist, M., Petrzika, M., Gassmann, B., and Brigelius-Flohe, R. (1995). Novel urinary metabolite of alpha-tocopherol, 2,5,7,8-tetramethyl-2(2'-carboxyethyl)-6-hydroxychroman, as an indicator of an adequate vitamin E supply? *Am J Clin Nutr 62*, 1527S-1534S.

Serbinova, E., Kagan, V., Han, D., and Packer, L. (1991). Free radical recycling and intramembrane mobility in the antioxidant properties of alpha-tocopherol and alpha-tocotrienol. *Free Radic Biol Med 10*, 263–275.

Sheets, J.J. and Mason, J.I. (1984). Ketoconazole: A potent inhibitor of cytochrome P-450-dependent drug metabolism in rat liver. *Drug Metab Dispos 12*, 603–606.

Shrader, W.D., Amagata, A., Barnes, A., Enns, G.M., Hinman, A., Jankowski, O., Kheifets, V., Komatsuzaki, R., Lee, E., Mollard, P. et al. (2011). alpha-Tocotrienol quinone modulates oxidative stress response and the biochemistry of aging. *Bioorg Med Chem Lett 21*, 3693–3698.

Sontag, T.J. and Parker, R.S. (2002). Cytochrome P450 omega-hydroxylase pathway of tocopherol catabolism. Novel mechanism of regulation of vitamin E status. *J Biol Chem 277*, 25290–25296.

Sontag, T.J. and Parker, R.S. (2007). Influence of major structural features of tocopherols and tocotrienols on their omega-oxidation by tocopherol-omega-hydroxylase. *J Lipid Res 48*, 1090–1098.

Stocker, A. and Baumann, U. (2003). Supernatant protein factor in complex with RRR-alpha-tocopherylquinone: A link between oxidized vitamin E and cholesterol biosynthesis. *J Mol Biol 332*, 759–765.

Stocker, A., Tomizaki, T., Schulze-Briese, C., and Baumann, U. (2002). Crystal structure of the human supernatant protein factor. *Structure 10*, 1533–1540.

Strott, C.A. and Higashi, Y. (2003). Cholesterol sulfate in human physiology: What's it all about? *J Lipid Res 44*, 1268–1278.

Swanson, J.E., Ben, R.N., Burton, G.W., and Parker, R.S. (1999). Urinary excretion of 2,7, 8-trimethyl-2-(beta-carboxyethyl)-6-hydroxychroman is a major route of elimination of gamma-tocopherol in humans. *J Lipid Res 40*, 665–671.

Tanito, M., Itoh, N., Yoshida, Y., Hayakawa, M., Ohira, A., and Niki, E. (2004). Distribution of tocopherols and tocotrienols to rat ocular tissues after topical ophthalmic administration. *Lipids 39*, 469–474.

Then, S.M., Mazlan, M., Mat Top, G., and Wan Ngah, W.Z. (2009). Is vitamin E toxic to neuron cells? *Cell Mol Neurobiol 29*, 485–496.

Totta, P., Acconcia, F., Virgili, F., Cassidy, A., Weinberg, P.D., Rimbach, G., and Marino, M. (2005). Daidzein-sulfate metabolites affect transcriptional and antiproliferative activities of estrogen receptor-beta in cultured human cancer cells. *J Nutr 135*, 2687–2693.

Traber, M.G. (2007). Vitamin E regulatory mechanisms. *Annu Rev Nutr 27*, 347–362.

Traber, M.G. Rallis, M., Podda, M., Weber, C., Maibach, H.I., and Packer, L. (1998). Penetration and distribution of alpha-tocopherol, alpha- or gamma-tocotrienols applied individually onto murine skin. *Lipids 33*, 87–91.

Traber, M.G., Siddens, L.K., Leonard, S.W., Schock, B., Gohil, K., Krueger, S.K., Cross, C.E., and Williams, D.E. (2005). Alpha-tocopherol modulates Cyp3a expression, increases gamma-CEHC production, and limits tissue gamma-tocopherol accumulation in mice fed high gamma-tocopherol diets. *Free Radic Biol Med 38*, 773–785.

Traber, M.G. and Sies, H. (1996). Vitamin E in humans: Demand and delivery. *Annu Rev Nutr 16*, 321–347.

Tsuzuki, W., Yunoki, R., and Yoshimura, H. (2007). Intestinal epithelial cells absorb gamma-tocotrienol faster than alpha-tocopherol. *Lipids 42*, 163–170.

Uto, H., Kiyose, C., Saito, H., Ueda, T., Nakamijra, T., Igarashi, O., and Kondo, K. (2004). Gamma-tocopherol enhances sodium excretion as a natriuretic hormone precursor. *J Nutr Sci Vitaminol (Tokyo) 50*, 277–282.

Viola, V., Pilolli, F., Piroddi, M., Pierpaoli, E., Orlando, F., Provinciali, M., Betti, M., Mazzini, F., and Galli, F. (2011). Why tocotrienols work better: Insights into the in vitro anti-cancer mechanism of vitamin E. *Genes Nutr 7*, 29–41.

Wang, X., Ni, J., Hsu, C.L., Johnykutty, S., Tang, P., Ho, Y.S., Lee, C.H., and Yeh, S. (2009). Reduced expression of tocopherol-associated protein (TAP/Sec14L2) in human breast cancer. *Cancer Invest 27*, 971–977.

Wang, Y., Moreland, M., Wagner, J.G., Ames, B.N., Illek, B., Peden, D.B., and Jiang, Q. (2011). Vitamin E forms inhibit IL-13/STAT6-induced eotaxin-3 secretion by up-regulation of PAR4, an endogenous inhibitor of atypical PKC in human lung epithelial cells. *J Nutr Biochem* [epub ahead of print].

Wechter, W.J., Kantoci, D., Murray, E.D., Jr., D'Amico, D.C., Jung, M.E., and Wang, W.H. (1996). A new endogenous natriuretic factor: LLU-alpha. *Proc Natl Acad Sci USA 93*, 6002–6007.

Yang, Z., Lee, M.J., Zhao, Y., and Yang, C.S. (2011). Metabolism of tocotrienols in animals and synergistic inhibitory actions of tocotrienols with atorvastatin in cancer cells. *Genes Nutr 7*, 11–18.

Yap, S.P., Yuen, K.H., and Lim, A.B. (2003). Influence of route of administration on the absorption and disposition of alpha-, gamma- and delta-tocotrienols in rats. *J Pharm Pharmacol 55*, 53–58.

Yap, S.P., Yuen, K.H., and Wong, J.W. (2001). Pharmacokinetics and bioavailability of alpha-, gamma- and delta-tocotrienols under different food status. *J Pharm Pharmacol 53*, 67–71.

Yoshida, Y. and Niki, E. (2002). Antioxidant effects of alpha- and gamma-carboxyethyl-6-hydroxychromans. *Biofactors 16*, 93–103.

Yoshida, Y., Niki, E., and Noguchi, N. (2003). Comparative study on the action of tocopherols and tocotrienols as antioxidant: Chemical and physical effects. *Chem Phys Lipids 123*, 63–75.

Yoshida, H., Yusin, M., Ren, I., Kuhlenkamp, J., Hirano, T., Stolz, A., and Kaplowitz, N. (1992). Identification, purification, and immunochemical characterization of a tocopherol-binding protein in rat liver cytosol. *J Lipid Res 33*, 343–350.

You, C.S., Sontag, T.J., Swanson, J.E., and Parker, R.S. (2005). Long-chain carboxychromanols are the major metabolites of tocopherols and tocotrienols in A549 lung epithelial cells but not HepG2 cells. *J Nutr 135*, 227–232.

Zhao, Y., Lee, M.J., Cheung, C., Ju, J.H., Chen, Y.K., Liu, B., Hu, L.Q., and Yang, C.S. (2010). Analysis of multiple metabolites of tocopherols and tocotrienols in mice and humans. *J Agric Food Chem 58*, 4844–4852.

Zimmer, S., Stocker, A., Sarbolouki, M.N., Spycher, S.E., Sassoon, J., and Azzi, A. (2000). A novel human tocopherol-associated protein: Cloning, in vitro expression, and characterization. *J Biol Chem 275*, 25672–25680.

Zingg, J.M., Libinaki, R., Lai, C.Q., Meydani, M., Gianello, R., Ogru, E., and Azzi, A. (2010). Modulation of gene expression by alpha-tocopherol and alpha-tocopheryl phosphate in THP-1 monocytes. *Free Radic Biol Med 49*, 1989–2000.

4 Bioavailability of Tocotrienols and Interference of Their Bioavailability by α-Tocopherol Supplementation

Saiko Ikeda, Tomono Uchida, and Chisato Abe

CONTENTS

4.1 INTRODUCTION

Vitamin E is a fat-soluble antioxidant that inhibits lipid peroxidation in biological membranes. In nature, compounds with vitamin E activity are α-, β-, γ-, or δ-tocopherol and α-, β-, γ-, or δ-tocotrienol. α- and γ-tocopherol are abundant in dietary vitamin E while tocotrienol is only present in some plant sources, such as palm oil and rice bran. It is important to determine the distribution and metabolism of tocotrienol because it has some beneficial biological effects.

Dietary tocopherol and tocotrienol are absorbed in the small intestine and secreted with triacylglycerol-rich chylomicrons into lymph and blood (Kayden and Traber 1993; Traber and Sies 1996). After lipolysis of the triacylglycerol-rich chylomicrons in circulation, the dietary tocopherol and tocotrienol are transported to the liver (Abe et al. 2007a). Among vitamin E isoforms, α-tocopherol is preferentially incorporated into VLDL and transported to various tissues by lipoprotein (Traber and. Arai 1999; Traber et al. 2004) because of its high affinity for α-tocopherol transfer protein (αTTP; Hosomi et al. 1997). In contrast, the other vitamin E isoforms, γ-tocopherol and tocotrienol, are catabolized and excreted. Therefore, α-tocopherol has the highest bioavailability among the vitamin E isoforms.

4.2 TISSUE DISTRIBUTION OF TOCOTRIENOLS

However, some reports show peripheral tissue-specific accumulation of tocotrienol in animals. Hayes et al. (1993) reported that significant amounts of α- and γ-tocotrienol were found in adipose tissue of hamsters fed a diet containing α- and γ-tocotrienol. Podda et al. (1996) showed that α- and γ-tocotrienol were present in the skin of hairless mice fed a commercial diet containing a small amount of tocotrienol with a high amount of α-tocopherol. We also determined

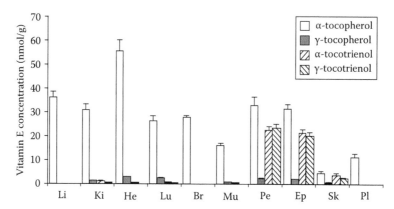

FIGURE 4.1 Tissue and plasma concentrations of α-, γ-tocopherol, α-, and γ-tocotrienol in rats fed a diet containing the vitamin isoforms for 8 weeks. The rats were deprived of food for 24 h before sacrifice. Li, liver; Ki, kidney; He, heart; Lu, lung; Br, brain; Mu, muscle; Pe, perirenal adipose tissue; Ep, epididymal fat; Sk, skin; Pl, plasma.

the tissue distribution of tocotrienol of rats to evaluate its bioavailability. Small amounts of α- and γ-tocotrienol could be detected in adipose tissue and skin, but not in the other tissues of rats fed a commercial diet containing <5 mg/kg of tocotrienol (Ikeda et al. 2001). Moreover, significant amounts of not only α-tocopherol but also α- and γ-tocotrienol accumulated in the adipose tissue and skin of rats fed a diet containing α- and γ-tocotrienol with α-tocopherol (Figure 4.1). Both tocopherol and tocotrienol quickly accumulated in liver, adrenal gland, lung, and heart; however, their accumulation in adipose tissue was very slow for 24 h after their administration by gavage (Uchida et al. 2012). This suggests that tocotrienol accumulation in adipose tissue was not due to its preferential uptake.

We also determined the retention capability of vitamin E in tissues. Rats were fed a vitamin E-rich diet containing α-tocopherol, α-, and γ-tocotrienol for 6 weeks, and then they were fed a vitamin E-free diet for 4 weeks. α-tocopherol and α-tocotrienol concentrations in the liver and heart decreased at 1 week after a change from a vitamin E-rich to a vitamin E-free diet, and the concentrations decreased to less than 44% at 4 weeks. In contrast, neither α-tocopherol nor α-tocotrienol concentrations in the adipose tissue decreased as a result of the 4 week vitamin E deficiency. Therefore, vitamin E slowly accumulates in adipose tissue compared with the other tissues but the vitamin E levels in adipose tissue are maintained without degradation for several weeks. Adipose tissue-specific accumulation of dietary tocotrienol is likely to be because of maintenance of the level without degradation.

4.3 INTERFERENCE OF TOCOTRIENOL ACCUMULATION BY α-TOCOPHEROL

The effect of α-tocopherol on the tissue concentration of tocotrienol was determined. Rats were fed a diet containing tocotrienol with or without α-tocopherol for 8 weeks and killed after deprivation for 24 h. Dietary α-tocopherol decreased α-tocotrienol concentration in the tissues; however, the γ-tocotrienol concentration was not decreased by α-tocopherol (Ikeda et al. 2003). The different effect of α-tocopherol on α- and γ-tocotrienol concentrations was observed in the rats without deprivation before sacrifice (Figure 4.2). In addition to α-tocotrienol, the γ-tocopherol concentration was also decreased in rats fed a diet containing γ-tocopherol and α-tocopherol. Because α-tocopherol, which has the highest affinity for αTTP in liver, is preferentially transported to extrahepatic tissues, the observed no effect level of dietary α-tocopherol on γ-tocotrienol concentration showed the possibility of a different transport system for γ-tocotrienol from the other vitamin E isoforms, such as liver-independent transport of γ-tocotrienol.

Then we determined tocotrienol uptake to tissues of rats at 8 h after oral administration of α- and γ-tocotrienol with or without α-tocopherol. Simultaneous administration of α-tocopherol decreased

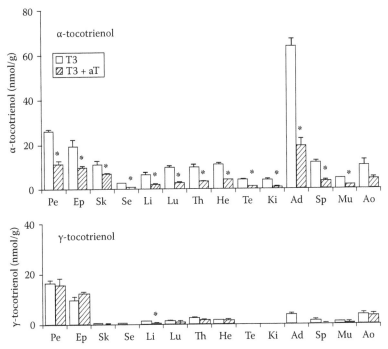

FIGURE 4.2 Tissue and serum concentrations of α- and γ-tocotrienol in rats fed a diet containing tocotrienol mixture (T3) or tocotrienol mixture with α-tocopherol (T3 + aT) for 7 weeks. The tocotrienol mixture contained α- and γ-tocotrienol, and tocopherol was undetectable in the mixture. The rats had free access to food until sacrifice. *Significantly different ($P < 0.05$) from the T3 group. Pe, perirenal adipose tissue; Ep, epididymal fat; Sk, skin; Se, serum; Li, liver; Lu, lung; Th, thymus; He, heart; Te, testis; Ki, kidney; Ad, adrenal gland; Sp, spleen; Mu, muscle; Ao, aorta.

the α-tocotrienol concentration in the serum and tissues (Figure 4.3). Surprisingly, the α-tocopherol administration also decreased the γ-tocotrienol concentration in the adipose tissue and skin. Thus, α-tocopherol inhibited tissue uptake of not only α-tocotrienol but also γ-tocotrienol after oral administration. Dietary γ-tocotrienol is likely to be transported to the tissues via the liver in the same manner as the other isoforms. However, the reason why dietary α-tocopherol does not affect the γ-tocotrienol concentration in tissues in diet studies remains unclear.

4.4 TOCOTRIENOL CATABOLISM TO CARBOXYETHYL-HYDROXYCHROMAN

All vitamin E isoforms undergo catabolism to phytyl short-chain carboxyethyl-hydroxychromans (CEHC) such as 2,5,7,8-tetramethyl-2(2′-carboxyethyl)-6-hydroxychroman (αCEHC), a metabolite of α-tocopherol and α-tocotrienol, and 2,7,8-trimethyl-2(2′-carboxyethyl)-6-hydroxychroman (γCEHC), and a metabolite of γ-tocopherol and γ-tocotrienol (Schultz et al. 1995; Swanson et al. 1999; Lodge et al. 2001). The catabolic pathway involves ω-hydroxylation of the phytyl chain and subsequently β-oxidation (Birringer et al. 2002; Parker et al. 2004). The rate-limiting step is ω-hydroxylation of vitamin E by cytochrome P450 (CYP) 4F2 in humans (Sontag and Parker 2002, 2007). CEHC is then conjugated with glucuronate in humans or with sulfate in rats and subsequently excreted into urine.

We determined total amounts of conjugated and unconjugated metabolites in rat tissues by HPLC with electrochemical detection, and 6-hydroxy-2,5,7,8-tetramethylchroman-2-carboxylic acid (trolox) was used as an internal standard (Uchida et al. 2011). At 24 h after oral administration of α- and γ-tocotrienol, both tocotrienols were present in all of the tissues examined (Figure 4.4).

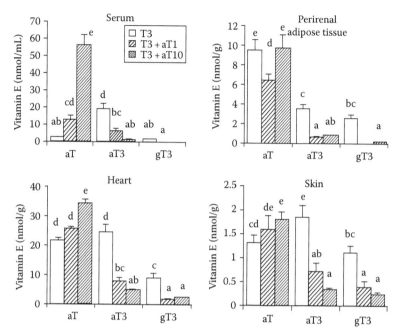

FIGURE 4.3 Concentrations of α-tocopherol (aT), α-tocotrienol (aT3), and γ-tocotrienol (gT3) in serum and tissues at 8 h after oral administration of 29.5 mg of tocotrienol mixture (T3), 29.5 mg of tocotrienol mixture with 1 mg of α-tocopherol (T3 + aT1), or 29.5 mg of tocotrienol mixture with 10 mg of α-tocopherol (T3 + aT10). The tocotrienol mixture (29.5 mg) contained 10 mg of α-tocotrienol and 14 mg of γ-tocotrienol. Means not sharing a letter differ at $P < 0.05$.

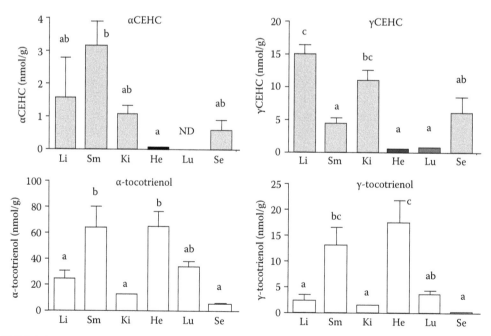

FIGURE 4.4 Tissue and serum distribution of α-, γ-tocotrienol, and their metabolites in rats at 24 h after oral administration of a tocotrienol mixture containing α- and γ-tocotrienol. Means not sharing a letter differ at $P < 0.05$. ND, not detected. (Modified from Uchida, T. et al., *J. Nutr. Sci. Vitaminol.*, 57, 326, 2011.)

However, αCEHC and γCEHC, metabolites of α- and γ-tocotrienol, mainly accumulated in the serum with limited deposits in the tissues including the liver, small intestine, and kidney. Their quantities in the heart, lung, adrenal gland, spleen, and brain were negligible or less than measurable amounts. Thus, CEHC was present as a few nanomoles per gram in tissue in not only the liver but also the kidney and small intestine after oral administration. The γCEHC concentration was higher than the γ-tocotrienol concentration in the liver and kidney. The high level of γCEHC in the kidney is interesting because γCEHC is an endogenous natriuretic factor that inhibits potassium channels in the thick ascending limb cells of kidney (Wechter et al. 1996). In addition, kidney highly expresses CYP4F2 in humans, suggesting that the kidney is capable of catabolizing vitamin E to CEHC.

Significant amounts of αCEHC and γCEHC were also present in the small intestine. We also found catabolic conversion of α- and γ-tocotrienol to their metabolites in human intestinal Caco-2 cells, although the conversion activity was weak (data not shown). Some dietary tocotrienol is likely to be catabolized to CEHC in the small intestine and is secreted into the circulatory system.

4.5 TOCOTRIENOL CATABOLISM AS A CRITICAL DETERMINANT OF ITS BIOAVAILABILITY

As mentioned earlier, the rate-limiting step of vitamin E catabolism to CEHC is ω-hydroxylation of vitamin E by CYP4F (Sontag and Parker 2002; Sontag and Parker 2007). Parker et al. (2000) showed that ketoconazole, a CYP inhibitor, inhibits catabolism of γ- and δ-tocopherol in HepG2 cells or α- and γ-tocopherol in rat hepatocytes. We determined the influence of catabolism to CEHC on the tissue tocotrienol concentration using ketoconazole (Abe et al. 2007b). Ketoconazole inhibited the urinary excretion of both αCEHC and γCEHC in rats administered α- and γ-tocotrienol by gavage. In addition, the inhibitor markedly elevated the α- and γ-tocotrienol concentrations in the various tissues, including liver, jejunum, kidney, adrenal gland, lung, heart, and spleen despite their low affinity for αTTP. Thus, CYP-dependent catabolism of tocotrienol is a critical determinant of its concentration in tissues.

We previously found that sesame seed and its lignan, such as sesamin and sesaminol, elevated α- and γ-tocopherol concentrations in rat tissues and decreased the urinary excretion of their metabolites (Ikeda et al. 2002; Uchida et al. 2007). Elevation of γ-tocopherol concentration by dietary sesame oil was also observed in humans (Lemcke-Norojärvi et al. 2001; Frank et al. 2008). We examined whether dietary sesame seed also elevates tocotrienol concentration in rat tissues (Ikeda et al. 2001). Dietary sesame seed elevated α- and γ-tocotrienol concentrations in limited tissues including adipose tissue and the skin of rats fed a diet containing α-tocopherol, α, and γ-tocotrienol, while the tocotrienol concentration in the other tissues was negligible (Figure 4.5). These data suggest that sesame lignan elevates both tocopherol and tocotrienol concentrations by inhibiting their catabolism to CEHC. Frank et al. (2008) reported that consumption of muffins containing sesame lignan decreased plasma γCEHC concentration and its urinary excretion in men, suggesting the improvement of tocotrienol bioavailability in humans, especially in adipose tissue, by dietary sesame seed.

4.6 ENHANCEMENT OF TOCOTRIENOL ABSORPTION USING CYCLODEXTRIN

We found that Triton WR1339, an inhibitor of the catabolism of triacylglycerol-rich lipoprotein by lipoprotein lipase, completely inhibits vitamin E transport to the liver and causes its accumulation in the plasma of rats after vitamin E administration by gavage (Abe et al. 2007a). This indicates that the plasma vitamin E of the Triton WR1339-treated rats is nearly equivalent to the amount absorbed *in vivo*. The plasma α- and γ-tocotrienol concentrations of the Triton-treated rats after tocotrienol administration were much lower than the α-tocopherol concentration after α-tocopherol administration, suggesting poor absorption of tocotrienol.

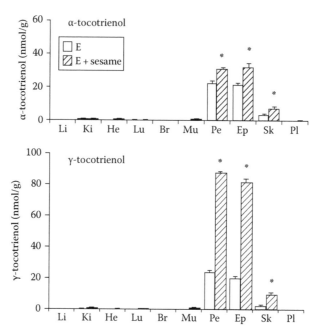

FIGURE 4.5 Effect of dietary sesame seed on α- and γ-tocotrienol concentrations in tissues and plasma. Rats were fed a diet containing α-, γ-tocopherol, α-, and γ-tocotrienol (E) or α-, γ-tocopherol, α-, and γ-tocotrienol with sesame seed (E + sesame) for 8 weeks. *Significantly different ($P < 0.05$) from the E group. Li, liver; Ki, kidney; He, heart; Lu, lung; Br, brain; Mu, muscle; Pe, perirenal adipose tissue; Ep, epididymal fat; Sk, skin; Pl, plasma.

γ-Cyclodextrin (γCD), consisting of 8 glucopyranoside units, can form an inclusion complex with hydrophobic molecules. Because formation of inclusion compounds improves water solubility of hydrophobic guest molecules, it was expected a complex of tocotrienol with γCD would improve its stability in the gastrointestinal tract. γCD is completely digested by salivary and pancreatic amylase, hence releasing gest molecules in the small intestine. Thus, we tried to enhance the intestinal absorption of tocotrienol using a γ-tocotrienol/γCD complex (Ikeda et al. 2010). Rats were administered by gavage an emulsion containing either γ-tocotrienol with γCD (not complexed) or a γ-tocotrienol/γCD complex. The administration of the γ-tocotrienol/γCD complex elevated the γ-tocotrienol concentration in plasma and some tissues compared with simultaneous administration of γ-tocotrienol and γCD (not complexed). To determine the effect of complexation on tocotrienol absorption, rats were injected with Triton WR1339 and then administered by oral gavage an emulsion containing either γ-tocotrienol with γCD (not complexed) or the tocotrienol/γCD complex. After pretreatment with Triton WR1339, the γ-tocotrienol absorption was increased by administration of the tocotrienol/γCD complex compared with γ-tocotrienol and γCD. However, dietary intake of the complex for 6 weeks did not affect the tissue accumulation of γ-tocotrienol. These results suggest that complexation of tocotrienol with γCD improves tocotrienol bioavailability for several hours after administration by enhancing intestinal absorption of tocotrienol. The complexation is likely to improve solubility and stability of tocotrienol in the gastrointestinal tract.

4.7   CONCLUSION

To evaluate tocotrienol bioavailability, we examined the tissue distribution of dietary tocotrienol and the effect of α-tocopherol, sesame lignan, and complexation with γ-cyclodextrin on the tocotrienol concentration in rats. α- and γ-tocotrienol concentrations in major tissues were very low compared with α-tocopherol, but we found significant amounts of dietary α- and γ-tocotrienol in adipose tissue by feeding a tocotrienol-rich diet for several weeks. Tocotrienol uptake to adipose tissue after its administration by gavage was very slow, showing no preferential uptake occurred. The adipose tissue–specific accumulation of dietary tocotrienol is likely to be because of maintenance of the level without degradation. Dietary α-tocopherol decreased the α-tocotrienol but not the γ-tocotrienol concentration in rat tissues. After oral administration, α-tocopherol inhibited tissue uptake of not only α-tocotrienol but also γ-tocotrienol, suggesting that γ-tocotrienol along with the other vitamin E isoforms is transported to the tissues via an αTTP-dependent transport system. We believe that tocotrienol bioavailability can be improved by regulating its catabolism to CEHC and its stability in the gastrointestinal tract.

REFERENCES

Abe, C., Ikeda, S., Uchida, T., Yamashita, K., Ichikawa, T. 2007a. Triton WR1339, an inhibitor of lipoprotein lipase, decreases vitamin E concentration in some tissues of rats by inhibiting its transport to liver. *J. Nutr.* 137: 345–350.

Abe, C., Uchida, T., Ohta, M., Ichikawa, T., Yamashita, K., Ikeda, S. 2007b. Cytochrome P450-dependent metabolism of vitamin E isoforms is a critical determinant of their tissue concentrations in rats. *Lipids* 42: 637–645.

Birringer, M., Pfluger, P., Kluth, D., Landes, N., Brigelius-Flohé, R. 2002. Identities and differences in the metabolism of tocotrienols and tocopherols in HepG2 cells. *J. Nutr.* 132: 3113–3118.

Frank, J., Lee, S., Leonard, S. W., Atkinson, J. K., Kamal-Eldin, A., Traber, M. G. 2008. Sex differences in the inhibition of γ-tocopherol metabolism by a single dose of dietary sesame oil in healthy subjects. *Am. J. Clin. Nutr.* 87: 1723–1729.

Hayes, K. C., Pronczuk, A., Liang, J. S. 1993. Differences in the plasma transport and tissue concentrations of tocopherols and tocotrienols: Observations in humans and hamsters. *Proc. Soc. Exp. Biol. Med.* 202: 353–359.

Hosomi, A., Arita, M., Sato, Y. et al. 1997. Affinity for α-tocopherol transfer protein as a determinant of the biological activities of vitamin E analogs. *FEBS Lett.* 409: 105–108.

Ikeda, S., Tohyama, T., Yamashita, K. 2002. Dietary sesame seed and its lignans inhibit 2,7,8-trimethyl-2(2′-carboxyethyl)-6-hydroxychroman excretion into urine of rats fed γ-tocopherol. *J. Nutr.* 132: 961–966.

Ikeda, S., Tohyama, T., Yoshimura, H., Hamamura, K., Abe, K., Yamashita, K. 2003. Dietary α-tocopherol decreases α-tocotrienol but not γ-tocotrienol concentration in rats. *J. Nutr.* 133: 428–434.

Ikeda, S., Toyoshima, K., Yamashita, K. 2001. Dietary sesame seeds elevate α- and γ-tocotrienol concentrations in skin and adipose tissue of rats fed the tocotrienol-rich fraction extracted from palm oil. *J. Nutr.* 131: 2892–2897.

Ikeda, S., Uchida, T., Ichikawa, T. et al. 2010. Complexation of tocotrienol with γ-cyclodextrin enhances intestinal absorption of tocotrienol in rats. *Biosci. Biotechnol. Biochem.* 74: 1452–1457.

Kayden, H. J., Traber, M. G. 1993. Absorption, lipoprotein transport, and regulation of plasma concentrations of vitamin E in humans. *J. Lipid Res.* 34: 343–358.

Lemcke-Norojärvi, M., Kamal-Eldin, A., Appelqvist, L. A., Dimberg, L. H., Ohrvall, M., Vessby, B. 2001. Corn and sesame oils increase serum γ-tocopherol concentrations in healthy Swedish women. *J. Nutr.* 131: 1195–1201.

Lodge, J. K., Ridlington, J., Leonard, S., Vaule, H., Traber, M. G. 2001. α- and γ-tocotrienols are metabolized to carboxyethyl-hydroxychroman derivatives and excreted in human urine. *Lipids* 36: 43–48.

Parker, R. S., Sontag, T. J., Swanson, J. E. 2000. Cytochrome P4503A-dependent metabolism of tocopherols an inhibition by sesamin. *Biochem. Biophys. Res. Commun.* 277: 531–534.

Parker, R. S., Sontag, T. J., Swanson, J. E., McCormick, C. 2004. Discovery, characterization, and significance of the cytochrome P450 ω-hydroxylase pathway of vitamin E catabolism. *Ann. NY Acad. Sci.* 1031: 13–21.

Podda, M., Weber, C., Traber, M. G., Packer, L. 1996. Simultaneous determination of tissue tocopherols, tocotrienols, ubiquinols, and ubiquinones. *J. Lipid Res.* 37: 893–901.

Schultz, M., Leist, M., Petrzika, M., Gassmann, B., Brigelius-Flohé, R. 1995. Novel urinary metabolite of α-tocopherol, 2,5,7,8-tetramethyl-2(2′-carboxyethyl)-6-hydroxychroman, as an indicator of an adequate vitamin E supply? *Am. J. Clin. Nutr.* 62: 1527S–1534S.

Sontag, T. J., Parker, R. S. 2002. Cytochrome P450 ω-hydroxylase pathway of tocopherol catabolism: Novel mechanism of regulation of vitamin E status. *J. Biol. Chem.* 277: 25290–25296.

Sontag, T. J., Parker, R. S. 2007. Influence of major structural features of tocopherols and tocotrienols on their ω-oxidation by tocopherol-ω-hydroxylase. *J. Lipid Res.* 48: 1090–1098.

Swanson, J. E., Ben, R. N., Burton, G. W., Parker, R. S. 1999. Urinary excretion of 2,7,8-trimethyl-2-(β-carboxyethyl)-6-hydroxychroman is a major rout of elimination of γ-tocopherol in humans. *J. Lipid Res.* 40: 665–671.

Traber, M. G., Arai, H. 1999. Molecular mechanisms of vitamin E transport. *Annu. Rev. Nutr.* 19: 343–355.

Traber, M. G., Burton, G. W., Hamilton, R. L. 2004. Vitamin E trafficking. *Ann. NY Acad. Sci.* 1031: 1–12.

Traber, M. G., Sies, H. 1996. Vitamin E in humans: Demand and delivery. *Annu. Rev. Nutr.* 16: 321–347.

Uchida, T., Abe, C., Nomura, S., Ichikawa, T., Ikeda, S. 2012. Tissue distribution of α- and γ-tocotrienol and γ-tocopherol in rats and interference with their accumulation by α-tocopherol. *Lipids* 47: 129–139.

Uchida, T., Ichikawa, T., Abe, C., Yamashita, K., Ikeda, S. 2007. Dietary sesame seed decreases urinary excretion of α- and γ-tocopherol metabolites in rats. *J. Nutr. Sci. Vitaminol.* 53: 372–376.

Uchida, T., Nomura, S., Ichikawa, T., Abe, C., Ikeda, S. 2011. Tissue distribution of vitamin E metabolites in rats after oral administration of tocopherol or tocotrienol. *J. Nutr. Sci. Vitaminol.* 57: 326–332.

Wechter, W. J., Kantoci, D., Murray, Jr. E. D., D'Amico, D. C., Jung, M. E., Wang, W. H. 1996. A new endogenous natriuretic factor: LLU-α. *Proc. Natl. Acad. Sci. USA* 93: 6002–6007.

5 Alpha-Tocopherol
A Detriment to Tocotrienol Benefits

Anne M. Trias and Barrie Tan

CONTENTS

5.1 INTRODUCTION

Alpha-tocopherol was discovered in 1922 by Evans and Bishop as the first of at least eight variations of vitamin E (Evans and Bishop 1922). It was determined to be a vital nutrient for the prevention of fetal resorption, as well as the maintenance of red blood cells (Horwitt 1960). Alpha-tocopherol and its closely related isomers, beta-, gamma-, and delta-tocopherols display a less-flexible larger structure with a longer-saturated phytyl tail, while their less closely related isomers, alpha-, beta-, gamma-, and delta-tocotrienols, have a shorter, more flexible unsaturated farnesyl tail. Tocotrienol's flexible and shorter lipophilic tail allows it to traverse a larger membrane area for added protection (Serbinova and Packer 1994; Atkinson et al. 2008).

Until a decade ago, alpha-tocopherol was believed to be the most important form of vitamin E. While still valuable in fetal and hematological protection, its antioxidant activity is surpassed by tocotrienol's manifold benefits that include superior antioxidant and anti-inflammatory capabilities, cholesterol/triglyceride management, and cellular health.

Although research clearly delineates tocotrienol's cholesterol-lowering properties, studies have had inconsistent outcomes. A review of the literature suggests that this variance points to fluctuating amounts of alpha-tocopherol in supplement compositions given to study populations. Alpha-tocopherol has been shown to interfere with the functions and benefits of tocotrienol. This chapter critically reviews the mechanisms of alpha-tocopherol interference and aims to document its role in the mitigation of tocotrienol functions. Studies are compared with regard to varying amounts of alpha-tocopherol content in tocotrienol mixtures and are found to yield better results if alpha-tocopherol is low or absent.

5.2 BACKGROUND AND CONTEXT

5.2.1 SUMMARY OF TOCOTRIENOL FUNCTIONS

Tocotrienol's first differentiated properties from tocopherols came from the University of Wisconsin in the 1980s (Qureshi et al. 1986), when alpha-tocotrienol was discovered in barley. Shortly thereafter, vitamin E–rich palm oil was identified as a mixture of 75% tocotrienols, predominantly gamma-tocotrienol, and 25% tocopherols, predominantly alpha-tocopherol (Tan 1989; Tan and Brzuskiewicz 1989). Studies of individual tocopherol and tocotrienol isomers ensued in the 1990s by the University of Wisconsin and Bristol-Myers Squibb (Pearce et al. 1992, 1994; Parker et al. 1993). Results confirmed the superior cholesterol-suppressive action of delta- and gamma-tocotrienol as well as alpha-tocopherol's inactivity (Table 5.1).

In general, delta- and gamma-tocotrienols are the most potent isomers for the majority of applications with the exception that alpha-tocotrienol appears to have some unique neurological benefits (Park et al. 2011a; Rink et al. 2011). We have previously defined "desmethyl tocotrienols" (DMT3) to highlight the C-5 *unsubstituted* position of vitamin E (Figure 5.1), namely, delta- and gamma-tocotrienol and delta- and gamma-tocopherol (Tan 2005). Interestingly, when tocopherols were studied apart from tocotrienols, delta- and gamma-tocopherol were clearly indicated to be of significantly greater potency than alpha-tocopherol in antioxidant protection (Muller et al. 2010), cancer prevention/treatment (McIntyre et al. 2000; Hsieh et al. 2010; Li et al. 2011; Park et al. 2011), antiangiogenesis (Wells et al. 2010), and inflammation protection (Jiang et al. 2000; Wang et al. 2011). The lack of substitution at the C-5 position of the *entire* vitamin E series is decidedly important.

Nonetheless, research reviewed in the latter parts of this chapter suggests that tocopherol interference may be limited to C-5-*substituted* tocopherol, namely, alpha-tocopherol. Alpha- and beta-isomers are the only two C-5-substituted vitamin Es. Because beta-tocopherol and beta-tocotrienol abundance in nature is insignificant (Eitenmiller and Lee 2004), interference is thus limited to the readily abundant alpha-tocopherol. Furthermore, alpha-tocopherol is the most commonly supplemented vitamin E form and is often taken at dosages 10–30 times higher than the daily value.

5.2.2 ADVENT AND RISE OF "TOCOTRIENOL-RICH FRACTION"

The phrase "tocotrienol-rich fraction" (TRF) was originally ascribed to palm tocotrienols, where the descriptive "tocotrienol-rich" emphasis came about because plants ordinarily produce a tocopherol mixture with only traces of tocotrienol (Tan 1989). Later, the term was broadened to include rice TRF (Qureshi et al. 2000). Palm and rice tocotrienol sources typically contain 25%–50% tocopherols—mainly as alpha-tocopherol—and although they are relatively correct as "tocotrienol-rich" mixtures, it is an arbitrary and imprecise designation. Among the current sources, annatto is the only tocopherol-free vitamin E composed solely of delta- and gamma-tocotrienol (Figure 5.2).

TABLE 5.1

Hypocholesterolemic Properties of Tocotrienol Isomers

- Delta- and gamma-tocotrienol are the most potent vitamin E inhibitors of endogenous cholesterol synthesis; whenever there is a difference, delta- is better than gamma-tocotrienol
- When combined, delta- and gamma-tocotrienol are synergistic
- Alpha-tocotrienol is the least potent cholesterol reducer and is 5× less active than delta- and gamma-tocotrienol
- Tocopherol is completely inactive as cholesterol biosynthesis inhibitors
- C-5-unsubstituted position on the vitamin E molecule is critical for activity

---

Position of methyl group	Tocopherols	Tocotrienols
5,7,8-Trimethyl	α-T	α-T3
5,8-Dimethyl	β-T	β-T3
7,8-Dimethyl	γ-T	γ-T3
8-Monomethyl	δ-T	δ-T3

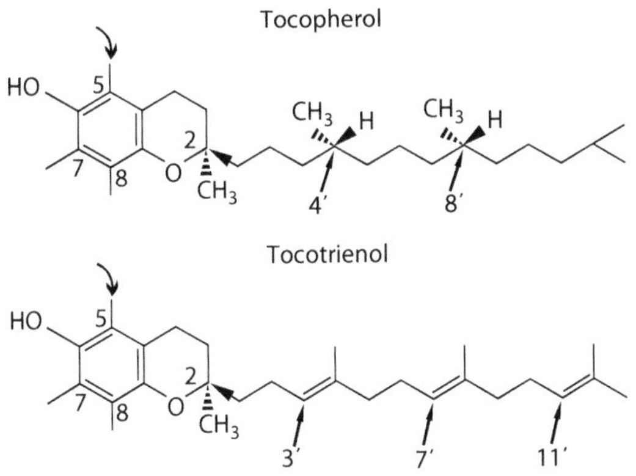

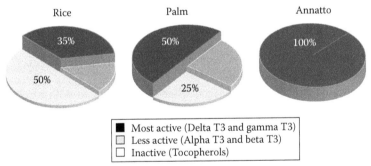

FIGURE 5.1 Chemical structures of vitamin E tocopherols and tocotrienols. Both tocopherols and tocotrienols have a chroman ring, the site of antioxidant action. The molecules differ in the length of the side chain, where tocopherol has a longer-saturated phytyl tail, and tocotrienol has a shorter unsaturated farnesyl tail. Methyl substitution on the chroman ring determines whether a vitamin E belongs to the alpha-, beta-, gamma-, or delta-isoform. Lack of substitution at the C-5 position (curvy arrow) of the entire vitamin E series is decidedly important for superior function. (Modified from Tan, B. and Brzuskiewicz, L., *Anal. Biochem.*, 180(2), 368, 1989.)

FIGURE 5.2 Tocotrienol sources and composition. The three major sources of tocotrienols are rice, palm, and annatto. The ratio of tocopherol-to-tocotrienol in each is 50:50, 25:75, and 0.1:99.9, respectively. Therefore, rice and palm contain 25%–50% tocopherols. The most recently discovered source—annatto tocotrienol—is naturally tocopherol-free and only contains delta- and gamma-tocotrienols.

Confusion arose when the tocopherol–tocotrienol ratios were unspecified, varied, or altered in studies, and the possibility of understanding the benefits of tocotrienol (beyond tocopherol) is unclear. A thorough review of this research suggests that the antiquated "TRF" designation should be avoided, and "tocopherol–tocotrienol mixture" with identified ratios and concentrations should be used instead. In an effort to harness the full benefits of tocotrienols derived from palm oil, some research was undertaken to reduce the amount of alpha-tocopherol in the mixture to a minimum and differentiate it as "tocotrienol-enhanced fraction" (TEF) rather than TRF (Gapor 2005). To date, TEF has not been adopted by the industry and TRF persists as the practice.

As of recent, alpha-tocopherol's antagonistic effects on tocotrienols have become increasingly pinpointed (Gee 2011), and many research groups have reduced alpha-tocopherol content in their studies or ceased its use altogether. A phase I clinical trial studying tocotrienol's effect on pancreatic cancer is utilizing pure delta-tocotrienol and excludes tocopherols—especially alpha-tocopherol—in order to achieve maximum benefits (Malafa and Sebti 2008; Husain et al. 2011). At the Second International Conference on Tocotrienols and Chronic Diseases (Las Vegas, NV; July 13–14, 2011), researchers presented study concepts favoring tocotrienol use over tocopherol–tocotrienol mixtures, including continuation of a clinical breast cancer trial with pure gamma-tocotrienol in place of the tocopherol–tocotrienol mixture used previously (Nesaretnam et al. 2011). In addition, a clinical study on alpha-tocopherol-free tocotrienols (delta-tocotrienol:gamma-tocotrienol of 1:1 ratio) on cholesterol homeostasis is underway at the UCLA Center for Human Nutrition (Heber 2011). This is a follow-up study to an earlier pilot study using this DMT3 formula (Zaiden et al. 2010).

5.3 MECHANISMS OF ALPHA-TOCOPHEROL INTERFERENCE

5.3.1 COMPROMISING CHOLESTEROL REDUCTION

Evidence collected as early as 1996 suggests that tocotrienols are more potent hypocholesterolemic agents when administered along with the lowest alpha-tocopherol content possible (Qureshi et al. 1996). In this novel research, a chicken model was utilized because the lipogenic activities of humans and avians are similar in that they are predominantly located in the liver (Shrago et al. 1971; Leveille et al. 1975). Lipogenic activities of rodents, however, are less similar to those of humans and are shared between the liver and adipose tissues (Yu et al. 2006). Chickens were fed varying amount of alpha-tocopherol and/or gamma-tocotrienol in a soy diet (15% alpha-tocopherol). The group that received no additional alpha-tocopherol and was given only gamma-tocotrienol had the greatest reduction in lipid parameters, while the group with the largest supplemented amount of alpha-tocopherol (without tocotrienol) showed increased activity of the rate-limiting enzyme responsible for cholesterol production (HMGR; 3-hydroxy-3-methyl-glutaryl-CoA reductase) with resultant elevation of cholesterol. Tested combinations showed alpha-tocopherol attenuating gamma-tocotrienol's cholesterol-lowering properties in a dose-dependent manner (Figure 5.3). For tocotrienols to effect cholesterol reduction, the alpha-tocopherol content should not be more than 15%.

It was later confirmed that alpha-tocopherol, when coadministered with tocotrienols, attenuated the inhibitory effect of tocotrienols on HMGR in guinea pigs (Khor and Ng 2000), where tocotrienol administration alone inhibited the enzyme's activity by 48%. When alpha-tocopherol was added, HMGR inhibition was only 13%. Clearly, alpha-tocopherol compromises tocotrienol's ability to reduce cholesterol.

5.3.2 ATTENUATING CANCER INHIBITION

Interestingly, alpha-tocopherol compromises tocotrienol's potency on cancer cells as well. Recently published data show that all tocopherols—especially alpha-tocopherol—attenuate delta-tocotrienol-induced apoptosis of human colorectal adenocarcinoma cells (Shibata et al. 2010). Previously, delta-tocotrienol was shown to be the most potent antiangiogenic agent of the vitamin E family, while tocopherol was without effect (Nakagawa et al. 2007). The suppression of activity occurred by cotreatment with alpha-tocopherol in a dose-dependent manner. Alpha-tocopherol also blocked delta-tocotrienol's induction and expression of genes involved in cell-cycle arrest and apoptosis.

Evidence of alpha-tocopherol's interference in other vitamin E cancer benefits has been observed in its hampering of the anticancer signaling and tumor growth arrest that gamma-tocopherol caused in mice bearing human breast cancer xenografts (Yu et al. 2009; Galli and Azzi 2010). Alpha-tocopherol also mitigated tamoxifen's function in estrogen receptor-positive breast cancer cells (Guthrie et al. 1997). Fifty percent inhibitory concentrations (IC50) of breast cancer cells were

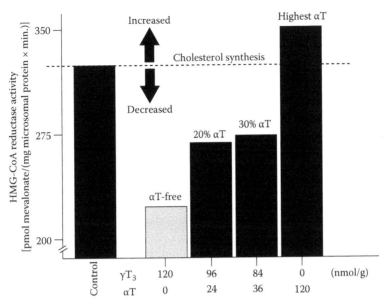

FIGURE 5.3 Alpha-tocopherol attenuation of tocotrienol functions in cholesterol management. Alpha-tocopherol (alpha-T) and/or gamma-tocotrienol (gamma-T3) were given to chickens at various concentrations, and HMGR activity was measured. The group receiving gamma-tocotrienol alone showed the greatest reduction in HMGR activity, while the group with the highest alpha-tocopherol supplementation had increased HMGR activity, resulting in higher cholesterol levels. (Modified from Qureshi, A.A. et al., *J. Nutr.*, 126(2), 389, 1996.)

125, 6, 4, 2, and 2 μg/mL for alpha-tocopherol, alpha-tocotrienol, TRF, gamma-tocotrienol, and delta-tocotrienol, respectively, while tamoxifen (TXF) was more potent at an IC50 of 0.04 μg/mL. Hence, the order of vitamin E potency in breast cancer reduction was delta-tocotrienol = gamma-tocotrienol > TRF > alpha-tocopherol ≫ alpha-tocopherol. Delta- and gamma-tocotrienol were 63× more potent than alpha-tocopherol and worked twice as well as TRF in breast cancer inhibition. When individual tocotrienol isomers were combined with TXF, only gamma- and delta-tocotrienol were synergistic, reducing the IC50 to 0.01 and 0.003 μg/mL, respectively. With alpha-tocopherol or TRF in combination with TXF, however, the IC50 increased to 47 and 0.5 μg/mL, respectively (Figure 5.4). The mitigation of TXF by alpha-tocopherol was more than 1000-fold, while TRF reduced the effectiveness of TXF by a factor of 13. Gamma- and delta-tocotrienol, on the other hand, improved the effectiveness of TXF by a factor of 4× and 13×, respectively. Hence, alpha-tocopherol combination with TXF—whether as stand-alone or as contained in TRF—reduces TXF function on estrogen receptor-positive breast cancer cells. Perhaps, these results present an underlying rationale for future breast cancer studies utilizing only gamma- and/or delta-tocotrienol rather than a tocopherol–tocotrienol mixture.

5.3.3 BLOCKING ABSORPTION AND DEPLETING TISSUE UPTAKE

The concept of absorption interference is not novel. In the class of lipid-soluble carotenoids, beta-carotene has been shown to interfere with the absorption of lutein and vice versa (Kostic et al. 1995; Albanes et al. 1997; van den Berg 1998). A major reason for alpha-tocopherol's attenuation of tocotrienol function appears to be due to blocked absorption. Ikeda et al. (2003) showed that alpha-tocotrienol given to rats in the absence of alpha-tocopherol accumulated in plasma and other tissues, while gamma-tocotrienol in the absence of alpha-tocopherol accumulated preferentially in adipose tissue and the skin. Alpha-tocotrienol concentration decreased if alpha-tocopherol was administered in combination, which may be due to alpha-tocopherol's high affinity to the alpha-tocopherol

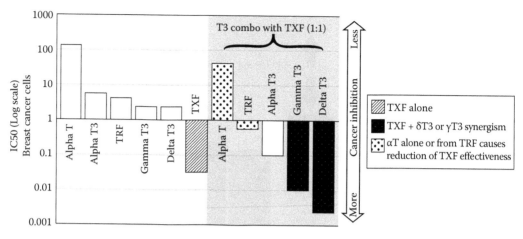

FIGURE 5.4 Tocotrienol inhibition of estrogen receptor-positive breast cancer cells. Fifty percent inhibitory concentration (IC50) was determined for all tocotrienol isomers, TRF, and TXF on MCF-7 breast cancer cells. Inhibition of MCF-7 cells by vitamin E isomers decreased in the order of delta-tocotrienol = gamma-tocotrienol > TRF > alpha-tocotrienol, while alpha-tocopherol did not work. Although TXF inhibited MCF-7 cells more efficiently than the various vitamin Es, synergism was observed when TXF was combined with delta- or gamma-tocotrienol. TXF combination with alpha-tocopherol or TRF, on the other hand, reduced the effectiveness of TXF. (Modified from Guthrie, N. et al., *J. Nutr.,* 127, 544S, 1997.)

transport protein (ATTP). Alpha-tocotrienol's affinity for ATTP is only 12% that of alpha-tocopherol, with other tocotrienol isomers having negligible affinity for the protein. When gamma-tocotrienol was administered with alpha-tocopherol, concentrations of this tocotrienol isomer did not decrease in the adipose tissue or skin, as might have been expected. The authors suggest that alpha- and gamma-tocotrienols may have accumulated in adipose tissue and skin prior to ATTP discrimination in the liver. Presently, however, the Ikeda group shows in this book that alpha-tocopherol administration also decreased the gamma-tocotrienol concentration in the adipose tissue and skin, thus inhibiting not only alpha-tocotrienol, but also gamma-tocotrienol tissue uptake (Chapter 4, Ikeda et al., 2012).

In human organs and tissues, vitamin Es besides alpha-tocopherol are often accumulated at much higher concentrations (Khanna et al. 2005), and alpha-tocopherol may negatively affect the "true bioavailability" of tocotrienols. Bioavailability refers to the organ distribution of an intended compound. It has been repeatedly demonstrated that all vitamin Es are absorbed through the gut with meals or adequate fat (Yap et al. 2001; Khosla et al. 2006) such that blood elevation should affect the kinetics—not the absorption—of tocotrienols. Elevated blood levels, as brought about by some novel delivery systems, merely alter the pharmacokinetics to accelerate blood appearance. This, in addition to alpha-tocopherol coadministration, could negatively affect the intended tissue deposition. For example, alpha-tocopherol was shown to lower gamma-tocopherol concentrations in rats (Behrens and Madere 1987) and increased its urinary excretion (Kiyose et al. 2001). Alpha-tocopherol was also shown to reduce serum levels of both gamma- and delta-tocopherol in humans (Handelman et al. 1985; Huang and Appel 2003) and depleted gamma-tocopherol uptake into blood and tissues in both animals and humans (Hensley et al. 2004; Galli and Azzi 2010). Orally supplemented alpha-tocotrienol was shown to effectively deliver to most tissues and vital organs, including the skin, adipose, ovaries, heart, liver, central nervous system, spinal cord, brain, lung, testes, and skeletal muscle. However, mechanisms for transporting alpha-tocopherol and alpha-tocotrienol appeared to compete in a fashion that favored alpha-tocopherol transport. Thus, cosupplementation of alpha-tocopherol and alpha-tocotrienol is likely to compromise tissue delivery of alpha-tocotrienol (Khanna et al. 2005).

More recently, alpha-tocopherol coadministration was shown to decrease uptake of delta-tocotrienol into cancer cells in a dose-dependent manner, hence attenuating delta-tocotrienol's apoptotic mechanism (Shibata et al. 2010). The result is tantalizing in that alpha-tocopherol abrogates cancer cytotoxicity solely by suppressing cellular delta-tocotrienol uptake.

5.3.4 Inducing Catabolism

Although it was previously shown that alpha-tocopherol does not appear to increase urinary excretion of gamma-tocotrienol (Ikeda et al. 2003), later investigations demonstrate that alpha-tocopherol is a positive effector of cohydroxylation of other vitamin Es, including the tocotrienol isomers (Sontag and Parker 2007). Here, researchers found a stimulatory catabolic effect of alpha-tocopherol toward all tocopherols and tocotrienols except alpha-tocopherol itself. Moreover, presence of double bonds in the side chain and position of methyl groups around the chromanol ring are determinant of tocopherol-ω-hydroxylation. Side-chain unsaturation in tocotrienols increases catabolism, while substitution of a methyl group at the C-5 position of the chromanol ring (as in the alpha-isomers) decreases the molecule's catabolism. Hence, tocotrienols are naturally catabolized faster with the desmethyl delta- and gamma-tocotrienols being most susceptible, and addition of alpha-tocopherol would stimulate this catabolism further (Figure 5.5). This hepatic construct for DMT3 destruction is exceedingly compelling.

5.3.5 Causing Drug Metabolism

All vitamin E isomers are metabolized by degradation of the molecules' side chains, involving an initial ω-oxidation followed by repeated cycles of β-oxidation. This catabolism causes shortening of the phytyl or farnesyl tail to produce water-soluble urinary carboxyethylhydroxychroman (CEHC) metabolites (Brigelius-Flohe and Traber 1999; Lodge et al. 2001; You et al. 2005; Sontag and Parker 2007; Yang et al. 2011). The mechanism is catalyzed by a cytochrome P450 enzyme and induced by nuclear pregnane X receptor (PXR), the same receptor that is activated by a large number of xenobiotics (such as polyaromatic hydrocarbons and antibiotics). While both tocopherols and tocotrienols activate this receptor *in vitro*, alpha-tocopherol *alone* activates PXR *in vivo*. Therefore, alpha-tocopherol may be responsible for the quicker metabolism and elimination of tocotrienols from the body. It has been speculated that alpha-tocopherol could interfere with prescription drugs, since it would catalyze drug metabolism by binding to and activating PXR (Brigelius-Flohe 2005, 2007). This theory is consistent with alpha-tocopherol's increase of tocotrienol catabolism (Sontag and Parker 2007).

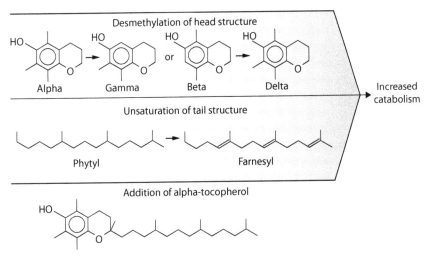

FIGURE 5.5 Vitamin E catabolism. Catabolism of vitamin Es is influenced by desmethylation of the head structure and unsaturation of the tail structure. Less methyl substitutions on the molecule's head and increased unsaturation of the tail result in a smaller molecule and increased catabolism. Addition of alpha-tocopherol also increases catabolism of the other vitamin E isomers. (Summarized from Sontag, T.J. and Parker, R.S., *J. Lipid Res.*, 48(5), 1090, 2007.)

5.3.6 Increasing Cholesterol and Blood Pressure

When given in high doses, alpha-tocopherol has been shown to increase HMGR activity with subsequently elevated cholesterol levels. A review of the literature indicates that tocopherols were shown to have either no effect or a slightly stimulatory cholesterolemic effect in human studies (Howard et al. 1982; Khor et al. 1995). At high dosages, tocopherols also showed a stimulatory effect on HMGR activity in guinea pigs and hamsters (Khor et al. 1995; Khor and Chieng 1997). Studies showed that isolated corn oil triglycerides (COTG) lowered serum total and LDL-cholesterol as well as triglycerides, but when supplemented with alpha-tocopherol, these lipids were raised (Khor and Ng 2000). The researchers recognized alpha-tocopherol's dose-dependent effect on HMGR, where low doses in COTG were still able to inhibit HMGR, while higher doses inhibited HMGR less, and the highest dose stimulated HMGR activity, thus increasing cholesterol and triglyceride levels. Alpha-tocopherol was also found to attenuate the HMGR inhibitory effect of tocotrienol at 33% composition. Ten milligrams of tocotrienols given to guinea pigs inhibited HMGR activity by 48%, but when 5 mg alpha-tocopherol was added to the mixture, inhibition was only 13%.

In a chicken study, where animals were given increasing dosages of alpha-tocopherol along with gamma-tocotrienol, the group receiving the highest amount of alpha-tocopherol in their feed showed increased HMGR activity (Qureshi et al. 1996).

In one animal study, high doses of alpha-tocopherol (2.6 g/day human equivalent) also increased blood pressure in spontaneously hypertensive rats (Miyamoto et al. 2009). Put together, alpha-tocopherol not only directly mitigates (Sections 5.3.1 through 5.3.4) but also indirectly opposes tocotrienol cardiovascular benefits (Sections 5.3.5 and this section), where alpha-tocopherol in large doses increases cholesterol and blood pressure.

5.4 EXAMINING LITERATURE OF TOCOTRIENOL'S LIPID-LOWERING BENEFITS

5.4.1 Studies Addressing Alpha-Tocopherol Interference

Mixed study outcomes, where interpretations of tocotrienol's lipid-lowering benefits varied due to inconsistent alpha-tocopherol content in research samples, have led to much confusion. Aware of alpha-tocopherol's liability to tocotrienol functions, several studies aimed to examine alpha-tocopherol interference more closely. The first-published clinical study on tocotrienol's hypolipidemic effect was carried out in 1991 by Qureshi et al. (1991) and divided into two parts. In the first part, patients received a tocotrienol mixture high in DTM3 (i.e., delta- and gamma-tocotrienols) and also containing 15%–20% of alpha-tocopherol. Total and LDL-cholesterol decreased a moderate average of 14% and 6%, respectively. Triglyceride levels, on the other hand, did not drop. In a cross-over (second part of the study), patients that failed to show cholesterol reduction on tocopherol–tocotrienol mixture were given tocopherol-free gamma-tocotrienol. The change in the supplement's composition caused a much greater effect on lipid levels than previously seen with the tocopherol–tocotrienol mixture. Total and LDL-cholesterol dropped 31% and 27%, respectively, and triglyceride dropped by 15%. The researchers concluded that gamma-tocotrienol worked better than tocopherol–tocotrienol mixtures for hypolipidemic application. In a similar two-part clinical study with patients randomized into a tocopherol–tocotrienol mixture and a tocopherol-free group, it was confirmed that alpha-tocopherol attenuated tocotrienol's lipid-lowering benefits (Qureshi et al. 1995). Here, patients on gamma-tocotrienol supplementation showed a quicker and slightly increased response in cholesterol-lowering versus the tocopherol–tocotrienol group.

Some studies are difficult to interpret, since tocopherol and tocotrienol composition of samples are not specified clearly. For example, in a clinical study, the decrease in total and LDL-cholesterol was found to vary widely, from 5% to 36% and 1% to 37%, respectively, and triglycerides remained unchanged (Tan et al. 1991). Inconsistencies may be due to high alpha-tocopherol levels in the supplements, disclosed as 30% tocopherols and 70% tocotrienols. A breakdown of isomers, however, was not described.

One of the most instructive studies on alpha-tocopherol interference with tocotrienols was published in 1996 and compared varying amounts of alpha-tocopherol and gamma-tocotrienol in combination given to chickens (Qureshi et al. 1996). The investigators found that the group with the highest gamma-tocotrienol concentration and minimal alpha-tocopherol (15% contributed through feed) had the greatest reduction in HMGR activity. It was noted that alpha-tocopherol mitigation was due to HMGR modulation. Increasing alpha-tocopherol causes HMGR—the critical step in cholesterol synthesis—to increase. Compellingly, the group receiving the highest amount of alpha-tocopherol showed an increase in HMGR activity and cholesterol production (Figure 5.3). This led to the conclusion that alpha-tocopherol in the tocopherol–tocotrienol mixture should not exceed 15%.

A two-part study in hamsters was also designed to compare the sole properties of tocotrienols with those of a tocopherol–tocotrienol mixture (Khor and Ng 2000). In the first part of the study, hamsters received only tocotrienols, and HMGR activity was reduced by 48%. In the second part of the study, researchers added 33% alpha-tocopherol to the tocotrienol mixture, and HMGR activity was reduced less—by 13% only—as compared to 48% in the tocopherol-free group. The conclusion was reached that tocotrienol alone works well in HMGR reduction, but the effect was attenuated by adding alpha-tocopherol to the mixture.

To distinguish the efficacy of various tocotrienols, Yu et al. (2006) studied separate isomers in a chicken model and found that delta- and gamma-tocotrienol were about equally effective in their hypolipidemic effect, with delta-tocotrienol showing a slight advantage. Alpha-tocotrienol and palm-derived tocopherol–tocotrienol mixture were approximately similar and less effective, while alpha-tocopherol was ineffective.

More recently, the lipid-lowering capabilities of the potent delta- and gamma-tocotrienols were tested in cell lines, animals, and clinical trials (Zaiden et al. 2010). The results varied significantly based on the study design. In cell lines, the mix of delta- and gamma-tocotrienol suppressed upstream regulators of cholesterol homeostasis genes including HMGR. These two compounds also reduced cholesterol and triglycerides in mice by 28% and 19%, respectively. In an 8 week clinical study, supplementation of the mixture only lowered triglycerides by 28%. Although the researchers speculate that delta- and gamma-tocotrienol's short half-life and low doses may be responsible for the lack of cholesterol reduction in humans, it is important to note that VLDL and chylomicrons were reduced. Since VLDL is a carrier of cholesterol, reduction of these lipids may be imminent and may require extended study duration. A clinical study is now underway at UCLA (Heber 2011) to clarify the effectiveness of tocopherol-free delta- and gamma-tocotrienol (50:50 ratio) in lipid management.

5.4.2 STUDIES THAT WORKED

When examining the lipid-lowering properties of tocotrienols, the best study outcomes are achieved when alpha-tocopherol is either low or absent, or when tocotrienols are used as single isomers (Table 5.2). In 1992, the first study to test separate tocotrienol isomers was performed in cell lines when tocotrienols were considered as drug candidates for Bristol-Myers Squibb (Pearce et al. 1992). The order of potency for tocotrienol effect on HMGR activity was determined to be delta- ≥ gamma- > alpha-tocotrienol, while alpha-tocopherol did not work. A binary mixture of delta- and gamma-tocotrienol was synergistic, whereas alpha-tocotrienol had no additional benefits and was at least 5× less active than the other isomers. Fifteen years later, a study at the University of Texas validated and extended the 1992 Bristol-Myers Squibb landmark paper (Song and DeBose-Boyd 2006). The investigators confirmed that delta- and gamma-tocotrienol are the two most active tocotrienols and showed that delta-tocotrienol not only downregulates but also degrades HMGR.

Qureshi et al., who pioneered tocotrienol research, performed several clinical and animal studies with reduced alpha-tocopherol and was the first to note the alpha-tocopherol attenuation problems.

TABLE 5.2
Studies That Worked for Lipid Lowering at Alpha-T Concentration < 9%

References	Study Subject	Supplementation			Outcome				Conclusion/Remarks
		Alpha-T	T3	DMT3	Total Cholesterol	LDL	Triglycerides	Other	
Pearce et al. (1992)	Cell line	Separate isomers	Separate isomers						Delta-T3 ≥ gamma-T3 > alpha-T3; Alpha-T does not work
Song and DeBose-Boyd (2006)	Cell line		Separate isomers						Delta- and gamma-T3 most active
Qureshi et al. (2001a)	Swine	4.5%	66.3%	48.3%	→	→			Low alpha-T
Qureshi et al. (2001b)	Mice	5.8%	57.5%	40.7%	→	→		Atherosclerotic lesions↓	Low alpha-T
Qureshi and Peterson (2001)	Chickens	7%	50%	35%	22%↓	42%↓	19%↓	apoB↓	Low alpha-T, lovastatin-T3 synergism
Qureshi et al. (2001c)	Humans	8.7%	61.7%	44.6%	20%↓	25%↓	18%↓		Low alpha-T; lovastatin-T3 synergism
Qureshi et al. (2002)	Humans	8.7%	61.7%	44.6%	→	→			Low alpha-T; daily dosage of 100 mg T3 optimal
Qureshi et al. (2011)	Chickens	—	100%	100%	23%↓	45%↓	45%↓	NO, TNF-alpha↓	Delta-T3 only; additive effect with quercetin/riboflavin combo
Tan et al. (2008)	Humans	—	100%	100%	15%–20%↓	15%–20%↓	15%–20%↓		No alpha-T, 100% delta- and gamma-T3

Note: ↓, decrease.

Two studies, one in swine and one in mice, utilized tocotrienol mixtures containing only 4%–6% alpha-tocopherol and 57%–67% tocotrienols. In both studies, lipid parameters decreased significantly, while, in the mice, atherosclerotic lesions were also reduced (Qureshi et al. 2001b). The lab group also tested tocotrienol synergism with lovastatin in chickens and humans, where alpha-tocopherol in the tocotrienol mixture was 7%–9% (Qureshi and Peterson 2001; Qureshi et al. 2001c). Lipid parameters, including triglycerides, in both animal and the human study decreased significantly, while tocotrienol–lovastatin synergism was also shown. A dose-dependence study in humans administering a tocotrienol supplement with 9% alpha-tocopherol content showed a daily dosage of 100 mg tocotrienols as optimal (Qureshi et al. 2002). With an alpha-tocopherol-free source of tocotrienols available from annatto, Qureshi et al. began utilizing pure delta-tocotrienol or mixtures of delta- and gamma-tocotrienol. Most recently, their study in chickens using 100% delta-tocotrienol exhibited a profound lipid-lowering effect, where total- and LDL-cholesterol were reduced 23% and 45%, respectively, and triglycerides dropped 45% (Qureshi et al. 2011). In addition, significant anti-inflammatory benefits were observed with reduced nitric oxide and TNF-α. When delta-tocotrienol was combined with quercetin and riboflavin, these levels were reduced even further.

A tocopherol-free mixture of delta- and gamma-tocotrienol was also tested in two small open-label studies (Tan and Mueller 2008). Patients received 75 mg of the supplement, and total and LDL-cholesterol levels dropped 15%–20% with a similar decrease in triglycerides.

Overall, tocopherol-free tocotrienol or mixtures with reduced alpha-tocopherol content (<15%) fared much better in producing a lipid-lowering effect than mixtures with higher alpha-tocopherol content.

5.4.3 STUDIES THAT DID NOT WORK

A thorough review of the literature clarifies that tocotrienol mixtures containing more than 20% alpha-tocopherol do not exhibit lipid-lowering benefits (Table 5.3). For example, two clinical studies using a tocotrienol supplement with ≥30% alpha-tocopherol content did not lower lipids (Wahlqvist et al. 1992; Mensink et al. 1999). Similarly, when patients were given a tocotrienol mixture containing 29% alpha-tocopherol, lipid levels remained unchanged, although an improvement in atherosclerosis was detected (Tomeo et al. 1995).

Patients in a randomized clinical study with three groups were given three different tocotrienol mixtures (Mustad et al. 2002). Groups 1 and 2 received supplements with an alpha-tocopherol content of 23% or higher, while Group 3 received a specialized "P25 Complex" containing 11 mg/g of alpha-tocopherol, few other tocotrienols, and an unspecified amount of the novel P25 didesmethyl tocotrienol. In all groups, lipid lowering did not occur, which in part could be attributed to high alpha-tocopherol levels.

The longest clinical study on tocotrienol's effect on atherosclerosis was completed after 4 years and also measured lipid parameters in patients (Kooyenga et al. 2001). Supplements throughout the 4 years changed from palm- to rice-derived tocotrienols, both of which contain significant amounts of alpha-tocopherol (~30%). An effect was seen on carotid atherosclerosis reduction, but total cholesterol only decreased 14%, and only in the fourth year. The delayed and reduced effects are likely due to high levels of alpha-tocopherol given to subjects.

It is thought that a high fat and/or a high cholesterol diet promote atherosclerosis (Black et al. 2000; Qureshi et al. 2001b). When tocotrienol was used to test the progression of atherosclerotic lesions, pure tocotrienol was more effective than tocopherol–tocotrienol mixture (with 30% alpha-tocopherol) and alpha-tocopherol (without tocotrienol; Figure 5.6). It is clear that alpha-tocopherol is at best less effective in cholesterol/atherosclerotic lesion reduction, and it may be speculated that alpha-tocopherol attenuates, thereby delaying or reducing the effects of tocotrienol on atherosclerosis. This may in part explain the delayed and reduced effect on cholesterol reduction in the 4 year clinical study.

TABLE 5.3
Studies That Did Not Work for Lipid Lowering at Alpha-T Concentration ≥ 23%

References	Study Subject	Supplementation			Outcome				Conclusion/Remarks
		Alpha-T	T3	DMT3	Total Cholesterol	LDL	Triglycerides	Other	
Wahlqvist et al. (1992)	Humans	30%			—	—	—	—	Alpha-T too high
Mensink et al. (1999)	Humans	33%	67%		—	—	—	—	Alpha-T too high
Tomeo et al. (1995)	Humans	29%	71%		—	—	—	Improvement of atherosclerosis	Alpha-T too high
Mustad et al. (2002)	Humans	23%–24%	48%–76%	39%	—	—	—	—	Alpha-T too high
Kooyenga et al. (2001)	Humans	33%	Varied	Varied	14%↓ at 4th year	—	—	Reduced carotid atherosclerosis	High alpha-T may have attenuated lipid reduction in earlier years of the study
Rasool et al. (2006)	Humans	26.2%	74.2%	39.6%	—	—	—	Blood pressure ↓ and improved antioxidant status	High alpha-T may have attenuated lipid reduction
Rasool et al. (2008)	Humans	24%	77%	53%	—	—	—	Improved arterial compliance	High alpha-T may have attenuated lipid reduction

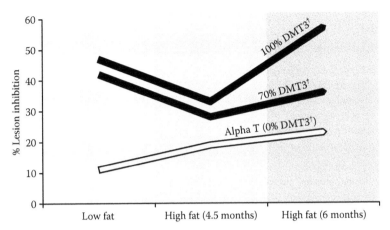

FIGURE 5.6 Tocotrienol effect on atherosclerotic lesion formation. Tocotrienol (100%), tocopherol–tocotrienol mixture (containing 30% alpha-tocopherol), and alpha-tocopherol were tested on atherosclerotic lesion protection in mice on a high fat or high cholesterol diet. Pure tocotrienol was more effective than tocopherol–tocotrienol mixture and alpha-tocopherol. [†]DMT3 = DeltaT3 and GammaT3. (Summarized from Black, T.M. et al., *J. Nutr.*, 130, 2420, 2000; Qureshi, A.A. et al., *J. Nutr.*, 131(10), 2606, 2001.)

In two clinical studies that demonstrated improved antioxidant status and arterial compliance with tocotrienols, no change in lipid parameters was seen (Rasool et al. 2006, 2008). The alpha-tocopherol composition used in these studies was 24%–26%, which could account for tocotrienol's ineffectiveness in lipid lowering. In an animal study using high alpha-tocopherol supplementation, blood pressure was raised (Miyamoto et al. 2009). If tocopherol-free DMT3 had been used instead, the effect to lower blood pressure may have been more evident in these spontaneously hypertensive rats, as was observed in previous studies where tocotrienol decreased blood pressure (Newaz and Nawal 1999; Newaz et al. 2003).

In general, studies on tocotrienol's lipid-lowering effects did not work if alpha-tocopherol content was greater than 20%.

5.5 CONCLUSION

Despite the popularity and early support of alpha-tocopherol, studies published in recent years bring no good news for vitamin E. While some studies suggest that alpha-tocopherol is being underdosed, with 2.1 g of the vitamin needed to suppress oxidation in humans (Roberts et al. 2007), large-scale meta-analyses reveal possible vitamin E toxicity in patients treated with high doses of alpha-tocopherol (Miller et al. 2005; Bjelakovic et al. 2007; Galli and Azzi 2010). Worthy of careful examination, the interventional Selenium and Vitamin E Cancer Prevention Trial (SELECT) showed that alpha-tocopherol supplemented at 400 IU/day did not prevent prostate cancer after 5.5 years (Lippman et al. 2009) and actually increased the risk of prostate cancer by 17% (Klein et al. 2011). However, evidence of the inactivity or even harm of alpha-tocopherol is nothing new, as studies over the last 30–40 years have documented that alpha-tocopherol increases cholesterol levels in humans (Dahl 1974; Farrell and Bieri 1975; Tsai et al. 1978; Schwartz and Rutherford 1981; Howard et al. 1982; Bierenbaum et al. 1985). Instead of the "superstar" it once claimed to be, alpha-tocopherol has now been downgraded to being nothing more than an antioxidant (Traber and Atkinson 2007).

Although early *in vitro* and *in vivo* studies clearly delineate tocotrienol's powerful lipid-lowering effect, many reports returned with ambiguity. Several research groups acknowledge that alpha-tocopherol poses a road block to tocotrienol benefits, especially in cholesterol lowering, and more recently cancer apoptosis. Others have even begun to explore possible mechanisms for the interference. Alpha-tocopherol is thought to interfere with tocotrienol benefits directly by compromising cholesterol

---

TABLE 5.4

Alpha-Tocopherol Interferences with Tocotrienol Functions

Direct interference by alpha-tocopherol
- Compromising cholesterol reduction
- Attenuating cancer cell inhibition
- Blocking absorption
- Depleting tissue uptake
- Inducing tocotrienol catabolism

Indirect interference by alpha-tocopherol
- Causing premature metabolism of prescription drugs
- Increasing cholesterol
- Increasing blood pressure
- Possible toxicity as revealed in large-scale clinical trials and meta-analyses
- Increasing prostate cancer

---

reduction, attenuating cancer cell inhibition, blocking absorption, and inducing its catabolism. Indirectly, alpha-tocopherol also leads to other predicaments, potentially causing the premature metabolism of prescription drugs, increasing cholesterol and blood pressure, and causing prostate cancer (Table 5.4).

Two of the three major sources of tocotrienol, namely, palm-derived and rice-derived tocotrienol mixtures, contain 25%–50% alpha-tocopherol, respectively, and only annatto supplies 100% delta- and gamma-tocotrienols free of tocopherol. High alpha-tocopherol content in palm and rice tocotrienols may pose a dilemma to both successful research trials and consumers alike. This review concludes that the alpha-tocopherol concentration should be ≤15% of the tocopherol–tocotrienol mixtures to be effective.

Latest R&D efforts either reduce alpha-tocopherol concentration in tocotrienol mixtures or remove it altogether. For nutritional supplement application, however, it is cost-prohibitive to adjust alpha-tocopherol content in tocotrienol mixtures, leaving consumers with limited choices.

More studies need to be conducted to further investigate the mechanisms by which alpha-tocopherol is not just innocuous, but unquestionably conflicts with tocotrienol functions. This review concludes that alpha-tocopherol is a liability and should be minimized or not combined with tocotrienols if the benefits of the latter are to be highlighted.

REFERENCES

Albanes, D., J. Virtamo et al. (1997). Effects of supplemental beta-carotene, cigarette smoking, and alcohol consumption on serum carotenoids in the Alpha-Tocopherol, Beta-Carotene Cancer Prevention Study. *Am J Clin Nutr* 66(2): 366–372.

Atkinson, J., R. F. Epand et al. (2008). Tocopherols and tocotrienols in membranes: A critical review. *Free Radic Biol Med* 44(5): 739–764.

Behrens, W. A. and R. Madere (1987). Mechanisms of absorption, transport and tissue uptake of RRR-alpha-tocopherol and D-gamma-tocopherol in the white rat. *J Nutr* 117(9): 1562–1569.

van den Berg, H. (1998). Effect of lutein on beta-carotene absorption and cleavage. *Int J Vitam Nutr Res* 68(6): 360–365.

Bierenbaum, M. L., F. J. Noonan et al. (1985). The effect of supplemental vitamin E on serum parameters in diabetics. Post coronary and normal subjects. *Nutr Res Int* 31(6): 1171–1180.

Bjelakovic, G., D. Nikolova et al. (2007). Mortality in randomized trials of antioxidant supplements for primary and secondary prevention: Systematic review and meta-analysis. *JAMA* 297(8): 842–857.

Black, T. M., P. Wang et al. (2000). Palm tocotrienols protect ApoE +/− mice from diet-induced atheroma formation. *J Nutr* 130: 2420–2426.

Brigelius-Flohe, R. (2005). Induction of drug metabolizing enzymes by vitamin E. *J Plant Physiol* 162(7): 797–802.

Brigelius-Flohe, R. (2007). Adverse effects of vitamin E by induction of drug metabolism. *Genes Nutr* 2(3): 249–256.

Brigelius-Flohe, R. and M. G. Traber (1999). Vitamin E: Function and metabolism. *FASEB J* 13(10): 1145–1455.

Dahl, S. (1974). Letter: Vitamin E in clinical medicine. *Lancet* 1(7855): 465.

Eitenmiller, R. R. and J. Lee (2004). Analysis of tocopherols and tocotrienols in food. *Vitamin E: Food Chemistry, Composition, and Analysis*. New York, Marcel Dekker, Inc.: pp. 364–366.

Evans, H. M. and K. S. Bishop (1922). On the existence of a hitherto unrecognized dietary factor essential for reproduction. *Science* 56: 650–651.

Farrell, P. M. and J. G. Bieri (1975). Megavitamin E supplementation in man. *Am J Clin Nutr* 28(12): 1381–1386.

Galli, F. and A. Azzi (2010). Present trends in vitamin E research. *Biofactors* 36(1): 33–42.

Gapor, A. (2005). Production of palm-based tocotrienols-enriched fraction (TEF). *MPOB* 290(287): 287–290.

Gee, P. T. (2011). Unleashing the untold and misunderstood observations on vitamin E. *Genes Nutr* 6(1): 5–16.

Guthrie, N., A. Gapor et al. (1997). Inhibition of proliferation of estrogen receptor-negative MDA-MB-435 and -positive MCF-7 human breast cancer cells by palm oil tocotrienols and tamoxifen, alone and in combination. *J Nutr* 127: 544S–548S.

Handelman, G. J., L. J. Machlin et al. (1985). Oral alpha-tocopherol supplements decrease plasma gamma-tocopherol levels in humans. *J Nutr* 115(6): 807–813.

Heber, D. (2011). Tocotrienols and cholesterol homeostasis: Basic and clinical research perspectives. *2nd International Conference on Tocotrienols & Chronic Diseases*, Las Vegas, NV, pp. 4–5.

Hensley, K., E. J. Benaksas et al. (2004). New perspectives on vitamin E: gamma-tocopherol and carboxyelth-ylhydroxychroman metabolites in biology and medicine. *Free Radic Biol Med* 36(1): 1–15.

Horwitt, M. K. (1960). Vitamin E and lipid metabolism in man. *Am J Clin Nutr* 8: 451–461.

Howard, D. R., C. A. Rundell et al. (1982). Vitamin E and serum lipids: A non-correlation. *Am J Clin Pathol* 77: 243–244.

Hsieh, T. C., S. Elangovan et al. (2010). Differential suppression of proliferation in MCF-7 and MDA-MB-231 breast cancer cells exposed to alpha-, gamma- and delta-tocotrienols is accompanied by altered expression of oxidative stress modulatory enzymes. *Anticancer Res* 30(10): 4169–4176.

Huang, H. Y. and L. J. Appel (2003). Supplementation of diets with alpha-tocopherol reduces serum concentrations of gamma- and delta-tocopherol in humans. *J Nutr* 133(10): 3137–3140.

Husain, K., R. A. Francois et al. (2011). Vitamin E {delta}-tocotrienol augments the anti-tumor activity of Gemcitabine and suppresses constitutive NF-{kappa}B activation in pancreatic cancer. *Mol Cancer Ther* 10(12): 2363–2372.

Ikeda, S., T. Tohyama et al. (2003). Dietary alpha-tocopherol decreases alpha-tocotrienol but not gamma-tocotrienol concentration in rats. *J Nutr* 133(2): 428–434.

Jiang, Q., I. Elson-Schwab et al. (2000). Gamma-tocopherol and its major metabolite, in contrast to alpha-tocopherol, inhibit cyclooxygenase activity in macrophages and epithelial cells. *Proc Natl Acad Sci USA* 97(21): 11494–11499.

Khanna, S., V. Patel et al. (2005). Delivery of orally supplemented alpha-tocotrienol to vital organs of rats and tocopherol-transport protein deficient mice. *Free Radic Biol Med* 39(10): 1310–1319.

Khanna, S., S. Roy et al. (2005). Neuroprotective properties of the natural vitamin E alpha-tocotrienol. *Stroke* 36(10): 2258–2264.

Khor, H. T. and D. Y. Chieng (1997). Lipidaemic effects of tocotrienols, tocopherols and squalene: Studies in the hamster. *Asia Pac J Clin Nutr* 6(1): 36–40.

Khor, H. T., D. Y. Chieng et al. (1995). Tocotrienols: A dose-dependent inhibitor for HMGCoA reductase. In *Nutrition, Lipids, Health, and Disease*. A. S. H. Ong, E. Niki, and L. Packer (Eds.), Champaign, IL: AOCS Press, pp. 104–108.

Khor, H. T. and T. T. Ng (2000). Effects of administration of alpha-tocopherol and tocotrienols on serum lipids and liver HMG CoA reductase activity. *Int J Food Sci Nutr* 51 (Suppl): S3–S11.

Khosla, P., V. Patel et al. (2006). Postprandial levels of the natural vitamin E tocotrienol in human circulation. *Antioxid Redox Signal* 8(5–6): 1059–1068.

Kiyose, C., H. Saito et al. (2001). Alpha-tocopherol affects the urinary and biliary excretion of 2,7,8-trimethyl-2 (2′-carboxyethyl)-6-hydroxychroman, gamma-tocopherol metabolite, in rats. *Lipids* 36(5): 467–472.

Klein, E. A., I. M. Thompson, Jr. et al. (2011). Vitamin E and the risk of prostate cancer: The Selenium and Vitamin E Cancer Prevention Trial (SELECT). *JAMA* 306(14): 1549–1556.

Kooyenga, D. K., T. R. Watson et al. (2001). Antioxidants modulate the course of carotid atherosclerosis: A four-year report. In *Micronutrients and Health*. K. Nesaretnam and L. Packer (Eds.), Champaign, IL: AOCS Press, pp. 366–375.

Kostic, D., W. S. White et al. (1995). Intestinal absorption, serum clearance, and interactions between lutein and beta-carotene when administered to human adults in separate or combined oral doses. *Am J Clin Nutr* 62(3): 604–610.

Leveille, G. A., D. R. Romsos et al. (1975). Lipid biosynthesis in the chick. A consideration of site of synthesis, influence of diet and possible regulatory mechanisms. *Poult Sci* 54(4): 1075–1093.

Li, G. X., M. J. Lee et al. (2011). Delta-tocopherol is more active than alpha- or gamma-tocopherol in inhibiting lung tumorigenesis in vivo. *Cancer Prev Res (Phila)* 4(3): 404–413.

Lippman, S. M., E. A. Klein et al. (2009). Effect of selenium and vitamin E on risk of prostate cancer and other cancers: The Selenium and Vitamin E Cancer Prevention Trial (SELECT). *JAMA* 301(1): 39–51.

Lodge, J. K., J. Ridlington et al. (2001). Alpha- and gamma-tocotrienols are metabolized to carboxyethyl-hydroxychroman derivatives and excreted in human urine. *Lipids* 36(1): 43–48.

Malafa, M. P. and S. Sebti (2008). *Delta-Tocotrienol Treatment and Prevention of Pancreatic Cancer*. US, Lee Moffitt Cancer Center & Research Institute, University of South Florida, Tampa, FL.

McIntyre, B. S., K. P. Briski et al. (2000). Antiproliferative and apoptotic effects of tocopherols and tocotrienols on preneoplastic and neoplastic mouse mammary epithelial cells. *Proc Soc Exp Biol Med* 224(4): 292–301.

Mensink, R. P., A. C. van Houwelingen et al. (1999). A vitamin E concentrate rich in tocotrienols had no effect on serum lipids, lipoproteins, or platelet function in men with mildly elevated serum lipid concentrations. *Am J Clin Nutr* 69(2): 213–219.

Miller, E. R., 3rd, R. Pastor-Barriuso et al. (2005). Meta-analysis: High-dosage vitamin E supplementation may increase all-cause mortality. *Ann Intern Med* 142(1): 37–46.

Miyamoto, K., M. Shiozaki et al. (2009). Very-high-dose alpha-tocopherol supplementation increases blood pressure and causes possible adverse central nervous system effects in stroke-prone spontaneously hypertensive rats. *J Neurosci Res* 87(2): 556–566.

Muller, L., K. Theile et al. (2010). In vitro antioxidant activity of tocopherols and tocotrienols and comparison of vitamin E concentration and lipophilic antioxidant capacity in human plasma. *Mol Nutr Food Res* 54(5): 731–742.

Mustad, V. A., C. A. Smith et al. (2002). Supplementation with 3 compositionally different tocotrienol supplements does not improve cardiovascular disease risk factors in men and women with hypercholesterolemia. *Am J Clin Nutr* 76(6): 1237–1243.

Nakagawa, K., A. Shibata et al. (2007). In vivo angiogenesis is suppressed by unsaturated vitamin E, tocotrienol. *J Nutr* 137(8): 1938–1943.

Nesaretnam, K., P. Meganathan et al. (2011). Tocotrienols and breast cancer: The evidence to date. *Genes Nutr* 7(1): 3–9.

Newaz, M. A. and N. N. Nawal (1999). Effect of gamma-tocotrienol on blood pressure, lipid peroxidation and total antioxidant status in spontaneously hypertensive rats (SHR). *Clin Exp Hypertens* 21(8): 1297–1313.

Newaz, M. A., Z. Yousefipour et al. (2003). Nitric oxide synthase activity in blood vessels of spontaneously hypertensive rats: Antioxidant protection by gamma-tocotrienol. *J Physiol Pharmacol* 54(3): 319–327.

Park, H. A., N. Kubicki et al. (2011a). Natural vitamin E alpha-tocotrienol protects against ischemic stroke by induction of multidrug resistance-associated protein 1. *Stroke* 42(8): 2308–2314.

Park, S. K., B. G. Sanders et al. (2011b). Tocotrienols induce apoptosis in breast cancer cell lines via an endoplasmic reticulum stress-dependent increase in extrinsic death receptor signaling. *Breast Cancer Res Treat* 124(2): 361–375.

Parker, R. A., B. C. Pearce et al. (1993). Tocotrienols regulate cholesterol production in mammalian cells by post-transcriptional suppression of 3-hydroxy-3-methylglutaryl-coenzyme A reductase. *J Biol Chem* 268(15): 11230–11238.

Pearce, B. C., R. A. Parker et al. (1992). Hypocholesterolemic activity of synthetic and natural tocotrienols. *J Med Chem* 35(20): 3595–3606.

Pearce, B. C., R. A. Parker et al. (1994). Inhibitors of cholesterol biosynthesis. 2. Hypocholesterolemic and antioxidant activities of benzopyran and tetrahydronaphthalene analogues of the tocotrienols. *J Med Chem* 37(4): 526–541.

Qureshi, A. A., B. A. Bradlow et al. (1995). Response of hypercholesterolemic subjects to administration of tocotrienols. *Lipids* 30(12): 1171–1177.

Qureshi, A. A., W. C. Burger et al. (1986). The structure of an inhibitor of cholesterol biosynthesis isolated from barley. *J Biol Chem* 261(23): 10544–10550.

Qureshi, A. A., H. Mo et al. (2000). Isolation and identification of novel tocotrienols from rice bran with hypocholesterolemic, antioxidant, and antitumor properties. *J Agric Food Chem* 48(8): 3130–3140.

Qureshi, A. A., B. C. Pearce et al. (1996). Dietary alpha-tocopherol attenuates the impact of gamma-tocotrienol on hepatic 3-hydroxy-3-methylglutaryl coenzyme A reductase activity in chickens. *J Nutr* 126(2): 389–394.

Qureshi, A. A. and D. M. Peterson (2001). The combined effects of novel tocotrienols and lovastatin on lipid metabolism in chickens. *Atherosclerosis* 156(1): 39–47.

Qureshi, A. A., D. M. Peterson et al. (2001a). Novel tocotrienols of rice bran suppress cholesterogenesis in hereditary hypercholesterolemic swine. *J Nutr* 131(2): 223–230.

Qureshi, A. A., N. Qureshi et al. (1991). Lowering of serum cholesterol in hypercholesterolemic humans by tocotrienols (palmvitee). *Am J Clin Nutr* 53(4 Suppl): 1021S–1026S.

Qureshi, A. A., J. C. Reis et al. (2011). Delta-tocotrienol and quercetin reduce serum levels of nitric oxide and lipid parameters in female chickens. *Lipids Health Dis* 10: 39.

Qureshi, A. A., W. A. Salser et al. (2001b). Novel tocotrienols of rice bran inhibit atherosclerotic lesions in C57BL/6 ApoE-deficient mice. *J Nutr* 131(10): 2606–2618.

Qureshi, A. A., S. A. Sami et al. (2001c). Synergistic effect of tocotrienol-rich fraction (TRF(25)) of rice bran and lovastatin on lipid parameters in hypercholesterolemic humans. *J Nutr Biochem* 12(6): 318–329.

Qureshi, A. A., S. A. Sami et al. (2002). Dose-dependent suppression of serum cholesterol by tocotrienol-rich fraction (TRF25) of rice bran in hypercholesterolemic humans. *Atherosclerosis* 161(1): 199–207.

Rasool, A. H., A. R. Rahman et al. (2008). Arterial compliance and vitamin E blood levels with a self emulsifying preparation of tocotrienol rich vitamin E. *Arch Pharm Res* 31(9): 1212–1217.

Rasool, A. H., K. H. Yuen et al. (2006). Dose dependent elevation of plasma tocotrienol levels and its effect on arterial compliance, plasma total antioxidant status, and lipid profile in healthy humans supplemented with tocotrienol rich vitamin E. *J Nutr Sci Vitaminol (Tokyo)* 52(6): 473–478.

Rink, C., G. Christoforidis et al. (2011). Tocotrienol vitamin E protects against preclinical canine ischemic stroke by inducing arteriogenesis. *J Cereb Blood Flow Metab* 31(11): 2218–2230.

Roberts, L. J., 2nd, J. A. Oates et al. (2007). The relationship between dose of vitamin E and suppression of oxidative stress in humans. *Free Radic Biol Med* 43(10): 1388–1393.

Schwartz, P. L. and I. M. Rutherford (1981). The effect of tocopherol on high-density lipoprotein cholesterol. *Am J Clin Pathol* 76(6): 843–845.

Serbinova, E. A. and L. Packer (1994). Antioxidant properties of alpha-tocopherol and alpha-tocotrienol. *Methods Enzymol* 234: 354–366.

Shibata, A., K. Nakagawa et al. (2010). Alpha-tocopherol attenuates the cytotoxic effect of delta-tocotrienol in human colorectal adenocarcinoma cells. *Biochem Biophys Res Commun* 397(2): 214–219.

Shrago, E., J. A. Glennon et al. (1971). Comparative aspects of lipogenesis in mammalian tissues. *Metabolism* 20(1): 54–62.

Song, B. L. and R. A. DeBose-Boyd (2006). Insig-dependent ubiquitination and degradation of 3-hydroxy-3-methylglutaryl coenzyme a reductase stimulated by delta- and gamma-tocotrienols. *J Biol Chem* 281(35): 25054–25061.

Sontag, T. J. and R. S. Parker (2007). Influence of major structural features of tocopherols and tocotrienols on their omega-oxidation by tocopherol-omega-hydroxylase. *J Lipid Res* 48(5): 1090–1098.

Tan, B. (1989). Palm carotenoids, tocopherols and tocotrienols. *J Am Oil Chem Soc* 66: 770–776.

Tan, B. (2005). Appropriate spectrum vitamin E and new perspectives on desmethyl tocopherols and tocotrienols. *JANA* 8(1): 35–42.

Tan, B. and L. Brzuskiewicz (1989). Separation of tocopherol and tocotrienol isomers using normal- and reverse-phase liquid chromatography. *Anal Biochem* 180(2): 368–373.

Tan, D. T., H. T. Khor et al. (1991). Effect of a palm-oil-vitamin E concentrate on the serum and lipoprotein lipids in humans. *Am J Clin Nutr* 53(4 Suppl): 1027S–1030S.

Tan, B. and A. M. Mueller (2008). Tocotrienols in cardiometabolic diseases. In *Tocotrienols: Vitamin E beyond Tocopherol*. R. Watson and V. Preedy (Eds.), Boca Raton, FL: CRC Press, pp. 257–273.

Tomeo, A. C., M. Geller et al. (1995). Antioxidant effects of tocotrienols in patients with hyperlipidemia and carotid stenosis. *Lipids* 30(12): 1179–1183.

Traber, M. G. and J. Atkinson (2007). Vitamin E, antioxidant and nothing more. *Free Radic Biol Med* 43(1): 4–15.

Tsai, A. C., J. J. Kelley et al. (1978). Study on the effect of megavitamin E supplementation in man. *Am J Clin Nutr* 31(5): 831–837.

Wahlqvist, M. L., Z. Krivokuca-Bogetic et al. (1992). Differential serum responses to tocopherols and tocotrienols during vitamin E supplementation in hypercholesterolemic individuals without change in coronary risk factors. *Nutr Res* 12: S181–S201.

Wang, Y., M. Moreland et al. (2012). Vitamin E forms inhibit IL-13/STAT6-induced eotaxin-3 secretion by up-regulation of PAR4, an endogenous inhibitor of atypical PKC in human lung epithelial cells. *J Nutr Biochem* 23(6): 602–608.

Wells, S. R., M. H. Jennings et al. (2010). Alpha-, gamma- and delta-tocopherols reduce inflammatory angiogenesis in human microvascular endothelial cells. *J Nutr Biochem* 21(7): 589–597.

Yang, Z., M. J. Lee et al. (2011). Metabolism of tocotrienols in animals and synergistic inhibitory actions of tocotrienols with atorvastatin in cancer cells. *Genes Nutr* 7(1): 11–18.

Yap, S. P., K. H. Yuen et al. (2001). Pharmacokinetics and bioavailability of alpha-, gamma- and delta-tocotrienols under different food status. *J Pharm Pharmacol* 53(1): 67–71.

You, C. S., T. J. Sontag et al. (2005). Long-chain carboxychromanols are the major metabolites of tocopherols and tocotrienols in A549 lung epithelial cells but not HepG2 cells. *J Nutr* 135(2): 227–232.

Yu, W., L. Jia et al. (2009). Anticancer actions of natural and synthetic vitamin E forms: RRR-alpha-tocopherol blocks the anticancer actions of gamma-tocopherol. *Mol Nutr Food Res* 53(12): 1573–1581.

Yu, S. G., A. M. Thomas et al. (2006). Dose-response impact of various tocotrienols on serum lipid parameters in 5-week-old female chickens. *Lipids* 41(5): 453–461.

Zaiden, N., W. N. Yap et al. (2010). Gamma delta tocotrienols reduce hepatic triglyceride synthesis and VLDL secretion. *J Atheroscler Thromb* 17(10): 1019–1032.

6 Antiangiogenic Effects of Tocotrienol

Takahiro Eitsuka, Kiyotaka Nakagawa, and Teruo Miyazawa

CONTENTS

6.1 INTRODUCTION

Angiogenesis is a complex process of sprouting new capillaries from the preexisting blood vessels. It happens in normal physiological processes, such as embryonic development, the female menstrual cycle, bone remodeling, and wound healing. On the other hand, angiogenesis also plays a crucial role in many pathological conditions, including tumor growth, diabetic retinopathy, psoriasis, rheumatoid arthritis, and atherosclerosis (Carmeliet and Jain, 2000; Folkman, 1995). The role of angiogenesis in tumor growth was first described by Folkman (1971). Without the supplement of blood circulation, the tumor size is restricted. Once a tumor becomes vascularized, the tumor mass expands rapidly (Hanahan and Folkman, 1996). These newly formed vessels not only promote tumor growth but also cause the tumor cells to become more malignant and metastatic (Fidler and Ellis, 1994). Evidence shows that inhibition of angiogenesis can suppress the progression of these associated diseases. Thus, angiogenesis has become a potential target, and a wide variety of therapies directed at interfering with this process are now in development (Scappaticci, 2002). Since some antiangiogenic agents are available in foods (Fang et al., 2007; Fassina et al., 2004; Mantell et al., 2000; Min et al., 2004; Tsuzuki et al., 2007), even if these agents possess moderate antiangiogenic effect, daily consumption of these compounds may help prevent angiogenic disorders.

On the basis of this background, it is of high interest to know whether tocotrienol (T3) suppresses cancers through its inhibitory effect on tumor angiogenesis. We have hypothesized that the suppressive effect of T3 on cancer may be attributable to the antiangiogenic activity of T3, and we have carried out a series of investigations (Eitsuka et al., 2006; Inokuchi et al., 2003; Miyazawa et al., 2004, 2009; Nakagawa et al., 2004, 2007; Shibata et al., 2008a,b, 2009). In our previous review of *Tocotrienols: Vitamin E Beyond Tocopherols* (Nakagawa et al., 2008), we discussed the antiangiogenic effect of T3 and its mechanism from the fundamental data of *in vitro* cell studies, DNA chip analysis, and *in vivo* egg and animal models. In this review, we introduce our current research on the antiangiogenic effect of T3 and its underlying molecular mechanisms.

6.2 *IN VITRO* STUDY OF ANGIOGENESIS INHIBITION BY T3

Since angiogenic processes are involved in endothelial cell proliferation, migration, and tube formation, modulation of these processes serves as a good strategy for preventing angiogenic disorders. It is well known that various growth factors have a major role in neovascularization, and one of the most important factors is vascular endothelial growth factor (VEGF; Ferrara and Gerber, 2001). We therefore examined the effect of T3 on VEGF-induced proliferation, migration, and tube formation of human umbilical vein endothelial cells (HUVEC). T3 at a low micromolar range inhibited HUVEC proliferation (Figure 6.1A), with the following order of inhibitory potency: δ-T3 > β-T3 > γ-T3 > α-T3 (Shibata et al., 2009). The ranking order was similar to the incorporation of each T3 isomers into HUVEC (Shibata et al., 2009). Structurally, δ-T3 lacks the 5- and 7-methyl groups attached onto its chroman ring, so it is allowed to pass easily through cell membranes. The better incorporation of δ-T3 into HUVEC would be the reason for its greater proliferation inhibitory effect. δ-T3 remarkably suppressed migration (Figure 6.1B) and tube formation (Figure 6.1C) in HUVEC, and the amount of δ-T3 required for inhibiting either cell migration (2 μM) or tube formation (2.8 μM) was lower than that required for attenuating cell proliferation (5 μM; Shibata et al., 2009). These findings suggest that the main antiangiogenic effect of δ-T3 would be the suppression of migration and tube formation in HUVEC. In contrast, α-tocopherol (α-Toc) did not exhibit any effects on VEGF-induced HUVEC proliferation, migration or tube formation, even at a high concentration of 50 μM (Shibata et al., 2009). These results suggest that δ-T3 is the more bioactive compound than α-Toc in term of the angiogenesis inhibitor.

6.3 MOLECULAR MECHANISM FOR ANGIOGENESIS INHIBITION BY T3

Because of inadequate blood supply, highly aggressive and rapidly growing tumors are exposed to hypoxia. Hypoxia is the major pathophysiological condition regulating angiogenesis (Pugh and Ratcliffe, 2003). Indeed, several types of tumors secrete angiogenetic factors like VEGF, which are promoted by hypoxic conditions (Mizukami et al., 2005). Increased angiogenesis in response to hypoxia is part of an adaptive response mediated by the key transcription factor, hypoxia-inducible factor (HIF)-1α (Pugh and Ratcliffe, 2003). HIF-1α activates expression of the VEGF gene by binding to hypoxia response element (HRE) in VEGF promoter region (Paul et al., 2004). HIF-1 expression is elevated in many human cancers (Ke and Costa, 2006), thus supporting the notion that the hypoxia/HIF-1 system is a potential molecular target in cancer therapeutics (Semenza, 2003). We, therefore, examined the effect of T3 on mRNA expression of HIF-1α and VEGF in DLD-1 cells (human colorectal adenocarcinoma) under normoxic and hypoxic conditions. DLD-1 cells incubated in hypoxic conditions had greater VEGF mRNA expression than cultures in normoxia. δ-T3 suppressed the hypoxia-induced VEGF mRNA expression (Figure 6.2A; Shibata et al., 2008b). Whereas hypoxic conditions did not affect HIF-1α mRNA expression, both hypoxic and δ-T3 treatment in combo reduced HIF-1α mRNA expression (Figure 6.2B; Shibata et al., 2008b). To further analyze the mechanism by which T3 regulates HIF-1α transcription factor, we measured the expression level of HIF-1α protein and performed transient transfections of DLD-1 cells with luciferase-plasmid constructs containing HRE. Western blotting revealed that hypoxia markedly increased the HIF-1α protein level, while δ-T3 reduced hypoxia-induced HIF-1α protein accumulation (Figure 6.2C; Shibata et al., 2008b). Hypoxia elicited an increase in luciferase activity expressed by an HRE-luciferase reporter construct, and the transcriptional activity was inhibited by δ-T3 (Figure 6.2D; Shibata et al., 2008b). These results indicate that δ-T3 suppresses HIF-1α through both transcriptional and post-transcriptional mechanisms and thereby inhibits VEGF transcriptional activation.

VEGF exerts its biologic effect through interaction with receptors present on the cell surface. These receptor tyrosine kinases include VEGF receptor (VEGFR)-1 and VEGFR-2, which are predominantly present on vascular endothelial cells (Terman et al., 1992). VEGFR-2 is the main receptor responsible for mediating the proangiogenic effects of VEGF in tumor-associated

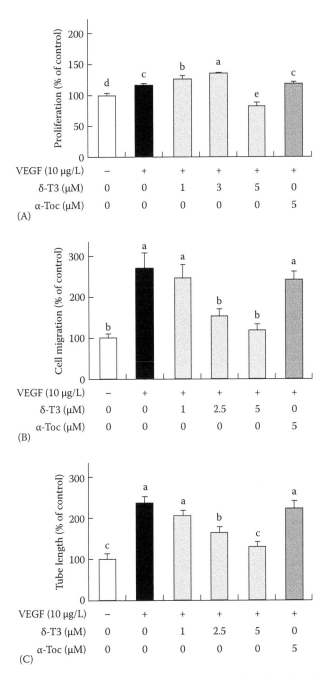

FIGURE 6.1 Effects of δ-T3 and α-Toc on VEGF-induced HUVEC proliferation, migration, and tube formation. (A) HUVEC were incubated for 24 h in medium-containing VEGF and either δ-T3 or α-Toc at concentrations from 0 to 5 μM. The viable cells were then evaluated by WST-1 assay. Values are mean ± SD, $n = 6$. (B) The migration assays were carried out in a modified Boyden chamber consisting of a cell culture insert membrane (3 μm pore membrane coated with fibronectin). HUVECs were suspended in 500 μL of medium-containing 1% FBS and either δ-T3 or α-Toc and were then added to the top chamber. The lower chamber was filled with 750 μL of medium-containing 1% FBS and 10 μg/L VEGF. The whole chamber was incubated for 22 h, and the number of cells that had migrated to the lower side of the filter was quantified. Values are mean ± SD, $n = 4$. (C) HUVECs were suspended in 500 μL of test medium-containing 10 μg/L VEGF and either δ-T3 or α-Toc. Following incubation of the cell suspension on the Matrigel plate for 18 h, tube lengths were quantified by photography using an optical microscopy. Values are mean ± SD, $n = 4$. Means without a common letter differ, $P < 0.05$.

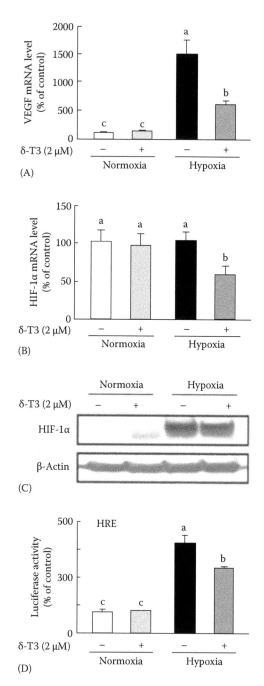

FIGURE 6.2 Effects of δ-T3 on hypoxia/HIF-1 system in DLD-1 cells and VEGF signaling in HUVEC. DLD-1 cells were cultured with δ-T3 (0 or 2 μM) under normoxic or hypoxic conditions for 24 h. The mRNA expression levels of VEGF (A) and HIF-1α (B) were measured by real-time RT-PCR. Values are mean ± SD, $n = 6$. Means without a common letter differ, $P < 0.05$. (C) Effect of δ-T3 on HIF-1α protein in DLD-1 cells under normoxic or hypoxic conditions for 24 h, followed by western blot analysis. (D) DLD-1 cells were transfected with the PGL3 reporter vector containing a tandem repeat of HIF-1α-binding site (HRE) and SV40 promoter. After transfection for 24 h, the cells were treated with or without δ-T3 under normoxic or hypoxic conditions for 24 h, and luciferase activity was then evaluated using the Luc assay system. Values are mean ± SD, $n = 3$. Means without a common letter differ, $P < 0.05$.

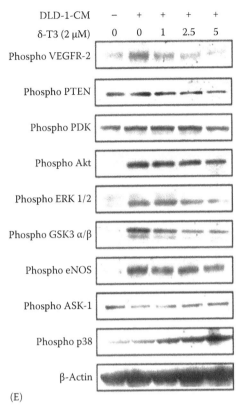

(E)

FIGURE 6.2 (continued) (E) HUVECs were treated with 0–5 μM δ-T3 for 6 h and then stimulated with DLD-1-CM for 10 min. The intracellular proteins associated with VEGF-signaling pathway were detected by western blot analysis.

endothelium (Waltenberger et al., 1994). VEGFR-2 activates multiple downstream signaling cascades, such as PI3K/PDK/Akt pathway (Cross et al., 2003). Considering the critical role of these signaling molecules in angiogenesis, we investigate whether the antiangiogenic effect of T3 is mediated through pathway modulation. Stimulation of HUVEC with tumor-cell-cultured medium (CM) containing certain growth factors as angiogenic stimuli was accompanied by increased phosphorylation of VEGFR-2 and PI3K/PDK/Akt pathway proteins like PDK, Akt, and PTEN. When δ-T3 was added to CM, VEGFR-2 and PI3K/PDK/Akt pathway protein phosphorylation were suppressed (Figure 6.2E; Shibata et al., 2008a). We next examined the effect of δ-T3 on signals related to PI3K/PDK/Akt, such as endothelial nitric oxide synthase (eNOS), glycogen synthase kinase 3 (GSK3) α/β, and extracellular-signal-regulated kinase (ERK) 1/2, all of which are involved in cell proliferation and survival. CM stimulation resulted in activation of eNOS, GSK3 α/β, and ERK 1/2, and the changes were reduced to basal (nonstimulated) levels by δ-T3 treatment (Figure 6.2E; Shibata et al., 2008a). We also found that a relatively high dose of δ-T3 increased the phosphorylation of stress response proteins such as ASK-1 and p38 mitogen-activated protein kinase (Figure 6.2E; Shibata et al., 2008a), which are involved in apoptosis induction in endothelial cells. Considering these findings, the following mechanism is conceivable for the antiangiogenic effect of T3. In tumor cells, T3 inhibits hypoxia-induced HIF-1α protein accumulation, leading to reduction of VEGF mRNA expression. Furthermore, in endothelial cells, T3 downregulates VEGFR-2 and PI3K/PDK/Akt signaling pathway, thereby attenuating cell survival and tube formation, resulting in angiogenesis inhibition (Figure 6.3). In case of relatively high dose, T3 not only blocks Akt and inhibits downstream survival signals, but also enhances the ASK-1 and p38 pathway, thereby eliciting an apoptotic effect in endothelial cells (Figure 6.3).

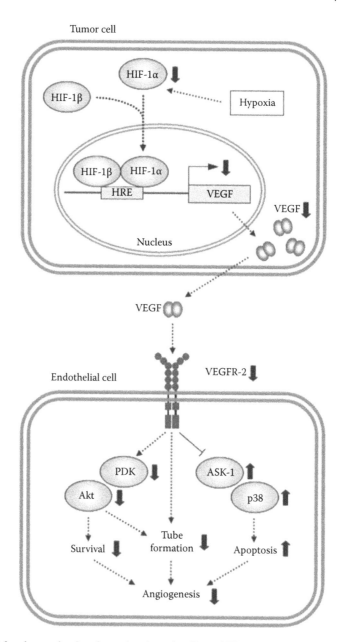

FIGURE 6.3   Molecular mechanism for antiangiogenic effect of T3.

6.4   *IN VIVO* STUDY OF ANGIOGENESIS INHIBITION BY T3

To evaluate the effect of T3 on *in vivo* tumor angiogenesis, we conducted Matrigel plug assay using nude mice, because numerous studies reported the usability of its assay to assess the *in vivo* efficacy of inhibitors for tumor-associated angiogenesis (Fang et al., 2007; Kong et al., 2007). The DLD-1-Matrigel-implanted control mice appeared to show significant neovascularization (as judged by hemoglobin (Hb) content in Matrigel plug, 3.9 ± 1.2 µg Hb/mg Matrigel), compared with mice injected with Matrigel alone (0.6 ± 0.2 µg Hb/mg Matrigel; Figure 6.4; Shibata et al., 2008a). The suppression of vessel formation in mice implanted with the DLD-1-Matrigel-containing δ-T3 (20 µg) was clearly observed (1.3 ± 0.6 µg Hb/mg Matrigel; Figure 6.4;

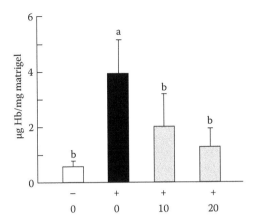

FIGURE 6.4 Effect of δ-T3 on DLD-1-induced vessel formation in the Matrigel plug assay. DLD-1 cells were suspended in serum-free RPMI-1640 medium. Aliquots of the cell suspension were mixed with Matrigel-containing 0–20 μg δ-T3, and the mixture was injected into flanks of nude mice. The Matrigel plugs were removed 14 days after the implantation and subjected to the measurement of hemoglobin content. Values are mean ± SD, $n = 6$. Means without a common letter differ, $P < 0.05$.

Shibata et al., 2008a). Histological analysis of the DLD-1-Matrigel plug of control mice indicated an obvious angiogenic response (Shibata et al., 2008a). The CD31/platelet endothelial cell adhesion molecule-1 (PECAM-1) positive endothelial cells and the red blood cells dyed by hematoxylin and eosin were clearly present, indicating that endothelial cells had infiltrated the DLD-1-Matrigel. In contrast, the DLD-1-Matrigel-containing δ-T3 showed a low number of both CD31/PECAM-1-positive and erythroid cells (Shibata et al., 2008a), suggesting that δ-T3 inhibited the endothelial cell invasion and neovessel formation. Therefore, these results may be due to the inhibitory effects of δ-T3 on endothelial signaling of proangiogenic factors, such as VEGF. It is also possible that the *in vivo* antiangiogenic effect of δ-T3 is not only due to its direct action on endothelial cells, but also to the consequent effects on both endothelial cells and other cell types such as macrophages, leukocytes, and tumor cells.

6.5 INFLUENCE OF COADMINISTRATION OF Toc ON THE ANTICANCER EFFECT OF T3

Toc is widely present in a variety of foods, whereas T3-containing foods are limited. Recent studies have demonstrated that T3 is superior to Toc for cancer chemoprevention (Miyazawa et al., 2009). However, there is little information concerning the influence of the coadministration of Toc on the anticancer properties of T3. In an attempt to clarify whether Toc affects the antiproliferative activity of T3, DLD-1 cells were treated with both Toc isomers and δ-T3. All Toc isomers, especially α-Toc, diminished δ-T3-induced cytotoxicity to DLD-1 cells (Shibata et al., 2010b). Coadministration of α-Toc dose dependently decreased δ-T3 uptake into DLD-1 cells (Shibata et al., 2010b). These results indicate that α-Toc is not only less cytotoxic to cancer cells, but it also reduces the cytotoxicity of δ-T3 by inhibiting its cellular uptake. Our findings therefore raise concerns about the chemopreventive activity of T3 *in vivo* because α-Toc is ubiquitously present as the predominant vitamin E molecule in animals. It has been shown that dietary supplementation of pure T3 can effectively suppress tumor growth in a mouse xenograft model (Hiura et al., 2009), suggesting a high dose of purified T3 may overcome the inhibitory effects of endogenous α-Toc. T3 daily intake in Japanese population was estimated around 1.86–2.15 mg/day/person, which appeared relatively low compared with Toc (9 mg Toc/day/person; Sookwong et al., 2010). Thus, additional amounts of T3 or Toc-free T3 might be necessary for therapeutic performance of T3.

6.6 CONCLUSION

An understanding of the fundamental mechanisms of angiogenesis had allowed the discovery of inhibitors targeting VEGF for use in cancer therapy, as well as in the prevention of angiogenic disorders such as diabetic retinopathy (Kim et al., 1993). Several antiangiogenic agents are available from natural sources. For instance, tea catechin (epigallocatechin gallate) and red wine polyphenol (resveratrol) have antiangiogenic effects via modulation of gene expression or signal transduction of VEGF (Zhang et al., 2005; Zhu et al., 2007). Although these compounds, as well as T3, are natural products, questions regarding their safety and toxicity must be addressed. In case of T3, there was no critical loss or adverse events in animals in preclinical studies (Nakamura et al., 2001). T3 is absorbed through the intestine (Ikeda et al., 1996) and is distributed into the bloodstream of humans, suggesting that T3 is bioavailable. T3 reached a concentration of 1.6 μmol/L in human plasma after T3 oral administration (~700 mg/day; Fairus et al., 2006). In our cell culture studies, the concentrations of T3 were high enough to inhibit *in vitro* angiogenic factor secretion and signal transduction. It is thus tempting to speculate that the inclusion of T3 in diets may have anticancer effects through angiogenesis inhibition.

We also demonstrated that the inhibitory effect of T3 on tumor angiogenesis was via reduction of cyclooxygenase 2 (COX-2) and interleukin (IL; Shibata et al., 2008b). It is well known that these molecules can act as not only angiogenic factors but also inflammatory inducers. We therefore investigated the effect of T3 on skin inflammation *in vitro* and *in vivo* and found that T3 has a potent anti-inflammatory action through downregulation of COX-2 and IL (Nakagawa et al., 2010; Shibata et al., 2010a). Our findings will provide new insights into the application of T3 for anti-inflammatory purposes.

In this review, we described our current research on the angiogenesis-inhibitory effect of T3 and its related mechanism for cancer prevention. A series of experimental data from cell studies and an animal model demonstrated that T3 performed potent antiangiogenic function *in vitro* and *in vivo*. The antiangiogenic effect of T3 was attributable to the regulation of hypoxia/HIF-1 system in tumor cells and VEGF signaling in endothelial cells. These findings indicate that T3 is a promising anticancer agent for minimizing tumor angiogenesis. The experimental data shown in this review warrant its testing in other models of cancer prevention, with a realistic prospect of its use for preventive and therapeutic approaches in humans.

REFERENCES

Carmeliet, P., Jain, R.K. 2000. Angiogenesis in cancer and other diseases. *Nature*, 407, 249–257.

Cross, M.J., Dixelius, J., Matsumoto, T., Claesson-Welsh, L. 2003. VEGF-receptor signal transduction. *Trends Biochem. Sci.*, 28, 488–494.

Eitsuka, T., Nakagawa, K., Miyazawa, T., 2006. Down-regulation of telomerase activity in DLD-1 human colorectal adenocarcinoma cells by tocotrienol. *Biochem. Biophys. Res. Commun.*, 348, 170–175.

Fairus, S., Nor, R.M., Cheng, H.M., Sundram, K. 2006. Postprandial metabolic fate of tocotrienol-rich vitamin E differs significantly from that of α-tocopherol. *Am. J. Clin. Nutr.*, 84, 835–842.

Fang, J., Zhou, Q., Liu, L.Z., Xia, C., Hu, X., Shi, X., Jiang, B.H. 2007. Apigenin inhibits tumor angiogenesis through decreasing HIF-1α and VEGF expression. *Carcinogenesis*, 28, 858–864.

Fassina, G., Venè, R., Morini, M., Minghelli, S., Benelli, R., Noonan, D.M., Albini, A. 2004. Mechanisms of inhibition of tumor angiogenesis and vascular tumor growth by epigallocatechin-3-gallate. *Clin. Cancer Res.*, 10, 4865–4873.

Ferrara, N., Gerber, H.P. 2001. The role of vascular endothelial growth factor in angiogenesis. *Acta Haematol.*, 106, 148–156.

Fidler, I.J., Ellis, L.M. 1994. The implications of angiogenesis for the biology and therapy of cancer metastasis. *Cell*, 79, 185–188.

Folkman, J. 1971. Tumor angiogenesis: therapeutic implications. *N. Engl. J. Med.*, 285, 1182–1186.

Folkman, J. 1995. Clinical applications of research on angiogenesis. *N. Engl. J. Med.*, 333, 1757–1763.

Hanahan, D., Folkman, J. 1996. Patterns and emerging mechanisms of the angiogenic switch during tumorigenesis. *Cell*, 86, 353–364.

Hiura, Y., Tachibana, H., Arakawa, R., Aoyama, N., Okabe, M., Sakai, M., Yamada, K. 2009. Specific accumulation of γ- and δ-tocotrienols in tumor and their antitumor effect in vivo. *J. Nutr. Biochem.*, 20, 607–613.

Ikeda, I., Imasato, Y., Sasaki, E., Sugano, M. 1996. Lymphatic transport of α-, γ- and δ-tocotrienols and α-tocopherol in rats. *Int. J. Vitam. Nutr. Res.*, 66, 217–221.

Inokuchi, H., Hirokane, H., Tsuzuki, T., Nakagawa, K., Igarashi, M., Miyazawa, T. 2003. Anti-angiogenic activity of tocotrienol. *Biosci. Bitechnol. Biochem.*, 67, 1623–1627.

Ke, Q., Costa, M. 2006. Hypoxia-inducible factor-1 (HIF-1). *Mol. Pharmacol.*, 70, 1469–1480.

Kim, K.J., Li, B., Winer, J., Armanini, M., Gillett, N., Phillips, H.S., Ferrara, N. 1993. Inhibition of vascular endothelial growth factor-induced angiogenesis suppresses tumour growth in vivo. *Nature*, 362, 841–844.

Kong, D., Li, Y., Wang, Z., Banerjee, S., Sarkar, F.H. 2007. Inhibition of angiogenesis and invasion by 3,3'-diindolylmethane is mediated by the nuclear factor-κB downstream target genes MMP-9 and uPA that regulated bioavailability of vascular endothelial growth factor in prostate cancer. *Cancer Res.*, 67, 3310–3319.

Mantell, D.J., Owens, P.E., Bundred, N.J., Mawer, E.B., Canfield, A.E. 2000. 1α,25-Dihydroxyvitamin D3 inhibits angiogenesis in vitro and in vivo. *Circ. Res.*, 87, 214–220.

Min, J.K., Han, K.Y., Kim, E.C., Kim, Y.M., Lee, S.W., Kim, O.H., Kim, K.W., Gho, Y.S., Kwon, Y.G. 2004. Capsaicin inhibits in vitro and in vivo angiogenesis. *Cancer Res.*, 64, 644–651.

Miyazawa, T., Shibata, A., Sookwong, P., Kawakami, Y., Eitsuka, T., Asai, A., Oikawa, S., Nakagawa, K. 2009. Antiangiogenic and anticancer potential of unsaturated vitamin E (tocotrienol). *J. Nutr. Biochem.*, 20, 79–86.

Miyazawa, T., Tsuzuki, T., Nakagawa, K., Igarashi, M. 2004. Antiangiogenic potency of vitamin E. *Ann. NY Acad. Sci.*, 1031, 401–404.

Mizukami, Y., Jo, W.S., Duerr, E.M., Gala, M., Li, J., Zhang, X., Zimmer, M.A. et al. 2005. Induction of interleukin-8 preserves the angiogenic response in HIF-1α-deficient colon cancer cells. *Nat. Med.*, 11, 992–997.

Nakagawa, K., Eitsuka, T., Inokuchi, H., Miyazawa, T. 2004. DNA chip analysis of comprehensive food function: inhibition of angiogenesis and telomerase activity with unsaturated vitamin E, tocotrienol. *Biofactors*, 21, 5–10.

Nakagawa, K., Shibata, A., Maruko, T., Sookwong, P., Tsuduki, T., Kawakami, K., Nishida, H., Miyazawa, T. 2010. γ-Tocotrienol reduces squalene hydroperoxide-induced inflammatory responses in HaCaT keratinocytes. *Lipids*, 45, 833–841.

Nakagawa, K., Shibata, A., Sookwong, P., Miyazawa, T. 2008. Chemistry of tocotrienols, Chapter 6: Angiogenesis inhibition. In *Tocotrienols: Vitamin E beyond Tocopherols*, eds. R.R. Watson and V.R. Preedy, pp. 79–84. Taylor & Francis, Boca Raton, FL.

Nakagawa, K., Shibata, A., Yamashita, S., Tsuzuki, T., Kariya, J., Oikawa, S., Miyazawa, T. 2007. In vivo angiogenesis is suppressed by unsaturated vitamin E, tocotrienol. *J. Nutr.*, 137, 1938–1943.

Nakamura, H., Furukawa, F., Nishikawa, A., Miyauchi, M., Son, H.Y., Imazawa, T., Hirose, M. 2001. Oral toxicity of a tocotrienol preparation in rats. *Food Chem. Toxicol.*, 39, 799–805.

Paul, S.A., Simons, J.W., Mebjeesh, N.J. 2004. HIF at the crossroads between ischemia and carcinogenesis. *J. Cell Physiol.*, 200, 20–30.

Pugh, C.W., Ratcliffe, P.J. 2003. Regulation of angiogenesis by hypoxia: Role of the HIF system. *Nat. Med.*, 9, 677–684.

Scappaticci, F.A. 2002. Mechanisms and future directions for angiogenesis-based cancer therapies. *J. Clin. Oncol.*, 20, 3906–3927.

Semenza, G.L. 2003. Targeting HIF-1 for cancer therapy. *Nat. Rev. Cancer*, 3, 721–732.

Shibata, A., Nakagawa, K., Kawakami, Y., Tsuzuki, T., Miyazawa, T. 2010a. Suppression of γ-tocotrienol on UVB induced inflammation in HaCaT keratinocytes and HR-1 hairless mice via inflammatory mediators multiple signaling. *J. Agric. Food Chem.*, 58, 7013–7020.

Shibata, A., Nakagawa, K., Sookwong, P., Tsuduki, T., Asai, A., Miyazawa, T. 2010b. α-Tocopherol attenuates the cytotoxic effect of δ-tocotrienol in human colorectal adenocarcinoma cells. *Biochem. Biophys. Res. Commun.*, 397, 214–219.

Shibata, A., Nakagawa, K., Sookwong, P., Tsuzuki, T., Oikawa, S., Miyazawa, T. 2008a. Tumor anti-angiogenic effect and mechanism of action of δ-tocotrienol. *Biochem. Pharmacol.*, 76, 330–339.

Shibata, A., Nakagawa, K., Sookwong, P., Tsuzuki, T., Oikawa, S., Miyazawa, T. 2009. δ-Tocotrienol suppressed VEGF induced angiogenesis whereas α-tocopherol does not. *J. Agric. Food Chem.*, 57, 8696–8704.

Shibata, A., Nakagawa, K., Sookwong, P., Tsuzuki, T., Tomita, S., Shirakawa, H., Komai, M., Miyazawa, T. 2008b. Tocotrienol inhibits secretion of angiogenic factors from human colorectal adenocarcinoma cells by suppressing hypoxia-inducible factor-1α. *J. Nutr.*, 138, 2136–2142.

Sookwong, P., Nakagawa, K., Yamaguchi, Y., Miyazawa, T., Kato, S., Kimura, F., Miyazawa. T. 2010. Tocotrienol distribution in foods: Estimation of daily tocotrienol intake of Japanese population. *J. Agric. Food Chem.*, 58, 3350–3355.

Terman, B.I., Dougher-Vermazen, M., Carrion, M.E., Dimitrov, D., Armellino, D.C., Gospodarowicz, D., Böhlen, P. 1992. Identification of the KDR tyrosine kinase as a receptor for vascular endothelial cell growth factor. *Biochem. Biophys. Res. Commun.*, 187, 1579–1586.

Tsuzuki, T., Shibata, A., Kawakami, Y., Nakagawa, K., Miyazawa, T. 2007. Conjugated eicosapentaenoic acid inhibits vascular endothelial growth factor-induced angiogenesis by suppressing the migration of human umbilical vein endothelial cells. *J. Nutr.*, 137, 641–646.

Waltenberger, J., Claesson-Welsh, L., Siegbahn, A., Shibuya, M., Heldin, C.H. 1994. Different signal transduction properties of KDR and Flt1, two receptors for vascular endothelial growth factor. *J. Biol. Chem.*, 269, 26988–26995.

Zhang, Q., Tang, X., Lu, Q.Y., Zhang, Z.F., Brown, J., Le, A.D. 2005. Resveratrol inhibits hypoxia-induced accumulation of hypoxia-inducible factor-1α and VEGF expression in human tongue squamous cell carcinoma and hepatoma cells. *Mol. Cancer Ther.*, 4, 1465–1474.

Zhu, B.H., Zhan, W.H., Li, Z.R., Wang, Z., He, Y.L., Peng, J.S., Cai, S.R., Ma, J.P., Zhang, C.H. 2007. (-)-Epigallocatechin-3-gallate inhibits growth of gastric cancer by reducing VEGF production and angiogenesis. *World J. Gastroenterol.*, 13, 1162–1169.

7 Mechanism of Delta-Tocotrienol on Colorectal Cancer

Sayori Wada and Yuji Naito

CONTENTS

7.1 INTRODUCTION

A recent study showed that colorectal cancer ranked third as the most common cancer for estimated new cases and fourth for estimated deaths in males (Jemal et al., 2011). For females, it was second for estimated new cases and third for estimated deaths. That study showed an estimate of over 1.2 million new colorectal cancer cases and 608,700 deaths worldwide in 2008. Environmental factors were responsible for 90%–95% of cancer causes, whereas genes were responsible for only 5%–10%, and 30%–35% of the environmental factors were associated with diet. Diet was strongly associated with cancer deaths in as many as 70% of colorectal cancer cases (Anand et al., 2008). A case-controlled study showed that a high intake of dietary vitamin E was associated with a reduced risk of distal colorectal cancer (relative risk 0.65; 95% confidence interval 0.48–0.89) in the Caucasian (Williams et al., 2010), and pooled analysis of cohort studies demonstrated that a high consumption of vitamin E from both food and supplements was associated with a reduced risk of colon cancer (relative risk 0.82; 95% confidence interval: 0.74–0.91; Park et al., 2010). Contrary, intake of vitamin E from food only, not supplements, had no correlation with colon cancer risk (relative risk 0.99; 95% confidence interval: 0.89–1.11; Park et al. 2010). Vitamin E was defined as α-tocopherol in these studies, and no study of tocotrienol has been reported.

Tocotrienols have been reported to have more tumor-suppressive potency than α-tocopherol in *in vitro* studies (McIntyre et al., 2000; Shah et al., 2003; He et al., 1997). The relative anti-proliferative potency among tocotrienol isoforms seems to be δ- > γ- > α- in various types of cancer cells, for example, breast and liver cancer cells (Yu et al., 1999; Wada et al., 2005). Conversely, few studies have focused on the anticancer effects of δ-tocotrienol on colorectal cancer, and the results are not widely known. In this study, we present an overview of the results obtained in studies on the properties and potency of δ-tocotrienol related to the prevention of colorectal cancer.

7.2 DISTRIBUTION AND CELLULAR UPTAKE OF δ-TOCOTRIENOL

In a human study conducted in Malaysia using healthy subjects, a 2 month oral administration protocol of tocotrienol-rich vitamin E increased the plasma level of α-, γ-, and δ-tocotrienol in a dose-dependent manner (Rasool et al., 2006). In that study, the ingestion of 80, 160, and 320 mg/day of tocotrienol-rich vitamin E (including 15% δ-tocotrienol) resulted in an increase of plasma δ-tocotrienol by approximately 30, 60, and 80 ng/mL, respectively, which was not detectable at the baseline. A significant difference was shown for this change between the placebo and treatment groups.

A study conducted on colon tissue showed results on the concentration of γ-tocotrienol alone and γ- and δ-tocotrienol together, but not δ-tocotrienol alone (Yang et al., 2012). The levels of γ-tocotrienol and its metabolites, γ-CEHC and γ-CMBHC, in the colon were reported to be 0.60 ± 0.14, 5.49 ± 0.80, and 37.02 ± 4.97 μmol/kg, respectively, in athymic nude mice after a 2-week-diet with 0.05% γ-tocotrienol. Ncr Nu/Nu mice, inoculated with human lung cancer H1299 cells, were fed with diets containing 0.1% γ-tocotrienol and 0.1% δ-tocotrienol together with tocopherols. After a 7 week administration protocol, the levels of tocotrienols were approximately 0.5 μmol/kg in the liver and >10 μmol/kg in the small intestine, colon, spleen, and kidney. The levels in the xenograft tumor and lung were in the range of 1–10 μmol/kg, and the serum level of γ- and δ-tocotrienol was 1.63 ± 0.61 and 0.59 ± 0.08 μM, respectively.

A mouse study showed specific accumulation of γ- and δ-tocotrienol (approximately 20 and 8 μg/g) in inoculated hepatoma MH134 tumor cells, but no distribution of γ- and δ-tocotrienol was detected in the liver or lung (Hiura et al., 2009). The effective concentrations of γ- and δ-tocotrienol for antiproliferation were approximately 20–30 μM in colon cancer cells (Yang et al., 2010). However, the concentration of γ- and δ-tocotrienol in plasma was approximately at most 300 and 80 ng/mL after a 2 month supplementation protocol (Rasool et al., 2006). The accumulation of tocotrienol in a tumor and long-term oral administration may be the key to this issue.

The intracellular concentrations of tocotrienol isomers were higher than those of tocopherol isomers in intestinal epithelial Caco2 cells (Tsuzuki et al., 2007). The concentrations of each of the tocotrienol isomers and those of each of the tocopherol isomers were nearly identical, but the concentrations of the δ-isomers (both tocopherol and tocotrienol) tended to be highest. The authors suggested that the structure of the phytyl chain (saturated or unsaturated) is much more critical for cellular uptake than that of the chromanol ring.

Interestingly, Shibata et al. (2010) demonstrated that the concurrent administration of α-tocopherol with δ-tocotrienol reduced the intracellular concentration of δ-tocotrienol, compared with the administration of δ-tocotrienol alone.

7.3 ACTION MECHANISM OF δ-TOCOTRIENOL FOR COLORECTAL CANCER PREVENTION

7.3.1 Anti-Proliferative Effects

A recent study showed that δ-tocotrienol inhibited cell proliferation in colon cancer cells (Yang et al., 2010). In that study, the 50% inhibitory concentration (IC_{50}) of δ-tocotrienol was 20 μM in human colon carcinoma HCT116 cells and 30 μM in human colon carcinoma HT-29 cells.

Another recent study showed that a mixture of δ-tocotrienol and a novel δ-tocotrienol peroxydimer, extracted from *Kielmeyera coriacea* root bark, suppressed cell growth in human colon cancer HCT-8 cells, and the IC_{50} value was 13.02 μg/mL (de Mesquita et al., 2011).

7.3.2 Induction of Apoptosis and Paraptosis

The tocotrienol-rich fraction (TRF), a fraction of palm oil including mainly α-, γ-, and δ-tocotrienols, together with some amount of α-tocopherol, also induced apoptosis through the activation of p53 and an increase in the Bax/Bcl-2 ratio in human colon carcinoma RKO cells (Agarwal et al., 2004). This effect was independent from the regulation of the cell cycle.

Another study showed that δ-tocotrienol at the concentration of 10 μM induced apoptosis in human colorectal adenocarcinoma DLD-1 cells (Shibata et al., 2010). Importantly, the concurrent administration of α-tocopherol with δ-tocotrienol attenuates these anti-proliferative and proapoptotic effects of δ-tocotrienol in DLD-1 cells. In that paper, the authors also showed that α-tocopherol diminishes the gene expression, including cell cycle arrest genes (CDKN1A, CDKN1B, and GADD45D) and apoptosis-inducing genes (CASP3, CASP7, CASP9, and APAF1). They also showed that α-tocopherol suppresses the protein expression induced by δ-tocotrienol, involving p21 and p27 (cell cycle arrest–related proteins), and cleaved caspase-7 and caspase-9 (apoptosis-inducing proteins). It was proposed that this attenuation of α-tocopherol may be due to the reduction of the cellular uptake of δ-tocotrienol.

Differing from apoptosis and necrosis, paraptosis is defined as a third form of cell death, which is a form of programmed cell death, but does not involve DNA fragmentation or traditional apoptotic body formation (Chen et al., 2002; Sperandio et al., 2000).

It was proposed that δ-tocotrienol induces paraptosis-like cell death in human colon carcinoma SW620 cells, and also that this effect is associated with downregulation of the Wnt signaling pathway involving cyclin D1, c-myc, c-jun, and matrix metalloproteinase-7 (MMP-7; Zhang et al., 2011).

7.3.3 Induction of Cell Cycle Arrest

One paper reported that δ-tocotrienol induced the expression of p21 and p27, both in the genes and protein level in human colorectal adenocarcinoma DLD-1 cells (Shibata et al., 2010). This was not a direct observation, but it demonstrated that δ-tocotrienol has the potency to cause cell cycle arrest on colorectal adenocarcinoma cells, since both p21 and p27 cause cell cycle arrest.

7.3.4 Telomerase Inhibition

The inhibition of telomerase is an anticancer target, since the reactivation of telomerase is detected in most cancer cells (Kim et al., 1994). Another study showed that δ-tocotrienol inhibited telomerase activity in DLD-1 cells in a dose- and time-dependent manner, possibly through the suppression of the mRNA level of human telomerase reverse transcriptase (hTERT) and c-myc via the inhibition of protein kinase C (PKC; Eitsuka et al., 2006).

7.3.5 Synergistic Actions with Anticancer Drugs

Atorvastatin is a statin used to reduce the level of cholesterol and low density lipoproteins through the inhabitation of the 3-hydroxy-3-methylglutaryl coenzyme A (HMG-CoA) reductase. It has been proposed that statin can improve a patient's outcome by reducing invasion and metastasis of colon cancer (Bardou et al., 2010).

Another study showed that δ-tocotrienol demonstrated a synergistic effect with atorvastatin in human colon cancer cells (Yang et al., 2010). In that study, the IC_{50} of δ-tocotrienol alone in HT29 and HCT119 was 30 and 20 μM, respectively, and in combination with atorvastatin, 9 and 3.9 μM, respectively (the ratios of atorvastatin/δ-tocotrienol were 1:1 and 1:5 in HT29 and HCT119, based on the IC_{50} values of atorvastatin alone and δ-tocotrienol alone).

7.3.6 Angiogenesis

The inhibition of angiogenesis is one of the strategies employed to reduce colorectal cancer growth, since neovascularization is necessary for cancer growth and metastasis (Giatromanolaki et al., 2006). In mice injected with human colorectal adenocarcinoma DLD-1 cells, the ingestion of 2.5 or 10 mg/day of tocotrienol extract from palm oil (Tocomin 50, which containing 14% α-tocopherol, 14% α-tocotrienol, 24% γ-tocotrienol, and 6% δ-tocotrienol) significantly reduced the angiogenesis index, which indicates the level of neovascularization in tumors in a dose-dependent manner (Nakagawa et al., 2007). In that paper, incubation with δ-tocotrienol reduced new blood vessel formation in chick embryos. The authors also demonstrated that δ-tocotrienol suppressed fibroblast growth factor (FGF)-induced human umbilical vein endothelial cells (HUVEC) proliferation, migration, and tube formation, which may be associated with both the modification of phosphatidylinositol-3 kinase/PDK/Akt signaling and the induction of apoptosis. Another study showed that δ-tocotrienol also suppressed vascular endothelial growth factor (VEGF)-induced HUVEC proliferation, migration, and tubular formation and induced HUVEC apoptosis, through the inhibition of VEGF receptor 2 signaling and the activation of caspase (Shibata et al., 2009).

Growth factors, such as VEGF and FGF, derived from human colorectal adenocarcinoma DLD-1 cells promoted HUVEC tube formation, proliferation, migration, and adhesion. δ-Tocotrienol at the concentration of 2.5–5 μM significantly suppressed these pro-angiogenetic effects (Shibata et al., 2008b). This effect was also shown in an in vivo study, where DLD-1-Matrigel-containing δ-tocotrienol implanted in mice showed less neovascularization compared with DLD-1-Matrigel alone, and it was proposed that the suppression of the infiltration of CD31/platelet adhesion molecule-1 (PECAM-1) positive endothelial cells was associated with the action mechanisms of δ-tocotrienol (Shibata et al., 2008b).

δ-Tocotrienol inhibited hypoxia-induced VEGF secretion from DLD-1 cells under hypoxic conditions, while normoxic conditions show less effect (Shibata et al., 2008a). The authors also demonstrated that δ-tocotrienol suppressed interleukin-8 (IL-8) in both mRNA and protein levels and COX-2 in the protein level, via inhibition of the hypoxia-inducible factor-1α (HIF-1α) protein expression or by increasing HIF-1α degradation in hypoxia conditions.

These results suggest that δ-tocotrienol has a potential for antiangiogenesis, not only through a direct effect on endothelial cells, but also through interactions between colorectal cancer cells and endothelial cells (Figure 7.1).

7.4 COMPARISON OF ITS BIOACTIVITY BETWEEN TOCOTRIENOL ISOFORMS

Few studies have compared the bioactivity of the various tocotrienol isoforms in colorectal cancer cells. However, one study showed that the IC_{50} of γ- and δ-tocotrienol were 17.5 and 20 μM in human colon carcinoma HCT116 cells and 30 and 30 μM in human colon carcinoma HT-29 cells, respectively (Yang et al., 2010).

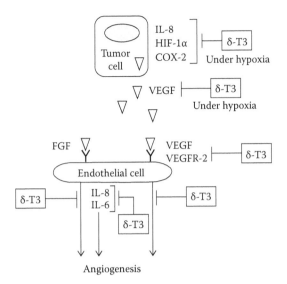

FIGURE 7.1 Anti-angiogenetic effects of δ-tocotrienol. δ-Tocotrienol suppresses endothelial-cell proliferation, which is induced by either FGF or VEGF. δ-Tocotrienol also reduces VEGFR-2 protein expression and
suppresses IL-8 and IL-6 in HUVEC cells. In human colorectal adenocarcinoma DLD-1 cells, δ-tocotrienol
suppresses VEGF secretion and decreases mRNA expression of IL-8 and HIF-1α and protein expression of
HIF-1α and COX-2 under hypoxia condition. Abbreviations: T3, tocotrienol; FGF, fibroblast growth factor;
VEGF, vascular endothelial growth factor; VEGFR-2, vascular endothelial growth factor receptor 2; HUVEC,
human umbilical vein endothelial cells; IL-8, interleukin-8; HIF-1α, hypoxia-inducible factor-1α; COX-2,
cyclooxygenase-2; IL-6, interleukin-6.

Both β- and δ-tocotrienol, but not α- and γ-tocotrienol, had a significant telomerase inhibitory
effect in human colorectal adenocarcinoma DLD-1 cells, and δ-tocotrienol showed a greater effect
than β-tocotrienol (Eitsuka et al., 2006).

A comparison study was conducted on the tumor necrosis factor-α (TNF-α) suppression activity
among α-, γ-, and δ-tocotrienol (Qureshi et al., 2010). In that study, δ-tocotrienol showed the most
significant reducing effect on TNF-α concentration, both in macrophage culture supernatant and
in mice serum.

A study employing an oral administration of γ- and δ-tocotrienol reduced the volume of the
injected tumors, and δ-tocotrienol had more significant effects in male C3H/HeN mice (Hiura et al.,
2009).

In regard to the inhibitory effect of angiogenesis, all of the tocotrienol isomers had an antiproliferative effect on HUVEC proliferation, which is induced by FGF. IC$_{50}$ of α-, β-, γ-, and
δ-tocotrienol were 13.1 ± 0.2, 9.4 ± 0.2, 9.4 ± 0.2, and 5.5 ± 0.1 μmol/L, respectively (Nakagawa
et al., 2007), and δ-tocotrienol showed the most significant suppressive effect.

Similarly, δ-tocotrienol showed the most significant potency for the inhibition of VEGF-
induced HUVEC proliferation (Shibata et al., 2009). After 72 h of incubation of HUVEC with
each of the isoforms, δ-tocotrienol tended to suppress cell proliferation most significantly, followed
by β-tocotrienol and γ-, and α-tocotrienol showed the weakest effect, but it was still significant.
The tocotrienol uptake of α-, β-, γ-, and δ-tocotrienol was 6.0 ± 0.5, 7.4 ± 1.2, 7.6 ± 0.3, and 7.9 ±
0.8 nmol/mg protein of HUVEC, when the cells were incubated with 1 μM of the tocotrienol isoforms. The authors of that paper proposed a correlation between the degree of the anti-angiogenesis
property and the intracellular concentration of the tocotrienols.

In another study, also employing HUVEC cells, δ-tocotrienol showed the most suppressive potency
for pro-angiogenic cytokine, IL-8 and IL-6, followed by γ-tocotrienol and TRF (Selvaduray et al., 2012).

Under hypoxia conditions, the VEGF suppressive potency was δ- > β- > γ- > α-tocotrienol in
DLD-1 cells (Shibata et al., 2008a).

7.5 PROPOSED MECHANISM OF δ-TOCOTRIENOL FOR THE PREVENTION OF COLORECTAL CANCER

δ-Tocotrienol and its included compounds demonstrated a suppressive effect on colorectal cancer, and the induction of cell death, telomerase inhibition, antiangiogenesis, and anti-inflammation were the proposed mechanisms. There are other proposed action mechanisms for δ-tocotrienol related to colorectal cancer therapy, but to date, these have not been proven directly.

7.5.1 MODIFICATION OF MICROFLORA

It has been reported that gut microbiota play an important role in carcinogenesis, and the increasing number of bifidobacterium is associated with a reduced colorectal cancer risk (Roberfroid et al., 2010). The ingestion of vitamin E (2 g α-tocopherol/kg basal diet) increased the fecal bifidobacteria concentration, compared with a nontreatment group in D-galactose-induced hepatic Balb/cJ mice (Chen et al., 2011). Since α-tocopherol was administered as an antioxidant positive control, tocotrienols may show the same property to some extent.

Albermann et al. (2008) reported the biosynthesis of δ-tocotrienol in recombinant *Escherichia coli*, which are nonphotosynthetic microorganisms, although in general, tocochromanols are synthesized in photosynthetic organisms.

7.5.2 MODIFICATION OF IMMUNITY

The oral administration of TRF enhanced the antitumor activity of dendritic cell vaccines in mice, which were inoculated with murine metastatic mammary gland tumor 4T1 cells (Hafid et al., 2010). In that paper, dendritic cell vaccines with tumor lysate from 4T1 cells together with TRF ingestion showed the most significant tumor-suppressive effect through increasing the population of natural killer cells and CD8 cells.

7.5.3 MODIFICATION OF TUMOR–STROMAL INTERACTION

It has been proposed that stromal cells, such as macrophages or fibroblasts, play a critical role in colorectal carcinogenesis. The suppression of TNF-α is an important strategy for colorectal cancer prevention, since it has been proposed that a high TNF-α expression in colorectal cancer cells is associated with positive lymph node status and recurrence of the tumor in patients (Grimm et al., 2010).

TNF-α derived from colon cancer cells activated stromal macrophages, and then it induced colony-stimulating factor-1 (CSF-1) and TNF-α in macrophages and enhanced its own TNF-α expression. CSF-1 derived from macrophages stimulated the expression of MMP-2 and VEGF-A through CSF-1 receptors. These interactions between cancer cells and stromal macrophages stimulate colon carcinogenesis at least partially, since TNF-α, MMP-2, and VEGF-A promote macrophage recruitment, extracellular matrix remodeling, and endothelial cell proliferation, respectively (Zins et al., 2007).

From these results, the reduction of TNF-α may be an effective chemopreventive approach. Qureshi et al. (2010) demonstrated that δ-tocotrienol inhibited TNF-α, both in vitro and in vivo, and it decreased the TNF-α concentration in lipopolysaccharide (LPS)-stimulated murine macrophage RAW 264.7 cells and reduced the serum level of TNF-α in LPS-stimulated BALB/c mice. Cyclooxygenase-2 (COX-2) derived from macrophages promotes tumorigenic progression of intestinal epithelial cells, through the induction of its COX-2 expression and cell proliferation, as well as the suppression of cell-to-cell contact inhibition, membranous E-cadherin, and the transforming growth factor-β type II receptors (TGF-β RII; Ko et al., 2002). TRF inhibited the LPS-induced COX-2 expression, but not COX-1 in human monocyte cells (Wu et al., 2008).

7.5.4 Prevention of Cachexia

There is an association between the serum level of acute-phase response proteins and cytokines, including TNF-α, and prognosis of colorectal cancer patients (Kemik et al., 2010). The authors of that study suggested that body weight loss was inversely correlated to the serum level of adiponectin, which may be downregulated by TNF-α. The treatment of TNF-α reduction may prevent cachexia, and one paper stated that supplementation of δ-tocotrienol (125 μM/kg) for 4 weeks reduced the serum level of TNF-α and nitric oxide in female chicken (Qureshi et al., 2011).

7.5.5 Suppression of Cancer Stem Cells

Ricci-Vitiani et al. (2007) demonstrated that colorectal cancer is created and propagated by CD133[+] cells, which have lost their differentiation properties and whose proportion in the tumor cells is about 2.5%. In prostate cancer, γ-tocotrienol downregulates the expression of prostate cancer stem cell markers (Luk et al., 2011). These data may suggest that tocotrienols are also inhibitory for colorectal cancer stem cells.

7.6 EFFECTIVE INTAKE OF δ-TOCOTRIENOL FROM DAILY FOODS

It has been proposed that α-tocopherol reduces the anti-proliferative effect of δ-tocotrienol on colorectal cancer through reducing cellular uptake (Shibata et al., 2010). Most natural resources of δ-tocotrienol, for example, brown rice or safflower oil, contain α-tocopherol, and the concentration of α-tocopherol is much higher than δ-tocotrienol (Franke et al., 2007; Sookwong et al., 2010). The daily food intake of tocotrienol may possibly attenuate its properties by α-tocopherol within the food. Adzuki beans, which are often consumed in Japan as sweets, have a unique ratio of vitamin E, containing 4.44 ± 0.04 mg/kg of δ-tocotrienol, but α-tocopherol was not detectable (Sookwong et al., 2010). GPNO2016 brown rice has a high concentration of δ-tocotrienol (31.84 μg/g), but it has a rather low concentration of α-tocopherol (1.89 μg/g; Min et al., 2011). Applying these foods in a human trial may be one strategy to study the reduction of the interference of α-tocopherol to δ-tocotrienol uptake.

7.7 CONCLUSION

δ-Tocotrienol demonstrated anticancer properties through several action mechanisms, such as the induction of apoptosis and paraptosis-like cell death, telomerase inhibition, and the suppression of angiogenesis in *in vitro* studies (Table 7.1), and it seems that δ-tocotrienol is the most potent agent between the isoforms with regard to the prevention of colorectal cancer. However, few animal studies have been conducted, and no data have demonstrated direct tumor-suppressive effects against colorectal cancer (Table 7.2). The data accumulated to date is not sufficient to completely reveal the effects of δ-tocotrienol and its mechanisms, especially for clinical application. In addition, the distribution of δ-tocotrienol to colon tissue has not yet been clearly elucidated. In colorectal cancer, unlike other types of cancer, δ-tocotrienol may possibly have an effect both hematogenously and via gut lumen. The uptake interference of α-tocopherol was suggested, but other interactions have not been investigated yet. After these other interactions have been clarified to some extent, human trials will be conducted employing δ-tocotrienol to examine its effect as preventive treatment for colorectal cancer. The World Cancer Research Fund and American Institute for Cancer Research concluded that the evidence of vitamin E protecting against colorectal cancer is not sufficient (World Cancer Research Fund, 2007) up to the date of 2007. A lot of progress in tocotrienol research has been made within the last few years, and these results suggest that tocotrienol, especially δ-tocotrienol, is a promising agent for the prevention of colorectal cancer.

TABLE 7.1

Anticancer Effect of δ-Tocotrienol in In Vitro Studies

Effective Isoforms	No or Slight Effect	Type of Tumor	Action Mechanism	Reference
Antiproliferation				
γ-T3 > δ-T3		Human colon carcinoma HCT116 cells	IC_{50}: γ-T3 17.5 μM, δ-T3 20 μM	Yang et al. (2010)
γ-T3 = δ-T3		Human colon carcinoma HT-29 cells	IC_{50}: γ-T3 30 μM, δ-T3 30 μM	Yang et al. (2010)
δ-T3 and δ-T3 peroxy-dimer		Human colon cancer HCT-8	IC_{50}: mixture of δ-T3 and δ-T3 peroxy-dimer 13.2 μM	de Mesquita et al. (2011)
Proapoptosis				
TRF		Human colon carcinoma RKO cells	Activated p53, increased Bax/Bcl-2 ratio	Agarwal et al. (2004)
δ-T3		Human colorectal adenocarcinoma DlD-1 cells	Induced caspase-3, -7, and -9	Shibata et al. (2010)
Paraptosis-like cell death				
δ-T3		Human colon carcinoma SW620 cells	Reduced β-catenin, Wnt, cyclin D1, c-jun, and MMP-7	Zhang et al. (2011)
Cell cycle arrest				
δ-T3		Human colorectal adenocarcinoma DlD-1 cells	Induced p21 and p27	Shibata et al. (2010)
Telomerase inhibition				
δ-T3 > β-T3	α-, γ-T3	Human colorectal adenocarcinoma DlD-1 cells	Suppressed mRNA expression of hTERT and c-myc via inhibition of PKC	Eitsuka et al. (2006)
Antiangiogenesis				
δ-T3 > β-, γ-T3 > α-T3		HUVEC cells	Suppressed FGF-induced cell proliferation	Nakagawa et al. (2007)
δ-T3		HUVEC cells	Suppressed FGF-induced migration and tube formation	Nakagawa et al. (2007)
δ-T3		HUVEC cells treated with conditioned medium of human colorectal adenocarcinoma DLD-1 cells	Suppressed VEGF-induced cell proliferation, migration, tube formation, and adhesion	Shibata et al. (2008b)
δ-T3 > β-T3 > γ-T3 > α-T3		HUVEC cells	Suppressed VEGF-induced cell proliferation	Shibata et al. (2009)
δ-T3 > γ-T3 > TRF		HUVEC cells	Suppressed proangiogenic cytokine, IL-8, and IL-6	Selvaduray et al. (2012)
δ-T3 > β-T3 > γ-T3 > α-T3		Human colorectal adenocarcinoma DLD-1 cells	Suppressed VEGF secretion under hypoxia condition	Shibata et al. (2008a)

TABLE 7.1 (continued)
Anticancer Effect of δ-Tocotrienol in In Vitro Studies

Effective Isoforms	No or Slight Effect	Type of Tumor	Action Mechanism	Reference
δ-T3		Human colorectal adenocarcinoma DLD-1 cells	Suppressed IL-8, HIF-1α, and COX-2 under hypoxia condition	Shibata et al. (2008a)
Anti-inflammation				
δ-T3 > γ-T3 > β-T3	α-T3	Macrophage RAW 264 cells	Suppressed TNF-α	Qureshi et al. (2010)

Abbreviations: T3, tocotrienol; IC50, 50% inhibitory concentration; TRF, tocotrienol-rich fraction; MMP-7, matrix metalloproteinase; hTERT, human telomerase reverse transcriptase; PKC, protein kinase C; HUVEC, human umbilical vein endothelial cells; FGF, fibroblast growth factor; VEGF, vascular endothelial growth factor; IL-8, interleukin-8; HIF-1α, hypoxia-inducible factor-1α; COX-2, cyclooxygenase-2; TNF-α, tumor necrosis factor-α.

TABLE 7.2
Anticancer Effects of δ-Tocotrienol in Animal Studies

Effective Isoforms	No or Slight Effect	Effect	Reference
Tumor volume reduction			
δ-T3 > γ-T3		Suppressed the growth of tumor (implanted murine hepatoma MG134 cells) in C3H/HeN mice	Hiura et al. (2009)
Suppression of vessel formation			
Tocotrienol extract from palm oil (14% α-tocopherol, 14% α-tocotrienol, 24% γ-tocotrienol, and 6% δ-tocotrienol)	α-T1	Suppressed neovascularization of tumor (implanted colorectal adenocarcinoma DLD-1 cells) in ICR mice	Nakagawa et al. (2007)
δ-T3		Increased the frequency of avascular zone of chick embryos	Nakagawa et al. (2007)
δ-T3		Inhibited tumor (implanted colorectal adenocarcinoma DLD-1 cells) induced angiogenesis in nude mice	Shibata et al. (2008b)
δ-T3	α-T1	Inhibited tumor (implanted colorectal adenocarcinoma DLD-1 cells, which were treated with VEGF) induced angiogenesis in nude mice	Shibata et al. (2009)
Anti-inflammation			
δ-T3 > γ-T3 > β-T3	α-T3	Suppressed serum level of TNF-α in LPS-stimulated BALC/c mice	Qureshi et al. (2010)
δ-T3		Reduced serum level of TNF-α and NO in female chicken	Qureshi et al. (2011)

Abbreviations: T3, tocotrienol; T1, tocopherol; VEGF, vascular endothelial growth factor; TNF-α, tumor necrosis factor-α; LPS, lipopolysaccharide; NO, nitric oxide.

REFERENCES

Agarwal, M. K., Agarwal, M. L., Athar, M., and Gupta, S., 2004. Tocotrienol-rich fraction of palm oil activates p53, modulates Bax/Bcl2 ratio and induces apoptosis independent of cell cycle association. *Cell Cycle* 3 (2):205–211.

Albermann, C., Ghanegaonkar, S., Lemuth, K. et al., 2008. Biosynthesis of the vitamin E compound delta-tocotrienol in recombinant Escherichia coli cells. *Chembiochem* 9 (15):2524–2533.

Anand, P., Kunnumakkara, A. B., Sundaram, C. et al., 2008. Cancer is a preventable disease that requires major lifestyle changes. *Pharm Res* 25 (9):2097–2116.

Bardou, M., Barkun, A., and Martel, M., 2010. Effect of statin therapy on colorectal cancer. *Gut* 59 (11):1572–1585.

Chen, Y., Douglass, T., Jeffes, E. W. et al., 2002. Living T9 glioma cells expressing membrane macrophage colony-stimulating factor produce immediate tumor destruction by polymorphonuclear leukocytes and macrophages via a "paraptosis"-induced pathway that promotes systemic immunity against intracranial T9 gliomas. *Blood* 100 (4):1373–1380.

Chen, H. L., Wang, C. H., Kuo, Y. W., and Tsai, C. H., 2011. Antioxidative and hepatoprotective effects of fructo-oligosaccharide in d-galactose-treated Balb/cJ mice. *Br J Nutr* 105 (6):805–809.

de Mesquita, M. L., Araujo, R. M., Bezerra, D. P. et al., 2011. Cytotoxicity of delta-tocotrienols from Kielmeyera coriacea against cancer cell lines. *Bioorg Med Chem* 19 (1):623–630.

Eitsuka, T., Nakagawa, K., and Miyazawa, T., 2006. Down-regulation of telomerase activity in DLD-1 human colorectal adenocarcinoma cells by tocotrienol. *Biochem Biophys Res Commun* 348 (1):170–175.

Franke, A. A., Murphy, S. P., Lacey, R., and Custer, L. J., 2007. Tocopherol and tocotrienol levels of foods consumed in Hawaii. *J Agric Food Chem* 55 (3):769–778.

Giatromanolaki, A., Sivridis, E., and Koukourakis, M. I., 2006. Angiogenesis in colorectal cancer: prognostic and therapeutic implications. *Am J Clin Oncol* 29 (4):408–417.

Grimm, M., Lazariotou, M., Kircher, S. et al., 2010. Tumor necrosis factor-alpha is associated with positive lymph node status in patients with recurrence of colorectal cancer - indications for anti-TNF-alpha agents in cancer treatment. *Anal Cell Pathol (Amst)* 33 (3):151–163.

Hafid, S. R., Radhakrishnan, A. K., and Nesaretnam, K. 2010. Tocotrienols are good adjuvants for developing cancer vaccines. *BMC Cancer* 10:5.

He, L., Mo, H., Hadisusilo, S., Qureshi, A. A., and Elson, C. E. 1997. Isoprenoids suppress the growth of murine B16 melanomas in vitro and in vivo. *J Nutr* 127 (5):668–674.

Hiura, Y., Tachibana, H., Arakawa, R. et al., 2009. Specific accumulation of gamma- and delta-tocotrienols in tumor and their antitumor effect in vivo. *J Nutr Biochem* 20 (8):607–613.

Jemal, A., Bray, F., Center, M. M. et al., 2011. Global cancer statistics. *CA Cancer J Clin* 61 (2):69–90.

Kemik, O., Sumer, A., Kemik, A. S. et al., 2010. The relationship among acute-phase response proteins, cytokines and hormones in cachectic patients with colon cancer. *World J Surg Oncol* 8:85.

Kim, N. W., Piatyszek, M. A., Prowse, K. R. et al., 1994. Specific association of human telomerase activity with immortal cells and cancer. *Science* 266 (5193):2011–2015.

Ko, S. C., Chapple, K. S., Hawcroft, G. et al., 2002. Paracrine cyclooxygenase-2-mediated signalling by macrophages promotes tumorigenic progression of intestinal epithelial cells. *Oncogene* 21 (47):7175–7186.

Luk, S. U., Yap, W. N., Chiu, Y. T. et al., 2011. Gamma-tocotrienol as an effective agent in targeting prostate cancer stem cell-like population. *Int J Cancer* 128 (9):2182–2191.

McIntyre, B. S., Briski, K. P., Gapor, A., and Sylvester, P. W. 2000. Antiproliferative and apoptotic effects of tocopherols and tocotrienols on preneoplastic and neoplastic mouse mammary epithelial cells. *Proc Soc Exp Biol Med* 224 (4):292–301.

Min, B., McClung, A. M., and Chen, M. H., 2011. Phytochemicals and antioxidant capacities in rice brans of different color. *J Food Sci* 76 (1):C117–C126.

Nakagawa, K., Shibata, A., Yamashita, S. et al., 2007. In vivo angiogenesis is suppressed by unsaturated vitamin E, tocotrienol. *J Nutr* 137 (8):1938–1943.

Park, Y., Spiegelman, D., Hunter, D. J. et al. 2010. Intakes of vitamins A, C, and E and use of multiple vitamin supplements and risk of colon cancer: a pooled analysis of prospective cohort studies. *Cancer Causes Control* 21 (11):1745–1757.

Qureshi, A. A., Reis, J. C., Papasian, C. J., Morrison, D. C., and Qureshi, N., 2010. Tocotrienols inhibit lipopolysaccharide-induced pro-inflammatory cytokines in macrophages of female mice. *Lipids Health Dis* 9:143.

Qureshi, A. A., Reis, J. C., Qureshi, N. et al., 2011. delta-Tocotrienol and quercetin reduce serum levels of nitric oxide and lipid parameters in female chickens. *Lipids Health Dis* 10:39.

Rasool, A. H., Yuen, K. H., Yusoff, K., Wong, A. R., and Rahman, A. R., 2006. Dose dependent elevation of plasma tocotrienol levels and its effect on arterial compliance, plasma total antioxidant status, and lipid profile in healthy humans supplemented with tocotrienol rich vitamin E. *J Nutr Sci Vitaminol (Tokyo)* 52 (6):473–478.

Ricci-Vitiani, L., Lombardi, D. G., Pilozzi, E. et al., 2007. Identification and expansion of human colon-cancer-initiating cells. *Nature* 445 (7123):111–115.

Roberfroid, M., Gibson, G. R., Hoyles, L. et al., 2010. Prebiotic effects: metabolic and health benefits. *Br J Nutr* 104(Suppl 2):S1–S63.

Selvaduray, K. R., Radhakrishnan, A. K., Kutty, M. K., and Nesaretnam, K., 2012. Palm tocotrienols decrease levels of pro-angiogenic markers in human umbilical vein endothelial cells (HUVEC) and murine mammary cancer cells. *Genes Nutr* 7(1):53–61.

Shah, S., Gapor, A., and Sylvester, P. W. 2003. Role of caspase-8 activation in mediating vitamin E-induced apoptosis in murine mammary cancer cells. *Nutr Cancer* 45 (2):236–246.

Shibata, A., Nakagawa, K., Sookwong, P. et al., 2008a. Tocotrienol inhibits secretion of angiogenic factors from human colorectal adenocarcinoma cells by suppressing hypoxia-inducible factor-1alpha. *J Nutr* 138 (11):2136–2142.

Shibata, A., Nakagawa, K., Sookwong, P. et al., 2008b. Tumor anti-angiogenic effect and mechanism of action of delta-tocotrienol. *Biochem Pharmacol* 76 (3):330–339.

Shibata, A., Nakagawa, K., Sookwong, P. et al., 2009. delta-Tocotrienol suppresses VEGF induced angiogenesis whereas alpha-tocopherol does not. *J Agric Food Chem* 57 (18):8696–8704.

Shibata, A., Nakagawa, K., Sookwong, P. et al., 2010. alpha-Tocopherol attenuates the cytotoxic effect of delta-tocotrienol in human colorectal adenocarcinoma cells. *Biochem Biophys Res Commun* 397 (2):214–219.

Sookwong, P., Nakagawa, K., Yamaguchi, Y. et al., 2010. Tocotrienol distribution in foods: estimation of daily tocotrienol intake of Japanese population. *J Agric Food Chem* 58 (6):3350–3355.

Sperandio, S., de Belle, I., and Bredesen, D. E., 2000. An alternative, nonapoptotic form of programmed cell death. *Proc Natl Acad Sci USA* 97 (26):14376–14381.

Tsuzuki, W., Yunoki, R., and Yoshimura, H., 2007. Intestinal epithelial cells absorb gamma-tocotrienol faster than alpha-tocopherol. *Lipids* 42 (2):163–170.

Wada, S., Satomi, Y., Murakoshi, M. et al., 2005. Tumor suppressive effects of tocotrienol in vivo and in vitro. *Cancer Lett* 229 (2):181–191.

Williams, C. D., Satia, J. A., Adair, L. S. et al. 2010. Antioxidant and DNA methylation-related nutrients and risk of distal colorectal cancer. *Cancer Causes Control* 21 (8):1171–1181.

World Cancer Research Fund & American Institute for Cancer Research (2007). Cancers; Colon and rectum, In: *Food, Nutrition, Physical Activity, and the Prevention of Cancer: A Global Perspective*. American Institute for Cancer Research: Washington, DC.

Wu, S. J., Liu, P. L., and Ng, L. T., 2008. Tocotrienol-rich fraction of palm oil exhibits anti-inflammatory property by suppressing the expression of inflammatory mediators in human monocytic cells. *Mol Nutr Food Res* 52 (8):921–929.

Yang, Z., Lee, M. J., Zhao, Y., and Yang, C. S., 2012. Metabolism of tocotrienols in animals and synergistic inhibitory actions of tocotrienols with atorvastatin in cancer cells. *Genes Nutr* 7(1):11–18.

Yang, Z., Xiao, H., Jin, H. et al., 2010. Synergistic actions of atorvastatin with gamma-tocotrienol and celecoxib against human colon cancer HT29 and HCT116 cells. *Int J Cancer* 126 (4):852–863.

Yu, W., Simmons-Menchaca, M., Gapor, A., Sanders, B. G., and Kline, K., 1999. Induction of apoptosis in human breast cancer cells by tocopherols and tocotrienols. *Nutr Cancer* 33 (1):26–32.

Zhang, J. S., Li, D. M., He, N. et al., 2011. A paraptosis-like cell death induced by delta-tocotrienol in human colon carcinoma SW620 cells is associated with the suppression of the Wnt signaling pathway. *Toxicology* 285 (1–2):8–17.

Zins, K., Abraham, D., Sioud, M., and Aharinejad, S., 2007. Colon cancer cell-derived tumor necrosis factor-alpha mediates the tumor growth-promoting response in macrophages by up-regulating the colony-stimulating factor-1 pathway. *Cancer Res* 67 (3):1038–1045.

8 Targeted Prostate Cancer Chemoprevention Trial with Tocotrienols

William L. Stone, Victoria P. Ramsauer,
Sharon E. Campbell, and Koymangalath Krishnan

CONTENTS

8.1 INTRODUCTION

Over the last two decades, an enormous amount of scientific effort has been devoted to studying the relationship between vitamin E and prostate cancer. This effort is well justified, since prostate cancer remains the most common cancer in American men after skin cancer and is the second leading cause of cancer deaths: over 220,000 men will develop prostate each year (U.S. Cancer Statistics Working Group 2011). Nevertheless, large-scale, well-designed clinical intervention studies have not shown that alpha-tocopherol prevents prostate cancer or cancer in general (Lippman et al. 2009; Ju et al. 2010; Wada 2012). Alpha-tocopherol is the primary form of vitamin E in the plasma of fasting subjects and the primary form of vitamin E in most vitamin supplements. Gamma-tocopherol is, however, the primary dietary form of vitamin E. Vitamin E is a term that refers to at least eight different compounds that fall into two general categories: tocopherols and tocotrienols. Tocotrienols are normally not present in human plasma at detectable levels, yet the evidence for their role in preventing prostate cancer is both extensive and compelling (Conte et al. 2004; Srivastava and Gupta 2006; McAnally et al. 2007; Barve et al. 2009; Campbell et al. 2011; Luk et al. 2011). Excellent reviews are available on the general anticancer effects of tocotrienols (Wada 2009, 2012; Ju et al. 2010). It is unlikely that an anticancer effect could be achieved by consuming a tocotrienol rich diet, and instead a supplement—possibly in the form of a soft gel—would be necessary. Despite the ever-increasing data supporting the antiprostate cancer role of tocotrienols, a well-designed chemoprevention trial has yet to be conducted. Given the negative results with alpha-tocopherol chemoprevention trials, a future prostate cancer chemoprevention trial with another isoform of vitamin E must be well justified and designed. Moreover, the cost effectiveness of any future tocotrienol chemoprevention trial must be given high priority.

This chapter will focus on the issues, obstacles, and research gaps related to the design of a future prostate cancer chemoprevention trial for tocotrienols. William et al. (2009) have provided an excellent review of the key concepts involved in the design of cost-effective chemoprevention trials. The framework established by these investigators, particularly with respect to molecular targets for cancer, is central to the design presented here. As will be detailed later, the synergistic ability of tocotrienols and statins to suppress the level and activity of 3-hydroxy-3-methylglutaryl (HMG)-CoA reductase provides a powerful therapeutic strategy for reducing the risk of both prostate cancer and cardiovascular disease. Before discussing the various aspects of a tocotrienol prostate cancer chemoprevention trial, it is first important to make a clear distinction between tocopherols and tocotrienols.

8.2 VITAMIN E IS BOTH TOCOPHEROLS AND TOCOTRIENOLS

Most early research linking vitamin E with cancer did not carefully distinguish between the different isoforms of this lipid-soluble vitamin. More recent research has, for the most part, been fairly explicit about the particular isoform of vitamin E used in an investigation, but superficial summaries and press releases typically refer only to "vitamin E" without specifying a particular isoform. This nomenclature issue is very problematic in the case where a large-scale clinical trial reports a negative result for one vitamin E isoform (e.g., all racemic-alpha-tocopherol), which is then extrapolated to all isoforms. Even the National Cancer Institutes webpage "Antioxidants and Cancer Prevention: Fact Sheet" (see http://www.cancer.gov/cancertopics/factsheet/prevention/antioxidants) fails to specify the particular isoform of vitamin E used in a particular investigation.

8.2.1 Vitamin E Isoforms Have Distinct Chemical, Biological, and Anticancer Properties

The first task of this review will be to point out the critical differences in the structure, biological properties, and anticancer effects of the vitamin E isoforms. Vitamin E's function has historically been associated with its antioxidant properties. It is now recognized, however, that vitamin E has important non-antioxidant roles, can function as a pro-oxidant under some circumstances, and can mediate cell signaling and gene expression (Azzi and Stocker 2000; Azzi et al. 2004). Vitamin E refers to at least four tocopherols (alpha-, beta-, gamma-, and delta) and four corresponding tocotrienols. Figure 8.1 shows the structural elements of the eight naturally occurring vitamin E isoforms with particular attention to the correct stereochemistry and the atom numbering on the chroman head (Moss). Tocopherols have a phytyl tail that is fully saturated with no double bonds whereas tocotrienols have an unsaturated farnesyl isoprenoid tail with three double bonds. The position and

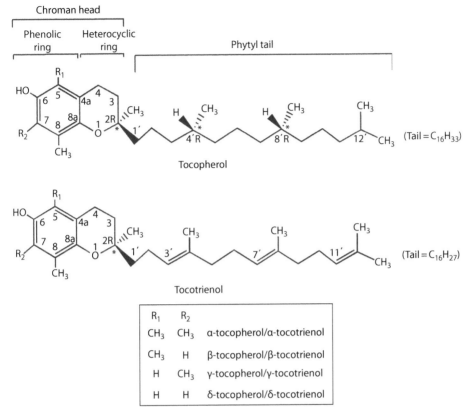

FIGURE 8.1 Structure of vitamin E.

number of the methyl groups on the chromanol ring determine the alpha-, beta-, gamma-, or delta-designation for both tocopherols and tocotrienols.

Although the structural differences between the various vitamin E isoforms may seem minor, they are nevertheless quite important in determining marked differences in their chemistry and biological properties (Cooney et al. 1993, 1995; Devaraj and Traber 2003; Stone and Papas 2003). The only difference between alpha-tocopherol and gamma-tocopherol is the lack of a methyl group at position 5 on the chromanol ring (see Figure 8.1), yet this results in major differences in chemical reactivity, particularly with respect to reactive nitric oxide species (RNOS; Cooney et al. 1993).

Peroxynitrite (ONOO–) is a RNOS formed by the very rapid reaction between nitric oxide (NO) and the superoxide radical, $O2^{\bullet-}$. ONOO– can undergo a heterolytic cleavage to form a nitronium ion, which subsequently nitrates protein tyrosine residues forming 3-nitrotyrosine. The level of 3-nitrotyrosine on proteins is a measure of *in vivo* peroxynitrite formation. Jiang et al. (2002) found that gamma-tocopherol inhibits 3-nitrotyrosine formation in rats with inflammation, an effect attributed to gamma-tocopherol's ability to trap peroxynitrite to form 5-nitro-gamma-tocopherol. This reaction is not possible with alpha-tocopherol, which has a methyl group at the 5-position (Christen et al. 1997; Jiang et al. 2002). The process of inflammation and the formation of 3-nitrotyrosine are relevant to prostate cancer. Floriano-Sánchez et al. (2009) found 3-nitrotyrosine levels to be about fivefold higher in paraffin-embedded prostate tissues from prostate cancer subjects compared to subjects with benign prostatic hyperplasia. Although not yet reported in the literature, it would also be expected that gamma-tocotrienol would have a chromanol ring chemistry similar to that of gamma-tocopherol.

In addition to unique chemistries, the different isoforms of tocopherol have different anticancer effects (Stone and Papas 1997; Campbell et al. 2003, 2006; Stone et al. 2004). This is well illustrated by the work of Yu et al. (2009) who found that RRR-alpha-tocopherol (the isoform used in many chemoprevention trials) not only did not have an anticancer effect, but actually inhibited the *in vitro* and *in vivo* anticancer effects of RRR-gamma-tocopherol.

8.2.2 TOCOTRIENOLS, BUT NOT TOCOPHEROLS, ARE FARNESYLATED BENZOPYRANS AND HAVE UNIQUE EFFECTS ON ISOPRENOID AND CHOLESTEROL SYNTHESIS

The alterations in the biological properties of vitamin E isoforms caused by differences between the phytyl tail and the farnesyl tail are just as profound as those caused by differences in the number and position of the methyl groups on the chromanol ring. Tocotrienols with a farnesyl tail induce prenyl pyrophosphate pyrophosphatase, which catalyzes the dephosphorylation of farnesyl diphosphate to form farnesol (Theriault et al. 1999; Mo and Elson 2004). Farnesol, in turn, downregulates the activity of HMGCoA reductase by a posttranscriptional mechanism.

HMGCoA reductase is the committed step for the biosynthesis of isoprenoids and sterols such as cholesterol. Tocotrienols, by decreasing the level of HMGCoA reductase, decrease plasma total cholesterol levels and low-density lipoprotein (LDL)-cholesterol in humans and animal models (Qureshi et al. 1986, 2001, 2002). Tocopherols with a phytyl tail exhibit none of these remarkable alterations in cholesterol metabolism. Moreover, Qureshi et al. (1996) found that alpha-tocopherol attenuates the ability of gamma-tocotrienol to suppress HMGCoA reductase and to lower plasma cholesterol levels in a chicken model. Qureshi et al. (1996) did not distinguish between RRR-alpha-tocopherol, the natural form found in foods, and all-racemic-alpha-tocopherol, the synthetic form found in most soft-gel supplements. Khor and Ng (2000) were able to reproduce the results of Qureshi et al. (1996) using male hamsters, where tocotrienols caused hypocholesterolemia and suppressed HMGCoA reductase—effects that were attenuated by alpha-tocopherol.

As first suggested by Qureshi et al. (1996), the alterations in farnesyl metabolism caused by tocotrienols are a key to understanding some of its anticancer effects. It is also remarkable that tocotrienols can reduce atherosclerotic lesions in the apoE(−/−) mouse model (with a low fat diet) to a fourfold higher extent than alpha-tocopherol (Qureshi et al. 2002).

Statins are widely prescribed drugs for treating hyperlipidemia that inhibit HMGCoA reductase, but by binding to the active site and blocking substrate access. In hypercholesterolemic humans, tocotrienols plus lovastatin act synergistically to lower serum total cholesterol and LDL-cholesterol, whereas alpha-tocopherol does nothing more to lipid parameters than lovastatin alone (Qureshi et al. 2001). As will be discussed later, the synergy between tocotrienols and statins in lowering serum cholesterol is paralleled by a synergistic anticancer effect.

8.2.3 ALPHA-TOCOPHEROL CAN INTERFERE WITH THE ANTICANCER EFFECTS OF TOCOTRIENOLS

Shibata et al. (2010) recently investigated the ability of alpha-tocopherol to attenuate the cytotoxic effects of delta-tocotrienol on colorectal adenocarcinoma cells. Delta-tocotrienol alone induced cell-cycle arrest and proapoptotic gene/protein expression, all of which were attenuated by the presence of alpha-tocopherol. The investigators also looked into a possible mechanism for this attenuation and found that alpha-tocopherol decreased the cellular uptake of delta-tocotrienol in a dose-dependent manner (Shibata et al. 2010). This result needs to be tested in other cancer cell lines and in appropriate animal models. Many commercial preparations of tocotrienols have high levels of alpha-tocopherol, which could severely diminish the anticancer and hypocholesterolemic effects of the tocotrienols. This is an important consideration in the design of a future prostate cancer chemoprevention trial.

8.3 TOCOTRIENOLS AND TARGETED CHEMOPREVENTION FOR PROSTATE CANCER

Tocotrienols hold the promise of being very cost-effective chemopreventive agents that could be consumed as a dietary supplement over a long time period with minimal side effects. Chemoprevention is the "Holy Grail" for preventing prostate cancer, which is primarily a disease of aging and is unique in having a long latency period during which cancer growth is slow, causes few symptoms, and provides a long window of opportunity for intervention. Prostate cancer is preceded by prostatic intraepithelial neoplasia (PIN) that is characterized by an increased proliferative ability of prostate gland cells and morphological alterations. Chemopreventive agents are particularly well suited for decreasing prostate cancer mortality by extending the time during which PIN progresses to prostate cancer. In the United States, only about 15% of men diagnosed with prostate cancer actually die from prostate cancer. The notion that men with prostate cancer are more likely to die "with prostate cancer" rather than "because of prostate cancer" has recently been challenged by new data from the United Kingdom showing that, in this population, prostate cancer causes about 50% of the deaths of men diagnosed with this disease (Chustecka 2011). The difference between the U.S. data and the U.K. data may, at least in part, be attributable to the higher prevalence of prostate specific antigen (PSA) screening in asymptomatic U.S. men compared to U.K. men, thereby leading to a higher rate of prostate cancer diagnoses in the United States as well as diagnosis at an earlier stage of the disease (Chustecka 2011). Nevertheless, in both the United States and the United Kingdom, cardiovascular disease is a primary cause of death for men as well as the primary cause of death for men with prostate cancer. Tocotrienols could extend the life expectancy and the quality of life for aging men by exerting both a chemopreventive effect on prostate cancer and by lowering plasma levels of atherogenic LDL-cholesterol.

A "targeted" approach to chemoprevention, as outlined in Figure 8.2, would first identify a high-risk population as well as environmental factors and genetic/protein biomarkers to help predict

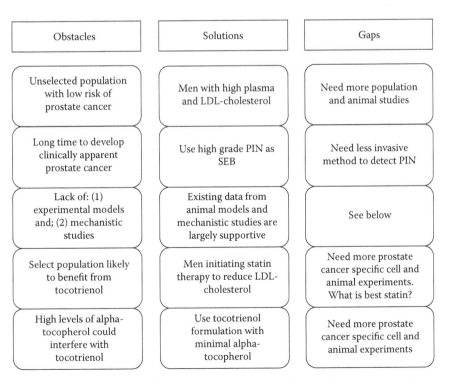

Obstacles	Solutions	Gaps
Unselected population with low risk of prostate cancer	Men with high plasma and LDL-cholesterol	Need more population and animal studies
Long time to develop clinically apparent prostate cancer	Use high grade PIN as SEB	Need less invasive method to detect PIN
Lack of: (1) experimental models and; (2) mechanistic studies	Existing data from animal models and mechanistic studies are largely supportive	See below
Select population likely to benefit from tocotrienol	Men initiating statin therapy to reduce LDL-cholesterol	Need more prostate cancer specific cell and animal experiments. What is best statin?
High levels of alpha-tocopherol could interfere with tocotrienol	Use tocotrienol formulation with minimal alpha-tocopherol	Need more prostate cancer specific cell and animal experiments

FIGURE 8.2 Prospective tocotrienol chemoprevention trial: obstacles, solutions, and research gaps.

which individuals would be responders to a given chemopreventive regimen (William et al. 2009). For a tocotrienol chemoprevention trial for prostate cancer, both these tasks may not be as daunting as first assumed.

8.3.1 HIGH LEVEL OF LOW-DENSITY LIPOPROTEIN–CHOLESTEROL IS A RISK FACTOR FOR PROSTATE CANCER

In a hospital-based case–control study, Magura et al. (2008) found that hypercholesterolemia (50–74 years old men) is significantly associated with prostate cancer (an odds ratio of 1.64). High levels of LDL were associated with a 60% increased risk for prostate cancer (Magura et al. 2008). The association between cholesterol and prostate cancer actually goes back to 1942 when Swyer (1942) noted an increased cholesterol content in prostatic adenomas compared to normal tissue. The important molecular interrelationships between tocotrienols, cholesterol metabolism, and prostate cancer will be further detailed later.

Since most men above the age of 20 have a lipid profile measured at least once every 5 years (as recommended by the National Institutes of Health), it is logistically quite easy to identify a large cohort of men with elevated plasma cholesterol and elevated LDL-cholesterol.

8.3.2 MEN TAKING A STATIN FOR HIGH LDL-CHOLESTEROL WOULD LIKELY RESPOND TO TOCOTRIENOL CHEMOPREVENTION FOR PROSTATE CANCER

Having a high LDL-cholesterol level and being older than 55 are risk factors for cardiovascular disease in men and indications for prescribing a statin for lowering LDL-cholesterol (http://www.mayoclinic.com/health/statins/CL00010). This is particularly important since there is strong evidence suggesting that tocotrienols and statins act synergistically as anticancer agents (Wali and Sylvester 2007; Sylvester et al. 2011; Sylvester 2012). Men who are initiating statin therapy for hyperlipidemia are very likely, therefore, to benefit from the prostate chemoprevention effects of tocotrienols. Additional experiments testing the synergistic effects of tocotrienols and statins on prostate cancer in an animal model are critically needed (see Figure 8.2). Nevertheless, statins are amongst the most widely prescribed drugs, and identifying a large cohort of men with high LDL-cholesterol who are initiating statin therapy is not a clinical obstacle. In order to design the best prospective tocotrienol–statin chemoprevention trial, it would be advantageous to (1) include two additional arms, that is, one with statin alone and one with tocotrienols alone and (2) predetermine which members of the statin family of drugs have an optimal synergy with tocotrienol in preventing prostate cancer cell growth.

8.3.3 HIGH-GRADE PROSTATIC INTRAEPITHELIAL NEOPLASIA AS A SURROGATE ENDPOINT BIOMARKER FOR PROSTATE CANCER

In order for a chemoprevention trial to be cost effective, it is necessary to utilize surrogate endpoint biomarkers (SEBs) rather than reduced cancer mortality. This enables the trials to be smaller and shorter in duration (Bostwick and Aquilina 1996; William et al. 2009). As detailed by Bostwick and Aquilina (1996), high-grade PIN is the ideal SEB since it (1) is a very likely precursor to prostate cancer; (2) is routinely found in needle biopsies from men without prostate cancer; and (3) decreases with androgen deprivation therapy. Needle biopsies are generally performed in men with an abnormal digital rectal exam (DRE) and/or an elevated PSA level or PSA velocity. A large number of men have one or more indications that support a second biopsy. These would include (1) a suspicious DRE; (2) persistently rising PSA levels; (3) a low free PSA; and (4) the presence of PIN in the previous biopsy. The progression of high-grade PIN between biopsies can, therefore, provide an excellent outcome parameter for a tocotrienol chemoprevention trial.

8.4 TOCOTRIENOLS AND PROSTATE CANCER MOLECULAR AND CELLULAR TARGETS

Before embarking on a chemoprevention trial, it is imperative (see Figure 8.2) that the underlying molecular mechanisms are fairly well understood and that data from appropriate cell and animal models are supportive. These data are reviewed later.

8.4.1 HIGH-GRADE PROSTATIC INTRAEPITHELIAL NEOPLASIA, TOCOTRIENOLS, AND THE TRAMP ANIMAL MODEL

The transgenic adenocarcinoma of the mouse prostate (TRAMP; Hurwitz et al. 2001) model is useful for evaluating the efficacy of prostate cancer chemopreventive agents. Prostate cancer progression in the TRAMP mouse model closely resembles that in human prostate cancer with a time-dependent increase in high-grade PIN, adenocarcinomas, and metastatic lesions. Recent work by Barve et al. (2010) using the TRAMP model is significant, since it demonstrates that dietary mixed tocotrienols reduce the levels of high-grade PIN as well as the incidence of tumor formation compared to controls. The molecular mechanism most likely involves increased expression of the Bcl-XL/Bcl-2-associated death promoter protein (BAD), apoptosis, and the modulation of cell-cycle regulatory proteins (Barve et al. 2010).

8.4.2 PRACTICAL ASPECTS OF TOCOTRIENOL SUPPLEMENTATION

The positive results detailed earlier with the TRAMP model (Barve et al. 2010) suggest that inhibiting the presence of high-grade PIN could be a useful SEB for a tocotrienol prostate chemoprevention trial. On a practical level, it would be important to know which isomer(s) of tocotrienol are the most potent in reducing high-grade PIN and/or inducing apoptosis in prostate cancer cells. There are no *in vivo* data addressing this issue, but recent studies show that both 2R-delta-tocotrienol and 2R-gamma-tocotrienol are potent inhibitors of LnCAP and PC-3 cell proliferation (Yap et al. 2008; Campbell et al. 2011). Yap et al. (2008) found 2R-delta-tocotrienol to be somewhat more effective than 2R-gamma-tocotrienol at inhibiting the growth of LNCaP cells, whereas Campbell et al. (2011) found both 2R-gamma and 2R-delta-tocotrienols to have similar potencies. For PC-3 cells, Campbell et al. (2011) found 2R-delta-tocotrienol to be more effective at inhibiting cell proliferation than 2R-gamma-tocotrienol, but Yap et al. (2008) found the reverse.

Despite these differences, it is clear that either 2R-delta-tocotrienol or 2R-gamma-tocotrienol is a potent inhibitor of androgen-dependent prostate cancer cell growth (LnCAP) or androgen-independent prostate cancer cell growth (PC-3). Moreover, neither of these isoforms inhibits the growth of primary human prostate epithelial cells (Campbell et al. 2011) or an immortalized human prostate epithelial cell line (Yap et al. 2008). RRR-alpha-tocopherol exhibits no growth inhibitory properties with either LnCAP or PC-3 cells, which is consistent with the Selenium and Vitamin E Cancer Prevention Trial (SELECT) data (Yap et al. 2008; Campbell et al. 2011).

The composition of the mixed tocotrienols used in the Barve et al. (2010) study was RRR-alpha-tocotrienol (12%–14%), 2R-beta-tocotrienol (1%), 2R-gamma-tocotrienol (18%–20%), 2R-delta-tocotrienol (4%–6%), and RRR-alpha-alpha-tocotrienol (12%–14%). The predominant vitamin E isomers in the mixed tocotrienols were, therefore, 2R-gamma-tocotrienol and RRR-alpha-tocopherol, which were present in about equal amounts. The control animals (at 24 weeks) had about 20% low-grade PIN and 80% high-grade PIN, and 0.3% mixed tocotrienols significantly shifted this to about 50% low-grade PIN and 50% high-grade PIN (Barve et al. 2010). For human subjects to achieve this dose of mixed tocotrienols, a supplement of about 3 g/day would be required. Multiple gel capsules would have to be consumed daily, engendering less compliance than a single daily capsule. The ability of RRR-alpha-tocopherol to attenuate the anticancer and hypolipidemic effects of tocotrienols suggests that a commercial source of tocotrienol free of tocopherols would be superior, since a lower dose could be used. Fortunately, the tocotrienol-rich fraction from the Annatto bean is free of tocopherols and contains about 90% delta-tocotrienol and about 10% gamma-tocotrienol, i.e., the most potent anticancer isoforms. As will be detailed later, selecting a population of men initiating statin therapy may further reduce (by about half) the dose of tocotrienol required to affect a reduction in cancer cell growth.

8.4.3 MOLECULAR MECHANISMS UNDERLYING THE CHEMOPREVENTIVE EFFECTS OF TOCOTRIENOLS IN PROSTATE CANCER

The molecular mechanisms underlying the anticancer effects of tocotrienols have been well studied and are compelling. The primary purpose of this chapter is to outline the design of a targeted chemoprevention trial. We will, therefore, focus on anticancer effects related to the synergistic suppression of HMGCoA reductase by statins and tocotrienols since this is relevant to the chemoprevention trial outlined in Figure 8.2.

8.4.4 CHOLESTEROL, LIPID RAFTS, AND PROSTATE CANCER

The ability of tocotrienols to decrease the synthesis of mevalonate by enhancing the degradation of HMGCoA reductase is likely to be one of the broad mechanisms underlying their anticancer effects. Mevalonate is a precursor for cholesterol synthesis as well as a precursor for the isoprenoid intermediates essential for the isoprenylation of small GTP binding proteins and heterotrimeric G-protein gamma-subunit. Agents that inhibit HMGCoA reductase or reduce its level can affect cancer-relevant signal transduction events by (1) modulating the cholesterol content of lipid rafts or (2) decreasing the posttranslational isoprenylation of G-proteins. We will discuss the role of tocotrienols and statins in both. Lipid rafts are sphingolipid-cholesterol-rich microdomains found in the plasma membrane of all mammalian cells; they play a key role in signal transduction events, and increasing evidence suggests they are important determinants of prostate tumor growth and aggressiveness (Di Vizio et al. 2008).

In pioneering work, Zhuang et al. (2005) found that the statin drug simvastatin lowered the cholesterol content of lipid rafts in LNCaP prostate cancer cells, inhibited the Akt signaling pathway, and induced apoptosis. Activation of the Akt signaling pathway is a fundamental characteristic of many types of cancer and is a key determinant of cancer aggressiveness. Zhuang et al. (2005) found that replenishing cell membranes with cholesterol caused Akt reactivation and reversed the antiapoptotic effect. Particularly important was the observation that elevating plasma-cholesterol levels in a LNCaP xenograft mouse model (1) increased tumor growth; (2) increased Akt activation; (3) reduced xenograft apoptosis; and (4) increased the cholesterol content and protein tyrosine phosphorylation in lipid rafts isolated from xenograft tumors (Zhuang et al. 2005). Zhuang et al. (2005) suggest that lipid rafts are "a promising subcellular location for the identification of novel molecular targets involved in cholesterol-dependent tumor progression mechanisms."

Li et al. (2006) further investigated the role of cholesterol-depleting agents on lipid rafts and apoptosis in a variety of cancer cell lines. Li et al. (2006) found that elevated levels of cholesterol-rich lipid rafts correlated with apoptosis sensitivity caused by cholesterol-depleting agents (Li et al. 2006). Moreover, these investigators found that prostate cancer cell lines contained more lipid rafts and were more sensitive to apoptosis induced by cholesterol-depleting agents than a normal human prostate epithelial cell line (PZ-HPV7; Li et al. 2006). In agreement with the work of Zhuang et al. (2005), cholesterol depletion in lipid rafts resulted in decreased Akt activation and increased apoptosis (Li et al. 2006).

Li et al. (2006) used methyl-beta-cyclodextrin as a cholesterol-depleting agent. Cyclodextrins are cyclic oligosaccharides that deplete cellular cholesterol by sequestering the cholesterol molecule inside the cyclodextrin ring. Unlike statins or tocotrienols, which inhibit the mevalonate pathway and the subsequent synthesis of isoprenoids, methyl-beta-cyclodextrin does not directly influence cholesterol or isoprenoid biosynthesis. Therefore, the effects of methyl-beta-cyclodextrin on modulating lipid raft-dependent signal transduction pathways are due only to changes in lipid raft-cholesterol content rather than posttranslational modifications of lipid-raft proteins by isoprenoids. The fact that cholesterol repletion was found to replenish cell-surface rafts and restore Akt activation further supports the direct role of cholesterol in the pro-cancer effects of lipid rafts.

8.4.5 Akt1 and Lipid Rafts in Prostate Cancer Cells

Since the inactivation of Akt by cholesterol-lowering agents is now well established, it is important to know if this is a direct effect on Akt itself and/or an effect mediated by upstream components of the pathway. Adams et al. (2007) showed that a subpopulation of Akt1 could be found in the cholesterol rich lipid-raft fractions from human LNCaP prostate cancer cells. Moreover, removal of cholesterol from cholesterol-rich lipid rafts by methyl-beta-cyclodextrin-blocked Akt1 activation (Adam et al. 2007). These data strongly support a direct role of cholesterol in activating Akt1 in the cholesterol-rich lipid rafts of prostate cancer cells.

Since both tocotrienols and statins reduce cellular cholesterol synthesis and lower plasma-cholesterol levels, it is very likely that both these agents have anticancer effects, at least in part by lowering the cholesterol content of lipid rafts and inactivating Akt1. Surprisingly, the ability of tocotrienols to reduce the cholesterol content of lipid rafts in tumor cells has not been well investigated.

8.4.6 Tocotrienols and Statins Affect the Isoprenylation of G-Protein Regulatory Proteins

By inhibiting HMGCoA reductase, both tocotrienols and statins could reduce the levels of intermediates (e.g., farnesyl pyrophosphate, geranylgeranyl pyrophosphate) in the mevalonate cascade that are important in the isoprenylation of the Ras superfamily of small GTP-binding proteins (small G-proteins) as well as the gamma-subunit of heterotrimeric G-proteins. G-proteins are important in regulating cell growth and play key roles is prostate cancer and cancer in general (Kue and Daaka 2000; Sahai and Marshall 2002; Hurst and Hooks 2009). Isoprenylation is required to activate G-proteins by hydrophobically anchoring them to the plasma membrane. Yano et al. (2005) have shown that a redox-silent derivative of alpha-tocotrienol (40 μM), but not alpha-tocotrienol itself, inhibits the growth of human lung adenocarcinoma cells and suppresses both Ras farnesylation and the geranylgeranylation of RhoA. These investigators did not examine either gamma- or delta-tocotrienol, which have a much greater anticancer effect than alpha-tocotrienol.

The potential synergistic action of statins and tocotrienols on isoprenylation is of particular interest for this chapter, but no information is yet available for prostate cancer cell lines. Nevertheless, studies with other cancer cell lines are very informative and consistent. Wali and Sylvester (2007) demonstrated a synergistic antiproliferative effect of gamma-tocotrienol and various statins with mammary tumor cells. Subeffective doses of statins and gamma-tocotrienol (2 μM) alone did not affect protein isoprenylation or mitogenic signaling, whereas combined treatment inhibited cancer cell growth and decreased the isoprenylation of Rap1A and Rab6 (small G-proteins), as well as MAPK signaling (Wali and Sylvester 2007).

Yang et al. (2010) studied the effects of atorvastatin (commercial name is Lipitor) and gamma-tocotrienol on the mevalonate cascade in two colon cancer cell lines. Atorvastatin and gamma-tocotrienol (or delta-tocotrienol) alone inhibited colon cancer cell growth and together exerted a synergistic growth inhibition (Yang et al. 2010). Neither gamma-tocopherol nor delta-tocopherol produced a growth inhibition significantly different from that produced by atorvastatin alone (Yang et al. 2010). For the colon cancer cell system studied by Yang et al. (2010), (1) growth inhibition by gamma-tocotrienol alone was independent of cholesterol and isoprenoid synthesis; (2) growth inhibition by atorvastatin alone or the combination of atorvastatin and gamma-tocotrienol was not dependent upon cholesterol synthesis or farnesyl pyrophosphate synthesis but was dependent upon geranylgeranyl pyrophosphate synthesis; and (3) the isoprenylation of RhoA, but not k-Ras, was identified as the key G-protein affected by atorvastatin and gamma-tocotrienol. The dysregulation of RhoA and other small G-proteins plays a key role in the progression of PIN to metastatic prostate cancer (Sahai and Marshall 2002).

The work of Yang et al. (2010) implicates the importance of geranylgeranyl pyrophosphate in modulating colon cancer cell killing and further suggests that an alternative gamma-tocotrienol mechanism for cancer cell killing exists that is not dependent upon inhibiting cholesterol or isoprenoid synthesis. It is significant, therefore, that Campbell et al. (2011) recently described a peroxisome proliferator activated receptor (PPAR)-gamma-dependent mechanism, whereby gamma- and delta-tocotrienols induce growth arrest in the PC3 prostate cancer cell lines. Gamma-tocotrienol (delta-tocotrienol was not tested) was able to induce apoptosis at levels as low as 1 μM.

It is also significant that Yang et al. (2010) found a synergistic action between atorvastatin, gamma-tocotrienol, and celecoxib in their ability to inhibit the growth of human colon cancer cell lines. Celecoxib is a sulfa nonsteroidal anti-inflammatory drug (NSAID) and selective inhibitor of cyclooxygenases-2 (COX-2), which converts arachidonic acid to prostaglandin H2 (PGH2), a precursor to prostaglandin E2 (PGE2), which in turn promotes the activation of Akt and the Ras/MAPK/ERK pathway. The use of some NSAIDS, for example, ibuprofen, naproxen, is associated with a modest reduction in the risk of prostate cancer. This, however, is not a universal finding with some studies reporting a risk reduction only when both a statin and NSAID are used together; epidemiological evidence in this area is still inconclusive (Coogan et al. 2010; Mahmud et al. 2011). It would, nevertheless, be important to document any concurrent use of NSAIDs and statins (dose and duration) in any future tocotrienol prostate cancer chemoprevention trial.

8.5 TOCOTRIENOLS, LIPID RAFTS, ErbB2, AND THE ANDROGEN RECEPTOR

The PI3 kinase-Akt, MAPK/ERK, and the androgen receptor (AR) pathways are the most relevant signaling cascades in prostate cancer. A recent study of 181 primary and 37 metastatic prostate tumors found that the PI3K-Akt signaling pathway was activated in 42% of the primary tumors examined, with pathway mutations in all of the metastatic samples (Taylor et al. 2010). The AR pathway has been extensively studied and constitutes the foundation for most of the prostate cancer therapies currently in use. A well-studied group of chemoprevention agents for prostate cancer are "5-alpha-reductase" inhibitors, which block the conversion of testosterone to the more active dihydrotestosterone form. Both dihydrotestosterone and testosterone are agonists for the AR transcription factor and both promote the transcriptional activation of AR and the subsequent balance between cell proliferation and apoptosis (cf. Heinlein and Chang [2004] for an excellent review). In the early stages of prostate cancer, androgen deprivation is therapeutically effective, but eventually all subjects develop a resistance to androgen deprivation and progress to more advanced tumors. Moreover, although the 5-alpha-reductase inhibitors (5-ARIs) reduce the incidence of prostate cancer diagnosis by about 24%, they unfortunately increase the incidence of high-grade prostate cancer (Theoret et al. 2011). The FDA has not, therefore, approved the use of 5-ARIs for the chemoprevention of prostate cancer.

There is a growing consensus that an optimal strategy is to prevent or slow the progression to androgen-resistant prostate cancer in the first place rather than attempting to "cure it" after its development [see Jathal et al. [2011] for a review]. In this respect, the factors that modulate the kinase signal transduction cascades that activate AR activity are key targets, with the receptor tyrosine kinases of the ErbB family being of particular interest, since they turn on the PI3K-Akt and MAPK/ERK pathways thought to be important in the transcriptional activation of the AR (Jathal et al. 2011). AR phosphorylation (or that of its coregulators) enables its transcriptional activation at very low levels of androgen, that is, an "androgen-independent" state (Heinlein and Chang 2004).

In prostate cancer, ErbB2 expression is known to be associated with androgen-independent receptor signaling (Mellinghoff et al. 2004; Gregory et al. 2005) and poor survival (Carles et al. 2004; Edwards et al. 2006). ErbB2 has exceptional features that distinguish it from other members of the ErbB kinase family. No soluble ligand has been identified for ErbB2; thus, the mechanism of activation differs from other ErbB family members, where the interaction with high-affinity soluble ligands induces a conformational change, which favors the formation of dimers and activation (Yarden and Sliwkowski 2001).

Work by Yeh et al. (1999) has shown that the overexpression of ErbB2 (also known as HER2) in LNCaP cells (androgen-dependent cell line) caused (1) increased cell growth and (2) a transcriptional activation of the AR that was only partially blocked by antiandrogen treatment. These authors present additional evidence showing the involvement of the MAPK pathway in the activation of the AR. Similarly, Craft et al. (1999) found that the overexpression of ErbB2 in androgen-dependent prostate cancer cell lines permitted androgen-independent growth. Conversely, siRNA knockdown of ErbB2 results in reduced prostate cancer cell growth and reduced transcriptional activation of the AR as evidenced by reduced PSA secretion (Mellinghoff et al. 2004).

The aforementioned results collectively suggest that therapeutic agents that suppress ErbB2 pathways could be useful in preventing prostate cancer and its progression to an androgen-independent stage. It is relevant, therefore, that Shin-Kang et al. (Shin-Kang et al. 2011) recently found that gamma- or delta-tocotrienols inhibit Akt and Erk activation and suppress the growth of pancreatic cancer cells by suppressing the ErbB2 pathway. Tocopherols did not exert any of these effects (Shin-Kang et al. 2011). Similar experiments have not yet been reported for prostate cancer cell lines. The role of ErbB2 in prostrate cancer is a very active area of investigation and is complicated by the finding that the enhanced sensitivity of the AR to low androgen levels is not modulated by ErbB2 alone, but a heterodimer formed with ErbB3 (Agus et al. 2002; Mellinghoff et al. 2004; Jathal et al. 2011).

Lipid rafts also play a key role in modulating the activities of ErbB proteins (Nagy et al. 2002; Chinni et al. 2008; Di Vizio et al. 2008). Chinni (2008) has studied the role of the C-X-C chemokine receptor type 4 (CXCR4, also known as fusin) and its only known ligand CXCL12 in the transactivation of ErbB2 localized to the lipid rafts of prostate cancer cells. Binding of the chemokine CXCL12 to its receptor CXCR4 initiates signaling events resulting in the expression of metalloproteinase-9 in prostate cancer bone metastasis. Both CXCR4 and ErbB2 are found in prostate cancer cell lipid rafts, and the CXCL12 chemokine causes a transactivation of lipid-raft ErbB2 and a subsequent activation of Akt (Chinni et al. 2008).

Quite significantly, agents that lower the lipid-raft cholesterol content also (1) inhibit lipid-raft CXCL12/CXCR4 transactivation of ErbB2; (2) decrease MMP-9 secretion; and (3) decrease the invasiveness of prostate cancer cells (Chinni et al. 2008). The ability of cholesterol-lowering agents to inhibit AR activation was not studied in this model system (Chinni et al. 2008). Nevertheless, these data suggest that tocotrienols and statins could inhibit the transactivation of ErbB2 by CXCL12/CXCR4 and perhaps even AR activation. Clearly, there is much to be done in this area.

8.6 CONCLUSION

This chapter has, hopefully, provided a reasonable framework for the design of a future prospective tocotrienol-statin chemoprevention trial with three arms: (1) tocotrienol alone; (2) statin alone; and (3) statin plus tocotrienol. As indicated in Figure 8.2, many of the obstacles associated with a targeted and cost-effective chemoprevention trial already have solutions. By utilizing a cohort of men initiating statin therapy for high LDL-cholesterol, it should be possible to select for a high prostate cancer risk group with a high likelihood of being responders by virtue of the synergistic anticancer effects of statins and delta- and/or gamma-tocotrienol. Utilizing a tocotrienol formulation with no tocopherols is also critical due to the attenuating effect tocopherols have on the anticancer effects of tocotrienols. Men taking a statin and delta- or gamma-tocotrienol should also have a lower

LDL-cholesterol and a lower cardiovascular risk than men taking a statin alone. The use of low-grade PIN to high-grade PIN is an excellent SEB for prostate cancer, and the TRAMP animal model has already validated the chemopreventive effects of mixed tocotrienols. The molecular mechanisms underlying the anticancer effects of tocotrienols are now fairly well documented: animal experiments looking at the potential synergistic chemopreventive effects of statins and tocotrienols in a prostate cancer model are a major research gap.

REFERENCES

Adam, R.M., Mukhopadhyay, N.K., Kim, J., Di Vizio, D., Cinar, B., Boucher, K., Solomon, K.R., and Freeman, M.R. 2007, Cholesterol sensitivity of endogenous and myristoylated Akt, *Cancer Research*, 67(13), 6238–6246.

Agus, D.B., Akita, R.W., Fox, W.D., Lewis, G.D., Higgins, B., Pisacane, P.I., Lofgren, J.A. et al. 2002, Targeting ligand-activated ErbB2 signaling inhibits breast and prostate tumor growth, *Cancer Cell*, 2(2), 127–137.

Azzi, A., Gysin, R., Kempna, P., Munteanu, A., Negis, Y., Villacorta, L., Visarius, T., and Zingg, J.M. 2004, Vitamin E mediates cell signaling and regulation of gene expression, *Annals of the New York Academy of Sciences*, 1031, 86–95.

Azzi, A. and Stocker, A. 2000, Vitamin E: Non-antioxidant roles, *Progress in Lipid Research*, 39(3), 231–255.

Barve, A., Khor, T.O., Nair, S., Reuhl, K., Suh, N., Reddy, B., Newmark, H., and Kong, A.N. 2009, Gamma-tocopherol-enriched mixed tocopherol diet inhibits prostate carcinogenesis in TRAMP mice, *International Journal of Cancer*, 124(7), 1693–1699.

Barve, A., Khor, T.O., Reuhl, K., Reddy, B., Newmark, H., and Kong, A.N. 2010, Mixed tocotrienols inhibit prostate carcinogenesis in TRAMP mice, *Nutrition and Cancer*, 62(6), 789–794.

Bostwick, D.G. and Aquilina, J.W. 1996, Prostatic intraepithelial neoplasia (PIN) and other prostatic lesions as risk factors and surrogate endpoints for cancer chemoprevention trials, *Journal of Cellular Biochemistry; Supplement*, 25, 156–164.

Campbell, S.E., Rudder, B., Phillips, R.B., Whaley, S.G., Stimmel, J.B., Leesnitzer, L.M., Lightner, J. et al. 2011, Gamma-tocotrienol induces growth arrest through a novel pathway with TGFbeta2 in prostate cancer, *Free Radical Biology and Medicine*, 50(10), 1344–1354.

Campbell, S.E., Stone, W.L., Lee, S., Whaley, S., Yang, H., Qui, M., Goforth, P., Sherman, D., McHaffie, D., and Krishnan, K. 2006, Comparative effects of RRR-alpha- and RRR-gamma-tocopherol on proliferation and apoptosis in human colon cancer cell lines, *BMC Cancer*, 6, 13.

Campbell, S.E., Stone, W.L., Whaley, S.G., Qui, M., and Krishnan, K. 2003, Gamma (gamma) tocopherol upregulates peroxisome proliferator activated receptor (PPAR) gamma (gamma) expression in SW 480 human colon cancer cell lines, *BMC Cancer*, 3, 25.

Carles, J., Lloreta, J., Salido, M., Font, A., Suarez, M., Baena, V., Nogue, M., Domenech, M., and Fabregat, X. 2004, Her-2/neu expression in prostate cancer: A dynamic process?, *Clinical Cancer Research: An Official Journal of the American Association for Cancer Research*, 10(14), 4742–4745.

Chinni, S.R., Yamamoto, H., Dong, Z., Sabbota, A., Bonfil, R.D., and Cher, M.L. 2008, CXCL12/CXCR4 transactivates HER2 in lipid rafts of prostate cancer cells and promotes growth of metastatic deposits in bone, *Molecular Cancer Research: MCR*, 6(3), 446–457.

Christen, S., Woodall, A.A., Shigenaga, M.K., Southwell-Keely, P.T., Duncan, M.W., and Ames, B.N. 1997, Gamma-tocopherol traps mutagenic electrophiles such as NO(X) and complements alpha-tocopherol: Physiological implications, *Proceedings of the National Academy of Sciences of the United States of America*, 94(7), 3217–3222.

Chustecka, Z. 2011, June 17, 2011-last update, Prostate cancer kills more men in the UK than in the US result of PSA testing? [Homepage of Medscape Medical News > Oncology], [Online]. Available at: http://www.medscape.com/viewarticle/744803

Conte, C., Floridi, A., Aisa, C., Piroddi, M., Floridi, A., and Galli, F. 2004, Gamma-tocotrienol metabolism and antiproliferative effect in prostate cancer cells, *Annals of the New York Academy of Sciences*, 1031, 391–394.

Coogan, P.F., Kelly, J.P., Strom, B.L., and Rosenberg, L. 2010, Statin and NSAID use and prostate cancer risk, *Pharmacoepidemiology and Drug Safety*, 19(7), 752–755.

Cooney, R.V., Franke, A.A., Harwood, P.J., Hatch-Pigott, V., Custer, L.J., and Mordan, L.J. 1993, Gamma-tocopherol detoxification of nitrogen dioxide: Superiority to alpha-tocopherol, *Proceedings of the National Academy of Sciences of the United States of America*, 90(5), 1771–1775.

Yang, Z., Xiao, H., Jin, H., Koo, P.T., Tsang, D.J., and Yang, C.S. 2010, Synergistic actions of atorvastatin with gamma-tocotrienol and celecoxib against human colon cancer HT29 and HCT116 cells, *International Journal of Cancer*, 126(4), 852–863.

Yano, Y., Satoh, H., Fukumoto, K., Kumadaki, I., Ichikawa, T., Yamada, K., Hagiwara, K., and Yano, T. 2005, Induction of cytotoxicity in human lung adenocarcinoma cells by 6-O-carboxypropyl-alpha-tocotrienol, a redox-silent derivative of alpha-tocotrienol, *International Journal of Cancer*, 115(5), 839–846.

Yap, W.N., Chang, P.N., Han, H.Y., Lee, D.T., Ling, M.T., Wong, Y.C., and Yap, Y.L. 2008, Gamma-tocotrienol suppresses prostate cancer cell proliferation and invasion through multiple-signalling pathways, *British Journal of Cancer*, 99(11), 1832–1841.

Yarden, Y. and Sliwkowski, M.X. 2001, Untangling the ErbB signalling network, *Nature Reviews Molecular Cell Biology*, 2(2), 127–137.

Yeh, S., Lin, H.K., Kang, H.Y., Thin, T.H., Lin, M.F., and Chang, C. 1999, From HER2/Neu signal cascade to androgen receptor and its coactivators: A novel pathway by induction of androgen target genes through MAP kinase in prostate cancer cells, *Proceedings of the National Academy of Sciences of the United States of America*, 96(10), 5458–5463.

Yu, W., Jia, L., Park, S.K., Li, J., Gopalan, A., Simmons-Menchaca, M., Sanders, B.G., and Kline, K. 2009, Anticancer actions of natural and synthetic vitamin E forms: RRR-alpha-tocopherol blocks the anticancer actions of gamma-tocopherol, *Molecular Nutrition and Food Research*, 53(12), 1573–1581.

Zhuang, L., Kim, J., Adam, R.M., Solomon, K.R., and Freeman, M.R. 2005, Cholesterol targeting alters lipid raft composition and cell survival in prostate cancer cells and xenografts, *The Journal of Clinical Investigation*, 115(4), 959–968.

9 δ-Tocotrienol
Demethylated Vitamin E with Hormetic Function and Therapeutic Application in Breast Cancer

Francesca Pilolli, Marta Piroddi, Elisa Pierpaoli,
Silvia Ciffolilli, Mauro Provinciali, and Francesco Galli

CONTENTS

9.1 INTRODUCTION

Tocotrienols (T3) are vitamin E forms with an isoprenyl side chain that are characterized by poor bioavailability and sustained metabolism, which may explain the very low tissue levels as well as the poor vitamin activity as assessed by the fetal resorption test. However, when used as supplements or tested *in vitro*, these forms show distinctive biological activities that are consistent with a series of health-promoting effects such as cholesterol-lowering, cytoprotection, and anticarcinogenic effects (reviewed in Aggarwal et al. [2010]). *In vitro* and *in vivo* experiments have demonstrated that these properties are dependent on specific signaling and metabolism (recently reviewed in Viola et al. [2012]) that clearly differentiate these vitamers from the most abundant forms of vitamin E in human tissues and body fluids, i.e., α- and γ-tocopherol (TOH). Obviously, these differences go far beyond the well-recognized antioxidant role that these vitamers may play in cell membranes and biological fluids

(Galli and Azzi 2010) and may suggest a revision of vitamin E definition to consider T3 as a distinct group of micronutrient vitamins within this family of compounds.

Over the last 2 decades, several studies have increasingly described the potential of desmethyl or hypomethylated configurations of T3 (HMT3) used alone or in combination with other treatments as anticancer agents. Consistent preclinical evidence of successful applications in the chemoprevention and chemotherapy of different human cancers such as those affecting prostate, breast, and colon (reviewed in Constantinou et al. [2008] and Viola et al. [2012]) has been obtained.

Structure–function studies have confirmed that cell responses associated with the anticancer effects of T3 are more pronounced when these vitamers contain hypo- (or des-)methylated chroman rings, which also produce the highest *in vitro* and *in vivo* detoxification response among the entire series of natural vitamin E forms with the order of magnitude: δ-T3 $\geq$ γ-T3 $\gg$ α-T3 $\geq$ γ-TOH $\geq$ δ-TOH $\gg$ α-TOH (reviewed in Galli et al. [2007] and Traber [2010]).

Importantly, in both the T3 and TOH subfamilies, gamma and delta configurations of the chroman ring, differing by just one methyl group, result in markedly different tumor- and concentration–specific anticancer activity (reviewed in Betti et al. [2006] and Pierpaoli et al. [2010]). δ-T3 was recently observed to be even more potent as hypoproliferative and pro-apoptotic agent in breast cancer cells than α-tocopherylsuccinate (α-TOS; Pierpaoli et al. 2010; Viola et al. 2010), which is the prototypal synthetic form of vitamin E with one of the highest anticancer activities so far demonstrated in literature. On the other hand, α-TOH was not only shown to lower anticancer potential, but it can lower also the biological activity and thus the anticancer potency of HM forms (Yu et al. 2009) possibly by interfering with uptake, metabolism, and signaling of these forms (these aspects are discussed in the recent review papers: Galli and Azzi 2010; Traber 2010; Viola et al. 2012).

In this context, we suggested that the anticancer signaling of HM vitamers is proportional and possibly associated with the extent of the metabolic and detoxification responses that these may produce in cancer cells (reviewed in Conte et al. [2004] and Galli et al. [2007]). In this sense, HMT3 behave as the most potent anticancer agents and cell-stressors within the E family. The latter property discussed below in this chapter, is the prerequisite for a role of HMT3 as hormetic agents that has been described for many other natural phenolics either with or without antioxidant activity (Galli 2007; Le Bourg 2009; Ristow et al. 2009). Actually, depending on uptake rates (Viola et al. 2011), HMT3 are observed to produce different kinds of responses: (1) a marked stress response that leads to the development of senescence-like phenotype with cell-cycle inhibition or even mitochondrial toxicity and apoptosis; (2) mild (submaximal) stress with subsequent induction of detoxification and antioxidant genes, which results in a higher extent of cell protection and improved capability of resistance against further stresses, i.e., the hormetic effect.

Underlying mechanisms of these responses are believed to include vitamer-specific, cell proteins and lipids that act as cell sensors and signaling effectors of T3 (Table 9.1).

This chapter describes these players and the mechanisms so far proposed to explain why γ-T3 and δ-T3 are the best candidates to find a pharmacological application as anticancer agents, particularly in breast cancer, one of the most prevalent forms of tumor in the female population worldwide. More advanced knowledge on these aspects are expected to help in planning the next generation of vitamin E trials that should provide clinical evidence to the anticipated therapeutic application of HMT3 in breast cancer as well as in other malignancies.

9.2   CELL TARGETS AND SIGNALING OF HMT3

9.2.1   ANTIOXIDANT AND REDOX-DERIVED EFFECTS

As reflected by structural similarity of tocopherols and tocotrienols, these show the same type of antioxidative effect (Kamal-Eldin and Appelqvist 1996). This is the result of either the electron transferring or hydrogen atom donating effect of the hydroxyl group in position 6 of the chroman ring. This chemistry makes them efficient antioxidants in radical and transition metal–catalyzed oxidation reactions

TABLE 9.1

Putative Biological Interactions and Signaling of T3

Context	Interactions and Responsive Genes[a]	Biological Response	References
Intracellular/ nuclear receptors and metabolism	Estrogen receptor β	Antagonizes ERα, tumor suppressor. Antiproliferative activity	Comitato et al. (2009)
	SXR	Steroid and xenobiotic receptor	Zhou et al. (2004)
	PXR (possible)	Drug (and vitamin E) metabolism and stress response	Brigelius-Flohe (2005), Traber (2007)
	Quinone reductase and heme-oxygenase Glutathione (GSH)-related enzymes (ARE-dependent)	DME, detoxification of xenobiotics, and antioxidant effects	Das et al. (2008), Hsieh and Wu (2008) Hsieh et al. (2010)
Binding proteins	α-TTP[b]	Uptake and trafficking of vitamin E forms in liver cells	Hosomi et al. (1997), Morley et al. (2008) Atkinson et al. (2008)
	α-TTP-like proteins such as TAP/Sec14L2 (low affinity binding)		
Plasmalemma	PUFA and cholesterol (colocalization and interaction) of membrane microdomains	Signaling (membrane rafts) and structural function by means of physical and chemical effects (such as fluidity, antioxidant protection, lipid–lipid, and lipid–protein interaction)	Atkinson et al. (2008, 2010)
Signaling			
Protein kinases	PKC	Regulation of membrane domains and several signaling pathways, cell growth, immune response, angiogenesis, etc.	Eitsuka et al. (2006)
	PI3K/Akt	As component of the PI3K/AKT/mTOR pathway promotes cell proliferation and thus cancer progression, apoptotic signaling inhibition, insulin signaling	Shah and Sylvester (2004), Shibata et al. (2008), Uto-Kondo et al. (2009)
	MAPKs	Survival and death pathways, proliferation and differentiation, stress, and inflammation	Sun et al. (2008), Then et al. (2009)
	JAK/STAT3	Proliferation, angiogenesis, and cell migration	Kannappan et al. (2010b)
	Cyclin-dependent kinases	Cell cycle regulation (cyclin D1/cdk4 and cyclin B1/cdk1)	Elangovan et al. (2008)
Cell cycle– related proteins	p53, p21, p16, p27, Rb/E2F	Cyclin kinase and senescence regulation mechanisms	Elangovan et al. (2008), Pierpaoli et al. (2010)
Mitochondrial proteins	Bcl2/Bax	Apoptotic signaling (intrinsic pathway)	Agarwal et al. (2004), Hsieh and Wu (2008), Then et al. (2009)
Transcription factors	Nrf2/Keap1	DME and antioxidant response (cellular protection)	Hsieh et al. (2010)
	NfkB/IkB	Cytokine production, oxidative stress, and control of proliferation/apoptosis	Sylvester et al. (2005), Ahn et al. (2007), Kuhad and Chopra (2009)

(continued)

TABLE 9.1 (continued)
Putative Biological Interactions and Signaling of T3

Context	Interactions and Responsive Genes[a]	Biological Response	References
Enzymes	HMG-CoA reductase (post-translational regulation)	Cholesterol biosynthesis and proposed role in inflammatory, endothelial, and cancer-cell signaling	Parker et al. (1993), Theriault et al. (2002), Song and DeBose-Boyd (2006)
	Telomerase (possible transcriptional regulation, downstream to PKC signaling)	T3-dependent control of cell proliferation and lifespan	Eitsuka et al. (2006)

[a] As transcripts or proteins.
[b] This binds α-TOH with an at least 10-fold higher affinity than HMT3 forms.

(Muller et al. 2010; Galli et al. 2011) and powerful chain breakers through the neutralization of peroxyl and alkoxyl radicals generated during lipid peroxidation (Kamal-Eldin and Appelqvist 1996). The presence of different methylation patterns and also that of an isoprenyl chain influence these properties regardless of the group in position 6 of the chroman ring. Indeed, the same kind of effect by these moieties is obtained when the OH group in this position is substituted with a NH_2 group (chromamines) to produce more effective antioxidant chroman derivatives without changing the antioxidant metabolism of vitamin E that results in the production of tocopherylquinone as one of the main byproducts (Galli et al. 2011).

The antioxidant properties of T3 have been demonstrated in several *in vitro* and *in vivo* model systems (reviewed in Suarna et al. [1993], Mensink et al. [1999], and Kamat and Devasagayam [2000]), and early studies by Serbinova et al. (1991) described that α-T3 shows a superior antioxidant effect compared to α-TOH in iron-catalyzed reactions of liver microsomes and cyt P-450 oxidation. It is now well established that structural characteristics of the side chain influence all the physical and chemical properties of vitamin E, including its propensity to produce an antioxidant effect when tested in different reaction environments and particularly in cell membranes (Atkinson et al. 2008). If compared with α-TOH, T3 with their unsaturated side chain show a higher recycling efficiency of chromanoxyl radicals (Suzuki et al. 1993) and a different repartition and spatial interaction with lipid components of cellular membranes and lipoproteins, which may influence the activity of these fat-soluble antioxidants. In this way, T3 could clusterize and produce different degrees of organization and channeling of the flux of hydroperoxyl radicals within the membrane.

Dietary T3 also become incorporated into circulating lipoproteins and are as efficient in scavenging peroxyl radicals as the corresponding TOH isomers (Suarna et al. 1993). α-T3, in particular, lowers the susceptibility of LDL to copper-induced oxidation *ex vivo*. Even if the tocotrienol concentrations within the LDL particle increased only marginally upon supplementation, T3 and particularly α-T3, were found to lower the susceptibility of LDL to copper-induced oxidation *ex vivo* (O'Byrne et al. 2000). The presence of the unsaturated side chain as a moiety responsible by itself of biologically relevant antioxidant effects cannot be excluded at least in some specific reactions (Yu et al. 2005).

Although the antioxidant effect has represented the former and more investigated biochemical interaction of vitamin E (and thus of HMT3) with cellular biomolecules, other and more complex levels of interaction have been demonstrated over the last decades, which may come from antioxidant-independent transcriptional effects of T3 (Viola et al. 2012). TOH and T3-responsive genes are under the control of both redox-sensitive and redox-independent components that constitute a multitargeted mechanism of transcriptional regulation that has been largely investigated both *in vitro* and *in vivo* (Galli and Azzi 2010). The available literature clearly demonstrates that function the HM conformation affects higher number of genes and produces more pronounced transcriptional responses than the fully methylated alpha conformation, but the latter shows highest antioxidant activity within the homologue series in both radical and transition metal reaction systems (Muller et al. 2010; Galli et al. 2011). This functional dichotomy suggests that antioxidant and signaling function of vitamin E forms could not overlap in many of the transcriptional effects reported in literature. Accordingly, signaling and neuro-protection effects of α-T3 appear to be independent of its antioxidant activity (Sen et al. 2000).

A redox-dependent component of T3 signaling is the membrane-associated transcription factor Nrf2 (Das et al. 2008; Hsieh and Wu 2008; Hsieh et al. 2010a,b) that controls drug-metabolizing enzyme (DME) and antioxidant genes described more in detail later. Besides HMT3, this transcriptional regulation is produced by several other hormetic agents such as food phenolics that, behaving as electrophilic stressors, train the cell to develop a higher level of metabolic capability and protection against further stressors (reviewed in Galli [2007]). Nrf2-activating food-derived phenolics include EGCG and resveratrol that synergize with the γ-T3-induced cell-cycle inhibition of estrogen receptor (ER)-positive MCF-7 breast cancer cells (Elangovan et al. 2008), suggesting that the DME/antioxidant response and the control of cell cycle may converge on common regulatory components 3. NFκB transcription activity is also influenced by the treatment of cells with HMT3 (Sylvester et al. 2005). This transcription factor is also under the influence of extracellular and intracellular fluxes of ROS, and its activity is responsible for the generation of inflammatory mediators and for the control of genes involved in cell proliferation, and senescence, as well as in the mitochondrial signaling of apoptosis.

9.2.2 CELL SIGNALING AND TRANSCRIPTIONAL RESPONSE

When compared with α-TOH and other vitamin E forms, T3 molecules show a distinctive cell signaling, possibly by the specific interaction with cellular sensors and receptors (Table 9.1). As introduced in the previous section, besides antioxidant effects and peroxyl radical scavenging, the chroman ring is believed to play a key role in vitamin E signaling (Galli and Azzi 2010). Indeed, the phenolic structure of chromans may dock into or interact with catalytic and regulatory pockets of enzymes (Chandra et al. 2002) and could mimic the steroid structure of estrogens (Comitato et al. 2009) and cholesterol that may facilitate lipid–lipid interactions in cell membranes together with the unsaturated side chain (Atkinson et al. 2008, 2010).

HMT3 are described to bind and activate signaling downstream of ERβ (Comitato et al. 2009). This means that HMT3 may behave as phytoestrogens. The same kind of response is generated by the soy isoflavon daidzein that in some subjects produces the bioactive metabolite equol, which has very close structural and functional homology with the hormone estradiol (reviewed in Galli [2007]). Soy isoflavons are reported to prevent oxidative stress and to produce a better control of insulin and cholesterol metabolism that results in lower cardiovascular morbidity and mortality (Mann et al. 2009; Clerici et al. 2011; Froyen and Steinberg 2011). Similar to estradiol (Santanam et al. 1998), phytoestrogenic substances at the physiologic concentrations observed in body fluids and tissues cannot behave as antioxidant molecules, but their transcriptional effects are well known to produce indirect antioxidant effects by the control of GSH-related defenses in liver cells and other tissues (reviewed in Galli [2007] and Clerici et al. [2011]). These effects demonstrate that ERβ ligands stimulate the same transcriptional elements that respond to HMT3, such as the aforementioned Nfr2/Keap1.

ERβ activation generates the transregulation of other receptors (Sanchez et al. 2010) that may help to explain the transcriptional response and the anticancer activity of T3. These include tyrosine-kinase receptors such as ErbBs that respond to growth factors and the overall activation of G protein-coupled receptors (GPCRs), as well as to chemokines and other ligands such as melatonin (reviewed in Luchetti et al. [2011]). Noteworthy, ErbBs include the ErbB2 (or HER2/neu) that regulates growth and proliferation of epidermal cells and is responsible for the expression of the proto-oncogene HER-2/neu. The latter is diagnosed in nearly 30% of breast tumor biopsies in association with negative prognosis and recidivation (Slamon et al. 1989; Ross and Fletcher 1999). Together with ERβ, these receptors regulate pathways such as the ERK-MAPK, p38, or Akt pathways that have been demonstrated to respond to T3 (Table 9.1) and the AC/cAMP/PKA pathway that can be affected secondarily to GPCRs as well as to cytokine receptors.

This signaling controls several responses to T3 supplementation in a vitamer- and concentration-dependent manner that include the same metabolic processing of T3 vitamers in hepatic and non-hepatic cells (see below). Again, this response is markedly expressed in the case of HMT3 and much less in the case of the fully methylated conformation.

9.3 METABOLISM AND TRANSFORMATION: THE DETOXIFICATION RESPONSE TO T3

9.3.1 T3 SIDE-CHAIN DEGRADATION AND CHROMAN METABOLITE FORMATION

Metabolism and biological activities of T3 suggest that this group of vitamers is not likely to provide classical vitamin E activity as α-TOH does, but rather, they appear to play other and distinct physiological functions that may extend to pharmacological effects and possibly to cancer therapy.

The former and more characterized consequence of the combination of an HM ring with the isoprenyl moiety is that of producing poor bioavailability of dietary vitamers and the highest response of transformation to hepatic metabolites. For the vitamin E molecules introduced with the diet, these responses depend on specific pathways converging in the hepatic α-tocopherol transfer protein (α-TTP), that is, the prototypal vitamin E binding protein regulating uptake and trafficking of all the vitamin E forms in liver cells as well as their blood transfering via nascent VLDL (Morley et al. 2008). The hepatic α-TTP binds the fully methylated and saturated form, i.e., α-TOH, with an at least 10-fold higher affinity than HM forms and all the T3 forms (Hosomi et al. 1997). While the bound vitamers are incorporated in the nascent VLDL for blood transfering and tissue distribution, the unbound forms undergo metabolic processing and biliary excretion.

The T3-derived induction of hepatic metabolism results in the formation of transformation metabolites with different chain length that can be measured in plasma and urine with well established analytical procedures reviewed in Galli et al. (2007) and Zhao et al. (2010). Metabolic processing of tocotrienol and tocopherol forms consists of an initial CYP450-dependent ω-hydroxylation followed by β-oxidation and resulting in the rapid formation of the endproduct carboxyethyl hydroxychroman (CEHC) acid. This is the main metabolite of vitamin E found *in vivo* in plasma and urine and is also considered the most useful indicator of vitamin E metabolism in humans and animals (Galli et al. 2002, 2003). Side-chain degradation starts with a hydroxylation of the ω-methyl group and is followed by five cycles of β-oxidation. All intermediates have been identified by MS analysis (Swanson et al. 1999; Schuelke et al. 2000; Birringer et al. 2002; Sontag and Parker 2002; Birringer 2010). Data from *in vitro* experiments performed with HepG2 cells have shown that in the case of γ-T3, all possible carboxylic acid intermediates of degradation, including γ-carboxydimethyldecadienyl hydroxychroman (γ-CDMD(en)$_2$HC), γ-carboxydimethyl-decyl hydroxychroman (γ-CDMDHC), γ-carboxydimethyloctenyl hydroxychroman (γ-CDMOenHC), γ-carboxymethylhexenyl hydroxychroman (γ-CMHenHC), γ-carboxymethylbutyl hedroxychroman (CMBHC), and γ-CEHC are released, whereas for α-tocotrienol, only the precursors, α-CEHC, α-CMBHC, α-CMHenHC, and α-CDMOenHC, but not α-CDMD(en)$_2$HC, are formed (Birringer et al. 2002). The identification of α- and γ-CMBHC—instead of a metabolite still containing the double bond present in the precursors α- and γ-CMHenHC—revealed that T3 metabolism involves a more complex mechanism compared to that of tocopherols and indicates that side-chain degradation follows the pathway of branched-chain fatty acids. In this case, auxiliary enzymes are required (Birringer et al. 2002).

9.3.2 DME RESPONSE TO T3

T3 represent the natural form of vitamin E with highest induction response of drug-metabolizing enzyme (DME) genes that include the phase I PXR-dependent Cyt P-450 isoenzyme CYP3A4, the form with broader drug-metabolizing activity in liver cells (Brigelius-Flohe 2005), and CYP4F2.

The latter is the main isoenzyme so far demonstrated to catalyze the ω-oxidation of the side chain as the first step of vitamin E metabolism (Sontag and Parker 2007) that has been described in detail the previous section. The *in vivo* and *in vitro* supplementation of T3 also stimulates the expression of phase II detoxification enzymes such as sulfo and glucuronyl transferases (Freiser and Jiang 2009). The γ-T3-induced inhibition of cell-cycle regulatory proteins in ER-positive MCF-7 human breast cancer cells is associated with redox changes and the induction of the phase II detoxification enzyme quinone reductase NQO2, which is controlled through the activation of the redox-sensitive transcription factors Nrf2-Keap1 (Hsieh et al. 2010). The transcription of other genes of relevance to anti-inflammatory and anticancer effects of T3 can be regulated by means of the redox-sensitive response of NFkB (Ahn et al. 2007). Other phase II and phase III genes involved in the coordinated response to α-TOH intake and metabolism are expected to be influenced by the highly metabolized HM-T3, such as the glutathione-*S*-transferase and biliary transporters that include *p*-glycoprotein (Belli et al. 2009) and other functional homologues identified in rats fed with diets high in α-TOH (Mustacich et al. 2009).

At the same time, DME genes can be influenced by T3 forms through direct effects on the same products of the DME response such as GST P1-1 that has been reported to be inhibited with an allosteric mechanism by physiological concentrations of α-TOC and γ-T3 (van Haaften et al. 2002). DME induction may suggest a risk of drug interactions. Hepatic metabolism and therapeutic efficacy of drugs when high doses of T3 are used as supplements to the diet (Brigelius-Flohe 2005).

At the same time, the DME response can be considered the cipher of T3 cytotoxicity and also a putative mechanism for the anticancer and cell-protection effects of these vitamers. Similar to drugs and other natural bioactive compounds and endogenous factors that fall into the concept of hormesis (reviewed in Galli [2007], Le Bourg [2009], and Ristow et al. [2009]), T3 show biphasic concentration-dependent effects that suggest a functional overlap between toxicity and therapeutic mechanisms.

In vitro studies carried out in different cell model systems have contributed to elucidate the relationship between cytotoxicity mechanisms and possible therapeutic effects of T3. Studies on primary cultures of cerebellar neurons and astrocytes exposed to high concentrations of γ-T3 (100 μM or higher) have shown marked effects of toxicity that were absent in the case of α-TOH (Mazlan et al. 2006; Then et al. 2009). This toxicity was associated with the activation of stress-dependent p38 MAPK and p53 (Then et al. 2009). On the other hand, at lower concentrations, γ-T3 was more potent than α-TOH in preventing H_2O_2 toxicity and the induction of the Bcl-2/Bax mitochondrial pathway of apoptosis.

It is noteworthy that phase II and III gene induction is a key event in drug resistance and may thus represent a problem in the application of T3 in cancer therapy. Although this aspect has been poorly investigated, anticancer effects of this form of vitamin E appear to involve multiple and specific mechanisms that may overcome resistance mechanisms of cancer cells at cell concentrations that are well tolerated in noncancerous cells. At the same time, the DME response to T3 could represent a facilitating component for other anticancer drugs that are directly or indirectly activated by the same enzymes that detoxify T3. These aspects could apply to the synergistic effects proposed for cotherapy regimens of γ-T3 and antioxidant phenolics as EGCG and resveratrol described earlier (Elangovan et al. 2008). It cannot be ruled out that this aspect may also influence the synergistic effects reported for statins and δ-T3 or γ-T3 (McAnally et al. 2007; Hussein and Mo 2009; Wali et al. 2009b), which primarily involves the inhibition of cholesterol biosynthesis (see in Section 9.5) or other drugs that may benefit from stress and senescence signaling of T3 (Table 9.1).

9.4 METABOLISM OR BIOACTIVATION PROCESS?

Vitamin E metabolites have been suggested to possess biological activities, which may have some relevance to the physiological function of this vitamin. It is anticipated that these activities may contribute to the anticancer role of T3 or other forms of vitamin E. Actually, pharmacological concentrations of CEHCs with gamma conformation have been demonstrated to stimulate the same anticancer signaling of the TOH and T3 precursors (Conte et al. 2004; Galli et al. 2004), and there is evidence that T3-responsive genes involved in vitamin E metabolism are also expressed in non-hepatic cancer cells, which produce chromanol metabolites (Conte et al. 2004; You et al. 2005; Yang et al. 2010). This metabolism may provide the conditions to reach high intracellular concentrations and peritumoral levels of CEHCs as well as of other metabolites.

Long-chain metabolites of T3 are formed in A549 type II alveolar epithelial cells, but not in HepG2 hepatocytes, thus suggesting the existence of cancer-specific differences in T3 metabolism (You et al. 2005). 9′-Carboxychromanol was identified as main metabolite in this lung carcinoma cell line, whereas 3′- and 5′-carboxychromanols predominated in HepG2 cells, and this difference was proposed to depend on a cell-specific inefficient conversion to 7′-carboxychromanols in the peroxisomal compartment of A549 cells.

More recent work by Freiser and Jiang (2009) demonstrated the accumulation of sulfated derivatives of long-chain intermediates both in A549 type II alveolar epithelial cells and *in vivo* in rats supplemented with γ-T3 or γ-TOH. Sulfated 9′-, 11′-, and 13′-carboxychromanols and their unconjugated counterparts were identified after *in vitro* supplementation in A549 cells and derivatization to sulfated forms was twofold faster in the case of γ-T3 than γ-TOH. The rapid (within 6 h from the supplementation) *in vivo* metabolization of these vitamers was consistent with the appearance in plasma of 13′-carboxychromanol and sulfated 9′-, 11′-, 13′-carboxychromanol, with the sulfated 11′-carboxychromanol as the most abundant long-chain metabolite in γ-T3-supplemented rats.

The finding that CEHCs possess discrete biological activities has suggested the existence of a relationship between metabolism and bioactivity of vitamin E forms (reviewed in Brigelius-Flohe [2006] and Galli et al. [2007]). CEHC metabolite bioactivity has so far been reported to include direct antioxidant and anti-inflammatory effects, mild natriuretic function, and even antiproliferative activity. More recent *in vitro* experiments have suggested a role of CEHCs in the control of PKC activity and superoxide anion generation of neutrophils (Varga et al. 2008). In the majority of these functions, γ-CEHC was described to possess higher bioactivity in the CEHC series.

CEHC have not been reported to bind nuclear receptors, such as PXR and PPAR, nor vitamin E binding proteins (reviewed in Traber [2004] and Brigelius-Flohe [2005]), which suggests that these short-chain metabolites may have limited relevance in the control of vitamin E–sensitive genes.

The existence of bioactive derivatives of vitamin E was confirmed in recent studies in which long-chain metabolites were investigated. These metabolites are rapidly processed by the metabolic machinery of liver cells to form the endproduct CEHC, and thus their levels in the circulation are extremely low, but their potency as *in vitro* anti-inflammatory and pro-apoptotic agents was proposed to be much stronger than that of CEHCs. Consistent with the proposed anti-inflammatory activity of T3 (Elangovan et al. 2008; Yam et al. 2009), long-chain metabolites, and particularly 13′-carboxychromanol, have been recently identified to inhibit effects on cyclooxygenase activity (Jiang and Yin 2008). At the same time, these metabolites promote oxidative stress and pro-apoptotic effects in HepG2 cells (Birringer et al. 2010).

Altogether, these pieces of evidence suggest that metabolites may sustain and even expand the function of vitamin E, also providing further insights into molecular mechanisms and possible applications of this vitamin in cancer therapy.

9.5 ANTICANCER MECHANISM OF HMT3: WHEN MORE TOXIC MEANS MORE EFFECTIVE

In vivo and *in vitro* anticancer mechanisms of T3 so far described in literature include antiproliferative effects by the inhibition of cell cycle, induction of apoptosis, antioxidant and anti-inflammatory effects, inhibition of angiogenesis, and suppression of 3-hydroxy-3-methylglutaryl coenzyme A (HMG CoA) reductase activity (reviewed in Wada [2009]).

This literature is consistent with the evidence that HMT3, i.e., the forms with highest *in vivo* metabolism and *in vitro* cytotoxicity effects—represent the most potent anticancer forms of vitamin E (reviewed in Constantinou et al. [2008] and Viola et al. [2012]). When investigated in cell model systems of breast and prostate cancer, which are two hormone-dependent cancers with expected susceptibility to vitamin E interventions, HMT3 show much stronger antiproliferative and pro-apoptotic activity than TOH and α-T3 (recently reviewed in Viola et al. [2012]). δ-T3 is the most potent form tested in pancreatic adenocarcinoma cells (Hussein and Mo 2009), while γ-T3 was recently described to be the vitamer with anticancer activity in colon cancer cells (Xu et al. 2009; Kannappan et al. 2010a), which is another cancer form tentatively proposed as preventable by vitamin E therapy (Stone et al. 2004) and in melanoma cells (Chang et al. 2009).

In both estrogen-sensitive (MCF-7 or ZR-75-1) and estrogen-insensitive cells (MDA-MB 435 or 231), T3 and particularly γ-T3 and δ-T3 were demonstrated to inhibit cell proliferation (Nesaretnam et al. 1998) with an estrogen-independent effect and synergistic activity with the antiestrogen drug tamoxifen (Guthrie et al. 1997; Nesaretnam et al. 2000). More recent work has demonstrated that cell-cycle inhibition by T3 occurs through the control of the Rb/cdk4/cyclin D pathway (Elangovan et al. 2008) that is also affected by the HM forms of tocopherols and particularly by γ-TOH (Betti et al. 2006). In the same cell models, T3 were demonstrated to induce apoptosis with δ-T3 as the most potent form (Yu et al. 1999) and with a mechanism that involves mitochondrial disruption and cyt c release (Takahashi and Loo 2004). As introduced earlier, recent studies by our group confirmed that δ-T3 is the most potent T3 form with pro-apoptotic activity higher than α-TOS in breast cancer cells (Pierpaoli et al. 2010). As described in the previous section, the activity of δ-T3 observed in this *in vitro* experimental model system can be partially explained by a high uptake rate that rapidly brings the cell content of this vitamer to the levels required to produce its *in vitro* anticancer activity.

However, experimental evidence clearly suggests the existence of a marked cell- and disease-related specificity for T3 effects that suggests other and more complex mechanisms than a simple increase in the uptake rate, and this appears to be true for the other forms of vitamin E as well (reviewed in Galli and Azzi [2010]). Intrinsic characteristics of cancer cells may sustain the therapeutic potential and specificity of action of T3. For instance, recent work has demonstrated that the α-TTP-like protein TAP/Sec14L2 normally expressed in non-neoplastic tissues as breast, prostate, and liver is lost or markedly decreased in expression after cancerogenic differentiation (Wang et al. 2009). This protein may thus represent a tumor suppressor with a physiological role in the antiproliferative activity of vitamin E molecules, which after downregulation may produce abnormal cell trafficking and metabolism of T3 in cancer cells, ultimately increasing T3 toxicity and leading to antiproliferative and cell death effects. Interestingly enough, this downregulation effect is observed in tissues that develop hormone-sensitive cancers responsive to T3 treatments such as prostate and breast. As a further example, malignant proliferation is associated with an increased HMG CoA reductase activity (Mo and Elson 2004), and T3 suppress this activity by either synthesis inhibition or accelerated degradation of the enzyme protein (Song and DeBose-Boyd 2006). Synergistic effects between statins and δ-T3 or γ-T3 have been demonstrated in *in vitro* antiproliferative activity tests carried out in diverse tumor cells (McAnally et al. 2007; Hussein and Mo 2009; Wali et al. 2009b).

The specificity of action of T3 in cancer cells may also involve other players. HM T3 forms are reported to produce the highest activation response of the caspase-dependent mitochondrial pathway of apoptosis (Sylvester 2007; Constantinou et al. 2009; Pierpaoli et al. 2010). In breast cancer cells, the γ-T3-induced apoptosisis is sustained by the endoplasmic reticulum stress signaling and caspase 12 activation (Wali et al. 2009). These vitamers, however, are also expected to activate the caspase-independent pathway (Constantinou et al. 2009), and we recently demonstrated a differential effect of δ-T3 with respect to α-TOS and other vitamin E forms on the induction of senescence-like cell genes, which further discloses the relationship between cell stress and antiproliferative mechanism of T3 in breast cancer cells (Pierpaoli et al. 2010). These genes include cell-cycle checkpoints such as the cyclin-dependent kinase (cdk) inhibitor p21 that regulates the activity of cyclin E and the oncogene p53. The same finding was obtained in ER-positive MCF-7 human breast cancer cells by Heisen et al. (2010). Growth suppression of these cells by γ-T3 was accompanied by a time- and dose-dependent modulation of cell cycle regulatory proteins such as the Rb/E2F complex, cyclin D1/cdk4, and cyclin B1/cdk1, which ultimately control Rb phosphorylation. Concomitantly, the Nrf2-dependent phase II enzyme quinone reductase 2 was induced, thus confirming the hypothesis of a functional link between the T3-dependent control of drug metabolism and anticancer pathways discussed in the previous sections.

A lower cancer incidence by the induction of the p21 signaling pathway has been suggested to be the underlying mechanism of the 15% increased lifespan of mice supplemented lifelong with α-TOH (Banks et al. 2010). Demethylated forms, and particularly the gamma form of TOH, have been observed to activate cellcycle regulators such as p27/Rb both *in vitro* (Betti et al. 2006) and *in vivo* (Lee et al. 2009). Therefore, p21 and other genes directly or indirectly involved in cellcycle control, such as p27 and p53, may represent the real effectors in the anticancer signaling of T3, influencing the balance between signals that drive the cell into the senescence-like pathway and cellcycle arrest or alternatively toward apoptotic cell death. Upstream elements in this signaling include PKC and the survival pathway ERK-MAPK that is known to influence the mitochondrial signaling in response to foreign stimuli and endobiotics such as hormones and redox-active metabolites (recently reviewed in Luchetti et al. [2011]). PKC was the former component in the cell signaling that was identified to be controlled by vitamin E (Galli and Azzi 2010) and is the earliest kinase that responds in a concentration and time-dependent manner to vitamin E, leading to signal transduction from the plasmalemma to downstream elements. Membrane translocation and activity of PKC are directly influenced by chromanols (Varga et al. 2008), which may provide a mechanism to explain the close correlation between kinetics profiles of antiproliferative signaling and uptake rate (i.e., relative concentration within the lipid bilayer) of vitamin E molecules (Betti et al. 2006).

Further anticancer mechanisms of T3 possibly associated with cell toxicity include the inhibition of angiogenesis that has been demonstrated both *in vitro* and *in vivo* (Miyazawa et al. 2004). This effect has been reported particularly in the case of δ-T3 with a mechanism that may involve the inhibition of the PI3K/PDK/Akt pathway and the inhibition of migration and adhesion of cancer cells onto endothelial cells and also the induction of endothelial cell stress (Shibata et al. 2008).

9.6 δ-T3: THE MOST POTENT ANTICANCER FORM OF VITAMIN E IN HER-2/neu-POSITIVE BREAST ADENOCARCINOMA

The superiority of T3 over TOH as anticancer agents in breast tumors has been established both *in vitro* and *in vivo* (Gould et al. 1991; McIntyre et al. 2000). Recent studies by our group in human SKBr3 and murine TUBO breast carcinoma cells have clearly demonstrated that δ-T3 can afford higher cell viability inhibition and apoptosis than other natural forms of vitamin E and α-TOS (Pierpaoli et al. 2010; Viola et al. 2012), that is, the synthetic and redox-silent derivative of vitamin E with one of the highest *in vitro* and *in vivo* anticancer activities so far reported in literature (reviewed in Zhao et al. [2009]). The extent of this *in vitro* anticancer signaling of δ-T3 follows that of the uptake rate of this form of T3 in cancer cells that is higher than that of any other form of vitamin E (Viola et al. 2012; Pierpaoli et al. manuscript in preparation).

As far as *in vivo* studies regards, Gould et al. (1991) were among the former to observe that T3, but not TOH, enhance tumor latency in a rat model of mammary cancer. T3-based therapy has also been successfully investigated in immunocompromised animals after ectopic implantation of breast cancer cells (Nesaretnam et al. 2004), confirming that HMT3 are the most efficient forms. However, the *in vivo* anticancer effects of δ-T3 in breast cancer, the most effective anticancer form of vitamin E *in vitro* (Pierpaoli et al. 2010; Viola et al. 2012), are still elusive. We recently investigated the antitumor activity of a T3 extract from Annatto seeds, a mixture of 90% δ-T3 and 10% γ-T3, in a genetically modified mice developing HER-2/neu-positive breast cancer (Pierpaoli et al. manuscript in preparation). Experimental data show that annatto-T3 administration delayed the development of tumor masses and drastically reduced the volume of mammary tumors compared to control mice. This effect was due to both senescence-like growth arrest and apoptotic cell death as determined by the analysis of cancer cells isolated from the tumor masses, while the immune system of these mice was not affected by the Anatto-T3 treatment. Supplementary data obtained from *in vitro* experiments demonstrate that human and mouse breast tumor cells exposed to increasing doses of annatto-T3 undergo growth arrest and apoptosis, modulating cell-cycle regulators like p53, p21[WAF1], and p27[kip1] and reducing the HER-2/neu RNA/protein expression, which is in agreement with the data obtained in the *in vitro* study on the anticancer mechanism of pure δ-T3 (Pierpaoli et al. 2010). Further preclinical investigation is awaited to establish the therapeutic potential of δ-T3 in HER-2/neu-positive breast cancer.

9.7   CELL UPTAKE: A CRITICAL ASPECT OF THE ANTICANCER ACTIVITY OF HMT3

Cell uptake rate and metabolic processing influence the *in vitro* bioactivity of different vitamin E forms. This is true for either cytoprotection or anticancer activity of T3, which shows concentration-dependent functional regulation of different signaling routes and groups of genes.

It has been recently observed that the difference between the *in vitro* cytoprotection function of α-T3 and α-TOH in glutamate toxicity originally shown in neuronal cells by Sen et al. (2000, 2004) may depend on the faster cell uptake rate of α-T3 rather than on vitamer-specific effects on cell signaling (Saito et al. 2010). Indeed, when T3 and TOH forms reached the same cell concentrations, the same level of activity was observed, suggesting higher potency of α-TOH in the prevention of glutamate cytotoxicity *in vivo* (Saito et al. 2010).

The same was demonstrated by our group comparing the antiproliferative activity of TOH forms on C6 glioblastoma cells (Betti et al. 2006). The HM form γ-TOH showed higher uptake rate and thus higher antiproliferative activity, but once the same cell content was reached, all the forms of TOH showed similar levels of activity.

The higher potency of T3 as compared to TOH forms as inhibitors of cell growth in preneoplastic and even more in neoplastic mouse mammary epithelial cells (McIntyre et al. 2000) has been attributed to a preferential uptake of T3. This rapidly provides the cell with levels of these vitamers that are critical for the generation of a stress response (Then et al. 2009). Recent data obtained in TUBO murine breast cancer cells showed that the anticancer effect of δ-T3, the most potent anticancer form in breast adenocarcinoma cells (Pierpaoli et al. 2010; Viola et al. 2012), follows the same cell uptake-dependent mechanism (Galli. F., unpublished data).

It is anticipated that a rapid and massive uptake of HM forms, and in particular of δ-T3, in cancer cells may influence the lipid structure and key functional domains of the plasmalemma (Atkinson et al. 2010). The differential cell uptake of vitamin E forms could involve specific transporters such as the organic anion transport system (Negis et al. 2007), but also direct membrane transfer and intramembrane diffusion, as well as interaction mechanisms that appear to favor uptake and bioactivity mechanisms of HMT3 forms (Palozza et al. 2006).

These aspects suggest that selective uptake and cellular distribution of T3 forms may contribute to the specificity of action of HMT3 in cancer tissues and also suggest a strategy to overcome limited efficacy of therapeutic protocols based on oral administration of these vitamers. Bypassing the liver metabolism with local and tumor-targeted administration procedures may enhance the anticancer potency and specificity of action of T3, thus providing higher pharmacokinetics and therapeutic efficacy.

9.8   *IN VITRO* AND *IN VIVO* STUDIES ON TOXICITY AND THERAPEUTIC WINDOW OF T3

Other key aspects in the application of T3 in cancer therapy concern the issues of efficacy and therapeutic window. The therapeutic window of a drug is the dose and blood concentration capable of maximizing positive therapeutic effects while excluding risks and side effects associated with toxicity and adverse reactions.

As far as toxicity and adverse reactions are concerned, oral vitamin E is considered to have very low toxicity in healthy humans (Hathcock et al. 2005; Galli and Azzi 2010); 1000 mg/day is the upper safe limit and 17 mg/kg bw/day, assuming a 60 kg person, is the tolerable upper intake level of α-TOH for adults as proposed by the Food and Nutrition Board, Institute of Medicine (Food and Nutrition Board 2000). Although a systematic investigation has not been performed, clinical studies on oral supplements and food rich in T3 are consistent with the absence of toxicity in humans. T3 is considered to be safe within the same window of dosage considered for α-TOH intake, that is, with UL of 1000 mg/day. Even T3-rich formulations with highest bioavailability (with plasma levels of a-T3 that increase up to ≈3 μM, i.e., up to threefold the levels obtained with normal T3 supplements) so far proposed for human supplementation, have been demonstrated to be safe (reviewed in Sen et al. [2007]).

Acute and chronic studies in animal models have confirmed low *in vivo* toxicity of T3 vitamers. Liver toxicity effects have been observed in mice, but only when these were feed with a diet very high in T3 (2% w/w, that is ~0.5 g/animal) (Tasaki et al. 2009).

As a consequence of this, palm oil-derived tocols, with T3 and α-TOH as the principal components, in all the ingredients and food intended for human use have recently obtained Generally Recognized As Safe certification by the US FDA board (FDA 2010).

The fact that similar potential and mechanisms of cytotoxicity of T3 could be proposed for other natural compounds with lipophilic nature such as carotenoids and their oxidation metabolites (Siems et al. 2009; both interfere with the cell redox and mitochondrial function), suggests to consider coadministrations as potentially hazardous. In humans, diets very high in palm oil intake have been reported to produce signs of liver sufferance, while a moderate intake of this oil, especially when used in the refined or red form (which is remarkably rich in T3 and carotenoids), has been proposed to be curative in different types of disorders (reviewed in Edem [2002]).

Based on the available evidence, it is possible to assume that T3 toxicity is prevented by the same mechanisms that control α-TOH metabolism and toxicity. The α-TTP-mediated selective restriction of liver uptake and the sustained metabolism of T3, which are described in detail in Section 9.3, provide the protection mechanism and, on the other hand, confirm the need for a prompt detoxification and the potential for toxicity effects in human cells.

Thus, once the toxicity of T3 is determined, what remains to be established is the dose within the UL that will produce highest bioactivity and therapeutic effects.

Neuroprotection and anticancer effects are two biological functions of T3 that can be considered to discuss this aspect. The former was defined by the original work of Sen et al. (2000) as the prevention activity that α-T3, but not α-TOH, has on glutamate-induced death of T4 hippocampal neuronal cells at nanomolar concentrations that are 4–10 times lower than the levels found in plasma. Indeed, α-T3 in human and animal plasma usually reaches maximum 1 μmol/L irrespective of the amount supplemented (Lodge et al. 2001; Mustad et al. 2002). Therefore, this cytoprotection effect is mediated by physiological T3 concentrations that produced c-Src-dependent stimulation of the survival pathway MAPK-ERK in these neuronal cells and decreased 12-LOX and eicosanoid pathway activation through a lowered depletion of intracellular glutathione (Sen et al. 2004). If such a tiny T3 concentration, as needed for neuronal cell protection, can be reached in the human brain by the oral supplementation of tocotrienols, remains to be conclusively demonstrated, but it is likely to occur (Khanna et al. 2005).

On the contrary, the well-recognized *in vitro* anticancer activity of most potent T3 forms, that is, HM forms, occurs at extracellular concentrations far from the physiological. Indeed, the majority of data obtained assessing the antiproliferative and pro-apoptotic activity of HM T3 in different breast cancer cell lines showed IC50 values between 3 and 30 μM, while, in nonmammary cells, IC50 values are between 20 and 70 μM (reviewed in Viola et al. [2012]). The lowest IC50 levels in breast cancer cells (McIntyre et al. 2000) were obtained by means of days of *in vitro* exposure to concentrations of HM T3 that are close to, but lower than, the levels of γ- and δ-T3 found in human and animal plasma after supplementation (Lodge et al. 2001; Mustad et al. 2002). Furthermore, half-life of all T3 investigated in humans (α, γ, δ) are 4.5–8.7 times shorter than those of α-TOH (Yap et al. 2001;

Schaffer et al. 2005), thus suggesting unfavorable pharmacokinetics of oral administration protocols by the sustained liver metabolism.

These aspects may lead to conclude that even at the highest dosages compatible with UL, oral T3 could not meet the extracellular levels required to generate main anticancer effects *in vivo*. Notwithstanding, levels and bioactivity of T3 could be higher and close to therapeutic efficacy thanks to local mechanisms, which could be further sustained by cancerogenic transformation (see above). Although tissue levels of T3 usually are very low (Podda et al. 1996), biodistribution studies in wild type and α-TTP null rodents have shown that supplemental T3 can be delivered to all organs (Khanna et al. 2005), thus suggesting the existence of α-TTP-independent mechanisms of tissue distribution for T3. Tissue-specific differences between α-T3 and α-TOH levels after standard or supplemented diets have been reported, with preferential uptake and higher levels of α-T3 than α-TOH in some tissues such as skin and possibly adipose tissues of these animals. Skin concentrations of α-T3 in the supplemented animals also showed a build up over time for regimens of prolonged supplementation, and tissue transport systems can be deactivated when animals are fed with diets deficient in T3 and rich in TOH, which suggests an interference of dietary α-TOH on T3 bioavailability and tissue distribution in animals supplemented with T3 (reviewed in Sen et al. [2007]).

Preliminary evidence suggests that T3 levels are lowered in the adipose tissue of breast lumps obtained from malignant breast cancer patients compared to benign patients (Nesaretnam et al. 2007). This evidence supports the idea that T3 may provide protection against breast cancer and that interventions aimed to increase T3 levels in the breast tissue may result in secondary prevention or even chemotherapeutic effects.

Based on this burden of knowledge, a therapeutic window for T3 might be proposed for the neuroprotective function that α-T3 can produce under conditions of glutamate-dependent cytotoxicity (this coincides with oral doses that maintain plasma levels of this form of T3 near to 1 μM), but not for the anticancer (chemoprevention) effect of HM T3 proposed by means of huge *in vitro* evidence.

In vivo studies so far performed in immunocompromised animals after ectopic implantation of breast cancer cells (Nesaretnam et al. 2004) as well as other studies that investigated tumor mass growth and vascularization in other models of ectopic implants (Nakagawa et al. 2007; Shibata et al. 2009; Weng-Yew et al. 2009) have not provided an affordable model system to clarify this point. These studies were based on the supplementation of high dosages (between 1 and 10 mg/day) of T3 under the form of palm oil–derived T3-rich fraction (TRF) that provided different contributions to the observed anticancer effects by the individual forms of T3 contained in this type of formulation. Moreover, information concerning bioavailability and tumor targeting of T3 in these studies was scant, and the models appear to be far from reflecting the conditions of human therapy. To our knowledge, *in vivo* studies on the anticancer effect of T3 in humans are missing. This lack of knowledge is a gap to fill before the next generation of clinical trials on T3 therapy of cancer will be proposed. Distribution, metabolism, and local activity in human tissues are poorly understood and deserve further investigation to confirm mechanisms, specificity of action, and therapeutic window of T3.

9.9 CONCLUSION AND FURTHER PERSPECTIVES

In conclusion, HMT3 are the more toxic forms of vitamin E that behave as cell stressors, mitocans, and pro-apoptotic agents. *In vitro* studies have demonstrated that all these effects are the key for the anticancer potential of T3 and may also provide a clue into the cell-protection mechanisms (hormetic effect) of T3 that involves the induction of drug metabolizing and stress-response genes.

Breast cancer is among the malignancies with highest responsiveness to T3 both *in vitro* and *in vivo*. Selective mechanisms of control of cell cycle and apoptosis in breast cancer cells have been identified. Highest levels of potency combined with this selectivity in the anticancer signaling have been observed for the HM form δ-T3 investigated both *in vitro* and *in vivo* in *HER-2/neu-positive breast adenocarcinoma*. More research is needed to confirm these preclinical findings and to translate them in the next generation of breast cancer chemoprevention and chemotherapy trials.

ACKNOWLEDGMENTS

Research work on vitamin E in the laboratory of FG has been supported by the national grant program PRIN of the Italian Ministry of University and Research (MIUR), grant code 20078TC4E5, and by the Italian Cystic Fibrosis Foundation (grant # FFC13/2008).

REFERENCES

Agarwal, M. K., M. L. Agarwal et al. (2004). Tocotrienol-rich fraction of palm oil activates p53, modulates Bax/Bcl2 ratio and induces apoptosis independent of cell cycle association. *Cell Cycle* 3(2): 205–211.

Aggarwal, B. B., C. Sundaram et al. (2010). Tocotrienols, the vitamin E of the 21st century: Its potential against cancer and other chronic diseases. *Biochem Pharmacol* 80(11): 1613–1631.

Ahn, K. S., G. Sethi et al. (2007). Gamma-tocotrienol inhibits nuclear factor-kappaB signaling pathway through inhibition of receptor-interacting protein and TAK1 leading to suppression of antiapoptotic gene products and potentiation of apoptosis. *J Biol Chem* 282(1): 809–820.

Atkinson, J., R. F. Epand et al. (2008). Tocopherols and tocotrienols in membranes: a critical review. *Free Radic Biol Med* 44(5): 739–764.

Atkinson, J., T. Harroun et al. (2010) The location and behavior of alpha-tocopherol in membranes. *Mol Nutr Food Res* 54(5): 641–651.

Banks, R., J. R. Speakman et al. (2010) Vitamin E supplementation and mammalian lifespan. *Mol Nutr Food Res* 54(5): 719–725.

Belli, S., P. M. Elsener et al. (2009). Cholesterol-mediated activation of P-glycoprotein: distinct effects on basal and drug-induced ATPase activities. *J Pharm Sci* 98(5): 1905–1918.

Betti, M., A. Minelli et al. (2006). Antiproliferative effects of tocopherols (vitamin E) on murine glioma C6 cells: Homologue-specific control of PKC/ERK and cyclin signaling. *Free Radic Biol Med* 41(3): 464–472.

Birringer, M. (2010) Analysis of vitamin E metabolites in biological specimen. *Mol Nutr Food Res* 54(5): 588–598.

Birringer, M., D. Lington et al. (2010). Proapoptotic effects of long-chain vitamin E metabolites in HepG2 cells are mediated by oxidative stress. *Free Radic Biol Med* 49: 1315–1322.

Birringer, M., P. Pfluger et al. (2002). Identities and differences in the metabolism of tocotrienols and tocopherols in HepG2 cells. *J Nutr* 132(10): 3113–3118.

Brigelius-Flohe, R. (2005). Induction of drug metabolizing enzymes by vitamin E. *J Plant Physiol* 162(7): 797–802.

Brigelius-Flohe, R. (2006). Bioactivity of vitamin E. *Nutr Res Rev* 19(2): 174–186.

Chandra, V., J. Jasti et al. (2002). First structural evidence of a specific inhibition of phospholipase A2 by alpha-tocopherol (vitamin E) and its implications in inflammation: Crystal structure of the complex formed between phospholipase A2 and alpha-tocopherol at 1.8 A resolution. *J Mol Biol* 320(2): 215–222.

Chang, P. N., W. N. Yap et al. (2009). Evidence of gamma-tocotrienol as an apoptosis-inducing, invasion-suppressing, and chemotherapy drug-sensitizing agent in human melanoma cells. *Nutr Cancer* 61(3): 357–366.

Clerici, C., E. Nardi et al. (2011). Novel soy germ pasta improves endothelial function, blood pressure, and oxidative stress in patients with type 2 diabetes. *Diabetes Care* 34(9): 1946–1948.

Comitato, R., K. Nesaretnam et al. (2009). A novel mechanism of natural vitamin E tocotrienol activity: Involvement of ERbeta signal transduction. *Am J Physiol Endocrinol Metab* 297(2): E427–E437.

Constantinou, C., J. A. Hyatt et al. (2009). Induction of caspase-independent programmed cell death by vitamin E natural homologs and synthetic derivatives. *Nutr Cancer* 61(6): 864–874.

Constantinou, C., A. Papas et al. (2008). Vitamin E and cancer: An insight into the anticancer activities of vitamin E isomers and analogs. *Int J Cancer* 123(4): 739–752.

Conte, C., A. Floridi et al. (2004). Gamma-tocotrienol metabolism and antiproliferative effect in prostate cancer cells. *Ann N Y Acad Sci* 1031: 391–394.

Das, M., S. Das et al. (2008). Caveolin and proteasome in tocotrienol mediated myocardial protection. *Cell Physiol Biochem* 22(1–4): 287–294.

Edem, D. O. (2002). Palm oil: Biochemical, physiological, nutritional, hematological, and toxicological aspects: A review. *Plant Foods Hum Nutr* 57(3–4): 319–341.

Eitsuka, T., K. Nakagawa et al. (2006). Down-regulation of telomerase activity in DLD-1 human colorectal adenocarcinoma cells by tocotrienol. *Biochem Biophys Res Commun* 348(1): 170–175.

Elangovan, S., T. C. Hsieh et al. (2008). Growth inhibition of human MDA-mB-231 breast cancer cells by delta-tocotrienol is associated with loss of cyclin D1/CDK4 expression and accompanying changes in the state of phosphorylation of the retinoblastoma tumor suppressor gene product. *Anticancer Res* 28(5A): 2641–2647.

FDA (2010). GRAS Notice (No. GRN 000307). C. OFAS.

Food and Nutrition Board, I. O. M., ed. (2000). Dietary Reference Intakes for Vitamin C, Vitamin E, Selenium, and Carotenoids. A report of the Panel on Dietary Antioxidants and Related Compounds, Subcommittees on Upper Reference Levels of Nutrients and Interpretation and Uses of Dietary Reference Intakes, and the Standing Committee on the Scientific Evaluation of Dietary Reference Intakes.. National Academy Press, Washington, DC.

Freiser, H. and Q. Jiang (2009). Gamma-tocotrienol and gamma-tocopherol are primarily metabolized to conjugated 2-(beta-carboxyethyl)-6-hydroxy-2,7,8-trimethylchroman and sulfated long-chain carboxychromanols in rats. *J Nutr* 139(5): 884–889.

Froyen, E. B. and F. M. Steinberg (2011). Soy isoflavones increase quinone reductase in hepa-1c1c7 cells via estrogen receptor beta and nuclear factor erythroid 2-related factor 2 binding to the antioxidant response element. *J Nutr Biochem* 22(9): 843–848.

Galli, F. (2007). Interactions of polyphenolic compounds with drug disposition and metabolism. *Curr Drug Metab* 8(8): 830–838.

Galli, F. and A. Azzi (2010). Present trends in vitamin E research. *Biofactors* 36(1): 33–42.

Galli, F., M. Cristina Polidori et al. (2007). Vitamin E biotransformation in humans. *Vitam Horm* 76: 263–280.

Galli, F., R. Lee et al. (2002). Gas chromatography mass spectrometry analysis of carboxyethyl-hydroxy-chroman metabolites of alpha- and gamma-tocopherol in human plasma. *Free Radic Biol Med* 32(4): 333–340.

Galli, F., R. Lee et al. (2003). Gamma-tocopherol biokinetics and transformation in humans. *Free Radic Res* 37(11): 1225–1233.

Galli, F., F. Mazzini et al. (2011). Tocotrienamines and tocopheramines: Reactions with radicals and metal ions. *Bioorg Med Chem* 19(21): 6483–6491.

Galli, F., A. M. Stabile et al. (2004). The effect of alpha- and gamma-tocopherol and their carboxyethyl hydroxy-chroman metabolites on prostate cancer cell proliferation. *Arch Biochem Biophys* 423(1): 97–102.

Gould, M. N., J. D. Haag et al. (1991). A comparison of tocopherol and tocotrienol for the chemoprevention of chemically induced rat mammary tumors. *Am J Clin Nutr* 53(4 Suppl): 1068S–1070S.

Guthrie, N., A. Gapor et al. (1997). Inhibition of proliferation of estrogen receptor-negative MDA-MB-435 and -positive MCF-7 human breast cancer cells by palm oil tocotrienols and tamoxifen, alone and in combination. *J Nutr* 127(3): 544S–548S.

Hathcock, J. N., A. Azzi et al. (2005). Vitamins E and C are safe across a broad range of intakes. *Am J Clin Nutr* 81(4): 736–745.

Hosomi, A., M. Arita et al. (1997). Affinity for alpha-tocopherol transfer protein as a determinant of the biological activities of vitamin E analogs. *FEBS Lett* 409(1): 105–108.

Hsieh, T. C., S. Elangovan et al. (2010a). Differential suppression of proliferation in MCF-7 and MDA-MB-231 breast cancer cells exposed to alpha-, gamma- and delta-tocotrienols is accompanied by altered expression of oxidative stress modulatory enzymes. *Anticancer Res* 30(10): 4169–4176.

Hsieh, T. C., S. Elangovan et al. (2010b). Gamma-tocotrienol controls proliferation, modulates expression of cell cycle regulatory proteins and up-regulates quinone reductase NQO2 in MCF-7 breast cancer cells. *Anticancer Res* 30(7): 2869–2874.

Hsieh, T. C. and J. M. Wu (2008). Suppression of cell proliferation and gene expression by combinatorial synergy of EGCG, resveratrol and gamma-tocotrienol in estrogen receptor-positive MCF-7 breast cancer cells. *Int J Oncol* 33(4): 851–859.

Hussein, D. and H. Mo (2009). d-Dlta-tocotrienol-mediated suppression of the proliferation of human PANC-1, MIA PaCa-2, and BxPC-3 pancreatic carcinoma cells. *Pancreas* 38(4): e124–e136.

Jiang, Q., X. Yin et al. (2008). Long-chain carboxychromanols, metabolites of vitamin E, are potent inhibitors of cyclooxygenases. *Proc Natl Acad Sci USA* 105(51): 20464–20469.

Kamal-Eldin, A. and L. A. Appelqvist (1996). The chemistry and antioxidant properties of tocopherols and tocotrienols. *Lipids* 31(7): 671–701.

Kamat, J. P. and T. P. Devasagayam (2000). Oxidative damage to mitochondria in normal and cancer tissues, and its modulation. *Toxicology* 155(1–3): 73–82.

Kannappan, R., J. Ravindran, et al. (2010a) Gamma-tocotrienol promotes TRAIL-induced apoptosis through reactive oxygen species/extracellular signal-regulated kinase/p53-mediated upregulation of death receptors. *Mol Cancer Ther* 9(8): 2196–2207.

Kannappan, R., V. R. Yadav et al. (2010b). {gamma}-Tocotrienol but not {gamma}-tocopherol blocks STAT3 cell signaling pathway through induction of protein tyrosine phosphatase SHP-1 and sensitizes tumor cells to chemotherapeutic agents. *J Biol Chem* 285(43): 33520–33528.

Khanna, S., V. Patel et al. (2005). Delivery of orally supplemented alpha-tocotrienol to vital organs of rats and tocopherol-transport protein deficient mice. *Free Radic Biol Med* 39(10): 1310–1319.

Kuhad, A. and K. Chopra (2009). Attenuation of diabetic nephropathy by tocotrienol: Involvement of NFkB signaling pathway. *Life Sci* 84(9–10): 296–301.

Le Bourg, E. (2009). Hormesis, aging and longevity. *Biochim Biophys Acta* 1790(10): 1030–1039.

Lee, H. J., J. Ju et al. (2009). Mixed tocopherols prevent mammary tumorigenesis by inhibiting estrogen action and activating PPAR-gamma. *Clin Cancer Res* 15(12): 4242–4249.

Lodge, J. K., J. Ridlington et al. (2001). Alpha- and gamma-tocotrienols are metabolized to carboxyethyl-hydroxychroman derivatives and excreted in human urine. *Lipids* 36(1): 43–48.

Luchetti, F., B. Canonico et al. (2011). Melatonin signaling and cell protection function. *FASEB J*: 24: 3603–3624.

Mann, G. E., B. Bonacasa et al. (2009). Targeting the redox sensitive Nrf2-Keap1 defense pathway in cardiovascular disease: protection afforded by dietary isoflavones. *Curr Opin Pharmacol* 9(2): 139–145.

Mazlan, M., T. Sue Mian et al. (2006). Comparative effects of alpha-tocopherol and gamma-tocotrienol against hydrogen peroxide induced apoptosis on primary-cultured astrocytes. *J Neurol Sci* 243(1–2): 5–12.

McAnally, J. A., J. Gupta et al. (2007). Tocotrienols potentiate lovastatin-mediated growth suppression in vitro and in vivo. *Exp Biol Med (Maywood)* 232(4): 523–531.

McIntyre, B. S., K. P. Briski et al. (2000). Antiproliferative and apoptotic effects of tocopherols and tocotrienols on preneoplastic and neoplastic mouse mammary epithelial cells. *Proc Soc Exp Biol Med* 224(4): 292–301.

Mensink, R. P., A. C. van Houwelingen et al. (1999). A vitamin E concentrate rich in tocotrienols had no effect on serum lipids, lipoproteins, or platelet function in men with mildly elevated serum lipid concentrations. *Am J Clin Nutr* 69(2): 213–219.

Miyazawa, T., T. Tsuzuki et al. (2004). Antiangiogenic potency of vitamin E. *Ann N Y Acad Sci* 1031: 401–404.

Mo, H. and C. E. Elson (2004). Studies of the isoprenoid-mediated inhibition of mevalonate synthesis applied to cancer chemotherapy and chemoprevention. *Exp Biol Med (Maywood)* 229(7): 567–585.

Morley, S., M. Cecchini et al. (2008). Mechanisms of ligand transfer by the hepatic tocopherol transfer protein. *J Biol Chem* 283(26): 17797–17804.

Muller, L., K. Theile et al. (2010). In vitro antioxidant activity of tocopherols and tocotrienols and comparison of vitamin E concentration and lipophilic antioxidant capacity in human plasma. *Mol Nutr Food Res* 54(5): 731–742.

Mustacich, D. J., K. Gohil et al. (2009). Alpha-tocopherol modulates genes involved in hepatic xenobiotic pathways in mice. *J Nutr Biochem* 20(6): 469–476.

Mustad, V. A., C. A. Smith et al. (2002). Supplementation with 3 compositionally different tocotrienol supplements does not improve cardiovascular disease risk factors in men and women with hypercholesterolemia. *Am J Clin Nutr* 76(6): 1237–1243.

Nakagawa, K., A. Shibata et al. (2007). In vivo angiogenesis is suppressed by unsaturated vitamin E, tocotrienol. *J Nutr* 137(8): 1938–1943.

Negis, Y., M. Meydani et al. (2007). Molecular mechanism of alpha-tocopheryl-phosphate transport across the cell membrane. *Biochem Biophys Res Commun* 359(2): 348–353.

Nesaretnam, K., R. Ambra et al. (2004). Tocotrienol-rich fraction from palm oil affects gene expression in tumors resulting from MCF-7 cell inoculation in athymic mice. *Lipids* 39(5): 459–467.

Nesaretnam, K., S. Dorasamy et al. (2000). Tocotrienols inhibit growth of ZR-75-1 breast cancer cells. *Int J Food Sci Nutr* 51(Suppl): S95–S103.

Nesaretnam, K., P. A. Gomez et al. (2007). Tocotrienol levels in adipose tissue of benign and malignant breast lumps in patients in Malaysia. *Asia Pac J Clin Nutr* 16(3): 498–504.

Nesaretnam, K., R. Stephen et al. (1998). Tocotrienols inhibit the growth of human breast cancer cells irrespective of estrogen receptor status. *Lipids* 33(5): 461–469.

O'Byrne, D., S. Grundy et al. (2000). Studies of LDL oxidation following alpha-, gamma-, or delta-tocotrienyl acetate supplementation of hypercholesterolemic humans. *Free Radic Biol Med* 29(9): 834–845.

Palozza, P., S. Verdecchia et al. (2006). Comparative antioxidant activity of tocotrienols and the novel chromanyl-polyisoprenyl molecule FeAox-6 in isolated membranes and intact cells. *Mol Cell Biochem* 287(1–2): 21–32.

Parker, R. A., B. C. Pearce et al. (1993). Tocotrienols regulate cholesterol production in mammalian cells by post-transcriptional suppression of 3-hydroxy-3-methylglutaryl-coenzyme A reductase. *J Biol Chem* 268(15): 11230–11238.

Pierpaoli, E., V. Viola et al. (2010). Gamma- and delta-tocotrienols exert a more potent anticancer effect than alpha-tocopheryl succinate on breast cancer cell lines irrespective of HER-2/neu expression. *Life Sci* 86(17–18): 668–675.

Podda, M., C. Weber et al. (1996). Simultaneous determination of tissue tocopherols, tocotrienols, ubiquinols, and ubiquinones. *J Lipid Res* 37(4): 893–901.

Ristow, M., K. Zarse et al. (2009). Antioxidants prevent health-promoting effects of physical exercise in humans. *Proc Natl Acad Sci USA* 106(21): 8665–8670.

Ross, J. S. and J. A. Fletcher (1999). The HER-2/neu oncogene: prognostic factor, predictive factor and target for therapy. *Semin Cancer Biol* 9(2): 125–138.

Saito, Y., K. Nishio et al. (2010). Cytoprotective effects of vitamin E homologues against glutamate-induced cell death in immature primary cortical neuron cultures: Tocopherols and tocotrienols exert similar effects by antioxidant function. *Free Radic Biol Med* 49(10): 1542–1549.

Sanchez, M., N. Picard et al. (2010). Challenging estrogen receptor beta with phosphorylation. *Trends Endocrinol Metab* 21(2): 104–110.

Santanam, N., R. Shern-Brewer et al. (1998). Estradiol as an antioxidant: Incompatible with its physiological concentrations and function. *J Lipid Res* 39(11): 2111–2118.

Schaffer, S., W. E. Muller et al. (2005). Tocotrienols: constitutional effects in aging and disease. *J Nutr* 135(2): 151–154.

Schuelke, M., A. Elsner et al. (2000). Urinary alpha-tocopherol metabolites in alpha-tocopherol transfer protein-deficient patients. *J Lipid Res* 41(10): 1543–1551.

Sen, C. K., S. Khanna et al. (2000). Molecular basis of vitamin E action. Tocotrienol potently inhibits glutamate-induced pp60(c-Src) kinase activation and death of HT4 neuronal cells. *J Biol Chem* 275(17): 13049–13055.

Sen, C. K., S. Khanna et al. (2004). Tocotrienol: the natural vitamin E to defend the nervous system? *Ann N Y Acad Sci* 1031: 127–142.

Sen, C. K., S. Khanna et al. (2007). Tocotrienols: the emerging face of natural vitamin E. *Vitam Horm* 76: 203–261.

Serbinova, E., V. Kagan et al. (1991). Free radical recycling and intramembrane mobility in the antioxidant properties of alpha-tocopherol and alpha-tocotrienol. *Free Radic Biol Med* 10(5): 263–275.

Shah, S. and P. W. Sylvester (2004). Tocotrienol-induced caspase-8 activation is unrelated to death receptor apoptotic signaling in neoplastic mammary epithelial cells. *Exp Biol Med (Maywood)* 229(8): 745–755.

Shibata, A., K. Nakagawa et al. (2008). Tumor anti-angiogenic effect and mechanism of action of delta-tocotrienol. *Biochem Pharmacol* 76(3): 330–339.

Shibata, A., K. Nakagawa et al. (2009). Delta-tocotrienol suppresses VEGF induced angiogenesis whereas alpha-tocopherol does not. *J Agric Food Chem* 57(18): 8696–8704.

Siems, W., C. Salerno et al. (2009). Beta-carotene degradation products - formation, toxicity and prevention of toxicity. *Forum Nutr* 61: 75–86.

Slamon, D. J., W. Godolphin et al. (1989). Studies of the HER-2/neu proto-oncogene in human breast and ovarian cancer. *Science* 244(4905): 707–712.

Song, B. L. and R. A. DeBose-Boyd (2006). Insig-dependent ubiquitination and degradation of 3-hydroxy-3-methylglutaryl coenzyme a reductase stimulated by delta- and gamma-tocotrienols. *J Biol Chem* 281(35): 25054–25061.

Sontag, T. J. and R. S. Parker (2002). Cytochrome P450 omega-hydroxylase pathway of tocopherol catabolism. Novel mechanism of regulation of vitamin E status. *J Biol Chem* 277(28): 25290–25296.

Sontag, T. J. and R. S. Parker (2007). Influence of major structural features of tocopherols and tocotrienols on their omega-oxidation by tocopherol-omega-hydroxylase. *J Lipid Res* 48(5): 1090–1098.

Stone, W. L., K. Krishnan et al. (2004). Tocopherols and the treatment of colon cancer. *Ann N Y Acad Sci* 1031: 223–233.

Suarna, C., R. L. Hood et al. (1993). Comparative antioxidant activity of tocotrienols and other natural lipid-soluble antioxidants in a homogeneous system, and in rat and human lipoproteins. *Biochim Biophys Acta* 1166(2–3): 163–170.

Sun, W., Q. Wang et al. (2008). Gamma-tocotrienol-induced apoptosis in human gastric cancer SGC-7901 cells is associated with a suppression in mitogen-activated protein kinase signalling. *Br J Nutr* 99(6): 1247–1254.

Suzuki, Y. J., M. Tsuchiya et al. (1993). Structural and dynamic membrane properties of alpha-tocopherol and alpha-tocotrienol: implication to the molecular mechanism of their antioxidant potency. *Biochemistry* 32(40): 10692–10699.

Swanson, J. E., R. N. Ben et al. (1999). Urinary excretion of 2,7, 8-trimethyl-2-(beta-carboxyethyl)-6-hydroxy-chroman is a major route of elimination of gamma-tocopherol in humans. *J Lipid Res* 40(4): 665–671.

Sylvester, P. W. (2007). Vitamin E and apoptosis. *Vitam Horm* 76: 329–356.

Sylvester, P. W., S. J. Shah et al. (2005). Intracellular signaling mechanisms mediating the antiproliferative and apoptotic effects of gamma-tocotrienol in neoplastic mammary epithelial cells. *J Plant Physiol* 162(7): 803–810.

Takahashi, K. and G. Loo (2004). Disruption of mitochondria during tocotrienol-induced apoptosis in MDA-MB-231 human breast cancer cells. *Biochem Pharmacol* 67(2): 315–324.

Tasaki, M., T. Umemura et al. (2009). Simultaneous induction of non-neoplastic and neoplastic lesions with highly proliferative hepatocytes following dietary exposure of rats to tocotrienol for 2 years. *Arch Toxicol* 83(11): 1021–1030.

Then, S. M., M. Mazlan et al. (2009). Is vitamin E toxic to neuron cells? *Cell Mol Neurobiol* 29(4): 485–496.

Theriault, A., J. T. Chao et al. (2002). Tocotrienol is the most effective vitamin E for reducing endothelial expression of adhesion molecules and adhesion to monocytes. *Atherosclerosis* 160(1): 21–30.

Traber, M. G. (2004). Vitamin E, nuclear receptors and xenobiotic metabolism. *Arch Biochem Biophys* 423(1): 6–11.

Traber, M. G. (2007). Vitamin E regulatory mechanisms. *Annu Rev Nutr* 27: 347–362.

Traber, M. G. (2010). Regulation of xenobiotic metabolism, the only signaling function of alpha-tocopherol? *Mol Nutr Food Res* 54(5): 661–668.

Uto-Kondo, H., R. Ohmori et al. (2009). Tocotrienol suppresses adipocyte differentiation and Akt phosphorylation in 3T3-L1 preadipocytes. *J Nutr* 139(1): 51–57.

van Haaften, R. I., G. R. Haenen et al. (2002). Tocotrienols inhibit human glutathione S-transferase P1-1. *IUBMB Life* 54(2): 81–84.

Varga, Z., E. Kosaras et al. (2008). Effects of tocopherols and 2,2′-carboxyethyl hydroxychromans on phorbol-ester-stimulated neutrophils. *J Nutr Biochem* 19(5): 320–327.

Viola, V., F. Pilolli et al. (2012). Why tocotrienols work better: Insights into the in vitro anti-cancer mechanism of vitamin E. *Genes Nutr* 7(1): 29–41.

Wada, S. (2009). Chemoprevention of tocotrienols: The mechanism of antiproliferative effects. *Forum Nutr* 61: 204–216.

Wali, V. B., S. V. Bachawal et al. (2009a). Endoplasmic reticulum stress mediates gamma-tocotrienol-induced apoptosis in mammary tumor cells. *Apoptosis* 14(11): 1366–1377.

Wali, V. B., S. V. Bachawal et al. (2009b). Suppression in mevalonate synthesis mediates antitumor effects of combined statin and gamma-tocotrienol treatment. *Lipids* 44(10): 925–934.

Wang, X., J. Ni et al. (2009). Reduced expression of tocopherol-associated protein (TAP/Sec14L2) in human breast cancer. *Cancer Invest*: 27: 971–977.

Weng-Yew, W., K. R. Selvaduray et al. (2009). Suppression of tumor growth by palm tocotrienols via the attenuation of angiogenesis. *Nutr Cancer* 61(3): 367–373.

Xu, W. L., J. R. Liu et al. (2009). Inhibition of proliferation and induction of apoptosis by gamma-tocotrienol in human colon carcinoma HT-29 cells. *Nutrition* 25(5): 555–566.

Yam, M. L., S. R. Abdul Hafid et al. (2009). Tocotrienols suppress proinflammatory markers and cyclooxygenase-2 expression in RAW264.7 macrophages. *Lipids* 44(9): 787–797.

Yang, W. C., F. E. Regnier et al. (2010). In vitro stable isotope labeling for discovery of novel metabolites by liquid chromatography-mass spectrometry: Confirmation of gamma-tocopherol metabolism in human A549 cell. *J Chromatogr A* 1217(5): 667–675.

Yap, S. P., K. H. Yuen et al. (2001). Pharmacokinetics and bioavailability of alpha-, gamma- and delta-tocotrienols under different food status. *J Pharm Pharmacol* 53(1): 67–71.

You, C. S., T. J. Sontag et al. (2005). Long-chain carboxychromanols are the major metabolites of tocopherols and tocotrienols in A549 lung epithelial cells but not HepG2 cells. *J Nutr* 135(2): 227–232.

Yu, F. L., A. Gapor et al. (2005). Evidence for the preventive effect of the polyunsaturated phytol side chain in tocotrienols on 17beta-estradiol epoxidation. *Cancer Detect Prev* 29(4): 383–388.

Yu, W., M. Simmons-Menchaca et al. (1999). Induction of apoptosis in human breast cancer cells by tocopherols and tocotrienols. *Nutr Cancer* 33(1): 26–32.

Yu, W., L. Jia et al. (2009). Anticancer actions of natural and synthetic vitamin E forms: RRR-alpha-tocopherol blocks the anticancer actions of gamma-tocopherol. *Mol Nutr Food Res* 53(12): 1573–1581.

Zhao, Y., J. Neuzil et al. (2009). Vitamin E analogues as mitochondria-targeting compounds: from the bench to the bedside? *Mol Nutr Food Res* 53(1): 129–139.

Zhao, Y., M.-J. Lee et al. (2010). Analysis of multiple metabolites of tocopherols and tocotrienols in mice and humans. *J Agric Food Chem* 58(8): 4844–4852.

Zhou, C., M. M. Tabb et al. (2004). Tocotrienols activate the steroid and xenobiotic receptor, SXR, and selectively regulate expression of its target genes. *Drug Metab Dispos* 32(10): 1075–1082.

10 Mevalonate-Suppressive Tocotrienols for Cancer Chemoprevention and Adjuvant Therapy

Huanbiao Mo, Manal Elfakhani, Anureet Shah, and Hoda Yeganehjoo

CONTENTS

10.1 INTRODUCTION

The tumor-suppressive activity of tocotrienols, vitamin E molecules with an unsaturated isoprenoid side chain, has been extensively reviewed in the previous edition of this book (Mo and Elson 2008). Tocotrienols at physiologically attainable concentrations suppress the proliferation of tumor cells derived from breast, liver, prostate, skin, colon, blood, lung, lymph gland, cervix, and nerve. Tocotrienol-mediated growth suppression is attributed to cell cycle arrest, mostly at the G1 phase of cell cycle, and apoptosis. Signaling pathways associated with promoting cell cycle progression, growth, and survival, including mitogen-activated protein kinases (MAPK), Ras, RhoA, Raf/MAPK kinase (MEK)/extracellular signal-regulated kinases (ERK), c-Jun, c-myc, cyclin D/cdk4, protein kinase C (PKC), phosphatidylinositol 3-kinase (PI3K), Akt, IκB kinase (IKK), IκB, nuclear factor κB (NFκB), c-Jun N-terminal kinase (JNK), Bcl-2, Bcl-xL, COX-2, matrix metalloproteinases (MMP), vascular endothelial growth factor (VEGF), FLIP, and telomerase, are suppressed by tocotrienols. On the other hand, signaling activities supporting growth arrest and apoptosis, including p21^{cip1WAF1}, transforming growth factor-β (TGF-β), p53, Fas, Bax, Apaf-1, caspases, and Bid fragmentation, are activated by tocotrienols. Animal models with chemically initiated carcinogenesis and implanted tumors confirmed the *in vitro* tumor-suppressive activity of tocotrienols. Differing from statins, the nondiscriminant competitive inhibitors of 3-hydroxy-3-methyglutaryl coenzyme A (HMG CoA) reductase, tocotrienols are downregulators of the activity of HMG CoA reductase. Dysregulation of HMG CoA reductase in tumors offers a unique target for tumor-specific intervention. Recent literature continues to support the potential of tocotrienols as tumor-targeted agents in cancer chemoprevention and/or therapy.

10.2 TUMOR-SUPPRESSIVE ACTIVITY OF TOCOTRIENOLS *IN VITRO*

Studies in the last 5 years confirmed the growth inhibitory activity of tocotrienols and their derivatives (Kashiwagi et al. 2008) in human MCF-7 (Choi and Lee 2009; Hsieh et al. 2010a,b; Pierpaoli et al. 2010; Yap et al. 2010b; Patacsil et al. 2011; Ramdas et al. 2011) and MDA-MB-231 (Elangovan et al. 2008; Hsieh et al. 2010a; Yap et al. 2010b; Patacsil et al. 2011) mammary adenocarcinoma cells, HL-60 leukemia cells (de Mesquita et al. 2011; Inoue et al. 2011), MDA-MB-435 melanoma cells (de Mesquita et al. 2011), DU145 (Kannappan et al. 2010b; Luk et al. 2011) and LNCaP (Yap et al. 2008; Jiang et al. 2011) prostate carcinoma cells, PC-3 prostate adenocarcinoma cells (Yap et al. 2008, 2010a; Kannappan et al. 2010b; Campbell et al. 2011; Jiang et al. 2011; Luk et al. 2011), HeLa cervical carcinoma cells (Wu and Ng 2010), HepG2 (Shibata et al. 2008b; Rajendran et al. 2011), C3A, SNU-387, and PLC/PRF5 (Rajendran et al. 2011) hepatocellular carcinoma cells, and A549 lung carcinoma cells (Kashiwagi et al. 2008). In addition, the list of tumor cells susceptible to tocotrienol-mediated growth inhibition has expanded to include human SGC-7901 gastric adenocarcinoma cells (Sun et al. 2008, 2009; Liu et al. 2010), MKN45 gastric cancer cells (Choi and Lee 2009), HT-29 (Xu et al. 2009, in press), SW620 (Zhang et al. 2011), HCT-8 (de Mesquita et al. 2011), and HCT116 (Choi and Lee 2009) colon cancer cells, DLD-1 colorectal adenocarcinoma cells (Shibata et al. 2008b), MIA PaCa-2 (Hussein and Mo 2009; Kannappan et al. 2010b; Kunnumakkara et al. 2010; Shin-Kang et al. 2011), and PANC-1 (Hussein and Mo 2009; Kunnumakkara et al. 2010), pancreatic carcinoma cells, BxPC-3 (Hussein and Mo 2009; Kunnumakkara et al. 2010), AsPC-1 (Kunnumakkara et al. 2010), and Panc-28 (Shin-Kang et al. 2011) pancreatic adenocarcinoma cells, NB-4 leukemia cells (Inoue et al. 2011), Raji lymphoma cells (Inoue et al. 2011), U266 multiple myeloma cells (Kannappan et al. 2010b), SY-5Y neuroblastoma cells (Inoue et al. 2011), SF-295 glioblastoma cells (de Mesquita et al. 2011), SKBR3 breast cancer cells (Pierpaoli et al. 2010), A375 (Fernandes et al. 2010), A2058 (Chang et al. 2009), G32 (Chang et al. 2009), and G361 (Chang et al. 2009) melanoma cells, NCI-H460 lung cancer cells (Choi and Lee 2009), MGH-U1 bladder cancer cells (Luk et al. 2011), murine 4T1 metastatic mammary tumor cells (Selvaduray et al. 2010), malignant + SA mammary epithelial cells (Samant et al. 2010; Shirode and Sylvester 2010), and MH134 hepatoma cells (Hiura et al. 2009).

Consistent with early studies, tocotrienols induced cell cycle arrest (Sun et al. 2008, 2009; Yap et al. 2008, 2010b; Hussein and Mo 2009; Xu et al. 2009; Fernandes et al. 2010; Kannappan et al. 2010a; Wu and Ng 2010; Li et al. 2011; Patacsil et al. 2011; Zhang et al. 2011) and apoptosis (Sun et al. 2008, 2009; Yap et al. 2008, 2010a; Chang et al. 2009; Hussein and Mo 2009; Xu et al. 2009; Fernandes et al. 2010; Kannappan et al. 2010a,b; Pierpaoli et al. 2010; Wu and Ng 2010; de Mesquita et al. 2011; Husain et al. 2011; Inoue et al. 2011; Ji et al. 2011; Jiang et al. 2011; Patacsil et al. 2011; Rajendran et al. 2011; Shin-Kang et al. 2011; Zhang et al. 2011) in the tumor cell lines. In addition, tocotrienols modulated signaling pathways and molecules regulating cell cycle, apoptosis, angiogenesis, invasion, and migration, such as NFκB (Ahn et al. 2007; Shibata et al. 2008b; Yap et al. 2008, 2010b; Chang et al. 2009; Xu et al. 2009; Kunnumakkara et al. 2010; Shirode and Sylvester 2010; Campbell et al. 2011; Husain et al. 2011), COX-2 (Ahn et al. 2007; Shibata et al. 2008b; Kunnumakkara et al. 2010; Shirode and Sylvester 2010; Ji et al. 2011), p21[cip1WAF1] (Pierpaoli et al. 2010), p53 (Kannappan et al. 2010a; Pierpaoli et al. 2010), p16 (Pierpaoli et al. 2010; Wu and Ng 2010), Raf/MEK/ERK (Nakagawa et al. 2007; Shibata et al. 2008a; Sun et al. 2008; Kannappan et al. 2010a; Yap et al. 2010b; Shin-Kang et al. 2011), phosphatase and tensin homolog (PTEN) (Shibata et al. 2008a), AKT (Nakagawa et al. 2007; Kashiwagi et al. 2008; Shibata et al. 2008a; Jiang et al. 2011; Rajendran et al. 2011), tyrosine kinase Src (Kashiwagi et al. 2008;

Rajendran et al. 2011), and downstream factors including mammalian target of rapamycin (mTOR), p-70 S6 kinase, and Foxo3a (Shirode and Sylvester 2010; Shin-Kang et al. 2011), glycogen synthase kinase 3 (GSK3; Shibata et al. 2008a), p38 (Nakagawa et al. 2007; Shibata et al. 2008a; Campbell et al. 2011), c-myc (Ahn et al. 2007; Sun et al. 2008; Kunnumakkara et al. 2010; Zhang et al. 2011), c-Jun (Yap et al. 2008, 2010b, Patacsil et al. 2011; Shin-Kang et al. 2011; Zhang et al. 2011), JNK (Yap et al. 2008, 2010b; Chang et al. 2009), cyclin D/cdk (Ahn et al. 2007; Nakagawa et al. 2007; Elangovan et al. 2008; Sun et al. 2008; Fernandes et al. 2010; Hsieh et al. 2010b; Kannappan et al. 2010b; Kunnumakkara et al. 2010; Samant et al. 2010; Wu and Ng 2010; Li et al. 2011; Patacsil et al. 2011; Rajendran et al. 2011; Zhang et al. 2011), cdk inhibitor p27^{kip1} (Samant et al. 2010), survivin (Ahn et al. 2007; Kannappan et al. 2010a,b; Kunnumakkara et al. 2010; Husain et al. 2011; Ji et al. 2011; Rajendran et al. 2011), Bid (Inoue et al. 2011), Bcl-xL (Ahn et al. 2007; Kannappan et al. 2010a,b; Husain et al. 2011; Ji et al. 2011; Rajendran et al. 2011), Bcl-2 (Ahn et al. 2007; Sun et al. 2008; Xu et al. 2009; Kannappan et al. 2010a,b; Kunnumakkara et al. 2010; Luk et al. 2011; Rajendran et al. 2011), Bax (Sun et al. 2008; Xu et al. 2009; Husain et al. 2011), caspases (Nakagawa et al. 2007; Sun et al. 2008; Yap et al. 2008, 2010b; Xu et al. 2009; Fernandes et al. 2010; Kannappan et al. 2010a,b; Husain et al. 2011; Inoue et al. 2011; Jiang et al. 2011; Luk et al. 2011; Patacsil et al. 2011; Rajendran et al. 2011; Shin-Kang et al. 2011), tumor necrosis factor–related apoptosis-inducing ligand (TRAIL) receptors death receptor (DR)-4 and DR-5 (Kannappan et al. 2010a), poly (ADP-ribose) polymerase (PARP) (Sun et al. 2008; Yap et al. 2008, 2010b; Hiura et al. 2009; Kannappan et al. 2010a,b; Husain et al. 2011; Jiang et al. 2011; Luk et al. 2011; Patacsil et al. 2011; Rajendran et al. 2011), TGF-β (Campbell et al. 2011; Patacsil et al. 2011), hypoxia-inducible factor-1α (HIF-1α) (Shibata et al. 2008b), VEGF (Ahn et al. 2007; Shibata et al. 2008a,b; Kannappan et al. 2010b; Kunnumakkara et al. 2010; Li et al. 2011; Rajendran et al. 2011), β-catenin (Yap et al. 2010b; Li et al. 2011; Xu et al. in press; Zhang et al. 2011), MMP-7 (Zhang et al. 2011), and MMP-9 (Ahn et al. 2007; Kunnumakkara et al. 2010; Liu et al. 2010; Ji et al. 2011; Li et al. 2011).

Signaling pathways and molecules newly emerged as targets of tocotrienols include Wnt (Zhang et al. 2011), signal transducer and activator of transcription 3 (STAT3) (Kannappan et al. 2010b), tumor suppressors including mitogen-induced genes 6 and 9 (Ramdas et al. 2011), retinoblastoma (Rb)/E2F complex (Elangovan et al. 2008; Hsieh et al. 2010b; Samant et al. 2010), members of Ras (Fernandes et al. 2010) oncogene family (RAP2A) (Ramdas et al. 2011), HGF-dependent Met activation (Ayoub et al. 2011), SMAD-2 (Campbell et al. 2011), ErbB2 (Shin-Kang et al. 2011), ErbB3 (Shin-Kang et al. 2011), HER-2/neu (Pierpaoli et al. 2010), Id1 (Yap et al. 2008, 2010b; Chang et al. 2009; Luk et al. 2011), epidermal growth factor receptor (EGFR) (Yap et al. 2008; Chang et al. 2009), oxidative stress modulatory enzymes including glutathione peroxidase, thioredoxin, and quinone reductase 2 (Hsieh et al. 2010a,b), Notch-1 (Ji et al. 2011), Hes-1 (Ji et al. 2011), estrogen receptor β (ERβ) (Comitato et al. 2009; Nesaretnam et al. 2011), and tyrosine phosphatase SHP-1 (Rajendran et al. 2011). Tocotrienols have also been shown to downregulate cancer stem cell markers, CD44 and CD133, in human PC-3 and DU145 prostate cancer cells (Luk et al. 2011), and cause accumulation of dihydroceramide and dihydrosphingosine in LNCaP prostate cancer cells (Jiang et al. 2011).

Recent studies confirmed the differential sensitivities of tumor and nontumor cells to tocotrienol-mediated growth suppression (Mo and Elson 2004, 2008). Human MCF7 estrogen-dependent breast cancer cells and MDA-MB231 estrogen-independent breast cancer cells were more sensitive than human MCF10A immortalized nontumorigenic breast epithelial cells to tocotrienol-mediated growth inhibition (Yap et al. 2010b; Patacsil et al. 2011) and apoptosis (Yap et al. 2010b). Parallel to this difference is the increased sensitivity of human MIA PaCa-2 (Husain et al. 2011; Shin-Kang et al. 2011) and PANC-1 (Shin-Kang et al. 2011) pancreatic carcinoma cells, Panc-28 (Shin-Kang et al. 2011), BxPC-3 (Shin-Kang et al. 2011), and ASPc-1 (Husain et al. 2011) pancreatic adenocarcinoma cells, and HPDE 6 C7-Kras cells to tocotrienols in comparison with human HPDE-E6E7 (Shin-Kang et al. 2011) and HPDE 6 C7 (Husain et al. 2011) normal pancreatic duct epithelial cells. Moreover, human LNCaP and PC-3 prostate tumor cells were more responsive to tocotrienols than PZ-HPV7 immortalized prostate epithelial cells (Yap et al. 2008).

Consistent with early studies showing the higher tumor-suppressive potencies of δ- and γ-tocotrienols (Guthrie et al. 1997; Yu et al. 1999; McIntyre et al. 2000a,b; Inokuchi et al. 2003; Conte et al. 2004), recent studies indicated that δ-(Hiura et al. 2009; Hsieh et al. 2010a; Pierpaoli et al. 2010; Selvaduray et al. 2010; Husain et al. 2011) and γ-(Hsieh et al. 2010b; Wu and Ng 2010; Yap et al. 2010b) tocotrienols are the most active vitamers in suppressing the growth of breast (Hsieh et al. 2010a,b; Pierpaoli et al. 2010; Selvaduray et al. 2010; Yap et al. 2010b), cervix (Wu and Ng 2010), liver (Hiura et al. 2009), and pancreatic (Husain et al. 2011) tumor cells.

10.3   TUMOR-SUPPRESSIVE ACTIVITY OF TOCOTRIENOLS *IN VIVO*

The growth-suppressive activity of tocotrienols in implanted mammary, prostate, skin, and spontaneous liver cancers has been reported. Progress on the *in vivo* tumor-suppressive activity of tocotrienols has been made using implanted models of breast cancer, transgenic models of prostate cancer, chemotherapeutic models of pancreatic cancer, and a model of implanted liver cancer.

A tocotrienol-rich fraction (TRF) significantly inhibited the incidence and volume of implanted 4T1 murine mammary tumors in BALB/c mice via suppression of VEGF expression and angiogenesis (Weng-Yew et al. 2009; Selvaduray et al. 2010). TRF and with higher potencies, γ- and δ-tocotrienols, upregulated IL-24 mRNA expression in tumor tissues (Selvaduray et al. 2010). Dietary γ-tocotrienol (250 mg/kg diet) inhibited the growth and lung metastases of murine 66cl-4-GFP mammary tumor cells implanted in BALB/c mice by suppressing Ki-67, inducing apoptosis and activating JNK and p38 MAPK (Park et al. 2010).

Pretreatment of PC-3 cells with 5 μg/mL of γ-tocotrienol prior to their orthotopic injection into SCID mice reduced tumor incidence and tumor size by 62% and >94%, respectively. Pre-feeding mice with 100 mg/kg/day γ-tocotrienol reduced tumor incidence and tumor size by 75% and >94%, respectively (Luk et al. 2011). Oral gavage feeding of γ-tocotrienol at 125 mg/kg body weight reduced the volume of subcutaneously (s.c.) injected LNCaP cells by 53% in male BALB/c nude mice (Jiang et al. 2011). The growth of implanted PC3-Luc cells in BALB/c athymic nude mice was inhibited by 50% with intraperitoneal (i.p.) injection of 50 mg/kg γ-tocotrienol (Yap et al. 2010a). Proliferation markers such as PCNA, Ki-67, and Id1 were inhibited by γ-tocotrienol and a γ-tocotrienol/docetaxel combination (Yap et al. 2010a). PARP cleavage and caspase-3 activation were enhanced by γ-tocotrienol and a γ-tocotrienol/docetaxel combination (Yap et al. 2010a). Dietary mixed tocotrienol (0.1%, 0.3% and 1%) containing 18%–20% of γ-tocotrienol and 4%–6% of δ-tocotrienol in a dose-dependent manner inhibited the incidence and weight of prostate tumors in TRAMP mice by upregulating apoptotic proteins (caspase-3 and BAD) and antigrowth proteins (p21[cip1WAF1] and p27[kip1]) and downregulating cyclins A and E (Barve et al. 2010).

γ-Tocotrienol suppressed the expression of Ki-67, COX-2, matrix metalloproteinase-9 (MMP-9), NFκB, and VEGF in orthotopically implanted MIA PaCa-2 tumor in male athymic nu/nu mice (Kunnumakkara et al. 2010). Oral gavage feeding of β-, γ-, and δ-tocotrienols (200 mg/kg twice daily) suppressed the growth of orthotopically implanted AsPc-1 pancreatic tumors in female SCID nude mice by upregulating the proapoptotic Bax and apoptosis marker CK18. δ-Tocotrienol also upregulated the cleavage of PARP1 and downregulated NFκB, surviving and Bcl-xL (Husain et al. 2011). Consistent with most *in vitro* studies, the potency of tocotrienols follows the descending order of δ-, γ-, β-, and α-tocotrienols (Husain et al. 2011).

Lastly, dietary δ- and γ-tocotrienols (0.1%) suppressed the growth of s.c. implanted murine MH134 hepatoma cells by 62% and 47%, respectively, in C3H/HeN mice (Hiura et al. 2009).

Concerns over the bioavailability of tocotrienols were dissipated by recent studies showing the high levels of tocotrienols in tissues and tumors. The concentrations of γ- and δ-tocotrienols in inoculated MH134 hepatomas reached 20 and 8 μg/g, respectively, in C3H/HeN mice fed diets containing 0.1% tocotrienols (Hiura et al. 2009). Female athymic nude mice fed 100 mg/kg δ-tocotrienol by oral gavage had peak plasma concentration of δ-tocotrienol at 57 μmol/L and peak tissue concentration of δ-tocotrienol at 14 and 32 nmol/g in the liver and pancreas, respectively (Husain et al. 2009). C57BL6 mice injected (i.p.) with 50 mg/kg γ-tocotrienol had a peak serum level of 250 mg γ-tocotrienol/L within 10 min; serum level maintained as high as 100 and 50 mg/L after 6 and 72 h, respectively (Yap et al. 2010a). These physiologically attainable levels of tocotrienol exceed the effective concentrations of tocotrienols *in vitro* and are accompanied with tumor-suppressive activities.

Tumor-suppressive doses of tocotrienols have been shown by early studies to be safe *in vivo*. More recently, i.p. injection of 50 mg/kg γ-tocotrienol in C57BL6 mice led to no detected toxicity shown by serum biomarkers including albumin, creatine, ALT, AST, urea, and ALP activity. Survival rate of mice did not change until the dose of 1000 mg/kg i.p. injection, 20-fold as high as the 50 mg/kg required for tumor suppression (Yap et al. 2010a). Another study determined the no-observed-adverse-effect level of tocotrienols in rats at 0.4% of diet (Tasaki et al. 2008), exceeding the efficacious dietary level (Hiura et al. 2009; Husain et al. 2011). Chronic (Yap et al. 2001) and short-term (Springett et al. 2011) administration of 800 mg/day δ-tocotrienol had no adverse effect in humans.

10.4 ANTIOXIDANT-INDEPENDENT MECHANISM OF ACTION

The differential effects of tocotrienols and tocopherols, vitamin E molecules with a saturated phytyl side chain, on tumor growth may provide insights on the mechanism of action for the tumor-suppressive activity of tocotrienols. Recent studies have shown that unlike tocotrienols, the tocopherols are either inactive or much less active than tocotrienols in suppressing the growth of pancreatic (Husain et al. 2011; Shin-Kang et al. 2011), mammary (Choi and Lee 2009; Ramdas et al. 2011), lung (Choi and Lee 2009), colon (Choi and Lee 2009), gastric (Choi and Lee 2009), and prostate (Yap et al. 2008) cancer cells. Tocotrienols, but not tocopherols, inhibited the proliferation, migration, and tube formation of HUVEC cells, and angiogenesis (Miyazawa et al. 2009; Shibata et al. 2009; Weng-Yew et al. 2009). α-Tocopherol has in fact been shown to attenuate the effects of tocotrienols on the proliferation of MDA-MB231 cells (Yap et al. 2010b) and human DLD-1 colorectal adenocarcinoma cells (Shibata et al. 2010) and Id1 and EGFR expression, PARP cleavage, and caspase activation in MDA-MB231 cells (Yap et al. 2010b). The Selenium and Vitamin E Cancer Prevention Trial (SELECT) showed that α-tocopheryl acetate supplement increased the risk of prostate cancer by 17% among healthy men (Klein et al. 2011).

The discrepancy in the tumor-suppressive activities of tocotrienols and tocopherols cannot be attributed to their antioxidant activities. Recent studies demonstrated that the side chain did not make any difference in antioxidant activity between tocopherols and tocotrienols (Yoshida et al. 2003; Muller et al. 2010; Saito et al. 2010). An ether derivative of tocotrienol, 6-*O*-carboxypropyl-α-tocotrienol, is redox-silent due to loss of the hydroxyl group on the chromanol ring of tocotrienol; 6-*O*-carboxypropyl-α-tocotrienol retains the tumor-targeted growth inhibitory activity of tocotrienols by inhibiting the growth of chemoresistant H28 mesothelioma cells, but not the nontumorigenic Met-5A mesothelial cell, through G2/M arrest, apoptosis, and inhibition of EGFR and STAT3 (Kashiwagi et al. 2009). Further, 6-*O*-carboxypropyl-α-tocotrienol also suppressed hypoxia response of A549 cells via inactivation of protein tyrosine kinase Src (Kashiwagi et al. 2008). Other redox-silent tocotrienol derivatives had much improved potency than their parent tocotrienols against +SA and MDA-MB-231 mammary tumor cells with no effect on immortalized normal mouse CL-S1 mammary epithelial cells (Behery et al. 2010); the derivatives also inhibited the migration of metastatic MDA-MB-231 mammary tumor cells. Additional studies have shown that the δ-tocotrienol-mediated upregulation of death receptors DR-4 and DR-5 and apoptosis (Kannappan et al. 2010a), anti-angiogenesis (Shibata et al. 2008a,b), and antimigration (Shibata et al. 2008a) activities require the production of reactive oxygen species.

10.5 DYSREGULATED HMG CoA REDUCTASE IN TUMORS SUPPORTS GROWTH

The differing impact of tocotrienols and tocopherols on cell proliferation is reminiscent of that on 3-hydroxy-3-methylglutaryl coenzyme A (HMG CoA) reductase, the rate-limiting enzyme of the mevalonate pathway (Goldstein and Brown 1990). The mevalonate pathway provides essential isoprenoid intermediates including prenyl pyrophosphates—the 15-carbon farnesyl pyrophosphate (FPP) and the 20-carbon geranylgeranyl pyrophosphate (GGPP)—and dolichol for cell survival and growth (Figure 10.1A). Prenyl pyrophosphates are covalently attached to the carboxy-terminal cysteine residue of the nuclear lamins (Hutchison et al. 1994; Moir et al. 2000; Maurer-Stroh

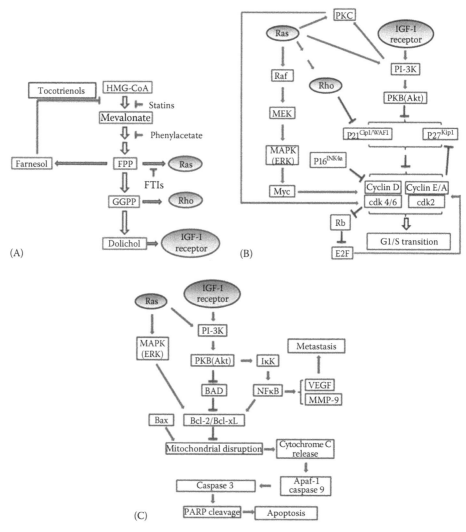

FIGURE 10.1 The mevalonate pathway provides essential intermediates for the posttranslational modification of Ras, Rho, and IGF-I receptor (oval shapes) (A), which initiate signaling pathways regulating cell cycle progression (B), apoptosis, and metastasis (C). The statins, FTIs, and phenylacetate inhibit HMG CoA reductase, farnesyl transferase, and mevalonate pyrophosphate decarboxylase, respectively (A), and suppress the downstream effects shown in B and C. Farnesol triggers the posttranscriptional downregulation of HMG CoA reductase (A). Tocotrienols mimic farnesol in specifically suppressing tumor reductase, but with higher potencies. Tocotrienols may offer tumor suppression without the toxicities associated with statins, FTIs, and phenylacetate.

et al. 2007) and members of the Ras and Rho families (Zhang and Casey 1996; Gelb 1997; Maurer-Stroh et al. 2007) and are essential to their membrane anchorage and biological function (Zhang and Casey 1996). Ras proteins involved in cell proliferation and survival are farnesylated, whereas Rho proteins that are responsible for actin-cytoskeletal dynamics, cell adhesion, and motility are geranylgeranylated (Zhang and Casey 1996). Dolichol is required for the N-linked glycosylation and membrane attachment of growth factor receptors including insulin-like growth factor I (IGF-I) receptor (Dricu et al. 1997) that promotes cell proliferation.

The Ras (Adjei 2001), Rho (Li et al. 2002), and IGF-I receptor (Dricu et al. 1997; McCampbell et al. 2006) proteins that rely on the mevalonate pathway for posttranslational modification and maturation play profound roles in cell cycle progression (Figure 10.1B), apoptosis, and metastasis (Figure 10.1C). Two pairs of regulators, cyclin D/cyclin-dependent kinase (cdk) 4/6 and cyclin E/A/cdk 2, promote cell cycle progression through the G1/S interface. Cyclin D/cdk 4/6 also promotes cyclin E/A/cdk 2 activity through a regulatory loop consisting of the tumor suppressor Rb protein and E2F (Figure 10.1B) (Massague 2004). The p16^{INK4a} protein suppresses the cyclin D/cdk4/6 activity (Sherr 2004). The cyclin/cdk activities are suppressed by p21$^{cip1/WAF1}$ and p27^{kip1} (Massague 2004), which are in turn suppressed by the Ras/Raf/ MEK/MAPK/ERKs/Myc (Gysin et al. 2005), Ras/Rac/Rho, and Ras/IGF-I receptor/PI3K/protein kinase B (PKB)/Akt pathways (Anderson and Harris 2001). The balance between the key players in regulating apoptosis, the anti-apoptotic Bcl-2/Bcl-xL and the proapoptotic Bax (Jiang and Wang 2004), is regulated by the Ras/Raf/MEK/MAPK (ERK) (Boucher et al. 2000) and IGF-I receptor/PI3K/PKB/Akt pathways (McCampbell et al. 2006) (Figure 10.1C), which also activate (Wang et al. 1999) NFκB, an anti-apoptotic (Holcomb et al. 2008) and pro-inflammatory molecule (Ralhan et al. 2009) that stimulates the activities of VEGF (Ferrara 2002; Ferrara et al. 2003) and MMP-9 (Gysin et al. 2005), two key activities in angiogenesis and metastasis (Figure 10.1C).

The extensive impact of statins on signaling activities associated with growth and apoptosis has been reviewed (Mo and Elson 2008). Parallel to the effect of statins on HMG CoA reductase and protein prenylation, the farnesyl transferase inhibitors (FTIs) (Ura et al. 1998; Weisz et al. 1999; End et al. 2001; Mizukami et al. 2001; Venkatasubbarao et al. 2005) and phenylacetate (Harrison et al. 1998), an inhibitor of mevalonate pyrophosphate decarboxylase (Figure 10.1A) that leads to the syntheses of prenyl pyrophosphates, suppress the growth of tumor cells by inducing G1 arrest and apoptosis (reviewed in Mo and Elson 2004).

In sterologenic tissues, the highly regulated HMG CoA reductase activity is modulated primarily through the sterol-feedback inhibition of the transcription of the reductase gene (Goldstein and Brown 1990). In the presence of a saturating concentration of sterols, a residual reductase activity maintains pools of FPP, GGPP and other nonsterol products. When those pools are saturated, *trans, trans* farnesol (farnesol), a nonsterol metabolite, is diverted from the sterologenic pathway and initiates posttranscriptional actions that further suppress reductase activity (Correll et al. 1994; Meigs and Simoni 1997).

HMG CoA reductase activity in tumor tissues, however, is dysregulated and elevated (Mo and Elson 2004). Adding to previously reviewed (Mo and Elson 2008) evidence that HMG CoA reductase is overexpressed in liver, prostate, pancreas, blood, lymphatic, gastric, colorectal, mammary, adrenal, brain, and nerve cancer cells is the recent finding that HMG CoA reductase and sterol biosynthesis enzymes are elevated in breast cancer cells (Monville et al. 2008).

10.6 TOCOTRIENOLS SUPPRESS HMG CoA REDUCTASE AND DOWNSTREAM GROWTH-SUPPORTIVE CELL SIGNALING

The initial finding of the hypocholesterolemic effect of tocotrienol via suppression of HMG CoA reductase (Qureshi et al. 1986) led to subsequent studies (Pearce et al. 1992; Parker et al. 1993) delineating the tocotrienol-mediated posttranscriptional downregulation of reductase. A recent study (Song and DeBose-Boyd 2006) suggested an additional transcriptional downregulation of reductase by δ-tocotrienol. Tocotrienols contain in their side chain a farnesol moiety, the signaling molecule that triggers the degradation of HMG CoA reductase (Correll et al. 1994; Meigs and Simoni 1997). Tocotrienol-mediated suppression of HMG CoA reductase activity leads to the suppression of cell proliferation, cell cycle arrest, and apoptosis. In human colon cancer HT-29 and HCT116 cells, γ-tocotrienol counteracted the atorvastatin-induced elevation of HMG CoA reductase expression (Yang et al. 2010). In +SA mammary tumor cells, γ-tocotrienol downregulated HMG CoA reductase in a concentration- and time-dependent manner (Wali et al. 2009b). γ-Tocotrienol and statins synergistically suppressed the proliferation of +SA cells via downregulation of the prenylation of Rap1A and Rab6 and ERK, p38 and cyclin D1 signaling; these effects were reversed by mevalonate (Wali et al. 2009c), the product of HMG CoA reductase. Supplemental mevalonate also attenuated δ-tocotrienol-mediated suppression of the proliferation of MIA PaCa-2, BxPC-3, and PANC-1 cells (Hussein and Mo 2009). A recent finding suggested that HIF-1α stimulates the transcription and enzyme activity of HMGR (Pallottini et al. 2008). Although tocotrienols have been reported to suppress HIF-1α (Shibata et al. 2008b), it is unknown whether HIF-1α mediates the suppressive impact of tocotrienols on HMG CoA reductase. Tocopherols do not modulate HMG CoA reductase activity (Pearce et al. 1992). In fact, studies showed that α-tocopherol may attenuate the impact of tocotrienol on HMG CoA reductase (Qureshi et al. 1996) or even augment HMG CoA reductase activity (Qureshi et al. 1989).

The aforementioned disparate effects of tocotrienols and tocopherols on HMG CoA reductase and cell proliferation are parallel to their divergent effects on cell signaling. γ-Tocotrienol, but not γ-tocopherol, suppressed the growth of PC-3 and LNCaP cells and potentiated the growth-suppressive activity of docetaxel (Yap et al. 2008) via downregulation of EGFR and NFκB and activation of caspases. α-Tocopherol attenuated the effects of δ-tocotrienol on human DLD-1 colorectal adenocarcinoma cell apoptosis, cell cycle proteins including p21[cip1WAF1], p27[kip1], and GADD45A, caspase activation, and cellular uptake of δ-tocotrienol (Shibata et al. 2010). α-Tocopherol attenuated γ-Tocotrienol-induced downregulation of Id-1, apoptosis, and loss of viability in CD133-depleted, but not CD133-enriched, PC-3 cells (Luk et al. 2011). Tocotrienols, but not tocopherols, inhibited the constitutive activation of STAT3 in U266 cells (Kannappan et al. 2010b), induced the expression of DR-4 and DR-5 in HCT-116 cells (Kannappan et al. 2010a), and upregulated IL-24 mRNA expression in implanted 4T1 murine mammary tumor tissues in BALB/c mice (Selvaduray et al. 2010).

The finding that tocotrienols, but not tocopherols, inhibited the constitutive and TNF-α-induced NFκB activation (Ahn et al. 2007) suggested that tocotrienols have anti-inflammatory activity (Nesaretnam and Meganathan 2011) as a consequence to suppression of HMG CoA reductase activity and mevalonate deprivation; the tocotrienol effect was reversed by mevalonate (Ahn et al. 2007). The FTI SCH6636 also inhibited NFκB activation in mammary and lung tumors and lymphoma (Takada et al. 2004). Tocotrienols, but not α-tocopherol, dose-dependently suppressed the secretion of TNF-α in LPS-stimulated RAW 264.7 cells and serum level of TNF-α and mRNA levels of TNF-α, IL-1b, IL-6, and iNOS in LPS-stimulated peritoneal macrophages of female BALB/c mice (Qureshi et al. 2010). TRF dose-dependently inhibited LPS-induced release of NO and PGE2 and expression of iNOS, COX-2, and NFκB (Wu et al. 2008).

10.7   POTENTIAL OF TOCOTRIENOLS IN ADJUVANT THERAPY

Several *in vitro* and *in vivo* studies have confirmed and extended our early observation (He et al. 1997; Mo and Elson 1999) that tocotrienols and mevalonate suppressors have synergistic impact on tumor growth. Blends of tocotrienols and statins synergistically suppressed the growth of A2058 melanoma cells (Fernandes et al. 2010), MIA PaCa-2 pancreatic carcinoma cells (Hussein and Mo 2009), +SA malignant mammary epithelial cells (Wali et al. 2009a; Sylvester 2011; Sylvester et al. 2011), and HT29 and HCT116 colon cancer cells (Yang et al. 2010). γ-Tocotrienol, atorvastatin, and a COX-2 inhibitor CXIB had synergistic effect on the growth of HT29 and HCT116 colon cancer cells via cell cycle arrest at G1 phase, p21[cip1WAF1] upregulation, and apoptosis (Yang et al. 2010).

Tocotrienols have also been shown to synergize with mevalonate suppressors including geranyl-geraniol (Katuru et al. 2011) and resveratrol (Cho et al. 2008; Hsieh and Wu 2008) in suppressing tumor cell growth. Dietary δ-tocotrienol and lovastatin synergistically suppressed the growth of implanted murine B16 melanoma cells in C57BL6 mice (McAnally et al. 2007).

Blends of tocotrienols and chemotherapeutic agents have synergistic impact on tumor growth and signaling. γ-Tocotrienol synergizes with celecoxib (Shirode and Sylvester 2010; Sylvester et al. 2011), erlotinib (Bachawal et al. 2010; Sylvester 2011), and gefitinib (Bachawal et al. 2010; Sylvester 2011) in suppressing the growth of murine malignant + SA mammary epithelial cells; blends with the latter two agents downregulated EGF-dependent mitogenic signaling (Bachawal et al. 2010; Sylvester 2011). γ-Tocotrienol and epigallocatechin gallate (EGCG) synergistically inhibited the growth of MCF-7 cells by upregulating cell cycle arrest and apoptotic proteins (Hsieh and Wu 2008). Tocotrienols, but not tocopherols, synergizes with docetaxel in inhibiting MDA-MB231 cell growth, activating caspases, and inhibiting NFκB activation and expression of EGFR and Id1 (Yap et al. 2010a). Combinations of gemcitabine and γ-(Kunnumakkara et al. 2010) or δ-(Husain et al. 2011) tocotrienols synergistically suppressed the growth of MIA PaCa-2 (Kunnumakkara et al. 2010; Husain et al. 2011), PANC-1 (Kunnumakkara et al. 2010), BxPC-3 (Kunnumakkara et al. 2010), and AsPC-1 (Kunnumakkara et al. 2010; Husain et al. 2011) pancreatic tumor cells via PARP1 cleavage, apoptosis, and upregulation of Bax. TRF mitigated cisplatin-induced activation of PI3K/AKT signaling and sensitized human H28 malignant mesothelioma cells to cisplatin-induced cytotoxicity (Nakashima et al. 2010). γ-Tocotrienol sensitized colon cancer cells to TNF-related apoptosis-inducing ligand (TRAIL) (Kannappan et al. 2010a) and potentiated the apoptotic effect of doxorubicin and paclitaxel in HepG2 cells (Rajendran et al. 2011). In addition, γ-tocotrienol potentiated chemotherapeutic drugs thalidomide and bortezomib in human U266 multiple myeloma cells (Kannappan et al. 2010a). γ-Tocotrienol, but not γ-tocopherol, suppressed the growth of PC-3 and LNCaP cells and potentiated the growth-suppressive activity of docetaxel (Yap et al. 2008) via downregulation of EGFR and NFκB and activation of caspases.

The growth of orthotopically implanted MIA PaCa-2 tumor cells was suppressed by a combination of daily gavage feeding of γ-tocotrienol (400 mg/kg) and i.p. injection of gemcitabine (25 mg/kg, twice weekly); growth suppression was accompanied by tumor apoptosis and reduced expression of NFκB-regulated cyclin D1, c-Myc, VEGF, MMP-9, and CXCR4 (Kunnumakkara et al. 2010). A combination of δ-tocotrienol (200 mg/kg oral gavage twice daily) and gemcitabine (100 mg/kg i.p. injection twice a week) synergistically suppressed the growth of orthotopically implanted AsPc-1 pancreatic tumors in female SCID nude mice by upregulating the proapoptotic Bax and cleavage of PARP1 and downregulating NFκB, survivin and Bcl-xL (Husain et al. 2011).

10.8   SUMMARY

The last few years has seen an increased interest in the tumor-suppressive activity of tocotrienols. Diverse signaling pathways regulating cell cycle progression and apoptosis are modulated by tocotrienols. The contrasting impact of tocotrienols and tocopherols on cell proliferation and cell signaling, independent of their antioxidant activity, may trace to their divergent effects on HMG CoA reductase activity, an activity that provides essential intermediates for the biological function of growth-related proteins. Tocotrienols and diverse mevalonate suppressors and chemotherapeutic agents have synergistic impact on tumor cell growth *in vitro* and *in vivo*. Clinical trials showing the anticancer activity of tocotrienols are underway (Nesaretnam et al. 2010, 2011; Springett et al. 2011). Fluorescent derivatives of tocotrienol (Mudit et al. 2010) have been developed to further define their mechanism of action. Recent efforts in creating tocotrienol derivatives with enhanced bioavailability and target delivery as well as higher tumor-suppressive potency (Nikolic and Agababa 2009; Ali et al. 2010; Elnagar et al. 2010) may afford novel approaches to cancer chemoprevention and/or therapy.

ACKNOWLEDGMENTS

This work was partially supported by the Agriculture and Food Research Initiative Grant 2009-02941 from the USDA National Institute for Food and Agriculture, Texas Department of Agriculture Food and Fiber Research Program, and Texas Woman's University Research Enhancement Program.

REFERENCES

Adjei, A. A. 2001. Blocking oncogenic Ras signaling for cancer therapy. *J. Natl. Cancer Inst. 93*, 1062–1074.

Ahn, K. S., G. Sethi, K. Krishnan and B. B. Aggarwal. 2007. γ-Tocotrienol inhibits nuclear factor-κB signaling pathway through inhibition of receptor-interacting protein and TAK1 leading to suppression of antiapoptotic gene products and potentiation of apoptosis. *J. Biol. Chem. 282*, 809–820.

Ali, H., A. B. Shirode, P. W. Sylvester and S. Nazzal. 2010. Preparation, characterization, and anticancer effects of simvastatin-tocotrienol lipid nanoparticles. *Int. J. Pharm. 389*, 223–231.

Anderson, K. M. and J. E. Harris. 2001. Selected features of nonendocrine pancreatic cancer. *Exp. Biol. Med. (Maywood) 226*, 521–537.

Ayoub, N. M., S. V. Bachawal and P. W. Sylvester. 2011. γ-Tocotrienol inhibits HGF-dependent mitogenesis and Met activation in highly malignant mammary tumour cells. *Cell Prolif. 44*, 516–526.

Bachawal, S. V., V. B. Wali and P. W. Sylvester. 2010. Combined γ-tocotrienol and erlotinib/gefitinib treatment suppresses Stat and Akt signaling in murine mammary tumor cells. *Anticancer Res. 30*, 429–437.

Barve, A., T. O. Khor, K. Reuhl, B. Reddy, H. Newmark and A. N. Kong. 2010. Mixed tocotrienols inhibit prostate carcinogenesis in TRAMP mice. *Nutr. Cancer 62*, 789–794.

Behery, F. A., A. Y. Elnagar, M. R. Akl, V. B. Wali, B. Abuasal, A. Kaddoumi, P. W. Sylvester and K. A. El Sayed. 2010. Redox-silent tocotrienol esters as breast cancer proliferation and migration inhibitors. *Bioorg. Med. Chem. 18*, 8066–8075.

Boucher, M. J., J. Morisset, P. H. Vachon, J. C. Reed, J. Laine and N. Rivard. 2000. MEK/ERK signaling pathway regulates the expression of Bcl-2, Bcl-X(L), and Mcl-1 and promotes survival of human pancreatic cancer cells. *J. Cell. Biochem. 79*, 355–369.

Campbell, S. E. et al. 2011. γ-Tocotrienol induces growth arrest through a novel pathway with TGFβ2 in prostate cancer. *Free Radic. Biol. Med. 50*, 1344–1354.

Chang, P. N., W. N. Yap, D. T. Lee, M. T. Ling, Y. C. Wong and Y. L. Yap. 2009. Evidence of γ-tocotrienol as an apoptosis-inducing, invasion-suppressing, and chemotherapy drug-sensitizing agent in human melanoma cells. *Nutr. Cancer 61*, 357–366.

Cho, I. J., J. Y. Ahn, S. Kim, M. S. Choi and T. Y. Ha. 2008. Resveratrol attenuates the expression of HMG-CoA reductase mRNA in hamsters. *Biochem. Biophys. Res. Commun. 367*, 190–194.

Choi, Y. and J. Lee. 2009. Antioxidant and antiproliferative properties of a tocotrienol-rich fraction from grape seeds. *Food Chem. 114*, 1386–1390.

Comitato, R., K. Nesaretnam, G. Leoni, R. Ambra, R. Canali, A. Bolli, M. P. Marino and F. Virgili. 2009. A novel mechanism of natural vitamin E tocotrienol activity: Involvement of ERβ signal transduction. *Am. J. Physiol. Endocrinol. Metab. 297*, E427–E437.

Conte, C., A. Floridi, C. Aisa, M. Piroddi and F. Galli. 2004. γ-Tocotrienol metabolism and antiproliferative effect in prostate cancer cells. *Ann. NY Acad. Sci. 1031*, 391–394.

Correll, C. C., L. Ng and P. A. Edwards. 1994. Identification of farnesol as the non-sterol derivative of mevalonic acid required for the accelerated degradation of 3-hydroxy-3-methylglutaryl-coenzyme A reductase. *J. Biol. Chem. 269*, 17390–17393.

Dricu, A., M. Carlberg, M. Wang and O. Larsson. 1997. Inhibition of N-linked glycosylation using tunicamycin causes cell death in malignant cells: Role of down-regulation of the insulin-like growth factor 1 receptor in induction of apoptosis. *Cancer Res. 57*, 543–548.

Elangovan, S., T. C. Hsieh and J. M. Wu. 2008. Growth inhibition of human MDA-MB-231 breast cancer cells by δ-tocotrienol is associated with loss of cyclin D1/CDK4 expression and accompanying changes in the state of phosphorylation of the retinoblastoma tumor suppressor gene product. *Anticancer Res. 28*, 2641–2647.

Elnagar, A. Y., V. B. Wali, P. W. Sylvester and K. A. El Sayed. 2010. Design and preliminary structure-activity relationship of redox-silent semisynthetic tocotrienol analogues as inhibitors for breast cancer proliferation and invasion. *Bioorg. Med. Chem. 18*, 755–768.

End, D. W. et al. 2001. Characterization of the antitumor effects of the selective farnesyl protein transferase inhibitor R115777 in vivo and in vitro. *Cancer Res. 61*, 131–137.

Fernandes, N. V., P. K. Guntipalli and H. Mo. 2010. D-δ-Tocotrienol-mediated cell cycle arrest and apoptosis in human melanoma cells. *Anticancer Res. 30*, 4937–4944.

Ferrara, N. 2002. VEGF and the quest for tumour angiogenesis factors. *Nat. Rev. Cancer 2*, 795–803.

Ferrara, N., H. P. Gerber and J. LeCouter. 2003. The biology of VEGF and its receptors. *Nat. Med. 9*, 669–676.

Gelb, M. H. 1997. Protein prenylation, et cetera: Signal transduction in two dimensions. *Science 275*, 1750–1751.

Goldstein, J. L. and M. S. Brown. 1990. Regulation of the mevalonate pathway. *Nature 343*, 425–430.

Guthrie, N., A. Gapor, A. F. Chambers and K. K. Carroll. 1997. Inhibition of proliferation of estrogen receptor-negative MDA-MB-435 and -positive MCF-7 human breast cancer cells by palm oil tocotrienols and tamoxifen, alone and in combination. *J. Nutr. 127*, 544S–548S.

Gysin, S., S. H. Lee, N. M. Dean and M. McMahon. 2005. Pharmacologic inhibition of RAF–>MEK–>ERK signaling elicits pancreatic cancer cell cycle arrest through induced expression of p27^{Kip1}. *Cancer Res. 65*, 4870–4880.

Harrison, L. E., D. C. Wojciechowicz, M. F. Brennan and P. B. Paty. 1998. Phenylacetate inhibits isoprenoid biosynthesis and suppresses growth of human pancreatic carcinoma. *Surgery 124*, 541–550.

He, L., H. Mo, S. Hadisusilo, A. A. Qureshi and C. E. Elson. 1997. Isoprenoids suppress the growth of murine B16 melanomas in vitro and in vivo. *J. Nutr. 127*, 668–674.

Hiura, Y., H. Tachibana, R. Arakawa, N. Aoyama, M. Okabe, M. Sakai and K. Yamada. 2009. Specific accumulation of γ- and δ-tocotrienols in tumor and their antitumor effect in vivo. *J. Nutr. Biochem. 20*, 607–613.

Holcomb, B., M. Yip-Schneider and C. M. Schmidt. 2008. The role of nuclear factor κB in pancreatic cancer and the clinical applications of targeted therapy. *Pancreas 36*, 225–235.

Hsieh, T. C., S. Elangovan and J. M. Wu. 2010a. Differential suppression of proliferation in MCF-7 and MDA-MB-231 breast cancer cells exposed to α-, γ- and δ-tocotrienols is accompanied by altered expression of oxidative stress modulatory enzymes. *Anticancer Res. 30*, 4169–4176.

Hsieh, T. C., S. Elangovan and J. M. Wu. 2010b. γ-Tocotrienol controls proliferation, modulates expression of cell cycle regulatory proteins and up-regulates quinone reductase NQO2 in MCF-7 breast cancer cells. *Anticancer Res. 30*, 2869–2874.

Hsieh, T. C. and J. M. Wu. 2008. Suppression of cell proliferation and gene expression by combinatorial synergy of EGCG, resveratrol and γ-tocotrienol in estrogen receptor-positive MCF-7 breast cancer cells. *Int. J. Oncol. 33*, 851–859.

Husain, K., R. A. Francois, S. Z. Hutchinson, A. M. Neuger, R. Lush, D. Coppola, S. Sebti and M. P. Malafa. 2009. Vitamin E δ-tocotrienol levels in tumor and pancreatic tissue of mice after oral administration. *Pharmacology 83*, 157–163.

Husain, K., R. A. Francois, T. Yamauchi, M. Perez, S. M. Sebti and M. P. Malafa. 2011. Vitamin E δ-tocotrienol augments the anti-tumor activity of gemcitabine and suppresses constitutive NFκB activation in pancreatic cancer. *Mol. Cancer Ther. 10*, 2363–2372.

Hussein, D. and H. Mo. 2009. D-δ-Tocotrienol-mediated suppression of the proliferation of human PANC-1, MIA PaCa2 and BxPC-3 pancreatic carcinoma cells. *Pancreas 38*, e124–e136.

Hutchison, C. J., J. M. Bridger, L. S. Cox and I. R. Kill. 1994. Weaving a pattern from disparate threads: Lamin function in nuclear assembly and DNA replication. *J. Cell Sci. 107 (Pt 12)*, 3259–3269.

Inokuchi, H., H. Hirokane, T. Tsuzuki, K. Nakagawa, M. Igarashi and T. Miyazawa. 2003. Anti-angiogenic activity of tocotrienol. *Biosci. Biotechnol. Biochem. 67*, 1623–1627.

Inoue, A., K. Takitani, M. Koh, C. Kawakami, T. Kuno and H. Tamai. 2011. Induction of apoptosis by γ-tocotrienol in human cancer cell lines and leukemic blasts from patients: Dependency on Bid, cytochrome c, and caspase pathway. *Nutr. Cancer 63*, 763–770.

Ji, X., Z. Wang, A. Geamanu, F. H. Sarkar and S. V. Gupta. 2011. Inhibition of cell growth and induction of apoptosis in non-small cell lung cancer cells by δ-tocotrienol is associated with notch-1 down-regulation. *J. Cell. Biochem. 112*, 2773–2783.

Jiang, Q., X. Rao, C. Y. Kim, H. Freiser, Q. Zhang, Z. Jiang and G. Li. 2011. Gamma-tocotrienol induces apoptosis and autophagy in prostate cancer cells by increasing intracellular dihydrosphingosine and dihydroceramide. *Int. J. Cancer 130*, 685–693.

Jiang, X. and X. Wang. 2004. Cytochrome C-mediated apoptosis. *Annu. Rev. Biochem. 73*, 87–106.

Kannappan, R., J. Ravindran, S. Prasad, B. Sung, V. R. Yadav, S. Reuter, M. M. Chaturvedi and B. B. Aggarwal. 2010a. γ-Tocotrienol promotes TRAIL-induced apoptosis through reactive oxygen species/extracellular signal-regulated kinase/p53-mediated upregulation of death receptors. *Mol. Cancer Ther. 9*, 2196–2207.

Kannappan, R., V. R. Yadav and B. B. Aggarwal. 2010b. γ-Tocotrienol but not γ-tocopherol blocks STAT3 cell signaling pathway through induction of protein-tyrosine phosphatase SHP-1 and sensitizes tumor cells to chemotherapeutic agents. *J. Biol. Chem. 285*, 33520–33528.

Kashiwagi, K., K. Harada, Y. Yano, I. Kumadaki, K. Hagiwara, J. Takebayashi, W. Kido, N. Virgona and T. Yano. 2008. A redox-silent analogue of tocotrienol inhibits hypoxic adaptation of lung cancer cells. *Biochem. Biophys. Res. Commun. 365*, 875–881.

Kashiwagi, K., N. Virgona, K. Harada, W. Kido, Y. Yano, A. Ando, K. Hagiwara and T. Yano. 2009. A redox-silent analogue of tocotrienol acts as a potential cytotoxic agent against human mesothelioma cells. *Life Sci. 84*, 650–656.

Katuru, R., N. V. Fernandes, M. Elfakhani, D. Dutta, N. Mills, D. L. Hynds, C. King and H. Mo. 2011. Mevalonate depletion mediates the suppressive impact of geranylgeraniol on murine B16 melanoma cells. *Exp. Biol. Med. (Maywood) 236*, 604–613.

Klein, E. A. et al. 2011. Vitamin E and the risk of prostate cancer. *JAMA 306*, 1549–1556.

Kunnumakkara, A. B. et al. 2010. γ-Tocotrienol inhibits pancreatic tumors and sensitizes them to gemcitabine treatment by modulating the inflammatory microenvironment. *Cancer Res. 70*, 8695–8705.

Li, X., L. Liu, J. C. Tupper, D. D. Bannerman, R. K. Winn, S. M. Sebti, A. D. Hamilton and J. M. Harlan. 2002. Inhibition of protein geranylgeranylation and RhoA/RhoA kinase pathway induces apoptosis in human endothelial cells. *J. Biol. Chem. 277*, 15309–15316.

Li, Y., W. G. Sun, H. K. Liu, G. Y. Qi, Q. Wang, X. R. Sun, B. Q. Chen and J. R. Liu. 2011. γ-Tocotrienol inhibits angiogenesis of human umbilical vein endothelia cell induced by cancer cell. *J. Nutr. Biochem. 22*, 1127–1136.

Liu, H. K., Q. Wang, Y. Li, W. G. Sun, J. R. Liu, Y. M. Yang, W. L. Xu, X. R. Sun and B. Q. Chen. 2010. Inhibitory effects of γ-tocotrienol on invasion and metastasis of human gastric adenocarcinoma SGC-7901 cells. *J. Nutr. Biochem. 21*, 206–213.

Luk, S. U. et al. 2011. Gamma-tocotrienol as an effective agent in targeting prostate cancer stem cell-like population. *Int. J. Cancer 128*, 2182–2191.

Massague, J. 2004. G1 cell-cycle control and cancer. *Nature 432*, 298–306.

Maurer-Stroh, S., M. Koranda, W. Benetka, G. Schneider, F. L. Sirota and F. Eisenhaber. 2007. Towards complete sets of farnesylated and geranylgeranylated proteins. *PLoS Comput. Biol. 3*, e66.

McAnally, J. A., J. Gupta, S. Sodhani, L. Bravo and H. Mo. 2007. Tocotrienols potentiate lovastatin-mediated growth suppression *in vitro* and *in vivo. Exp. Biol. Med. (Maywood) 232*, 523–531.

McCampbell, A. S., R. R. Broaddus, D. S. Loose and P. J. Davies. 2006. Overexpression of the insulin-like growth factor I receptor and activation of the AKT pathway in hyperplastic endometrium. *Clin. Cancer Res. 12*, 6373–6378.

McIntyre, B. S., K. P. Briski, A. Gapor and P. W. Sylvester. 2000a. Antiproliferative and apoptotic effects of tocopherols and tocotrienols on preneoplastic and neoplastic mouse mammary epithelial cells. *Proc. Soc. Exp. Biol. Med. 224*, 292–301.

McIntyre, B. S., K. P. Briski, M. A. Tirmenstein, M. W. Fariss, A. Gapor and P. W. Sylvester. 2000b. Antiproliferative and apoptotic effects of tocopherols and tocotrienols on normal mouse mammary epithelial cells. *Lipids 35*, 171–180.

Meigs, T. E. and R. D. Simoni. 1997. Farnesol as a regulator of HMG-CoA reductase degradation: Characterization and role of farnesyl pyrophosphatase. *Arch. Biochem. Biophys. 345*, 1–9.

de Mesquita, M. L. et al. 2011. Cytotoxicity of δ-tocotrienols from *Kielmeyera coriacea* against cancer cell lines. *Bioorg. Med. Chem. 19*, 623–630.

Miyazawa, T., A. Shibata, P. Sookwong, Y. Kawakami, T. Eitsuka, A. Asai, S. Oikawa and K. Nakagawa. 2009. Antiangiogenic and anticancer potential of unsaturated vitamin E (tocotrienol). *J. Nutr. Biochem. 20*, 79–86.

Mizukami, Y., H. Ura, T. Obara, A. Habiro, T. Izawa, M. Osanai, N. Yanagawa, S. Tanno and Y. Kohgo. 2001. Requirement of c-jun N-terminal kinase for apoptotic cell death induced by farnesyltransferase inhibitor, farnesylamine, in human pancreatic cancer cells. *Biochem. Biophys. Res. Commun. 288*, 198–204.

Mo, H. and C. E. Elson. 1999. Apoptosis and cell-cycle arrest in human and murine tumor cells are initiated by isoprenoids. *J. Nutr. 129*, 804–813.

Mo, H. and C. E. Elson. 2004. Studies of the isoprenoid-mediated inhibition of mevalonate synthesis applied to cancer chemotherapy and chemoprevention. *Exp. Biol. Med. (Maywood) 229*, 567–585.

Mo, H. and C. E. Elson. 2008. Role of the mevalonate pathway in tocotrienol-mediated tumor suppression. In *Tocotrienols: Vitamin E beyond Tocopherols*. eds. R. R. Watson and V. R. Preedy. Boca Raton, FL, CRC Press: pp. 185–207.

Moir, R. D., T. P. Spann, R. I. Lopez-Soler, M. Yoon, A. E. Goldman, S. Khuon and R. D. Goldman. 2000. Review: The dynamics of the nuclear lamins during the cell cycle—Relationship between structure and function. *J. Struct. Biol. 129*, 324–334.

Monville, F., L. Gaelle, N. Cervera, J. Wicinskij, J. Geneix, D. Birnbaum and E. Charafe-Jauffret. 2008. Sterol biosynthesis pathway is overexpressed in mammary tumorospheres. *Proc. Am. Assoc. Cancer Res.*, Abs# 2015.

Mudit, M., F. A. Behery, V. B. Wali, P. W. Sylvester and K. A. El Sayed. 2010. Synthesis of fluorescent analogues of the anticancer natural products 4-hydroxyphenylmethylene hydantoin and delta-tocotrienol.
Nat. Prod. Commun. 5, 1623–1626.

Muller, L., K. Theile and V. Bohm. 2010. In vitro antioxidant activity of tocopherols and tocotrienols and
comparison of vitamin E concentration and lipophilic antioxidant capacity in human plasma. *Mol. Nutr.
Food Res. 54*, 731–742.

Nakagawa, K., A. Shibata, S. Yamashita, T. Tsuzuki, J. Kariya, S. Oikawa and T. Miyazawa. 2007. In vivo
angiogenesis is suppressed by unsaturated vitamin E, tocotrienol. *J. Nutr. 137*, 1938–1943.

Nakashima, K., N. Virgona, M. Miyazawa, T. Watanabe and T. Yano. 2010. The tocotrienol-rich fraction from
rice bran enhances cisplatin-induced cytotoxicity in human mesothelioma H28 cells. *Phytother. Res. 24*,
1317–1321.

Nesaretnam, K. and P. Meganathan. 2011. Tocotrienols: Inflammation and cancer. *Ann. NY Acad. Sci. 1229*, 18–22.

Nesaretnam, K., P. Meganathan, S. D. Veerasenan and K. R. Selvaduray. 2011. Tocotrienols and breast cancer:
The evidence to date. *Genes Nutr. 7*, 3–9.

Nesaretnam, K., K. R. Selvaduray, G. Abdul Razak, S. D. Veerasenan and P. A. Gomez. 2010. Effectiveness
of tocotrienol-rich fraction combined with tamoxifen in the management of women with early breast
cancer: A pilot clinical trial. *Breast Cancer Res. 12*, R81.

Nikolic, K. and D. Agababa. 2009. Design and QSAR study of analogs of γ-tocotrienol with enhanced antiproliferative activity against human breast cancer cells. *J. Mol. Graph. Model. 27*, 777–783.

Pallottini, V., B. Guantario, C. Martini, P. Totta, I. Filippi, F. Carraro and A. Trentalance. 2008. Regulation of
HMG-CoA reductase expression by hypoxia. *J. Cell. Biochem. 104*, 701–709.

Park, S. K., B. G. Sanders and K. Kline. 2010. Tocotrienols induce apoptosis in breast cancer cell lines via an
endoplasmic reticulum stress-dependent increase in extrinsic death receptor signaling. *Breast Cancer
Res. Treat. 124*, 361–375.

Parker, R. A., B. C. Pearce, R. W. Clark, D. A. Gordon and J. J. Wright. 1993. Tocotrienols regulate cholesterol production in mammalian cells by post-transcriptional suppression of 3-hydroxy-3-methylglutaryl-coenzyme
A reductase. *J. Biol. Chem. 268*, 11230–11238.

Patacsil, D. et al. 2011. Gamma-tocotrienol induced apoptosis is associated with unfolded protein response in
human breast cancer cells. *J. Nutr. Biochem. 23*, 93–100.

Pearce, B. C., R. A. Parker, M. E. Deason, A. A. Qureshi and J. J. Wright. 1992. Hypocholesterolemic activity
of synthetic and natural tocotrienols. *J. Med. Chem. 35*, 3595–3606.

Pierpaoli, E., V. Viola, F. Pilolli, M. Piroddi, F. Galli and M. Provinciali. 2010. γ- and δ-tocotrienols exert
a more potent anticancer effect than α-tocopheryl succinate on breast cancer cell lines irrespective of
HER-2/neu expression. *Life Sci. 86*, 668–675.

Qureshi, A. A., W. C. Burger, D. M. Peterson and C. E. Elson. 1986. The structure of an inhibitor of cholesterol
biosynthesis isolated from barley. *J. Biol. Chem. 261*, 10544–10550.

Qureshi, A. A., B. C. Pearce, R. M. Nor, A. Gapor, D. M. Peterson and C. E. Elson. 1996. Dietary α-tocopherol
attenuates the impact of γ-tocotrienol on hepatic 3-hydroxy-3-methylglutaryl coenzyme A reductase
activity in chickens. *J. Nutr. 126*, 389–394.

Qureshi, A. A., D. M. Peterson, C. E. Elson, A. R. Mangels and Z. Z. Din. 1989. Stimulation of avian cholesterol metabolism by α-tocopherol. *Nutr. Rep. Int. 40*, 993–1001.

Qureshi, A. A., J. C. Reis, C. J. Papasian, D. C. Morrison and N. Qureshi. 2010. Tocotrienols inhibit lipopolysaccharide-induced pro-inflammatory cytokines in macrophages of female mice. *Lipids Health Dis. 9*, 143.

Rajendran, P., F. Li, K. A. Manu, M. K. Shanmugam, S. Y. Loo, A. P. Kumar and G. Sethi. 2011. γ-Tocotrienol is
a novel inhibitor of constitutive and inducible STAT3 signalling pathway in human hepatocellular carcinoma: Potential role as an antiproliferative, pro-apoptotic and chemosensitizing agent. *Br. J. Pharmacol.
163*, 283–298.

Ralhan, R., M. K. Pandey and B. B. Aggarwal. 2009. Nuclear factor-kappa B links carcinogenic and chemopreventive agents. *Front. Biosci. (Schol Ed) 1*, 45–60.

Ramdas, P., M. Rajihuzzaman, S. D. Veerasenan, K. R. Selvaduray, K. Nesaretnam and A. K. Radhakrishnan.
2011. Tocotrienol-treated MCF-7 human breast cancer cells show down-regulation of API5 and
up-regulation of MIG6 genes. *Cancer Genomics Proteomics 8*, 19–31.

Saito, Y., K. Nishio, Y. O. Akazawa, K. Yamanaka, A. Miyama, Y. Yoshida, N. Noguchi and E. Niki. 2010.
Cytoprotective effects of vitamin E homologues against glutamate-induced cell death in immature pri-
mary cortical neuron cultures: Tocopherols and tocotrienols exert similar effects by antioxidant function.
Free Radic. Biol. Med. 49, 1542–1549.

Samant, G. V., V. B. Wali and P. W. Sylvester. 2010. Anti-proliferative effects of γ-tocotrienol on mammary
tumour cells are associated with suppression of cell cycle progression. *Cell Prolif. 43*, 77–83.

Selvaduray, K. R., A. K. Radhakrishnan, M. K. Kutty and K. Nesaretnam. 2010. Palm tocotrienols inhibit pro-liferation of murine mammary cancer cells and induce expression of interleukin-24 mRNA. *J. Interferon Cytokine Res. 30*, 909–916.

Sherr, C. J. 2004. Principles of tumor suppression. *Cell 116*, 235–246.

Shibata, A., K. Nakagawa, P. Sookwong, T. Tsuduki, A. Asai and T. Miyazawa. 2010. α-Tocopherol attenuates the cytotoxic effect of δ-tocotrienol in human colorectal adenocarcinoma cells. *Biochem. Biophys. Res. Commun. 397*, 214–219.

Shibata, A., K. Nakagawa, P. Sookwong, T. Tsuduki, S. Oikawa and T. Miyazawa. 2009. δ-Tocotrienol sup-presses VEGF induced angiogenesis whereas α-tocopherol does not. *J. Agric. Food Chem. 57*, 8696–8704.

Shibata, A., K. Nakagawa, P. Sookwong, T. Tsuzuki, S. Oikawa and T. Miyazawa. 2008a. Tumor anti-angiogenic effect and mechanism of action of δ-tocotrienol. *Biochem. Pharmacol. 76*, 330–339.

Shibata, A., K. Nakagawa, P. Sookwong, T. Tsuduki, S. Tomita, H. Shirakawa, M. Komai and T. Miyazawa. 2008b. Tocotrienol inhibits secretion of angiogenic factors from human colorectal adenocarcinoma cells by suppressing hypoxia-inducible factor-1α. *J. Nutr. 138*, 2136–2142.

Shin-Kang, S., V. P. Ramsauer, J. Lightner, K. Chakraborty, W. Stone, S. Campbell, S. A. Reddy and K. Krishnan. 2011. Tocotrienols inhibit AKT and ERK activation and suppress pancreatic cancer cell proliferation by suppressing the ErbB2 pathway. *Free Radic. Biol. Med. 51*, 1164–1174.

Shirode, A. B. and P. W. Sylvester. 2010. Synergistic anticancer effects of combined γ-tocotrienol and cele-coxib treatment are associated with suppression in Akt and NFκB signaling. *Biomed. Pharmacother. 64*, 327–332.

Song, B. L. and R. A. DeBose-Boyd. 2006. Insig-dependent ubiquitination and degradation of 3-hydroxy-3-methylglutaryl coenzyme A reductase stimulated by δ- and γ-tocotrienols. *J. Biol. Chem. 281*, 25054–25061.

Springett, G. M., A. M. Neuger, B. A. Centeno, T. Hutchinson, H. Jump, R. Lush, S. Sebti and M. P. Malafa. 2011. A phase I dose-escalation study of the safety, PK, and PD of vitamin E δ-tocotrienol administered to subjects with resectable pancreatic exocrine neoplasia. *Proc. Am. Assoc. Cancer Res. 52*, Abs# 1299.

Sun, W., Q. Wang, B. Chen, J. Liu, H. Liu and W. Xu. 2008. γ-Tocotrienol-induced apoptosis in human gastric cancer SGC-7901 cells is associated with a suppression in mitogen-activated protein kinase signalling. *Br. J. Nutr. 99*, 1247–1254.

Sun, W., W. Xu, H. Liu, J. Liu, Q. Wang, J. Zhou, F. Dong and B. Chen. 2009. γ-Tocotrienol induces mitochon-dria-mediated apoptosis in human gastric adenocarcinoma SGC-7901 cells. *J. Nutr. Biochem. 20*, 276–284.

Sylvester, P. W. 2011. Synergistic anticancer effects of combined γ-tocotrienol with statin or receptor tyrosine kinase inhibitor treatment. *Genes Nutr. 7*, 63–74.

Sylvester, P. W., V. B. Wali, S. V. Bachawal, A. B. Shirode, N. M. Ayoub and M. R. Akl. 2011. Tocotrienol combination therapy results in synergistic anticancer response. *Front. Biosci. 17*, 3183–3195.

Takada, Y., F. R. Khuri and B. B. Aggarwal. 2004. Protein farnesyltransferase inhibitor (SCH 66336) abolishes NF-κB activation induced by various carcinogens and inflammatory stimuli leading to suppression of NF-κB-regulated gene expression and up-regulation of apoptosis. *J. Biol. Chem. 279*, 26287–26299.

Tasaki, M., T. Umemura, T. Inoue, T. Okamura, Y. Kuroiwa, Y. Ishii, M. Maeda, M. Hirose and A. Nishikawa. 2008. Induction of characteristic hepatocyte proliferation lesion with dietary exposure of Wistar Hannover rats to tocotrienol for 1 year. *Toxicology 250*, 143–150.

Ura, H., T. Obara, R. Shudo, A. Itoh, S. Tanno, T. Fujii, N. Nishino and Y. Kohgo. 1998. Selective cytotoxicity of farnesylamine to pancreatic carcinoma cells and Ki-ras-transformed fibroblasts. *Mol. Carcinog. 21*, 93–99.

Venkatasubbarao, K., A. Choudary and J. W. Freeman. 2005. Farnesyl transferase inhibitor (R115777)-induced inhibition of STAT3(Tyr705) phosphorylation in human pancreatic cancer cell lines require extracellular signal-regulated kinases. *Cancer Res. 65*, 2861–2871.

Wali, V. B., S. V. Bachawal and P. W. Sylvester. 2009a. Combined treatment of γ-tocotrienol with statins induce mammary tumor cell cycle arrest in G1. *Exp. Biol. Med. (Maywood) 234*, 639–650.

Wali, V. B., S. V. Bachawal and P. W. Sylvester. 2009b. Endoplasmic reticulum stress mediates γ-tocotrienol-induced apoptosis in mammary tumor cells. *Apoptosis 14*, 1366–1377.

Wali, V. B., S. V. Bachawal and P. W. Sylvester. 2009c. Suppression in mevalonate synthesis mediates antitumor effects of combined statin and γ-tocotrienol treatment. *Lipids 44*, 925–934.

Wang, W., J. L. Abbruzzese, D. B. Evans, L. Larry, K. R. Cleary and P. J. Chiao. 1999. The nuclear factor-κB RelA transcription factor is constitutively activated in human pancreatic adenocarcinoma cells. *Clin. Cancer Res. 5*, 119–127.

Weisz, B., K. Giehl, M. Gana-Weisz, Y. Egozi, G. Ben-Baruch, D. Marciano, P. Gierschik and Y. Kloog. 1999. A new functional Ras antagonist inhibits human pancreatic tumor growth in nude mice. *Oncogene 18*, 2579–2588.

Weng-Yew, W., K. R. Selvaduray, C. H. Ming and K. Nesaretnam. 2009. Suppression of tumor growth by palm tocotrienols via the attenuation of angiogenesis. *Nutr. Cancer 61*, 367–373.

Wu, S. J., P. L. Liu and L. T. Ng. 2008. Tocotrienol-rich fraction of palm oil exhibits anti-inflammatory property by suppressing the expression of inflammatory mediators in human monocytic cells. *Mol. Nutr. Food Res. 52*, 921–929.

Wu, S. J. and L. T. Ng. 2010. Tocotrienols inhibited growth and induced apoptosis in human HeLa cells through the cell cycle signaling pathway. *Integr. Cancer Ther. 9*, 66–72.

Xu, W., M. Du, Y. Zhao, Q. Wang, W. Sun and B. Chen. γ-Tocotrienol inhibits cell viability through suppression of β-catenin/Tcf signaling in human colon carcinoma HT-29 cells. *J. Nutr. Biochem.* (in press).

Xu, W. L., J. R. Liu, H. K. Liu, G. Y. Qi, X. R. Sun, W. G. Sun and B. Q. Chen. 2009. Inhibition of proliferation and induction of apoptosis by γ-tocotrienol in human colon carcinoma HT-29 cells. *Nutrition 25*, 555–566.

Yang, Z., H. Xiao, H. Jin, P. T. Koo, D. J. Tsang and C. S. Yang. 2010. Synergistic actions of atorvastatin with γ-tocotrienol and celecoxib against human colon cancer HT29 and HCT116 cells. *Int. J. Cancer 126*, 852–863.

Yap, W. N., P. N. Chang, H. Y. Han, D. T. W. Lee, M. T. Ling, Y. C. Wong and Y. L. Yap. 2008. γ-Tocotrienol suppresses prostate cancer cell proliferation and invasion through multiple-signalling pathways. *Br. J. Cancer 99*, 1832–1841.

Yap, S. P., K. H. Yuen and J. W. Wong. 2001. Pharmacokinetics and bioavailability of α-, γ- and δ-tocotrienols under different food status. *J. Pharm. Pharmacol. 53*, 67–71.

Yap, W. N., N. Zaiden, S. Y. Luk, D. T. Lee, M. T. Ling, Y. C. Wong and Y. L. Yap. 2010a. In vivo evidence of γ-tocotrienol as a chemosensitizer in the treatment of hormone-refractory prostate cancer. *Pharmacology 85*, 248–258.

Yap, W. N., N. Zaiden, Y. L. Tan, C. P. Ngoh, X. W. Zhang, Y. C. Wong, M. T. Ling and Y. L. Yap. 2010b. Id1, inhibitor of differentiation, is a key protein mediating anti-tumor responses of gamma-tocotrienol in breast cancer cells. *Cancer Lett. 291*, 187–199.

Yoshida, Y., E. Niki and N. Noguchi. 2003. Comparative study on the action of tocopherols and tocotrienols as antioxidant: Chemical and physical effects. *Chem. Phys. Lipids 123*, 63–75.

Yu, W., M. Simmons-Menchaca, A. Gapor, B. G. Sanders and K. Kline. 1999. Induction of apoptosis in human breast cancer cells by tocopherols and tocotrienols. *Nutr. Cancer 33*, 26–32.

Zhang, F. L. and P. J. Casey. 1996. Protein prenylation: Molecular mechanisms and functional consequences. *Annu. Rev. Biochem. 65*, 241–269.

Zhang, J. S., D. M. Li, N. He, Y. H. Liu, C. H. Wang, S. Q. Jiang, B. Q. Chen and J. R. Liu. 2011. A paraptosis-like cell death induced by δ-tocotrienol in human colon carcinoma SW620 cells is associated with the suppression of the Wnt signaling pathway. *Toxicology 285*, 8–17.

11 Potential of Tocotrienols in Lung Cancer

Xiangming Ji, Arvind Goja, and Smiti V. Gupta

CONTENTS

11.1 INTRODUCTION

11.1.1 CANCER

Cancer, the uncontrolled growth and spread of abnormal cells, results from the accumulation of numerous sequential mutations and alterations in nuclear and cytoplasmic molecules (Gescher et al. 2001). Cancer progression or tumorigenesis is considered to involve three key steps: initiation, in which a normal cell is transformed into an initiated or abnormal cell; promotion, by which the initiated cell is converted into a preneoplastic cell; and progression, the process whereby the cells become neoplastic (Thangapazham et al. 2006). Cancer may be initiated due to multiple factors including exposure to carcinogens, repeated genetic damage by oxidative stress, chronic inflammation, or hormonal imbalance. This, followed by a cascade of reactions triggered by multiple signaling molecules, makes it difficult to target a specific molecule responsible for the disease and thereby retard progression.

Lung cancer, a malignant tumor that forms in the lung tissue and usually in the cells lining air passages, is the most common cancer worldwide, accounting for 1.2 million new cases annually. According to the 2011 Cancer statistics, it is also the leading cause of cancer deaths in the United States with an estimated 221,130 new cases, and 156,940 deaths attributed to this cancer type. Based on histological differences, the two major types of lung cancer observed are the small cell lung cancer (SCLC), accounting for about 15% of lung cancer incidence, and the non-small cell lung cancer (NSCLC), which includes squamous cell carcinoma, adenocarcinoma, and large cell carcinoma. The latter accounts for approximately 85% of all lung cancers diagnosed (Wistuba and Gazdar 2006).

The common known causes of lung cancer include smoking, which accounts for 87% of cases, second-hand smoke, and exposure to substances such as arsenic, asbestos, radioactive dust (radon), environmental factors, and genetic changes.

The lung cancer death rate of 28% and 26% for men and women, respectively, is the highest mortality rate of all cancer types (Siegel et al. 2011). Thus, to reduce cancer incidence and mortality rate, and improve the survival time of lung cancer patients, new techniques and approaches must be developed to diagnose, prevent, and treat preinvasive lesions. In spite of extensive research and investment in different therapeutic approaches to treatment of lung cancer, at present no single drug has been found to be simultaneously effective and nontoxic. Most chemotherapeutic treatments suffer from adverse toxic reactions leading to acute and delayed nausea, mouth ulcerations, fatigue, nerve damage, blood clots, anemia, and mild impairments. Also, long-term chemotherapy treatments can amplify the risk for developing other types of cancers (Cross and Burmester 2006). Thus, it is important to develop effective preventative and/or therapeutic approaches either in the form of single agents or as combinations, which could potentially be both effective against lung cancer cell growth and relatively nontoxic.

11.1.2 Diet and Cancer

Various studies have shown that the predominance of chronic diseases including cancers is linked to certain lifestyles and environments. According to an analysis based on 206 human epidemiologic studies and 22 animal studies conducted in the last decade, a diet rich in fruits and vegetables correlated with a decrease in incidence of cancers of stomach, esophagus, lung, oral cavity and pharynx, endometrium, pancreas, and colon (Aggarwal and Shishodia 2006). Since cancer is a multifactorial disease, single target agents are now often considered to be less valuable for cancer prevention and/or treatment. Recent evidence supports that nonnutritive components in diet have therapeutic benefits attributable to their pleiotropic effects including downregulation of survival signaling and simultaneous activation of multiple death pathways in cancer cells. Thus, diet appears to have a major influence in cancer prevention, and specific dietary components may potentially play a key role in cancer therapy as well. In fact, more than 70% of the current anticancer drugs approved by the U.S. Food and Drug Administration (FDA) since 1970 can be traced back to having plant origin. Many of the original plants were used in traditional medicine for various ailments (Lam et al. 2009).

Over the recent years, many examples of nutrients acting as or on transcriptional factors that modify gene expression have bloomed in literature. Effects of various functional foods on various cancer types have been very well documented (Norman et al. 2004, Ogilvie 1998, Tapsell et al. 2006). Thus, isothiocyanates, bioactive compounds in cruciferous vegetables, were shown to reduce the risk of lung cancer by 22% in comparison to those who did not consume cruciferous vegetables (Lam et al. 2009).

The accumulating evidence of the beneficial role of dietary components has led into a new approach in cancer prevention and treatment with the goal to prevent carcinogenesis. Diet and dietary components can alter the risk of disease development by modulating multiple processes involved with onset, incidence, progression, and/or severity; food components can act on the human genome, either directly or indirectly, to alter the expression of genes and gene products; diet could potentially compensate for or accentuate effects of genetic polymorphisms; and the consequences of a diet are dependent on the balance of health and disease states and on an individual's genetic background (Trujillo 2006). Dietary agents have different roles depending on the source of the dietary agent. A particular dietary agent can show all or some of the properties necessary to cure or prevent the cancer. Dietary agent molecules may downregulate protein kinases, antiapoptotic proteins, molecules involved in metastasis and upregulate apoptotic proteins.

Bioactive substances can be accredited as a small quantity of compounds produced upon either *in vivo* or in the food-processing activities. Bioactive constituents of food are demonstrated to have physiological, behavioral, and immunological effects. Accumulating data from both epidemiological and animal studies have suggested chemopreventative roles for phytochemicals in certain forms of cancers and other diseases.

11.1.2.1 Dietary Component Vitamin E

Vitamin E refers to a group of fat-soluble compounds found in various types of foods such as eggs, meats, cereals, vegetables, and edible oils. Based on their chemical structures, vitamin E isoforms can be classified into two broad categories, the tocopherols and the tocotrienols, with the latter containing three *trans* double bonds in the farnesyl isoprenoid tail of the molecule. Based on the presence of the substituents on the chromanol ring or head group, both tocopherols and tocotrienols can be subdivided into α-, β-, γ-, δ-tocopherol and α-, β-, γ-, δ-tocotrienols, respectively (Sylvester et al. 2010). To date, approximately 90% of the literature on vitamin E is focused on the study of tocopherols, which are present at higher concentrations in natural sources than their tocotrienol counterparts. The interest in the relationship between vitamin E consumption and cancer can be traced as early as the 1930s (Davidson 1934). Since then, a number of studies supporting the anticancer activity of vitamin E, either directly as an antineoplastic agent or indirectly through the augmentation of chemotherapy effects were reported (Argyriou et al. 2006, Factor et al. 2000, Sylvester et al. 2010). *In vitro* studies have demonstrated that anticancer activity of vitamin E is associated with improved host immunity (Meydani et al. 1997, Zhang et al. 1995), inhibition of oncogenes (Turley et al. 1997), activation of tumor suppressor genes (Schwartz et al. 1993), reduction of DNA damage (Factor et al. 2000), and alteration of tumor cell proliferation pathways (Azzi et al. 1993). Some clinical studies have shown lower levels of serum vitamin E in cancer patients as compared with healthy controls (Choi et al. 1999, Kumagai et al. 1998, Malvy et al. 1997, Torun et al. 1995). For example, the mean serum values for vitamin E were found to be 10.2 μM in breast cancer patients and 25.7 μM in controls (Torun et al. 1995). Similarly, lower serum levels of vitamin A, vitamin E, and beta-carotene were associated with an increased risk of lung cancer (Kumagai et al. 1998).

However, there have been some contradictory reports documenting dietary vitamin E intake and different types of cancers, including breast cancer (Bohlke et al. 1999), gastric cancer (Hansson et al. 1994), larynx cancer (Negri et al. 2000), brain cancer (Hu et al. 1999), skin cancer (Stryker et al. 1990), ovarian cancer (Bidoli et al. 2001), and colon and lung cancer (Lee et al. 2005). Although there is a huge discrepancy on the relationship between vitamin E and cancer, these results should be considered cautiously for the following aspects. First, most of the case-control studies used the self-reporting method for vitamin E intake, which is vulnerable to recall bias. Second, a number of studies suffered from mismatched number of subjects between the patients and control groups, leading to statistical imperfections. Third, serum vitamin E level is likely to be affected by an individual's genetic status, which could in turn modify the vitamin E transportation and metabolism in the body. This could further introduce additional unexplained variability in the data. For example, α-tocopherol transfer protein (TPP) is the major transporter for vitamin E in humans (Arita et al. 1995). Patients with underexpression of TPP have remarkably low plasma levels of α-tocopherol (Krendel et al. 1987, Yokota et al. 1987). These observations support the notion that interindividual differences in the expression level or activity of TTP may determine the diversity in response to dietary vitamin E. A recent study reported that TTP could sensitize prostate cancer cells to the antiproliferative effects of vitamin E. This was attributed to the ability of the protein to increase the intracellular accumulation of the antioxidant (Morley et al. 2010). However, despite the array of possible explanations for the controversial data on the effects of vitamin E and various cancer types, the biological implications of these antagonistic findings must be resolved, which will require further in-depth investigations in establishing the role of vitamin E, especially tocopherols, in cancer. Moreover, it may be useful to turn our attention from vitamin E as a whole, consisting chiefly of the tocopherols to the minor, yet potentially beneficial fraction, the tocotrienols.

11.2 TOCOTRIENOLS AND CHRONIC DISEASE

Compared with tocopherols, tocotrienols account for only about 1% of the total published research on vitamin E because of their lower availability in nature and the fact that most research was not conducted using purified fractions of tocotrienols. Found in wheat germ, barley, some grains and vegetable oils, palm oil represents one of the richest natural sources of tocotrienols with 70% of its vitamin E being in the form of tocotrienols (Elson 1992, Sundram et al. 2003).

Identification of α-tocotrienol as an inhibitor of cholesterol biosynthesis started a spur of activity in tocotrienol research (Qureshi et al. 1986). Later, tocotrienols were found to regulate cholesterol production in mammalian cells by posttranscriptional suppression of 3-hydroxy-3-methylglutaryl-coenzyme A (HMG-CoA) reductase (Parker et al. 1993). Studies indicate that δ- and γ-tocotrienols enhance HMG-CoA reductase ubiquitination and degradation. In addition, δ-tocotrienol blocks the processing of sterol regulatory element-binding proteins (SREBPs) (Song and DeBose-Boyd 2006). This suppression of HMG-CoA activity is corroborated with a reported decrease in total cholesterol and low density lipoprotein plasma levels in hamsters (Raederstorff et al. 2002). Taken together, these reports suggest that dietary supplements of tocotrienols may represent a novel approach for the treatment of hypercholesterolemia.

In comparison to the tocopherols, tocotrienols have more potent antioxidant properties due to the presence of three double bonds in the hydrocarbon tail (Serbinova et al. 1991, Serbinova and Packer 1994). Overproduction of reactive oxygen and nitrogen species (RO/NS), leading to oxidative stress, is a well-established contributor to a multitude of chronic diseases, for example, cardiovascular, cancer, and neurodegeneration, as well as to the normal process of aging (Golden et al. 2002). Thus, agents that help to lower the burden of oxidative stress may be of benefit in preventing or delaying onset of these diseases. In line with their antioxidant capabilities, administration of tocotrienols, but not tocopherols, reduced the accumulation of protein carbonyls (indicators of oxidative damage during aging), and consequently extended the mean life span in *Caenorhabditis elegans* (Adachi and Ishii 2000). Very recently, it was observed that dietary supplementation with tocotrienols improved T-cell function in old mice (Ren et al. 2010).

Glutamate toxicity, associated with the Src pathway, has been considered as a major contributor to neurodegeneration (Smyth and Levey 1948, Yu and Salter 1998). In addition, it has been shown that 12-LOX, involved in the pathogenesis of Alzheimer disease, is phosphorylated by c-Src kinase in response to glutamate (Hall et al. 1995, Pratico et al. 2004). Therefore, inhibition of the Src pathway might play a vital role in prevention of neurodegenerative diseases. It has been shown that treatment of HT4 neuronal cells with α-tocotrienol blocked glutamate-induced death by suppressing glutamate-induced early activation of c-Src kinase (Sen et al. 2000). Furthermore, these *in vitro* results were substantiated with an animal study that demonstrated that α-tocotrienol is capable of diminishing neurodegeneration by inhibiting the Src and 12-Lox pathways (Rink et al. 2011). Taken together, α-tocotrienol appears to be a promising agent for prevention and/or treatment of neurodegenerative diseases.

11.2.1 TOCOTRIENOLS AND LUNG CANCER PREVENTION: POSSIBLE TARGETS AND MECHANISMS OF ACTION

The alteration of genes responsible for regulation of cell growth and differentiation transform a normal cell to a cancer cell, causing failure of cell growth regulation, ultimately resulting in cancer (Croce 2008). Accumulating evidence indicates that pathogenesis of cancer is a complex multistep process of sequential alterations in several oncogenes, tumor suppressor genes, or microRNA genes in cancer cells. Although α-tocotrienol seems to offer the most neuroprotection among all the vitamin E isomers, γ- and δ-tocotrienols have been shown to be superior to the other isomers in cancer prevention (Hsieh et al. 2010, Kannappan et al. 2010, Yap et al. 2008). One of the earlier studies investigating the anticancer effect of tocotrienols showed that α- and γ-tocotrienols were effective against sarcoma 180, Ehrlich carcinoma, and invasive mammary carcinoma (Komiyama et al. 1989). In addition, γ-tocotrienol showed a slight life-prolonging effect in mice with Meth A fibrosarcoma (Komiyama et al. 1989). However, no antitumor activity of tocotrienols was observed against P388 leukemia at doses of 5–40 mg/kg/day (Komiyama et al. 1989). Since then, there has been a tremendous interest in investigating the anticancer effects of tocotrienols. As such, tocotrienols have been shown to have antitumor effects on different human cancer cells including prostate, breast, colon, melanoma, and lung cancers (Kumar et al. 2006, McAnally et al. 2003, Sylvester and Shah 2005). Additionally, it has been shown that tocotrienols can induce apoptosis by inhibiting multiple signaling pathways such as EGFR, NF-κB, MAPK, and PI3K/AKT pathways (Shirode and Sylvester 2010).

11.2.1.1 Lung Cancer and the EGFR Pathway

Epidermal growth factor receptor (EGFR) is the cell-surface growth factor receptor that exists in an inactive monomer form inside the cell membrane. Upon ligand binding, EGFR may form homodimers of EGFR-EGFR or heterodimers with other ErbB family members, such as ErbB2 or ErbB3, by dimerization. EGFR dimerization stimulates its intrinsic intracellular tyrosine kinase activity, resulting in the autophosphorylation of the c-terminal tyrosine residue, which in turn upregulates the downstream signaling of EGFR via protein–protein interactions. This downstream signaling initiates signal transduction cascades, such as PI3K-AKT pathway, leading to DNA synthesis, cell proliferation, and migration. EGFR has been found to be overexpressed in many kinds of cancer, such as lung, breast, ovarian, head, and neck cancers (Chrysogelos and Dickson 1994, Hirsch et al. 2009, Maihle et al. 2002, Rogers et al. 2005). Moreover, the overexpression and activation of EGFR is considered to be a predictor of cancer progression and sensitivity to the tyrosine kinase inhibitors in NSCLC patients (Hirsch et al. 2009).

Erlotinib is a small molecule that inhibits EGFR tyrosine kinase by competitively binding at the receptor's ATP binding site. In clinical trials, American and Japanese patients with NSCLC responded differently to Erlotinib intervention with the rate of response between American and Japanese being 10% and 30%, respectively (Fukuoka et al. 2003, Kris et al. 2003). Overall, Asian, female, nonsmoking patients showed better drug response than other patients (Lynch et al. 2004). Further, gene sequencing data showed that somatic gene mutations coded for EGFR tyrosine kinase are responsible for Erlotinib's efficacy. Most of the EGFR beneficial mutations of NSCLC belong to two types: LREA deletion in exon 19 and L858R point mutation in exon 21 (Lynch et al. 2004, Paez et al. 2004, Pao et al. 2004). However, some patients who initially responded to Erlotinib showed acquired resistance to Erlotinib, which is associated with a secondary somatic mutation in T790M on exon 20 or by amplification of MET protein, another cell membrane receptor (Kobayashi et al. 2005, Pao et al. 2005). Further clinical data showed that about 50% of patients who developed Erlotinib resistance had T790M somatic mutation (Balak et al. 2006, Engelman et al. 2007, Kosaka et al. 2006). Additionally, MET amplification accounted for 20% of patients who developed Erlotinib resistance through ERBB3 (a membrane of the EGFR family)-dependent activation of PI3K pathway (Bean et al. 2008). It has been observed that almost all effective anticancer drugs have some side effects, which severely debilitate the patients, causing diarrhea, rash, and vomiting. Many groups are investigating solutions to this problem. In this respect, bioactive dietary agents such as δ-tocotrienol might have a significant impact in lung cancer prevention and/or therapy as a single agent or agent in combinatorial therapy.

11.2.1.2 Lung Cancer and Notch 1 Pathway

Notch proteins, the transmembrane receptors, are highly conserved in the development and the determination of cell fate (Artavanis-Tsakonas et al. 1999). As the ligand–receptor signaling pathway, notch signaling plays critical roles in mediating cell proliferation, survival, and apoptosis (Ohishi et al. 2003). Until now, four notch receptors have been found in mammals, namely, Notch1-4 (Mumm and Kopan 2000). Additionally, five notch ligands, including DLL-1, DLL-3, DLL-4, Jagged-1, and Jagged-2, have been identified (Bigas et al. 1998, Mumm and Kopan 2000). All the notch receptors and their lignads have been shown related to cancer (Miele et al. 2006). Once their ligands bind to the extracelluar domain, notch receptors undergo a series of proteolitic cleavages, releasing the intracellular notch, which then translocates into the nucleus (Oswald et al. 2001). There the active forms of notch in combination with other transcription factors that regulate the expression of target genes such as Hes-1, Bcl-X_L, and Survivin (Wang et al. 2006a,b) are involved in cell cycle growth and apoptosis. Since notch signaling regulates critical cell fate decisions, alterations in notch signaling are associated with tumorigenesis. It has been found that notch signaling is frequently dysregulated with increased expression in different types of cancers such as lung, colon, head and neck, and pancreatic (Buchler et al. 2005, Lin et al. 2010, Reedijk et al. 2008, Westhoff et al. 2009). Overexpression of Notch-1 has been shown to inhibit apoptosis in different types of cancers (Jundt et al. 2002, Miele and Osborne 1999), suggesting that notch could be considered as a therapeutic target. Clinical data have demonstrated that 30% of NSCLC patients have increased notch activity and another 10% have a gain-of-function mutation on the *Notch-1* gene (Westhoff et al. 2009). Recently, it has been reported that Notch-1 stimulates survival of NSCLC cells during hypoxia by activating the insulin-like growth factor pathway (Eliasz et al. 2010).

Data from our laboratory show that treatment of NSCLC cells (A549 and H1299) with δ-tocotrienol results in a dose- and time-dependent inhibition of cell growth, cell migration, tumor cell invasiveness, and induction of apoptosis (Ji et al. 2011). Real-time polymerase chain reaction(RT-PCR) and western blot analysis showed that antitumor activity by δ-tocotrienol was associated with a decrease in expression of Notch-1, Hes-1, Survivin, MMP-9, VEGF, and Bcl-XL. In addition, there was a decrease in NF-κB–DNA binding activity.

11.2.1.3   Lung Cancer and NF-κB

Nuclear factor-kappaB (NF-κB), another key apoptotic regulator, plays important roles in cancer cell transformation and development (Karin 2006). More and more data show that there is crosstalk between the Notch-1/Hes-1 pathways and the NF-κB pathway. Notch ligands have been shown to induce NF-κB activation in leukemia cells, with decreased Notch-1 expression accompanied with a decrease in NF-κB binding activity (Itoh et al. 2009). Moreover, Notch-1 has been found to induce sustained NF-κB activity by facilitating its nuclear retention (Shin et al. 2006). Specifically, NF-κB2 promoter activity is activated by Notch-1 pathway (Oswald et al. 1998). Recently, Notch-1/ Hes-1 pathways were found as the upstream mechanisms for maintainance of NF-κB activation in leukemia *in vivo* and *in vitro* (Espinosa et al. 2010). As Notch-1 downregulation showed antineoplastic effects *in vivo* and *in vitro* (Jundt et al. 2002, Miele and Osborne 1999, Nickoloff et al. 2003), the potential for treating certain cancers could be achieved by inhibiting notch signal transduction. The aforementioned literature reports in different cancer types corroborate our results in NSCLC cells in which we observed a concomitant decrease in NF-κB–DNA binding activity with decrease in Notch-1 expression upon treatment with δ-tocotrienol. Taken together, these results suggest that downregulation of Notch-1, via inhibition of NF-κB signaling pathways by δ-tocotrienol, could provide a potential novel approach for prevention of tumor progression and migration in NSCLC.

11.2.1.4   Lung Cancer and MicroRNA

To obtain a closer mechanistic insight into downregulation of Notch 1 by δ-tocotrienol, we turned our attention to the micro RNAs involved in this altered signaling. Micro RNAs (miRNA) are small noncoding RNAs that are involved in posttranscriptional gene regulation (Lee and Ambros 2001). These molecules silence their target genes' expression by directly interacting with the 3′-untranslated region (3′-UTR) of mRNA, promoting RNA degradation and thereby inhibiting transcription. Accumulating data demonstrate that miRNA play an important role in cancers by regulating the expression of various oncogenes and tumor suppressors genes (Caldas and Brenton 2005). For example, reduced expression of Let-7 microRNAs, the tumor suppressor gene, has been shown to be associated to with shortened postoperative survival in lung cancer patients (Takamizawa et al. 2004). Therefore, it is important to unravel the liaison, if any, between miRNA expression and Notch-1 signaling. It is also important to find novel agents that could regulate the specific miRNA expressions and Notch-1 pathway, which could then be potentially useful for the treatment of NSCLC patients in the future. More importantly, it has been suggested that dysregulation of specific miRNAs and their targets in various types of cancer is associated with the development and progression of cancers (Gironella et al. 2007, Volinia et al. 2006). Following up from our work on the effect of δ-tocotrienol on the Notch-1

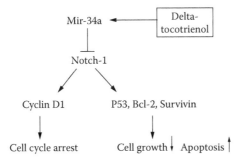

FIGURE 11.1   Molecular pathways induced by δ-tocotrienol via upregulation of a tumor suppressor gene, mir-34a, on NSCLC cells.

pathway in NSCLC cells, we hypothesized that tocotrienols, specifically δ-tocotrienol, will inhibit NSCLC cell growth and induce apoptosis by inhibition of Notch-1 signaling via alteration of specific miRNA expressions. Using microRNA microarray, we observed that downregulation of Notch-1 pathway by δ-tocotrienol correlated with upregulation of a tumor suppressor gene, mir-34a, in NSCLCs (Figure 11.1). Re-expression of mir-34a by transfection into A549 and H1650 cells resulted in a dose-dependent inhibition of cell growth, invasiveness, and induction of apoptosis in NSCLC cell lines. Cellular mechanism studies revealed that induction of mir-34a decreased the expression of Notch-1 and its downstream pathways including Hes-1, Cyclin D1, and Survivin. Our findings unveil δ-tocotrienol as an activator of a microRNA that can reduce the proliferation of NSCLC and offers a fresh starting point to design new and novel anticancer agents. Given the recently obtained generally recognized as safe (GRAS) status for tocotrienols, δ-tocotrienol may offer the coveted combination of effectiveness and nontoxicity as a potential agent against progression of NSCLC (Figure 11.1).

11.3   CONCLUSIONS AND PERSPECTIVES

In this chapter, we have attempted to summarize the role of tocotrienols in chronic diseases including cardiovascular, neurodegeneration, and aging in general, and their potential for prevention and/or treatment of lung cancer in particular.

Since cancer is a multifaceted disease, a number of drug targets from different signaling pathways have been identified in an effort to develop effective agents against its progression. As such, EGFR found to be overexpressed in many cancer types including lung, breast, ovarian, head, and neck cancers has been the focus of a number of pharmaceutical companies. In this regard, Erlotinib, a small molecule that inhibits EGFR tyrosine kinase activity, is currently the drug used as the first course of action against NSCLC. However, there is a great variability in interindividual response among patients or populations battling the disease, with certain subsets being either resistant or acquiring resistance to the drug. In addition, the problem of acute or sustained toxicity to normal tissues prevails, causing discomfort and secondary complications. Many research groups are investigating solutions to this problem. Recent data provide evidence in support of therapeutic benefits of nonnutritive dietary components. These have been attributable to their pleiotropic effects including downregulation of survival signaling and simultaneous activation of multiple death pathways in cancer cells. In addition, dietary agents have the added advantage of being relatively nontoxic at the levels consumed. Thus, diet appears to have a major influence in cancer prevention, and specific dietary components may potentially play a key role in cancer therapy as well.

Deregulation of notch proteins have been correlated with the development and progression of cancer and may be beneficial as biomarkers for diagnosis and prognosis, as well as targets for cancer therapy. More importantly, downregulation of Notch-1 pathway by natural dietary agents such as δ-tocotrienol could potentially be used for effective inhibition of the cell proliferation, induction of apoptosis, and reduction of invasion and migration in NSCLC.

It is our perspective that downregulation of the notch pathway by naturally occurring dietary agents including tocotrienols could be helpful for the potential prevention of tumor progression and/or treatment of human cancers. In view of the fact that natural agents are generally nontoxic, their use in the combat against cancer progression either as single agents or in synergism with current therapeutics would help alleviate at least some of the problems associated with toxic drug regimens.

REFERENCES

Adachi H, Ishii N 2000. Effects of tocotrienols on life span and protein carbonylation in *Caenorhabditis elegans. J Gerontol A Biol Sci Med Sci* 55: B280–B285.

Aggarwal BB, Shishodia S 2006. Molecular targets of dietary agents for prevention and therapy of cancer. *Biochem Pharmacol* 71: 1397–1321.

Argyriou AA, Chroni E, Koutras A, Iconomou G, Papapetropoulos S, Polychronopoulos P et al. 2006. A randomized controlled trial evaluating the efficacy and safety of vitamin E supplementation for protection against cisplatin-induced peripheral neuropathy: Final results. *Support Care Cancer* 14: 1134–1140.

Arita M, Sato Y, Miyata A, Tanabe T, Takahashi E, Kayden HJ et al. 1995. Human alpha-tocopherol transfer protein: cDNA cloning, expression and chromosomal localization. *Biochem J* 306: 437–443.

Artavanis-Tsakonas S, Rand MD, Lake RJ 1999. Notch signaling: Cell fate control and signal integration in development. *Science* 284: 770–776.

Azzi A, Boscoboinik D, Chatelain E, Ozer NK, Stauble B 1993. D-alpha-tocopherol control of cell proliferation. *Mol Aspects Med* 14: 265–271.

Balak MN, Gong Y, Riely GJ, Somwar R, Li AR, Zakowski MF et al. 2006. Novel D761Y and common secondary T790M mutations in epidermal growth factor receptor-mutant lung adenocarcinomas with acquired resistance to kinase inhibitors. *Clin Cancer Res* 12: 6494–6501.

Bean J, Riely GJ, Balak M, Marks JL, Ladanyi M, Miller VA et al. 2008. Acquired resistance to epidermal growth factor receptor kinase inhibitors associated with a novel T854A mutation in a patient with EGFR-mutant lung adenocarcinoma. *Clin Cancer Res* 14: 7519–7525.

Bidoli E, La Vecchia C, Talamini R, Negri E, Parpinel M, Conti E et al. 2001. Micronutrients and ovarian cancer: A case-control study in Italy. *Ann Oncol* 12: 1589–1593.

Bigas A, Martin DIK, Milner LA 1998. Notch1 and Notch2 inhibit myeloid differentiation in response to different cytokines. *Mol Cell Biol* 18: 2324–2333.

Bohlke K, Spiegelman D, Trichopoulou A, Katsouyanni K, Trichopoulos D 1999. Vitamins A, C and E and the risk of breast cancer: Results from a case-control study in Greece. *Br J Cancer* 79: 23–29.

Buchler P, Gazdhar A, Schubert M, Giese N, Reber HA, Hines OJ et al. 2005. The Notch signaling pathway is related to neurovascular progression of pancreatic cancer. *Ann Surg* 242: 791–800.

Caldas C, Brenton JD 2005. Sizing up miRNAs as cancer genes. *Nat Med* 11: 712–714.

Choi MA, Kim BS, Yu R 1999. Serum antioxidative vitamin levels and lipid peroxidation in gastric carcinoma patients. *Cancer Lett* 136: 89–93.

Chrysogelos SA, Dickson RB 1994. EGF receptor expression, regulation, and function in breast cancer. *Breast Cancer Res Treat* 29: 29–40.

Croce CM 2008. Oncogenes and cancer. *N Engl J Med* 358: 502–511.

Cross D, Burmester JK 2006. Gene therapy for cancer treatment: Past, present and future. *Clin Med Res* 4: 218–227.

Davidson JR 1934. An attempt to inhibit the development of tar-carcinoma in mice: Preliminary note. *Can Med Assoc J* 31: 486–487.

Trujillo E, Davis C, Milner J 2006. Nutrigenomics, proteomics, metabolomics, and the practice of dietetics. *J Am Diet Assoc* 106: 403–413.

Eliasz S, Liang S, Chen Y, De Marco MA, Machek O, Skucha S et al. 2010. Notch-1 stimulates survival of lung adenocarcinoma cells during hypoxia by activating the IGF-1R pathway. *Oncogene* 29: 2488–2498.

Elson CE 1992. Tropical oils: Nutritional and scientific issues. *Crit Rev Food Sci Nutr* 31: 79–102.

Engelman JA, Zejnullahu K, Mitsudomi T, Song Y, Hyland C, Park JO et al. 2007. MET amplification leads to gefitinib resistance in lung cancer by activating ERBB3 signaling. *Science* 316: 1039–1043.

Espinosa L, Cathelin S, D'Altri T, Trimarchi T, Statnikov A, Guiu J et al. 2010. The Notch/Hes1 pathway sustains NF-kappaB activation through CYLD repression in T cell leukemia. *Cancer Cell* 18: 268–281.

Factor VM, Laskowska D, Jensen MR, Woitach JT, Popescu NC, Thorgeirsson SS 2000. Vitamin E reduces chromosomal damage and inhibits hepatic tumor formation in a transgenic mouse model. *Proc Natl Acad Sci USA* 97: 2196–2201.

Fukuoka M, Yano S, Giaccone G, Tamura T, Nakagawa K, Douillard JY et al. 2003. Multi-institutional random-ized phase II trial of gefitinib for previously treated patients with advanced non-small-cell lung cancer (The IDEAL 1 Trial) [corrected]. *J Clin Oncol* 21: 2237–2246.

Gescher AJ, Sharma RA, Steward WP 2001. Cancer chemoprevention by dietary constituents: A tale of failure and promise. *Lancet Oncol* 2: 371–379.

Gironella M, Seux M, Xie MJ, Cano C, Tomasini R, Gommeaux J et al. 2007. Tumor protein 53-induced nuclear protein 1 expression is repressed by miR-155, and its restoration inhibits pancreatic tumor devel-opment. *Proc Natl Acad Sci USA* 104: 16170–16175.

Golden TR, Hinerfeld DA, Melov S 2002. Oxidative stress and aging: Beyond correlation. *Aging Cell* 1: 117–123.

Hall TJ, Schaeublin M, Jeker H, Fuller K, Chambers TJ 1995. The role of reactive oxygen intermediates in osteoclastic bone resorption. *Biochem Biophys Res Commun* 207: 280–287.

Hansson LE, Nyren O, Bergstrom R, Wolk A, Lindgren A, Baron J et al. 1994. Nutrients and gastric cancer risk. A population-based case-control study in Sweden. *Int J Cancer* 57: 638–644.

Hirsch FR, Varella-Garcia M, Cappuzzo F 2009. Predictive value of EGFR and HER2 overexpression in advanced non-small-cell lung cancer. *Oncogene* 28(Suppl 1): 32–37.

Hsieh TC, Elangovan S, Wu JM 2010. Differential suppression of proliferation in MCF-7 and MDA-MB-231 breast cancer cells exposed to alpha-, gamma- and delta-tocotrienols is accompanied by altered expres-sion of oxidative stress modulatory enzymes. *Anticancer Research* 30: 4169–4176.

Hu J, La Vecchia C, Negri E, Chatenoud L, Bosetti C, Jia X et al. 1999. Diet and brain cancer in adults: A case-control study in northeast China. *Int J Cancer* 81: 20–23.

Itoh M, Fu L, Tohda S 2009. NF-kappaB activation induced by Notch ligand stimulation in acute myeloid leukemia cells. *Oncol Rep* 22: 631–634.

Ji X, Wang Z, Geamanu A, Sarkar FH, Gupta SV 2011. Inhibition of cell growth and induction of apoptosis in non-small cell lung cancer cells by delta-tocotrienol is associated with Notch-1 down-regulation. *J Cell Biochem* 112: 2773–2783.

Jundt F, Anagnostopoulos I, Forster R, Mathas S, Stein H, Dorken B 2002. Activated Notch1 signaling pro-motes tumor cell proliferation and survival in Hodgkin and anaplastic large cell lymphoma. *Blood* 99: 3398–3403.

Kannappan R, Yadav VR, Aggarwal BB 2010. gamma-Tocotrienol but not gamma-tocopherol blocks STAT3 cell signaling pathway through induction of protein-tyrosine phosphatase SHP-1 and sensitizes tumor cells to chemotherapeutic agents. *J Biol Chem* 285: 33520–33228.

Karin M 2006. Nuclear factor-kappaB in cancer development and progression. *Nature* 441: 431–446.

Kobayashi S, Boggon TJ, Dayaram T, Janne PA, Kocher O, Meyerson M et al. 2005. EGFR mutation and resis-tance of non-small-cell lung cancer to gefitinib. *N Engl J Med* 352: 786–792.

Komiyama K, Iizuka K, Yamaoka M, Watanabe H, Tsuchiya N, Umezawa I 1989. Studies on the biological activity of tocotrienols. *Chem Pharm Bull (Tokyo)* 37: 1369–1371.

Kosaka T, Yatabe Y, Endoh H, Yoshida K, Hida T, Tsuboi M et al. 2006. Analysis of epidermal growth factor receptor gene mutation in patients with non-small cell lung cancer and acquired resistance to gefitinib. *Clin Cancer Res* 12: 5764–5769.

Krendel DA, Gilchrist JM, Johnson AO, Bossen EH 1987. Isolated deficiency of vitamin E with progressive neurologic deterioration. *Neurology* 37: 538–540.

Kris MG, Natale RB, Herbst RS, Lynch TJ, Jr., Prager D, Belani CP et al. 2003. Efficacy of gefitinib, an inhibi-tor of the epidermal growth factor receptor tyrosine kinase, in symptomatic patients with non-small cell lung cancer: A randomized trial. *JAMA* 290: 2149–2158.

Kumagai Y, Pi JB, Lee S, Sun GF, Yamanushi T, Sagai M et al. 1998. Serum antioxidant vitamins and risk of lung and stomach cancers in Shenyang, China. *Cancer Lett* 129: 145–149.

Kumar KS, Raghavan M, Hieber K, Ege C, Mog S, Parra N et al. 2006. Preferential radiation sensitization of prostate cancer in nude mice by nutraceutical antioxidant gamma-tocotrienol. *Life Sci* 78: 2099–2104.

Lam TK, Gallicchio L, Lindsley K, Shiels M, Hammond E, Tao XG et al. 2009. Cruciferous vegetable consumption and lung cancer risk: A systematic review. *Cancer Epidemiol Biomarkers Prev* 18: 184–195.

Lee RC, Ambros V 2001. An extensive class of small RNAs in *Caenorhabditis elegans*. *Science* 294: 862–864.

Lee IM, Cook NR, Gaziano JM, Gordon D, Ridker PM, Manson JE et al. 2005. Vitamin E in the primary pre-vention of cardiovascular disease and cancer: the Women's Health Study: A randomized controlled trial. *JAMA* 294: 56–65.

Lin JT, Chen MK, Yeh KT, Chang CS, Chang TH, Lin CY et al. 2010. Association of high levels of Jagged-1 and Notch-1 expression with poor prognosis in head and neck cancer. *Ann Surg Oncol* 17: 2976–2983.

Lynch TJ, Bell DW, Sordella R, Gurubhagavatula S, Okimoto RA, Brannigan BW et al. 2004. Activating mutations in the epidermal growth factor receptor underlying responsiveness of non-small-cell lung cancer to gefitinib. *N Engl J Med* 350: 2129–2139.

Maihle NJ, Baron AT, Barrette BA, Boardman CH, Christensen TA, Cora EM et al. 2002. EGF/ErbB receptor family in ovarian cancer. *Cancer Treat Res* 107: 247–258.

Malvy DJ, Arnaud J, Burtschy B, Sommelet D, Leverger G, Dostalova L et al. 1997. Assessment of serum antioxidant micronutrients and biochemical indicators of nutritional status in children with cancer in search of prognostic factors. *Int J Vitam Nutr Res* 67: 267–271.

McAnally JA, Jung M, Mo H 2003. Farnesyl-O-acetylhydroquinone and geranyl-O-acetylhydroquinone suppress the proliferation of murine B16 melanoma cells, human prostate and colon adenocarcinoma cells, human lung carcinoma cells, and human leukemia cells. *Cancer Lett* 202: 181–192.

Meydani SN, Meydani M, Blumberg JB, Leka LS, Siber G, Loszewski R et al. 1997. Vitamin E supplementation and in vivo immune response in healthy elderly subjects. A randomized controlled trial. *JAMA* 277: 1380–1386.

Miele L, Osborne B 1999. Arbiter of differentiation and death: Notch signaling meets apoptosis. *J Cell Physiol* 181: 393–409.

Miele L, Golde T, Osborne B 2006. Notch signaling in cancer. *Curr Mol Med* 6: 905–918.

Morley S, Thakur V, Danielpour D, Parker R, Arai H, Atkinson J et al. 2010. Tocopherol transfer protein sensitizes prostate cancer cells to vitamin E. *J Biol Chem* 285: 35578–35589.

Mumm JS, Kopan R 2000. Notch signaling: From the outside in. *Dev Biol* 228: 151–165.

Negri E, Franceschi S, Bosetti C, Levi F, Conti E, Parpinel M et al. 2000. Selected micronutrients and oral and pharyngeal cancer. *Int J Cancer* 86: 122–127.

Nickoloff BJ, Osborne BA, Miele L 2003. Notch signaling as a therapeutic target in cancer: A new approach to the development of cell fate modifying agents. *Oncogene* 22: 6598–6608.

Norman HA, Go VL, Butrum RR 2004. Review of the International Research Conference on Food, Nutrition, and Cancer, 2004. *J Nutr* 134: 3391S–3393S.

Ogilvie GK 1998. Interventional nutrition for the cancer patient. *Clin Tech Small Anim Pract* 13: 224–231.

Ohishi K, Katayama N, Shiku H, Varnum-Finney B, Bernstein ID 2003. Notch signalling in hematopoiesis. *Semin Cell Dev Biol* 14: 143–150.

Oswald F, Liptay S, Adler G, Schmid RM 1998. NF-kappaB2 is a putative target gene of activated Notch-1 via RBP-Jkappa. *Mol Cell Biol* 18: 2077–2088.

Oswald F, Tauber B, Dobner T, Bourteele S, Kostezka U, Adler G et al. 2001. p300 acts as a transcriptional coactivator for mammalian Notch-1. *Mol Cell Biol* 21: 7761–7774.

Paez JG, Janne PA, Lee JC, Tracy S, Greulich H, Gabriel S et al. 2004. EGFR mutations in lung cancer: Correlation with clinical response to gefitinib therapy. *Science* 304: 1497–1500.

Pao W, Miller VA, Politi KA, Riely GJ, Somwar R, Zakowski MF et al. 2005. Acquired resistance of lung adenocarcinomas to gefitinib or erlotinib is associated with a second mutation in the EGFR kinase domain. *PLoS Med* 2: 225–235.

Pao W, Miller V, Zakowski M, Doherty J, Politi K, Sarkaria I et al. 2004. EGF receptor gene mutations are common in lung cancers from "never smokers" and are associated with sensitivity of tumors to gefitinib and erlotinib. *Proc Natl Acad Sci USA* 101: 13306–13311.

Parker RA, Pearce BC, Clark RW, Gordon DA, Wright JJ 1993. Tocotrienols regulate cholesterol production in mammalian cells by post-transcriptional suppression of 3-hydroxy-3-methylglutaryl-coenzyme A reductase. *J Biol Chem* 268: 11230–11238.

Pratico D, Zhukareva V, Yao Y, Uryu K, Funk CD, Lawson JA et al. 2004. 12/15-lipoxygenase is increased in Alzheimer's disease: Possible involvement in brain oxidative stress. *Am J Pathol* 164: 1655–1662.

Qureshi AA, Burger WC, Peterson DM, Elson CE 1986. The structure of an inhibitor of cholesterol biosynthesis isolated from barley. *J Biol Chem* 261: 10544–10550.

Raederstorff D, Elste V, Aebischer C, Weber P 2002. Effect of either gamma-tocotrienol or a tocotrienol mixture on the plasma lipid profile in hamsters. *Ann Nutr Metab* 46: 17–23.

Reedijk M, Odorcic S, Zhang H, Chetty R, Tennert C, Dickson BC et al. 2008. Activation of Notch signaling in human colon adenocarcinoma. *Int J Oncol* 33: 1223–1229.

Ren Z, Pae M, Dao MC, Smith D, Meydani SN, Wu D 2010. Dietary supplementation with tocotrienols enhances immune function in C57BL/6 mice. *J Nutr* 140: 1335–1341.

Rink C, Christoforidis G, Khanna S, Peterson L, Patel Y, Abduljalil A et al. 2011. Tocotrienol vitamin E protects against preclinical canine ischemic stroke by inducing arteriogenesis. *J Cereb Blood Flow Metab* 31: 2218–2230.

Rogers SJ, Harrington KJ, Rhys-Evans P, O-Charoenrat P, Eccles SA 2005. Biological significance of c-erbB family oncogenes in head and neck cancer. *Cancer Metastasis Rev* 24: 47–69.

Schwartz J, Shklar G, Trickler D 1993. p53 in the anticancer mechanism of vitamin E. *Eur J Cancer B Oral Oncol* 29B: 313–318.

Sen CK, Khanna S, Roy S, Packer L 2000. Molecular basis of vitamin E action. Tocotrienol potently inhibits glutamate-induced pp60(c-Src) kinase activation and death of HT4 neuronal cells. *J Biol Chem* 275: 13049–13055.

Serbinova E, Kagan V, Han D, Packer L 1991. Free radical recycling and intramembrane mobility in the antioxidant properties of alpha-tocopherol and alpha-tocotrienol. *Free Radic Biol Med* 10: 263–275.

Serbinova EA, Packer L 1994. Antioxidant properties of alpha-tocopherol and alpha-tocotrienol. *Methods Enzymol* 234: 354–366.

Shin HM, Minter LM, Cho OH, Gottipati S, Fauq AH, Golde TE et al. 2006. Notch1 augments NF-kappaB activity by facilitating its nuclear retention. *EMBO J* 25: 129–138.

Shirode AB, Sylvester PW 2010. Synergistic anticancer effects of combined gamma-tocotrienol and celecoxib treatment are associated with suppression in Akt and NFkappaB signaling. *Biomed Pharmacother* 64: 327–332.

Siegel R, Ward E, Brawley O, Jemal A 2011. Cancer statistics, 2011: The impact of eliminating socioeconomic and racial disparities on premature cancer deaths. *CA Cancer J Clin* 61: 212–236.

Smyth CJ, Levey S 1948. Glutamic acid and its relationship to toxic symptoms following intravenous amino acid alimentation in men. *J Mich State Med Soc* 47: 530.

Song BL, DeBose-Boyd RA 2006. Insig-dependent ubiquitination and degradation of 3-hydroxy-3-methylglutaryl coenzyme a reductase stimulated by delta- and gamma-tocotrienols. *J Biol Chem* 281: 25054–25061.

Stryker WS, Stampfer MJ, Stein EA, Kaplan L, Louis TA, Sober A et al. 1990. Diet, plasma levels of beta-carotene and alpha-tocopherol, and risk of malignant melanoma. *Am J Epidemiol* 131: 597–511.

Sundram K, Sambanthamurthi R, Tan YA 2003. Palm fruit chemistry and nutrition. *Asia Pac J Clin Nutr* 12: 355–362.

Sylvester PW, Kaddoumi A, Nazzal S, El Sayed KA 2010. The value of tocotrienols in the prevention and treatment of cancer. *J Am Coll Nutr* 29: 324S–333S.

Sylvester PW, Shah S 2005. Intracellular mechanisms mediating tocotrienol-induced apoptosis in neoplastic mammary epithelial cells. *Asia Pac J Clin Nutr* 14: 366–373.

Takamizawa J, Konishi H, Yanagisawa K, Tomida S, Osada H, Endoh H et al. 2004. Reduced expression of the let-7 microRNAs in human lung cancers in association with shortened postoperative survival. *Cancer Res* 64: 3753–3756.

Tapsell LC, Hemphill I, Cobiac L, Patch CS, Sullivan DR, Fenech M et al. 2006. Health benefits of herbs and spices: The past, the present, the future. *Med J Aust* 185: S4–S24.

Thangapazham RL, Sharma A, Maheshwari RK 2006. Multiple molecular targets in cancer chemoprevention by curcumin. *AAPS J* 8: 443–449.

Torun M, Akgul S, Sargin H 1995. Serum vitamin E level in patients with breast cancer. *J Clin Pharm Ther* 20: 173–178.

Turley JM, Ruscetti FW, Kim SJ, Fu T, Gou FV, Birchenall-Roberts MC 1997. Vitamin E succinate inhibits proliferation of BT-20 human breast cancer cells: Increased binding of cyclin A negatively regulates E2F transactivation activity. *Cancer Res* 57: 2668–2675.

Volinia S, Calin GA, Liu CG, Ambs S, Cimmino A, Petrocca F et al. 2006. A microRNA expression signature of human solid tumors defines cancer gene targets. *Proc Natl Acad Sci USA* 103: 2257–2261.

Wang Z, Banerjee S, Li Y, Rahman KM, Zhang Y, Sarkar FH 2006a. Down-regulation of notch-1 inhibits invasion by inactivation of nuclear factor-kappaB, vascular endothelial growth factor, and matrix metalloproteinase-9 in pancreatic cancer cells. *Cancer Res* 66: 2778–2784.

Wang Z, Zhang Y, Li Y, Banerjee S, Liao J, Sarkar FH 2006b. Down-regulation of Notch-1 contributes to cell growth inhibition and apoptosis in pancreatic cancer cells. *Mol Cancer Ther* 5: 483–493.

Westhoff B, Colaluca IN, D'Ario G, Donzelli M, Tosoni D, Volorio S et al. 2009. Alterations of the Notch pathway in lung cancer. *Proc Natl Acad Sci USA* 106: 22293–22298.

Wistuba, II, Gazdar AF 2006. Lung cancer preneoplasia. *Annu Rev Pathol* 1: 331–348.

Yap WN, Chang PN, Han HY, Lee DT, Ling MT, Wong YC et al. 2008. Gamma-tocotrienol suppresses prostate cancer cell proliferation and invasion through multiple-signalling pathways. *Br J Cancer* 99: 1832–1841.

Yokota T, Wada Y, Furukawa T, Tsukagoshi H, Uchihara T, Watabiki S 1987. Adult-onset spinocerebellar syndrome with idiopathic vitamin E deficiency. *Ann Neurol* 22: 84–87.

Yu XM, Salter MW 1998. Gain control of NMDA-receptor currents by intracellular sodium. *Nature* 396: 469–474.

Zhang YH, Kramer TR, Taylor PR, Li JY, Blot WJ, Brown CC et al. 1995. Possible immunologic involvement of antioxidants in cancer prevention. *Am J Clin Nutr* 62: 1477S–1482S.

12 Tocotrienols and Atherosclerosis
Potential in Cardioprotection

Hapizah Mohd Nawawi

CONTENTS

12.1 INTRODUCTION

Atherosclerosis is defined as the presence of focal thickening (atheroma) of the tunica intima of large- and medium-sized elastic muscular arteries, leading to atherosclerosis-related clinical complications such as coronary artery disease (CAD), stroke, and peripheral vascular diseases. It is recognized as a chronic inflammatory disease in which an inflammatory response is the key event that leads to the formation of atheromatous plaques that develop in response to damage to the vessel wall, ultimately resulting in vascular occlusion (Ross 1999). It is associated with endothelial cell activation, oxidative stress, and accumulation of leucocytes in the walls of large arteries (Hansson et al. 1991). Atherogenesis can be influenced by multiple genetic and environmental factors that involve a complex interplay between blood components and the arterial wall. It is characterized by the infiltration of mononuclear blood cells into the intima, proliferation of vascular smooth muscle cells, and progressive deposition of extracellular matrix, which with time gives rise to characteristic fatty-fibrous lesions (Ross 1999).

The endothelium, which lines the inner surface of arteries, plays an important role in atherogenesis and is clearly related to cardiovascular diseases (CVD) (Ross 1993). Endothelial dysfunction (ED) occurs at the earliest stage of atherosclerosis. Dyslipidemia is one of the most important causes of ED, where oxidative stress promotes the formation of oxidized LDL (ox-LDL), a common initiating factor for clinical events (Nawawi 2003). ED is characterized by increased permeability of endothelial cells, procoagulant state, enhanced leucocyte adhesion due to increased endothelial expression of adhesion molecules such as intercellular adhesion molecule-1 (ICAM-1), and increased vascular tone due to reduction in nitric oxide (NO) production and proliferation of smooth muscle cells (Cines et al. 1998). ED is characterized by a shift in the actions of the endothelium toward reduced vasodilatation as well as proinflammatory and pro-thrombotic states (Harrison and Machin 1997). Once the endothelium has been injured, an immunologic cascade begins. Vascular injury induces upregulation of endothelial adhesion molecules such as soluble vascular cell adhesion molecule-1 (sVCAM-1), soluble intercellular cell adhesion molecule-1 (sICAM-1), selectins, and integrins (Cines et al. 1998). The continued inflammatory process enhances monocyte–endothelial cell adhesion, increases the number and emigration of monocytes from the blood into the tunica intima, and induces transformation into macrophages, which then engulf ox-LDL leading to foam cell formation, a key event in atherogenesis. The activation of these macrophages and lymphocytes leads to the release of hydrolytic enzymes, cytokines, chemokines, and growth factors. These will activate the classical and alternative complement pathways of the immune system, increase cell permeability and platelet activation, stimulate the proliferation and migration of smooth muscle cells, and promote fibrous tissue deposition into the vessel wall, leading to the formation and progression of fibrous plaque (Lusis and Aldons 2000). The lesions may evolve to contain large amounts of lipids, and if they become unstable or rupture, it may result in thrombotic occlusion of the overlying endothelium, leading to clinical events such as stroke and acute coronary syndrome. An unstable plaque that is prone to rupture and leads to clinical events has a greater lipid core and inflammation, but less amount of fibrous cap than a stable plaque (Koenig and Khuseyinova 2007).

CAD is the major cause of death in most developed and some developing countries (Srinath and Salim 1998). Although it predominates in affluent societies, high coronary risk profile has been identified even in the rural populations (Nawawi et al. 2002). A direct causative factor for the inflammatory response that induces ED has not been identified, but important contributions are suggested for ox-LDL-cholesterol, infectious agents, and hyperhomocysteinemia (Libby and Hansson 1991; Ross 1993). The major causal risk factors for atherosclerosis and CAD are cigarette smoking, hypertension, hypercholesterolemia, low serum levels of high density lipoprotein (HDL), and diabetes mellitus (Wilson et al. 1998). Other predisposing risk factors consist of obesity, insulin resistance, physical inactivity, family history of premature CAD, male gender, and possibly behavioral, socio-economic, and ethnic factors. Conditional risk factors associated with CAD include elevated serum levels of triglycerides, lipoprotein (a) [Lp(a)], small dense LDL particles, homocysteine, inflammatory status, and coagulant factors (e.g., fibrinogen and plasminogen activator inhibitor).

12.2 TOCOTRIENOLS

Vitamins are important among natural compounds and considered beneficial to human health. The vitamin E groups of compounds have been well recognized for their antioxidant and protective properties. Vitamin E comprises of tocopherols (T) and tocotrienols (T3), synthesized by plants and photosynthetic organisms. They are composed of a chromanol ring attached to an isoprenoid-derived hydrophobic tail (Theriault et al. 1999; Horvath et al. 2006). Structurally, these compounds are similar, except that tocotrienol has an unsaturated side chain with three trans double bonds at $3'$, $7'$, and $11'$ positions, whereas the T has a fully saturated aliphatic side chain (Kamal-Eldin and Appelqvist 1996). Both T and T3 have four different isomers (α, β, γ, and δ), which occur in nature. These isomers differ by the numbers and positions of methyl groups on the aromatic portion of the chromanol head group (Valentin and Qi 2005). The α-isomer contains three methyl groups, both β and γ have two, while the δ-isomer only has one methyl group on the aromatic ring. In the case of β- and γ-isomers, the methyl groups are at positions 5 and 8 or 7 and 8, respectively, of the chromanol head group. The α-, β-, γ-, and δ-isomers of the T and T3 are often referred to collectively as "tocochromanols" (Hunter and Cahoon 2007). The unsaturated side chain of tocotrienol allows for more efficient penetration into tissues that have saturated fatty layers such as the brain and liver, which leads to greater mobility and more uniform distribution in the membrane (Suzuki et al. 1993). T3 has other unique functional properties in contrast to T, including cholesterol-lowering properties and the potential to attenuate non-lipid-related risk factors for CVDs (Hood 1996).

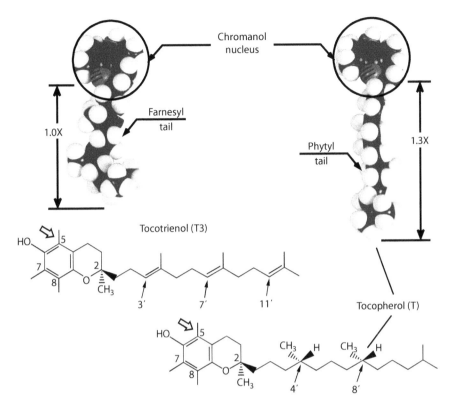

FIGURE 12.1 Structure of tocotrienols (T3) and tocopherols (T).

Out of the eight isomers, α-T is the main compound contained in most vitamin E supplements so far. It is commercially available in synthetic form, which does not come as a pure mixture (Setiadi et al. 2002). Figure 12.1 represents the chemical structures of tocopherols and tocotrienols.

12.2.1 Sources of Tocotrienols

Tocotrienol is the primary form of vitamin E found in the seed endosperm of most monocots, including agronomically important cereal grains such as wheat, rice, barley, and palm fruits (*Elensis guenensis*). These molecules are rarely found in vegetative tissues of plants. Humans and animals are unable to synthesize vitamin E, and therefore must obtain the isomers from plant sources (Mizushina et al. 2006). T is abundantly present in staple fruits such as peanut and walnut, and also in common vegetable oil such as sunflower and olive oils. On the other hand, T3 is only a minor constituent of plants and is found in high levels only in palm oil, cereal grains, and rice bran (Ong et al. 1993). Crude palm oil extracted from the fruits of *E. guenensis* contains a high amount of T3 (up to 800 mg/kg) mainly consisting of γ-T3 and α-T3 (Sen et al. 2007).

It is hypothesized that the biological activities of natural antioxidants and other phytochemicals in whole grains, in addition to digestion-resistant polysaccharides, contribute to risk reduction (Temple 2000). Primary sources of T include vegetable oils (olive, sunflower, and safflower oils), nuts, whole grains, and green leafy vegetables, while the primary source of T3 is in seed endosperms of most monocots, including cereal grains such as wheat, rice, and barley. Palm oil represents a major source of natural T3 (Patel et al. 2006; Sen et al. 2007). Subsequently, rice bran, palm, and annatto (90% delta and 10% gamma) oils were described as some of the richest sources of T3 by Tan and his coworkers. The T:T3 ratios in rice bran, palm, and annatto oils are 50:50, 25:75, and 0.1:99.9, respectively (Tan 2010).

12.2.2 Bioavailability of Tocotrienols

T3 have a variety of novel beneficial functions (Hood 1998; Theriault et al. 1999; Schaffer et al. 2005). Biological activities of tocols are generally believed to be due to their antioxidant action by inhibiting lipid peroxidation in biological membranes (Zieliński 2002). Most of the cardioprotective effects of T3 are mediated through their ability to inhibit a rate-limiting enzyme in cholesterol biosynthesis, as well as their antioxidant and anti-inflammatory activities (Aggarwal et al. 2010). Although T and T3 are structurally very similar and both are metabolized through similar mechanisms, T3 have been found to exhibit superior antioxidant activity (Serbinova et al. 1991; Pearce et al. 1994; Kamal-Eldin and Appelqvist 1996). Several mechanisms may account for the potency difference of T3 and T. First, because of structural differences, T3 may be more uniformly distributed in the lipid bilayer. Second, the chromanol ring of T3 may interact more efficiently with the lipid bilayer than that of T. Third, T3 may have a higher recycling efficiency (Serbinova and Packer 1994). Fourth, cellular uptake of T3 is 70 times higher than that of T (Saito et al. 2004). All of these factors may contribute to the greater efficacy of T3.

On the other hand, the bioavailability of orally taken T3 is lower than T (Sen et al. 2006). Hepatic α-T transfer protein (α-TTP), a critical regulator of vitamin E in mammals, selects T from tocochromanols in the liver. The presence of α-TTP that preferentially selects α-T explains why all other forms of vitamin E have lower biological activity compared to T. Even though T3 have potent free radical scavenging activities than T, they are less bioavailable after oral ingestion than T (Hosomi et al. 1997). It is suggested that with similar tissue levels, T3 would be a more effective antioxidant than T. It is important to note that T3 compared to T have a brief and transient metabolism and are inferior with regard to tissue retention and half-life. However, following oral ingestion, plasma T3 levels reach about 1 μM (Fairus et al. 2006), which is about a magnitude higher than that required to protect neurons with neurotoxic insults in cell culture studies (Khanna et al. 2003). Rats fed with α-T3 alone had higher bioavailability in some tissues (epididymal fat, perirenal adipose tissue, and skin) when compared to those fed equal amounts of α-T (Ikeda et al. 2003; Khanna et al. 2005). The binding affinity of α-TTP to natural α-T3 was reported to have 12.4% that of natural α-T (Hosomi et al. 1997). The bioavailability of α-T3 was significantly suppressed and always lower than α-T when rats were cosupplemented with equal amounts of α-T and α-T3 (Ikeda et al. 2003, 2005). There is direct evidence that α-T3 can be absorbed via an α-TTP independent pathway, such as by secretion into the small HDLs. Although α-T3 levels in the blood and liver are lower than those of α-T, higher levels of α-T3 than α-T were observed in adipose tissue, skin, vastus lateralis, heart, and spinal cord in mice.

12.2.3 Lipid-Lowering Effects of Tocotrienols

Hypercholesterolemia is often associated with increased oxidative stress and inflammation. Oxidative stress plays a major role in the pathogenesis of atherosclerosis and thus CAD (Naurooz-Zadeh et al. 2001). Endothelial cells, vascular smooth muscle cells, neutrophils, and monocytes can generate free radicals, leading to formation of ox-LDL, a highly atherogenic lipoprotein (Ridker 2003). Endothelium exposed to ox-LDL develops early signs of injury such as apoptosis and decreased endothelial cell nitric oxide synthase (eNOS) gene expression, leading to ED (Ridker et al. 2004). Ox-LDL induces the expression of adhesion molecules and attachment of monocytes and T-lymphocytes to the endothelial cells. Monocytes transmigrate into the tunica intima, transform into macrophages that generate reactive oxygen species (ROS), which convert ox-LDL to highly ox-LDL, and engulf ox-LDL via the scavenger receptors to form cells, a key event in atherogenesis (Mehta et al. 2001).

Elevated apolipoprotein B serum level is an independent risk factor for CAD (Albers et al. 1989). Clinical evidence has suggested that apoB is a better predictor of coronary risk than total or LDL-cholesterol (Sniderman et al. 1980). Lipoprotein (a) is a plasma lipoprotein with structural similarity to LDL, in which apoB is attached to apo(a) by a disulphide linkage and its elevated level is considered to be atherogenic (Scanu and Fless 1990). In isolated human liver cells, T3 (10 mM for 4 h) inhibited cholesterol synthesis by 32%. In addition, it is postulated that the three double bonds at the isoprenoid chain are essential for the inhibition of cholesterol synthesis (Qureshi et al. 1986, 1991a). Studies on the effects of γ-tocotrienol on apoB synthesis, degradation, and secretion in a human hepatocellular carcinoma cell line (HepG2) showed that the presence of γ-tocotrienol in the cells stimulated apoB degradation. It is postulated that the lack of cholesterol availability reduces the number of secreted apoB-containing lipoprotein by limiting apoB translocation into the endoplasmic reticulum lumen (Theriault et al. 1999). Several workers have also reported in epidemiological studies that T3 reduce the atherogenic apoB by 10%–15% (Qureshi et al. 1991a, 1995). A case-control study has reported that a rice-bran-derived TRF enriched with didesmethyl-tocotrienol, an isoform of tocotrienol with no methyl groups on the chromanol ring, decreased Lp(a) levels by 17% (Qureshi et al. 1995).

T3 affect the mevalonate pathway in mammalian cells by post-transcriptional suppression of HMG-CoA reductase, a rate-limiting enzyme involved in cholesterol synthesis. It was speculated that this effect is associated with the unique ability of the side chain to increase cellular farnesol, a mevalonate-derived product that signals proteolytic degradation of HMG-CoA reductase (Goldstein and Brown 1990; Rifkind 1998). *In vitro* cell culture experiments have elucidated the differential pharmacological effects between tocotrienol isomers, where γ- and δ-T3 that lack 5-methyl substitution are significantly more potent than α-tocotrienol in suppressing HMG-CoA reductase (Correll et al. 1994). It is also suggested that the farnesyl side chain and the methyl/hydroxy substitution pattern of γ-T3 execute a high level of HMG-CoA reductase suppression (Pearce et al. 1994). T3 cause post-transcriptional suppression of HMG-CoA reductase by a different pathway from the other inhibitors of cholesterol biosynthesis (Parker et al. 1993). *In vitro* studies have shown that γ-T3 exhibits a 30-fold greater cholesterol biosynthesis inhibition than α-T3. In addition, both the natural and synthetic T3 exhibit almost similar HMG-Co reductase suppression and cholesterol biosynthesis inhibition. Cell culture experiments showed that T3 inhibit the rate of acetate but not mevalonate incorporation into cholesterol in a dose- and time-dependent manner, with 50% inhibition at ~2 mM, maximal inhibition of ~80% within 6 h in HepG2 cells (Birringer 2002).

A key mechanism to suppress HMG-CoA reductase is via ubiquitination followed by rapid degradation by 26S proteosomes, a pathway that is activated with intracellular accumulation of sterols and nonsterol end products of the mevalonate metabolism. Sever (Sever et al. 2003) has demonstrated that Insig-1 and Insig-2, membrane-bound proteins of the ER, are required for sterol-accelerated ubiquitination of HMG-CoA reductase. More recently, it has been demonstrated that T3 stimulate ubiquitination and degradation of HMG-CoA reductase and block Sterol Regulatory Element Binding Protein (SREBP) processing, another sterol-mediated action of Insigs. It was also observed that γ-T3 is more selective in ubiquitination and degradation of HMG-CoA reductase rather than blocking SREBP processing. Both γ- and δ-T3 directly trigger ubiquitination without requiring further metabolism for their activity. More importantly, it was clearly shown that other forms of vitamin E neither enhance HMG-CoA reductase degradation nor block SREBP processing (Song and Debose-Boyd 2006).

In vivo research interest has been focused on T3 for their hypocholesterolemic action by inhibiting cholesterol biosynthesis (Qureshi et al. 1997; Hood 1998; Theriault et al. 1999). This action was reported in mice, chickens, and swine (Qureshi et al. 1991a,b; Qureshi and Peterson 2001). Hypercholesterolemic pigs fed on tocotrienol-rich fraction (TRF) supplement showed reduction in total serum cholesterol (44%), LDL-cholesterol (60%), apolipoprotein B (26%), thromboxane B2 (41%), and platelet factor 4 (PF4; 29%) (Qureshi et al. 1991a). T3 from both palm oil and rice bran origin have shown cholesterol-lowering properties (Pearce et al. 1992; Chen and Cheng 2006). Iqbal et al. (2003) showed that rice-bran-derived TRF reduced total cholesterol and LDL-cholesterol levels in rats through downmodulation of hepatic HMG-CoA reductase activity. In animal model experiments using rats, it was shown that rice bran oil (RBO) diet lowered plasma triglyceride, LDL-cholesterol, and hepatic triglyceride concentrations, but increased hepatic cholesterol 7-alpha-hydroxylase, hepatic LDL receptor, and HMG-CoA reductase mRNA. It was postulated that γ-T3 in RBO can lead to increased neutral sterol and bile acid excretion in feces via upregulation of cholesterol synthesis and catabolism (Chen et al. 2006).

Treatment with statins, inhibitors of-3-hydroxyl-3-methylglutaryl coenzyme (HMG-CoA) reductase, reduces serum cholesterol levels and ED, in addition to the incidence of cardiovascular events in patients with hypercholesterolemia (Nawawi et al. 2003a; Gresser and Gathof 2004). Furthermore, statins also have beyond lipid-lowering benefits including their effects on oxidative stress, inflammation, and endothelial activation (Nawawi et al. 2003b; Madamanchi et al. 2005). Both statins and T3 were demonstrated to have cholesterol-lowering properties in animals and humans, but with different mechanisms. A double-blind, placebo-controlled, cross-over clinical trial was performed in hypercholesterolemic subjects (serum TC > 5.7 mmol/L) to compare the efficacy between lovastatin alone (10 mg/day) versus lovastatin plus tocotrienol mixture (50 mg/day). It was shown that low dose tocotrienol mixture in combination with lovastatin was effective in lowering cholesterol levels, at the same time avoiding some adverse effects of statins (Qureshi 2001). Another double-blind cross-over study was conducted in hypercholesterolemic subjects (serum total cholesterol 6.2–8.0 mmol/L) to compare the cholesterol-lowering effects of palm oil TRF (200 mg palmvitee or 200 mg gamma-T3 capsules/day) and corn oil (300 mg/day). There was a 31% reduction in serum total cholesterol levels in seven of the hypercholesterolemic subjects after 4 weeks of 200 mg/day gamma-T3, suggesting the potent cholesterol inhibition of this T3 isomer (Qureshi et al. 1991b). However, α-T compromises the cholesterol reduction effect of T3 (Qureshi et al., 1996; Khor & Chieng 1996).

12.2.4 ANTIOXIDATIVE EFFECTS OF TOCOTRIENOLS

Lipid peroxidation plays an important role in atherogenesis. LDL oxidative modification leads to the formation of ox-LDL, which is preferentially taken up by macrophages via the scavenger receptors through an LDL receptor independent pathway. This pathway is unregulated and unsaturable, hence leading to enhanced foam cell formation, a key event in the pathogenesis of atherosclerosis (Steinberg et al. 1989). Peroxidation of membrane lipids modifies and inactivates cellular components leading to diseases. Antioxidants protect key cell components by scavenging free radicals before they cause lipid oxidation or DNA damage. The antioxidant activities of T3 depend primarily on the phenolic group in the chromanol ring, rather than the side chain. Several mechanisms were shown to contribute to the greater antioxidant activity of α-T3 than T: (a) a more uniform distribution of α-T3 within the membrane lipid bilayer, which enhances the interaction of chromanols with lipid radicals and (b) location of α-T3 nearer to the membrane surface, which facilitates recycling (Serbinova et al. 1991; Suzuki et al. 1993).

T3 have greater antioxidant activity than T in both *in vitro* and *in vivo* models (Nesaretnam et al. 1993). Kamal and Devasagayam (1995) reported that, α-T3 is 40-fold more effective than T in protecting rat liver microsomal membranes against lipid peroxidation, and also more potent in protecting cytochrome p450 and rat brain mitochondria from oxidative damage. The same study also reported that among the four isomers of T3, γ-T3 was the most effective followed by α and δ isomers. α-T3 was also found to exhibit greater peroxyl radical scavenging potency than α-T in liposomal membranes (Suzuki et al. 1993). Another *in vitro* study reported that palm-oil-derived TRF at concentrations in the range of 10–100 µg/mL (15–147 µM) consistently exhibits potent antioxidant activity in all three different *in vitro* assays, with the highest percent inhibition 96% at tocotrienol concentration of 10 µg/mL, using the ferric thiocyanate assay (Nawawi et al. 2005b). Recently, δ-T3 has been suggested as the best tocotrienol isomer in terms of lipid peroxidation inhibition compared to the other isomers (Palozza et al. 2006). δ-T3 is also the best isomer that reduces hydroperoxide-induced ROS formation in cultured fibroblast (Palozza et al. 2006). In that study, it has been suggested that the potent antioxidant activity is due to the methylation of the δ-T3 chromanol ring, which allows greater uptake by the cell membranes.

Suarna (Suarna et al.1993) reported that the oxidative protection to plasma in rats following supplementation with a T3/T mixture was comparable to that of the T preparation. Nafeeza et al. (2001) investigated the effect of TRF on the microscopic development of atherosclerosis and lipid peroxidation in the aortas of rabbits. After 10 weeks of treatment with TRF, cholesterol-fed rabbits had lower aortic contents of malondialdehyde, less intimal thickening, and greater preservation of the internal elastic lamina than untreated rabbits, suggesting that antioxidant activities of TRF could reduce experimental atherosclerosis. The supplementation of hyperlipidemic rats with TRF, in addition to lowering cholesterol, inhibited diene conjugated formation in LDL and TBARS production in liver microsomal membranes (Iqbal et al. 2004). Comparison among potent antioxidants on anti-atherosclerotic effect suggests that atheroprotective properties of T3 against hypercholesterolemia-induced atherosclerosis may not be solely linked to their antioxidant effect (Ozer and Azzi 2000). For example, one of the probucol analogues, bis (3,5-di-tert-butyl-4-hydroxyphenylether)propane, has failed to prevent atherosclerosis in rabbits despite its strong inhibition on LDL oxidation *in vitro* (Fruebis 1994). Minhajuddin (Minhajuddin et al. 2005) conducted a study to determine a minimum dose of TRF isolated from RBO, which leads to maximum reduction of malondialdehyde (MDA) levels in hypercholesterolemia-induced rats. In that study, it has been shown that different concentrations of TRF (4, 8, 12, 25, or 50 mg TRF/kg body wt/day in the hypercholesterolemia-induced rats reduced the MDA level after 1 week post-treatment. Interestingly, the optimal effect toward inhibition of TBARS production in hyperlipidemic rats was suggested at moderate TRF concentrations (8 mg TRF/kg body wt/day). Recently, Kawakami et al. (2007) reported that in rats given 0.8 mg/day, or equivalent to 48 mg/day of TRF if converted according to body weight of 60 kg in human, TRF had no effect on MDA level after 3 weeks post-treatment. This result is contradictory to results obtained from another study, where 40 mg/day of TRF was sufficient to significantly reduce the MDA level by 2 weeks post-treatment (Nawawi et al. 2005a). The difference of the result can be explained by the different composition of isomer contained in TRF in these two studies. Kawakami et al. (2007) has used TRF containing only gamma isomers, whereas palmvitee contains a mixture of α, β, γ, and δ isomers. The composition of the tocotrienol isomers in each palmvitee capsule are in the order of $\alpha > \gamma > \delta > \beta$ (42.3% > 34.6% > 20.2% > 2.9%). This suggests that TRF mixture may have stronger and more potent effect in reducing lipid peroxidation compared to TRF containing γ-T3 alone.

The presence of vitamin E in lipoproteins provides protection against free radical peroxidation. In humans, HDL and LDL are the major carriers of T. A randomized, double-blind, placebo-controlled clinical trial examined the effects of palm-oil TRF (300 mg palmvitee capsules/day), atorvastatin (10 mg/day), or palmvitee–atorvastatin combined therapy in subjects with non-familial hypercholesterolemia (NFH; serum total cholesterol > 6.5 mmol/L). The hypercholesterolemic subjects given palmvitee alone after 3 months had significant reduction in biomarkers of oxidative stress (serum MDA, ox-LDL, and isoprostane), inflammation (serum IL-6) and endothelial activation (serum ICAM-1), indicating beyond lipid-lowering properties of T3 and suggesting their great potential benefit in the prevention and treatment of atherosclerosis and CAD (Muid et al. 2007; Nawawi et al. 2007). Tomeo et al. (1995) has reported the significant decrease of TBARS after 12 months supplementation with palmvitee in patients with NFH compared to NC. In the same study, improvement of the blood flow in the carotid arteries was observed in 24% of study subjects. It was suggested that generation of MDA data might provide a clue about the mode of action of tocotrienol. Many studies supported the theory that antioxidants restrained the levels of blood lipid peroxides and blunt the formation of atherosclerotic lesions. Furthermore, Esterbauer (Esterbauer et al. 1991) has demonstrated that vitamin E was very effective in preventing *in vitro* oxidation of LDL. In addition, the need to investigate further roles of antioxidants such as tocotrienol in preventing and possibly reversing the natural course of carotid atherosclerosis has been highlighted (Tomeo et al. 1995).

Although α-T has been suggested to reduce the F_2-isoprostanes formation in hypercholesterolemia, reports on the effects of TRF on plasma F_2-isoprostane levels are scarce (Davi et al. 1997). Mustad (Mustad et al. 2002) have reported the nonbeneficial effects of tocotrienol (200 mg/day) toward reduction of F_2-isoprostanes among HC patients at 28 days posttreatment. However, these results are in disagreement with the finding from another study, where 12 weeks supplementation of 40 mg/day tocotrienol among NFH patients is found to sufficiently reduce the plasma F_2-isoprostanes levels (Nawawi et al. 2007). So far, clinical trials investigating the effect of TRF on isoprostanes levels among HC patients are lacking. However, beneficial effects of TRF in the reduction of isoprostane levels in animal studies with other CAD risks (hypertension and diabetes) were positive and promising. For example, Yoshida et al. (2007) has reported decreased levels of F_2-isoprostanes in a group of rats supplemented with α-tocotrienol for 1 month compared to control mice, which were given tocotrienol-free diet. Bayorh et al. (2005) have studied the effect of crude palm oil on F_2-isoprostane levels in hypertensive rats and found that crude palm oil potentially suppressed the F_2-isoprostane elevation in hypertensive salt-induced rats. In that study, it was suggested that the protective effect of palm oil might be related to the decrease in oxidative stress and preservation of endothelial function. However, in the same study it has been shown that the degree of oxidative stress in induced hypertensive rats was not completely reversed by palm oil. Another study reported the capacity of crude rice bran extract in lowering urinary F_2-isoprostanes and 8-OHdG levels compared to placebo on diabetic-induced rats. In that study, it was suggested that TRF contained in RBO may be more beneficial for human health than α-T alone (Kanaya et al. 2004).

12.2.5　Anti-Inflammatory and Anti-Endothelial Activation Properties of Tocotrienols

Atherosclerosis is recognized as a chronic inflammatory disease (Ross 1999). Pretreatment with T3 has been reported to reduce the induction of tumor necrosis factor (TNF) in mice, suggesting their potentially beneficial anti-inflammatory effects in atherosclerosis (Qureshi et al. 1993). Napolitano et al. (2007) evaluated the effects of T3 with a new compound FeAOX-6 on macrophage atherogenesis and its related functions, and reported that the combination resulted in dose-dependent reduction of cholesterol and cholesterol accumulation in human macrophages. The extent of reduction with α-T3 was greater than that induced by FeAOX-6.

The anti-inflammatory effects and mechanisms of action of palm-oil-derived TRF were investigated on lipopolysaccharide (LPS)-induced inflammatory response in human monocytic cells (Wu et al. 2008). It that study, it has been reported that TRF decreased the expression of proinflammatory cytokines and blocked the induction of iNOS and COX-2 expression mediated through nuclear factor kappa β (NFκB) deactivation. TRF at 1 µg/mL has significantly inhibited the production of IL-6 and nitric oxide, and only α-T3 reduced the TNF-α production. TRF and all isomers except for α-T downregulate the cyclooxygenase-2 gene expression.

T3 have been shown to reduce the stimulated endothelial cell expression of adhesion molecules (sVCAM-1, sICAM-1, and e-selectin) by blocking activation of NFκB. In addition, they also decrease monocyte–endothelial cell adhesion, which correlates with reduction in soluble adhesion molecule production in a dose-dependent manner (Theriault et al. 2002). Similar results have been reported by a group of investigators recently (Naito et al. 2005). However, the study was focused on the inhibitory effects of T3 on sVCAM-1 expression at both protein and mRNA levels in 25-hydroxy-cholesterol stimulated endothelial cells. Furthermore, in that study, the strongest inhibitory effect was shown by δ-T3 compared to α-T and α-, β-, and γ-T3 isomers. Cell culture experiments using endothelial cells showed that low to moderate concentration (0.3–5.0 mM) of palm TRF (tocotrienol enriched mixed fraction; T3:T ratio = 80:20%) led to reduction in gene and protein expression of sICAM-1, sVCAM-1, e-selectin, and IL6 production by stimulated endothelial cells, mediated via downregulation of NFκB and upregulation of eNOS (Nawawi et al. 2006a; Muid et al. 2009; see Figures 12.2 through 12.10). In addition, compared to palm TRF, pure T3 isomers have greater inhibition on inflammation, endothelial activation and NFκB, but elevate eNOS expression (Muid et al., 2012). Using an integrated AUC (area under the curve) of the concentration-response graph, among the pure TCT isomers, δ-T3 > α-T3 > γ-T3 >>> α-T in inhibition of NFκB gene expression, across a concentration range of 0.2–6.8 ug/ml (0.3–10.0 uM). It is interesting to note that γ-T3 isomer has potent inhibitory effect in NFκB gene expression at low (0.2–1.3 ug/ml), but not at high concentrations (1.7–6.8 ug/ml), while α-T is pro-inflammatory across all concentrations (Figure 12.13). Theriault et al. (2002) showed that palm-oil-derived α-T3 is a more potent and effective agent than α-T in inhibiting production of adhesion molecules (ICAM-1 and e-selectin). This may be due to the presence of the isoprenoid side chain in tocotrienol, which accounts for the superior activity of α-T3 over α-T. Furthermore, in cell culture and *in vitro* studies, it was observed that the optimal tocotrienol concentration as an antioxidant is much higher (about 100-fold) than that as an anti-inflammatory agent (Nawawi et al. 2006b).

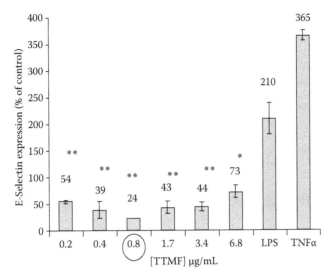

FIGURE 12.2 Effects of TTMF on e-selectin expression in LPS-stimulated cultured HUVECs. Incubation of HUVECs with TNF-α (10 ng/mL) was performed as positive control, incubation with LPS (1 μg/mL) alone was performed as negative control. Data are presented as changes of e-selectin expressed as a percentage of unstimulated HUVECs. Data are expressed as mean + SD. $*p < 0.05$, $**p < 0.01$ compared to LPS. TTMF: tocotrienol-tocopherol mixed fraction (tocotrienol:tocopherol ratio = 80:20%, tocotrienol concentration range: 0.2–6.8 μg/mL); LPS, lipopolysaccharide; HUVECs, human umbilical vein endothelial cells.

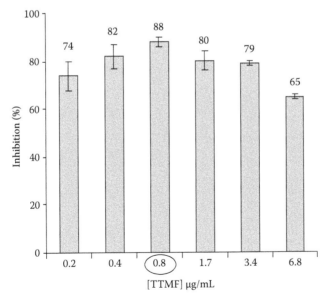

FIGURE 12.3 Bar graph shows inhibition of e-selectin expression by various concentrations of TTMF. Varying concentrations of tocotrienol were added to the HUVECs together with LPS (1 μg/mL) and incubated in a humidified incubator set at 37°C and 5% CO_2 for 16 h. Data are expressed as mean + SD. ANOVA $p < 0.0001$. TTMF: tocotrienol-tocopherol mixed fraction (tocotrienol:tocopherol ratio = 80:20%, tocotrienol concentration range: 0.2–6.8 μg/mL); LPS, lipopolysaccharide; HUVECs, human umbilical vein endothelial cells.

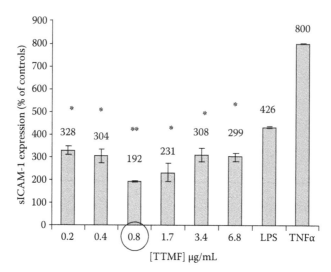

FIGURE 12.4 Effects of TTMF on s-ICAM expression in LPS stimulated cultured HUVECs. Incubation of HUVECs with TNF-α (10 ng/mL) was performed as positive control, incubation with LPS (1 μg/mL) alone was performed as negative control. Data are presented as changes of sICAM-1 expressed as a percentage of unstimulated HUVEC control. Data are expressed as mean + SD. *$p < 0.05$, **$p < 0.001$ compared to LPS. TTMF: tocotrienol-tocopherol mixed fraction (tocotrienol:tocopherol ratio = 80:20%, tocotrienol concentration range: 0.2–6.8 μg/mL); LPS, lipopolysaccharide; HUVECs, human umbilical vein endothelial cells; sICAM-1, soluble intercellular adhesion molecule.

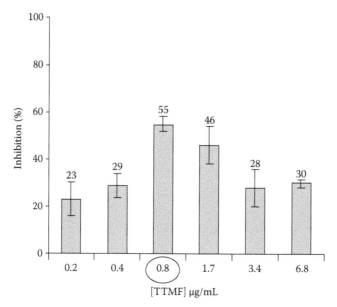

FIGURE 12.5 Inhibition of sICAM-1 expression by various concentrations of TTMF. Varying concentrations of tocotrienols were added to the HUVECs together with LPS (1 μg/mL) and incubated in a humidified incubator set at 37°C and 5% CO_2 for 16 h. Data are expressed as mean + SD. ANOVA $p < 0.05$. TTMF: tocotrienol-tocopherol mixed fraction (tocotrienol:tocopherol ratio = 80:20%, tocotrienol concentration range: 0.2–6.8 μg/mL); LPS, lipopolysaccharide; HUVECs, human umbilical vein endothelial cells; sICAM-1, soluble intercellular adhesion molecule.

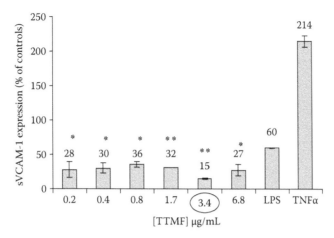

FIGURE 12.6 Effects of TTMF on s-VCAM expression in LPS stimulated cultured HUVECs. Incubation of HUVECs with TNF-α (10 ng/mL) was performed as positive control, incubation with LPS (1 μg/mL) alone was performed as negative control. Data are presented as changes of sVCAM-1 expressed as a percentage of unstimulated HUVECs. Data are expressed as mean + SD. $*p < 0.05$, $**p < 0.01$ compared to LPS. TTMF: tocotrienol-tocopherol mixed fraction (tocotrienol:tocopherol ratio = 80:20%, tocotrienol concentration range: 0.2–6.8 μg/mL); LPS, lipopolysaccharide; HUVECs, human umbilical vein endothelial cells.

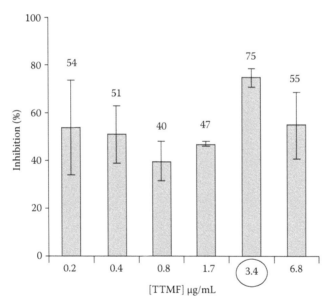

FIGURE 12.7 Inhibition of sVCAM-1 expression by various concentrations of TTMF. Varying concentrations of tocotrienols were added to the HUVECs together with LPS (1 μg/mL) and incubated in a humidified incubator set at 37OC and 5% CO_2 for 16 h. Data are expressed as mean + SD. ANOVA not significant. TTMF: tocotrienol-tocopherol mixed fraction (tocotrienol:tocopherol ratio = 80:20%, tocotrienol concentration range: 0.2–6.8 μg/mL); LPS, lipopolysaccharide; HUVECs, human umbilical vein endothelial cells; sVCAM-1, soluble vascular adhesion molecule.

12.2.6 ANTI-ATHEROSCLEROTIC EFFECTS OF TOCOTRIENOLS

Endothelial injury and dysfunction are fundamental stimuli responsible for the formation of atherosclerotic plaque, and vascular wall inflammation is pivotal in the etiology of atherosclerosis (Altman 2004). Dietary tocotrienol supplements have been shown to prevent atherosclerosis development in patients and animal models, including via their ability to reverse an arterial blockage.

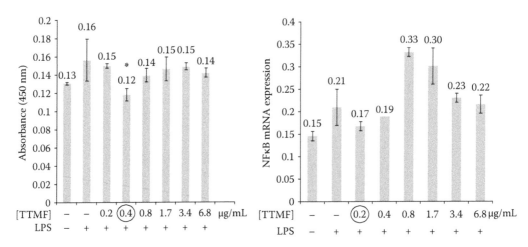

FIGURE 12.8 Effects of palm TTMF on NFκB p50 transcription factor in LPS stimulated cultured HUVECs. Varying concentrations of TTMF were added to the HUVECs together with LPS (1 μg/mL). Data are expressed as mean + SD. *$p < 0.05$ compared to LPS control. TTMF: tocotrienol-tocopherol mixed fraction (tocotrienol:tocopherol ratio = 80:20%, tocotrienol concentration range: 0.2–6.8 μg/mL); LPS, lipopolysaccharide; HUVECs, human umbilical vein endothelial cells.

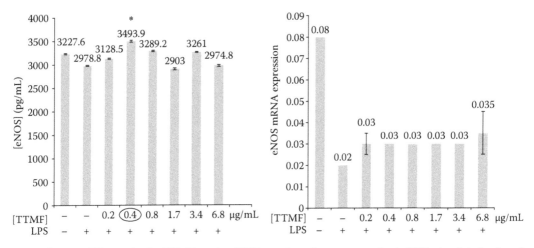

FIGURE 12.9 Effects of palm TTMF on the eNOS protein and gene expression in LPS stimulated cultured HUVECs. Varying concentrations of TTMF were added to the HUVECs together with LPS (1 μg/mL). Data are expressed as mean + SD. TTMF: tocotrienol-tocopherol mixed fraction (tocotrienol:tocopherol ratio = 80:20%, tocotrienol concentration range: 0.2–6.8 μg/mL); LPS, lipopolysaccharide; HUVECs, human umbilical vein endothelial cells; eNOS, endothelial nitric oxide synthase.

More recently, it has been elegantly demonstrated that palm TRF activate Peroxisome Proliferator-Activated Receptor-α (PPAR-α), PPAR-γ, and PPAR-δ. It is important to note that a TRF-rich diet reduced atherosclerosis development in ApoE-/- mice through PPAR target gene liver X receptor alpha (LXR alpha) and its downstream target genes apolipoproteins and cholesterol transporters, suggesting PPAR modulating activity as the most important aspect of *in vivo* action of T3 (Li et al. 2010). Black et al. (2000) suggested at least two mechanisms as to how palm T3 reduce lesions in atherosclerosis-prone apo E +/− mice: (1) antioxidant effect with no alterations in hepatic or serum cholesterol or lipoproteins and (2) effect independent of antioxidant action that may reflect the effects of T3 on foam cell formation, hepatic cholesterol secretion, and intestinal absorption. Most animal studies show significant anti-atherosclerotic effects with vitamin E, and the positive findings

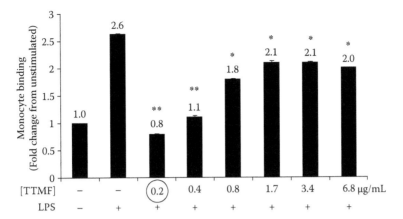

FIGURE 12.10 Effects of palm TTMF on the monocyte–endothelial cell binding in LPS stimulated cultured HUVECs. Varying concentrations of TTMF were added to the HUVECs together with LPS (1 μg/mL). Data are expressed as mean + SD. *$p < 0.05$, **$p < 0.01$ compared to LPS control. TTMF: tocotrienol-tocopherol mixed fraction (tocotrienol:tocopherol ratio = 80:20%, tocotrienol concentration range: 0.2–6.8 μg/mL); LPS, lipopolysaccharide; HUVECs, human umbilical vein endothelial cells.

were associated with starting vitamin E intervention at the same time as high fat diet or before development of the fatty-streak formation. Palm-derived TRF supplementation given before cholesterol feeding provides protection against development of early atherosclerotic lesions in rabbits with 10 weeks of continuous TRF supplementation (Omar et al. 2009; Razak et al. 2010). Nafeeza et al. (2001) investigated the effect of TRF on the microscopic development of atherosclerosis and lipid peroxidation, which showed lower aortic contents of MDA, less intimal thickening and greater preservation of the internal elastic lamina in the aortas of rabbits after 10 weeks of treatment with TRF.

However, the effect of T3 on atherosclerotic plaque has been controversial. Tocotrienol has been reported to have little effect on plasma lipids and atherosclerosis in cholesterol-fed rabbits (Hasselwander et al. 2002). Aishah et al. (2011) reported that TRF (T3:T ratio = 70:30%) supplementation in rabbits for 2 months prior to high cholesterol diet experimental induction of severe atherosclerosis led to significant reduction in atherosclerotic lesions and tissue biomarkers of inflammation and endothelial activation compared to placebo, suggesting a beneficial role of TRF in the prevention of atherosclerosis (Figures 12.11 and 12.12).

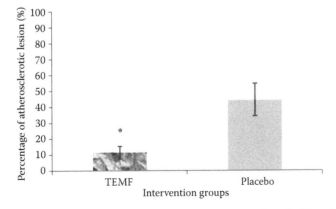

FIGURE 12.11 Percentage of atherosclerotic lesions in rabbits treated with TEMF or placebo in the groups for the prevention of established atherosclerosis. There was significant reduction in atherosclerotic lesions in TEMF-treated group compared to placebo (*$p < 0.05$). Data are expressed as mean ± SEM. TEMF, Tocotrienol-enriched mixed fraction (tocotrienol:tocopherol ratio = 70:30%, tocotrienols 15 mg/kg/day).

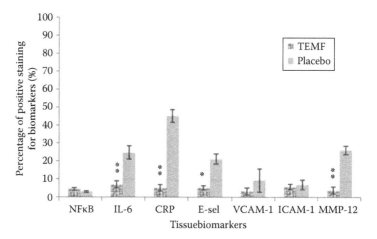

FIGURE 12.12 Immunocytochemical staining of tissue biomarkers for atherosclerosis in TEMF (tocotrienols 15 mg/kg/day) and placebo-treated groups for the prevention of established atherosclerosis. There were significant reduction in IL-6 ($p < 0.01$), CRP ($p < 0.01$), e-selectin ($p < 0.05$), and MMP-12 ($p < 0.01$) in the TEMF-treated compared to placebo group. Data are expressed as mean ± SEM. TEMF, Tocotrienol-enriched mixed fraction (tocotrienol:tocopherol ratio = 70:30%).

Another study using a rabbit experimental model demonstrated a dissociation of aortic lipid oxidation and lesion development, and suggests that vitamin E (T) does not prevent development of atherosclerotic lesions (Upston et al. 2001). Moreover, the literature relating to T has expanded enormously (Munteanu et al. 2004; Schneider 2005) while the natural T3 analogues have been poorly studied and received minimal public attention.

Epidemiological studies indicate an inverse relationship between vitamin E intake and CVD (Rimm et al. 1993). The initial enthusiasm for the clinical use of antioxidant vitamins in the

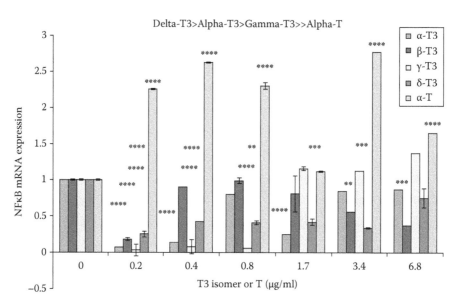

FIGURE 12.13 Effects of pure T3 isomers and α-T on the NFκB (p50) in LPS stimulated HUVECs. Varying concentrations of T3 isomers and α-T were added to the HUVECs together with LPS (1 µg/ml). Data are expressed as Mean ± SD. ****$p<0.0001$, ***$p<0.001$ and **$p<0.005$ compared to LPS control. T3: Tocotrienol, T: Tocopherol; T3 concentration range: 0.2–6.8 µg/ml; LPS: lipopolysaccharide; HUVECs: human umbilical vein endothelial cells.

prevention of CAD was derived from positive results in the preclinical setting (Prasad and Kalra 1993; Parker 1993). Stampfer et al. (1993) have suggested that the highest vitamin intake in men and women have shown reductions in the risk of coronary disease. Tocotrienol abridged blood levels of lipid peroxides with an apparent improved blood flow in patients with carotid atherosclerosis. Within 6 months of supplementation, 240 mg of palm tocotrienol complex per day, 92% of the patients had a regression in their carotid stenosis condition. In comparison, none of the placebo patients had any improvement and 4% of them had progression in the condition (Tomeo et al.1995).

In a meta-analysis that involved several clinical trials: (1) Cambridge Heart Anti-oxidant study (CHAOS), (2) MRC/BHF Heart Protection Study (HPS), (3) Gruppo Italiano per lo Studio della Soprawivenza nell'Infarto miocardico Prevention Study (GISSI), (4) Heart Outcomes Prevention Evaluation (HOPE) study, and (5) Primary Prevention Project (PPP), consumption of α-T as the main source of vitamin E has shown no significant benefit of α-T on all-cause mortality, cardiovascular death, and risk of stroke (Vivekananthan et al. 2003). The negative findings are postulated to be due to several factors such as timing of α-T intervention relative to the atherosclerotic process, preexisting antioxidant status of study participants, and the fact that results were driven by trials of α-T used as secondary prevention (Steinberg 2002). Another meta-analysis that has been performed recently to evaluate a potential dose-dependent effect of T supplementation (16.5–2000 IU/day with a median 400 IU/day, 267 mg/day) showed that all cause mortality progressively increased for dosages more than 150 IU/day or 100 mg/day (Miller et al. 2005). These data were based on the results reported on the various T-based vitamin E intervention clinical trials worldwide (Miller et al. 2005). It has to be emphasized that in this meta-analysis, almost all trials utilized α-T as the main source of vitamin E supplementation. It may not be appropriate to make such a conclusion on vitamin E, when all that has been tested for efficacy on a limited basis in clinical trials is α-T (Greenberg et al. 2005). Obviously, T is a form of vitamin E and not synonymous to vitamin E. T3, the other type of vitamin E, is not included as a main source of vitamin E in these meta-analyses, and thus should not be implicated in any randomized clinical trial using T to study the effects of vitamin E in CVD. More recently, a meta-analysis of human randomized controlled trials revealed that α-T supplementation increased all cause mortality at a 95% confidence interval (Bjelakovic et al. 2007; Ping 2011).

12.2.7 ANTI-ISCHEMIC EFFECTS OF TOCOTRIENOLS

Ischemic heart disease (IHD) is the most common form of CVD resulting in acute coronary syndrome including acute myocardial infarction (Lam and Lopaschuk 2007). Myocardial ischemia results from impairment of coronary blood supply, the majority of which is attributed to atherosclerosis. Apart from atherosclerotic plaques, oxidative stress plays an important role in IHD. By virtue of the excellent free radical scavenging activity of tocotrienols, attenuation of oxidative stress is expected to be more efficient in T3 than T. Hence, it is postulated that T3 may be considered a better therapeutic option in IHD. Ikeda et al. (2003) reported that, γ-T3 acts as a myocardial conditioning agent by activating the eNOS expression. eNOS enhances NO production, leading to vasodilatation and cardioprotection from ischemic phase.

Recently, T3 have been found to be effective in protecting the central nervous system compared to T, and tocotrienol inhibited glutamate-induced pp66 c-Src kinase activation in HT4 neuronal cells (Sen et al. 2000). A recent study showed the cardioprotection of palm TRF was linked to their ability to stabilize proteosomes (Das et al. 2005). Powell et al. (2005) have shown that the proteosome may become dysfunctional as a result of ischemia. TRF was observed to partially protect the proteosome, which may have facilitated the degradation of phosphor-c-Src (Das et al. 2005). γ-T3 has the most cardioprotective properties against myocardial ischemic injury compared to the other isomers. The molecular mechanisms afforded by T3 in cardioprotection are associated with their ability to stabilize the proteosome, allowing it to maintain a balance between prodeath and prosurvival signals (Das et al. 2008). In another study, resveratrol acts synergistically with γ-T3 to provide greater cardioprotection than either of them alone (Lekli et al. 2009). In addition, α-T3 is more potent in cardioprotection against oxidative stress induced by ischemia-reperfusion than α-T in rats (Nafeeza et al. 2001). One study reported that TRF was able to reduce myocardial infarction size, improve post-ischemic ventricular dysfunction, and ventricular arrhythmias. T3 consist of four different isomers. Although these isomers possess comparable antioxidant properties, their ability to potentiate signal transduction is different. In addition to being a more potent antioxidant than T, α-T3 in nanomolar concentration, but not α-T, have been shown to block glutamate-induced death by suppressing early activation of c-Src kinase (Sen et al. 2000).

12.2.8   EFFECTS OF TOCOTRIENOLS ON MONOCYTE–ENDOTHELIAL CELL ADHESION

Monocyte adherence to endothelial cells is mediated via adhesion molecules including ICAM-1, VCAM-1, and e-selectin (Carlos and Harlan 1994). Enhanced adhesion molecule expression has been shown to be a critical step in foam cell formation and the development of atherosclerosis.

α-T at 10 μM has been reported to inhibit the monocyte–endothelial cell adhesion (Theriault et al. 2002). Several studies have shown that pure T3 isomers and TTMF are more potent than α-T in terms of reducing monocyte–endothelial cell adhesion. (Theriault et al., 2002; Muid et al., 2011) have also shown the reduction of monocyte–endothelial cells adhesion was maximal at low concentrations of pure δ- (0.6 μm/L, 52.4% inhibition) and γ-T3 isomers (0.6 μm/L, 45.6% inhibition; Muid et al. 2001). Choa et al. (2002) reported that compared to α-T3, the γ-T3 isomers have a 1.5fold more profound inhibitory effect on monocyte cell binding using a 15 μM concentration within 24h, and suggested the role for prenylated protein in the regulation of monocyte adhesion. Studies on cell cultures have reported that δ-T3 is the most potent tocotrienol isomer in reducing monocyte–endothelial cell binding (Muid 2001; Naito et al. 2005).

12.2.9   ANTITHROMBOTIC EFFECTS OF TOCOTRIENOLS

An arterial thrombus is a solid mass of blood constituents formed within the vascular system consisting of aggregated platelets, adherent to the vessel wall and immobilized by fibrin. It is predisposed by abnormality of the arterial wall such as endothelial injury in atherosclerosis, abnormal blood flow such as stasis or turbulent blood flow, and abnormality in the blood component such as in hypercoagulable states. A thrombus may be dislodged and form an emboli leading to obstruction of the distal artery resulting in tissue ischemia or infarction (Hirsh 1987). Typically, a ruptured atheromatous plaque in a coronary artery will lead to thrombus formation and arterial occlusion resulting in acute myocardial infarction. The antithrombotic properties of T3 have been reported, where TRF and purified tocotrienol was shown to reduce the synthesis of an eicosanoid, thromboxane B2, and platelet factor 4. This is attributed by reduced activity of phospholipase A2, an enzyme that potentiates release of arachidonic acid from membrane-bound phospholipids to various eicosanoids (Douglas et al. 1986). More recently, Qureshi et al. (2011) reported that intravenously administered α-T3 is more potent than α-T in inhibiting platelet-mediated thrombus formation, and collagen and adenosine diphosphate (ADP)-induced platelet aggregation in stenosed coronary arteries of dogs. Thus, it is suggested that intravenously administered tocotrienol could potentially prevent pathological platelet thrombus formation, and thus provide a therapeutic benefit in conditions such as stroke and myocardial infarction.

12.3   CONCLUSION

Atherosclerosis is now recognized as a chronic inflammatory disease leading to atherosclerosis-related complications such as CAD. Several factors, including oxidative stress, inflammation, ED, and hypercholesterolemia play crucial roles in the pathogenesis of atherosclerosis and CAD. Therefore, by virtue of the lipid lowering, potent antioxidant, and anti-inflammatory properties of T3, as well as improvement in endothelial function with tocotrienol treatment, there is a strong potential role of T3 in the prevention and regression of atherosclerosis. In addition, tocotrienol inhibitory effects on monocyte–endothelial cell adhesion, a key event in atherogenesis, and their anti-ischemic and antithrombotic properties further render the cardioprotective potential of T3. Recent meta-analyses of randomized clinical trials using α-T supplementation revealed increment of all cause mortality, suggesting that α-T supplementation is undesirable as it does more harm than good. α-T supplementation depresses the bioavailability of other forms of the vitamin, especially T3 that has high chemopreventive and therapeutic capability. The dietary reference intake for vitamin E was made on the wrong assumption that the α-T isomer is the only relevant form of vitamin E. In view of the clear evidence that α-T supplementation increases all cause mortality and T3 can be absorbed in an α-TTP-dependent pathway, there is a strong need to critically review the dietary reference intake recommendations. Experimental data have clearly demonstrated that T3 have good chemoprotective and therapeutic potential against various degenerative diseases, including atherosclerosis and its complications such as CAD, whereas T is ineffective. In addition, T appears to inhibit both the cholesterol-lowering and pleiotrophic effects of T3. It is hence timely for T3 and TRF to be evaluated clinically to fully explore their chemopreventive and therapeutic potential in view of the numerous positive *in vitro* and *in vivo* studies, and to a very limited extent, human intervention trials. The high binding affinity of α-T to α-TTP poses a challenge to the bioavailability of T3. Hence, suitable materials for clinical evaluation are pure T3 preparations or those containing very minimal amount of α-T. Therefore, bigger and appropriate randomized clinical trials need to be conducted using TRFs and pure tocotrienol isomers to elucidate the benefits of T3 in the prevention and treatment of atherosclerosis and CAD.

ACKNOWLEDGMENTS

The author would like to express her greatest appreciation to Aishah Muhd, Suhaila Muid, and Thuhairah Rahman in the assistance rendered in the preparation of this chapter.

REFERENCES

Aggarwal BB, Sundaram C, Prasad S, Kannappan R (2010). Tocotrienols, the vitamin E of the 21st century: its potential against cancer and other chronic diseases. *Biochem Pharmacol* 80:1613–1631.

Aishah NM, Omar E, Thuhairah AR, Nawawi H (2011). Tocotrienol-tocopherol mixed fraction supplementation prevents inflammation in established atherosclerosis. *Atheroscler Suppl* 12 (Suppl 1):143.

Albers JJ, Brunzell JD, Knopp RH (1989). Apoprotein measurements and their clinical application in cholesterol screening. *Clin Lab Med* 34:4–8.

Altman R (2004). Risk factor in coronary atherosclerosis athero-inflammation: The meeting point. *Thromb J* 1:4–8.

Bayorh MA, Abukhalaf IK, Ganafa AA (2005). Effect of palm oil on blood pressure, endothelial function and oxidative stress. *Asia Pac J Clin Nutr* 14(4):325–339.

Birringer M, Pfluger P, Kluth D, Landes N, Brigelius-Flohe R (2002). Identities and differences in the metabolism of tocotrienols and tocopherols in HepG2 cells. *J Nutr* 132:3113–3118.

Bjelakovic G, Nikolova D, Glund LL, Simonetti RG, Glund C (2007). Mortality in randomized trials of antioxidant supplements for primary and secondary prevention–Systematic review and meta-analysis. *JAMA* 297:842–857.

Black TM, Wang P, Maed N, Coleman RA (2000). Palm tocotrienols protect ApoE 1/2 mice from diet-induced atheroma formation. *J Nutr* 130:2420–2426.

Carlos TM, Harlan JM (1994). Leukocyte-Endothelial adhesion molecules. *Blood* 84:2068–2101.

Chao J-T, Gapor A, Theriault A (2002). Inhibitory effect of δ-tocotrienol, a HMG CoA reductase inhibitor, on monocyte-endothelial cell adhesion. *J Nutr Sci Vitaminol* 48:332–337.

Chen CW, Cheng HH (2006). A rice bran oil diet increases LDL receptor and HMG-CoA reductase mRNA expressions and insulin sensitivity in rats with streptozotocin/nicotinamide induced type 2 diabetes. *J Nutr* 136:1472–1476.

Chen WY, Cheng BC, Jiang MJ, Hsieh MY, Chang MS (2006). IL-20 is expressed in atherosclerosis plaques and promotes atherosclerosis in apolipoprotein E-deficient mice. *Arterioscler Thromb Vasc Biol* 26:2090 –2095.

Cines DB, Pollak ES, Buck CA, Loscalzo J, Zimmerman GA, McEver RP, Pober JS, Wick TM (1998). Endothelial cells in physiology and in the pathophysiology of vascular disorders. *Blood* 91:3527–3561.

Correll CC, Ng L, Edwards PA (1994). Identification of farnesol as the non-sterol derivative of mevalonic acid required for the accelerated degradation of 3-hydroxy-3-methylglutaryl-coenzyme A reductase. *J Biol Chem* 269:17390–17393.

Das S, Powell SR, Wang P, Divald A, Nesaretnam K, Tosaki A, Cordis GA, Maulik N, Das DK (2006) Cardioprotection with palm tocotrienol: antioxidant activity of tocotrienol is linked with its ability to stabilize proteasomes. *Am J Physiol Heart Circ Physiol* 289:361–367.

Das S, Lekli I, Das M, Das DK (2008). Cardioprotection with palm oil tocotrienols: comparison of different isomers. *Am J Physiol Heart Circ Physiol* 294:970–978.

Davi G, Alessandrini P, Mezzetti A, Minotti G, Bucciarelli T, Costantini F, Cipollonne F, Bittolo Bon G, Ciabattoni G, Patrono C (1997). In vivo formation of 8-epi-prostaglandin F2α is increased in hypercholesterolemia. *Arterioscler Thromb Vasc Biol* 17:3230–3235.

Douglas CE, Chan AC, Choy PC (1986). Vitamin E inhibits platelet phospholipase A2. *Biochem Biophys Acta* 876:639–645.

Esterbauer H, Dieber-Rotheneder M, Striegl G, Waeg G (1991). Role of vitamin E in preventing the oxidation of low-density lipoprotein. *Am J Clin Nutr* 53:314S–321S.

Fairus S, Nor RM, Cheng HM, Sundram K (2006). Postprandial metabolic fate of tocotrienol-rich vitamin E differs significantly from that of a- tocopherol. *Am J Clin Nutr* 84:835–842.

Fruebis J, Silvestre M, Shelton D, Napoli C, Palinski W (1999). Inhibition of VCAM-1 expression in the arterial wall is shared by structurally different antioxidants that reduce early atherosclerosis in NZW rabbits. *J Lipid Res* 40:1958–1966.

Goldstein JL, Brown MS (1990). Regulation of the mevalonate pathway. *Nature* 343:425–430.

Greenberg ER (2005). Vitamin E supplements: good in theory, but is the theory good. *Ann Intern Med* 142:75–76.

Gresser U, Gathof BS (2004). Atorvastatin: gold standard for prophylaxis of myocardial ischemia and stroke - comparison of the clinical benefit of statins on the basis of randomized controlled endpoint studies. *Eur J Med Res* 9:1–17.

Hansson GK, Seifert PS, Bondjers G (1991). Immunohistochemical detection of macrophages and T-lymphocytes in atherosclerotic lesions of cholesterol-fed rabbits. *Arterioscler Thromb* 11:745–750.

Harrison CN, Machin SJ (1997). Essential thrombocythaemia and antiphospholipid antibodies. *Am J Med* 102:317–318.

Hasselwander O, Kramer K, Hoppe PP, Oberfrank U, Baldenius K, Schröder H, Kaufmann W, Bahnemann R, Nowakowsky B (2002). Effects of feeding various tocotrienol sources on plasma lipids and aortic atherosclerotic lesions in cholesterol-fed rabbits. *Food Res Int* 35(2002):245–251.

Hirsh J (1987). Hyperactive platelets and complications of coronary artery disease. *N Engl J Med* 316:1543–1544.

Hood RL (1996). Tocotrienols and cholesterol metabolism. In: Ong ASH, Niki E, Packer L, eds. *Nutrition, Lipids, Health, and Disease*. pp. 96–103. Champaign, IL: AOCS Press.

Hood RL (1998). Tocotrienols in metabolism. In: Bidlack WR, Omaye ST, Meskin MS, Jahner D, eds. *Phytochemicals—A New Paradigm*. pp. 33–51.Lancaster, PA: Technomic.

Horvath G, Wessjohann L, Bigirimana J, Jansen M, Guisez Y, Caubergs R (2006). Differential distribution of tocopherols and tocotrienols in photosynthetic and non-photosynthetic tissues. *Phytochemistry* 67:1185–1195.

Hosomi A, Arita M, Sato Y, Kiyose C, Ueda T, Igarashi O, Arai H, Inoue K. (1997). Affinity for a-tocopherol transfer protein as a determinant of the biological activities of vitamin E analogs. *FEBS Lett* 409:105–108.

Hunter SC, Cahoon EB (2007). Enhancing vitamin E in oilseeds: unravelling tocopherol and tocotrienol biosynthesis. *Lipids* 42:97–108.

Ikeda S, Tohyama T, Yoshimura H, Hamamura K, Abe K, Yamashita K (2003). Dietary alpha tocopherol decreases alpha-tocotrienol but not gamma-tocotrienol concentration in rats. *J Nutr* 133:428–434.

Iqbal J, Minhajuddin M, Beg ZH (2003). Suppression of 7, 12-dimethylbenz anthracene induced carcinogenesis and hypercholesterolaemia in rats by Tocotrienol rich fraction isolated from rice bran oil. *Eur J Cancer Prev* 12:447–453.

Iqbal J, Minhajuddin M, Beg ZH (2004). Suppression of diethylnitrosamine and 2 acetylaminofluorene induced hepatocarcinogenesis in rats by tocotrienol-rich fraction isolated from rice bran oil. *Eur J Cancer Prev* 13:515–520.

Kamal J, Devasagayam TPA (1995). Tocotrienols from palm oil as potent inhibitors of lipid peroxidation and protein oxidation in rat brain mitochondria. *Neurosci Lett* 195:179–182.

Kamal-Eldin A, Appelqvist LA (1996). The chemistry and antioxidant properties of tocopherols and tocotrienols. *Lipids* 31:671–701.

Kanaya Y, Doi T, Sasaki H, Fujita A, Matsuno S, Okamoto K (2004). Rice bran extract prevents the elevation of plasma peroxylipid in KKAy diabetic mice. *Diabetes Res Clin Pract* 66S:S157–S160.

Kawakami Y, Tsuzuki T, Nakagawa K, Miyazawa T (2007). Distribution of tocotrienols in rats fed a rice bran tocotrienol concentrate. *Biosci Biotechnol Biochem* 71:464–471.

Khanna S, Patel V, Rink C, Roy S, Sen K (2005). Delivery of oral supplemented tocotrienol to vital organs of rats and tocopherol-transfer protein deficient mice. *Free Radical Biol Med* 39:1310–1319.

Khanna S, Roy S, Ryu H, Bahadduri P, Swaan PW, Ratan RR, Sen CK (2003). Molecular basis of vitamin E action: tocotrienols modulates 12-lipoxygenase, a key mediator of glutamate induced neurodegeneration. *J Biol Chem* 278:43508–43515.

Khor HT, Chieng DY (1996). Effect of dietary supplementation of tocotrienols and tocopherols on serum lipids in the hamster. *Nutrition Research* 16(8):1393–1401.

Koenig W, Khuseyinova N (2007). Biomarkers of atherosclerotic plaque instability and rupture. *Arterioscler Thromb Vasc Biol* 27:15–26.

Lam A, Lopaschuk GD (2007). Anti-anginal effects of partial fatty acid oxidation inhibitors. *Curr Opin Pharmacol* 7:179–185.

Lekli I, Ray D, Mukherjee S, Gurusamy N, Ahsan MK, Jahasz B, Bak I, Tosaki A, Gherghiceanu M, Popescu LM, Das DK (2009). Coordinated autophagy with resveratrol and gamma-tocotrienol confers synergetic cardioprotection. *J Cell Mol Med* 14:2506–2518.

Li F, Tan W, Kang Z et al. (2010). Tocotrienol enriched palm oil prevents atherosclerosis through modulating the activities of peroxisome proliferators-activated receptors. *Atherosclerosis* 211:278–282.

Libby P, Hansson GK (1991). Involvement of the immune system in human atherogenesis: current knowledge and unanswered questions. *Lab Invest* 64:5–15.

Lusis AJ (2000). Atherosclerosis. *Nature* 407(6801):233–241.

Madamanchi NR, Vendrov A, Runge MS (2005). Oxidative stress and vascular disease. *Arterioscler Thromb Vasc Biol* 25:29–38.

Mehta JL, Li DY, Chen HJ (2001). Inhibition of LOX-1 by statins may relate to upregulation of eNOS. *Biochem Biophys Res Comm* 289:857–861.

Miller ER, Barriuso RP, Dalal D, Riemersma RA, Appel LJ, Guallar E (2005). Meta-analysis: High dosage vitamin E supplementation may increase all cause mortality. *Ann Intern Med* 142:37–46.

Minhajuddin M, Beg ZH, Iqbal J (2005). Hypolipidemic and antioxidant properties of tocotrienol rich fraction isolated from rice bran oil in experimentally induced hyperlipidemic rats. *Food Chem Toxicol* 43:747–753.

Mizushina Y, Nakagawa K, Shibata A, Awata Y, Kuriyama I, Shimazaki N et al. (2006). Inhibitory effect of tocotrienol on eukaryotic DNA polymerase lambda and angiogenesis. *Biochem Biophys Res Commun* 339(3):949–955.

Muid S, Froemming GRA, A. Manaf, Nawawi H (2009).Tocotrienol rich fraction upregulates endothelial nitric oxide synthase protein expression in stimulated endothelial cells. *Atherosclerosis* Suppl 10(2):580.

Muid S, Froemming GRA, Nawawi H (2011). Inhibitory effects of pure tocotrienol isomers on inflammation, endothelial activation and monocyte binding activity. *Atherosclerosis* Suppl 12(1):76.

Muid S, Froemming GRA, Nawawi H (2012). Inhibitory effects of pure tocotrienol isomers on inflammation, endothelial activation and monocyte binding activity. *Proceedings of XVI International Symposium on Atherosclerosis (ISA2012)*, Sydney, New South Wales, Australia, March 25–29, 2012.

Muid S, Yusoff K, Nawawi H (2007). Improvement in oxidative stress in patients with non-familial hypercholesterolaemia (NFH) treated with palm oil derived vitamin E. *Malaysian J Pathol* 29 (Suppl A):189.

Munteanu A, Zingg JM, Azzi A (2004). Anti-atherosclerotic effects of vitamin E-myth or reality? *J Cell Mol Med* 8:59–76.

Mustad VA, Smith CA, Ruey PP, Edens NK, DeMichele SJ (2002). Supplementation with 3 compositionally different tocotrienol supplements does not improve cardiovascular disease risk factors in men and women with hypercholesterolemia. *Am J Clin Nutr* 76:1237–1243.

Nafeeza MI, Norzana AG, Jalaluddin HL, Gapor MT (2001). The effects of a tocotrienol-rich fraction on experimentally induced atherosclerosis in the aorta of rabbits. *Malays J Pathol* 23:17–25.

Naito Y, Shimozawa M, Kuroda M, Nakabe N, Manabe H, Katada K, Kokura S, Ichikawa H, Yoshida N, Noguchi N, Yoshikawa T (2005). Tocotrienols reduce 25-hydroxycholesterol-induced monocyte-endothelial cell interaction by inhibiting the surface expression of adhesion molecules. *Atherosclerosis*180:19–25.

Napolitano M, Avanzi L, Manfredini S, Bravo E (2007). Effects of new combinative antioxidant FeAOX-6 and a-tocotrienol on macrophage atherogenesis related functions. *Vascular Pharmacol* 46:394–405.

Naurooz-Zadeh J, Smith CCT, Betteridge DJ (2001). Measures of oxidative stress in heterozygous familial hypercholesterolaemia. *Atherosclerosis* 156:435–441.

Nawawi H (2003). Dyslipidaemia and endothelial dysfunction. *J Asean Fed Endocr Soc* 21(1/2):5–16.

Nawawi H, Muid S, Annuar R, Yusoff K (2005a). Reduction in oxidative stress, inflammation, and endo-thelial dysfunction in patients with non familial hypercholesterolaemia treated with low dose statin. *Atherosclerosis* (Suppl) 6(1):72.

Nawawi H, Muid S, Manaf A, Yusoff K (2005b). Potent antioxidant activity of tocotrienol in in vitro assays. *Atherosclerosis* (Suppl) 6(1):168.

Nawawi H, Muid S, Manaf A, Yusoff K (2006a). Low to moderate tocotrienol concentrations exhibits optimal antioxidant activity and reduces production of inflammatory markers by endothelial cells. *Atherosclerosis* Suppl 7(3):224.

Nawawi H, Muid S, Manaf A, Yusoff K (2006b). Higher tocotrienol optimal concentration as an anti-oxidant than as an anti-inflammatory agent. *J Hypertens* Suppl 6(24):397.

Nawawi H, Muid S, Yusoff K (2007). Effects of palmvitee supplementation on Isoprotanes levels in patients with non familial hypercholesteroleamia. *Proceedings of the 2nd Research Workshop*, UiTM Hotel, Shah Alam, Selangor, Malaysia, pp. 54–54, ISBN 978-983-3644-45-2.

Nawawi H, Nor I, Noor I, Karim NA, Arshad F, Khan R, Yusoff K (2002). Current status of coronary risk fac-tors among rural Malays in Malaysia. *J Cardiovasc Risk* 9:17–22.

Nawawi H, Osman NS, Yusoff K, Khalid BAK (2003a). Reduction in serum levels of adhesion molecules, interleukin 6 and C-reactive protein following short-term low-dose atorvastatin treatment in patients with non familial hypercholesterolaemia. *Horm Metab Res* 35:1–8.

Nawawi H, Osman NS, Annuar R, Khalid BA, Yusoff K (2003b). Soluble intercellular adhesion molecule-1 and interleukin-6 levels reflect endothelial dysfunction in patients with primary hypercholesterolaemia treated with atorvastatin. *Atherosclerosis* 169(2):283–291.

Nesaretnam K, Devasagayam TPA, Singh BB, Basiron Y (1993). Influence of palm oil or its tocotrienol-rich fraction on lipid peroxidation potential on rat liver mitochondria and microsomes. *Biochem Mol Biol Int* 30:159–167.

Omar E, Azlina AR, Mahamad Rodi NH, Wan Rohaini WA, Vellayan S, Nawawi H (2009). Palm-derived tocotrienol-rich fraction protects against the development of early atherosclerotic lesions in rab-bits. *Proceedings of 1st Palm-International Nutra-Cosmoceutical Conference PINC*, Kuala Lumpur, Malaysia, p. 51.

Ong FB, Wan Ngah WZ, Shamaan NA, Md Top AG, Marzuki A, Khalid AK (1993). Glutathione S-transferase and gamma-glutamyl transpeptidase activities in cultured rat hepatocytes treated with tocotrienol and tocopherol. *Comp Biochem Physiol C* 1993;106:237–240.

Ozer NK, Azzi A (2000). Effect of vitamin E on the development of atherosclerosis. *Toxicology* 148 (2–3):179–185.

Palozza P, Verdecchia S, Avanzi L, Vertuani S, Serini S, Iannone A, Manfredini S (2006). Comparative anti-oxidant activity of tocotrienols and the novel chromanylpolyisoprenyl molecule FeAox-6 in isolated membranes and intact cells. *Mol Cell Biochem* 287:21–32.

Parker RA, Pearce BC, Clark RW, Gordon DA, Wright JJ (1993). Tocotrienols regulate cholesterol produc-tion in mammalian cells by post-transcriptional suppression of 3-Hydroxy-3-methylglutaryl-coenzyme A reductase. *J Biol Chem* 268:11230–11238.

Patel V, Khanna S, Roy S, Ezziddin O, Sen CK (2006). Natural vitamin E a-tocotrienol: Retention in vital organs in response to long-term oral supplementation and withdrawal. *Free Radic Res* July 40(7):763–771.

Pearce BC, Parker RA, Deason ME, Qureshi, AA, Kim Wright JJ (1992). Hypocholesterolemic activity of synthetic and natural tocotrienols. *J Med Chem* 35:3595–3606.

Pearce BC, Parker RA, Deason ME, Dischino DD, Gillespie E, Qureshi AA, Kim Wright JJ, Volk K (1994). Inhibitors of cholesterol biosynthesis-Hypocholesterolemic and antioxidant activities of benzopyran and tetrahydronaphthalene analogues of the tocotrienols. *J Med Chem* 37:526–541.

Ping TG (2011). Unleasing the untold and misunderstood observations on vitamin E. *Genes Nutr* 6:5–16.

Powell, Saul R, Wang P, Katzeff H et al. (2005). *Antioxid Redox Signal* 7(5–6):538–546.

Prasad K, Kalra J (1993). Oxygen free radicals and hypercholesterolemic atherosclerosis: effect of vitamin E. *Am Heart J* 125(4):958–973.

Qureshi AA, Pearce BC, Nor RM, Gapor A, Peterson DM, Elson, CE 1996. Dietary alphatocopherol attenuates the impact of gamma-tocotrienol on hepatic 3-hydroxy-3-methylglutaryl coenzyme A reductase activity in chickens. *J. Nutr.* 126:389–394.

Qureshi AA, Bradlow BA, Brace L, Manganello J, Peterson DM, Pearce BC, Wright JJ, Gapor A, Elson CE (1995). Response of hypercholesterolemic subjects to administration of tocotrienols. *Lipids* 30(12):1171–1177.

Qureshi AA, Bradlow BA, Salser WA, Brace LD (1997). Novel tocotrienols of rice bran modulate cardiovascu-lar disease risk parameters of hypercholesterolemic humans. *Nutr Biochem* 8:290–298.

Qureshi AA, Burger WC, Peterson DM, Elson CE (1986). The structure of an inhibitor of cholesterol biosynthesis isolated from barley. *J Biol Chem* 261:10544–10550.

Qureshi AA, Chaudhary V, Weber FE, Chicoye E, Qureshi N (1991a). Effects of brewer's grain and other cereals on lipid metabolism in chickens. *Nutr Res* 11:159–162.

Qureshi N, Hofman J, Qureshi AA (1993). Inhibition of LPS induced tumour necrosis factor synthesis and hypocholesterolaemic effect of novel tocotrienols. In *Proceedings of the PORIM International Palm Oil Congress*, Kaula Lampur, Malaysia, September 20–25, p. N16.

Qureshi AA, Karpen CW, Qureshi NP, Christopher J, Morrison DC, Folt JD (2011). Tocotrienols-induced inhibition of platelet thrombus formation and platelet aggregation in stenosed canine coronary arteries. *Lipids Health Dis* 10(58):1s–13s.

Qureshi AA, Peterson DM (2001). The combined effects of novel tocotrienols and lovastatin on lipid metabolism in chickens. *Atherosclerosis* 156:39–47.

Qureshi AA, Qureshi N, Hasler-Rapacz JO, Weber FE, Chaudhary V, Crenshaw TD, Gapor A et al. (1991b). Dietary tocotrienols reduce concentrations of plasma cholesterol, apolipoprotein B., thromboxane B2, and platelet factor 4 in pigs with inherited hyperlipidemias. *Am J Clin Nutr* 53:1042–1046.

Qureshi AA, Salser WA, Parmar R, Emeson EE (2001). Novel tocotrienols of rice bran inhibit atherosclerotic lesions in C57BL/6 ApoE-deficient mice. *J Nutr* 131:2606–2618.

Razak AA, Omar E, Muhammad NA, Mahamad Rodi NH, Nawawi H (2010). Tocotrienol-rich fraction supplementation before cholesterol feeding provides protection against early atherosclerosis. *Atherosclerosis* 2 (Suppl 11):188.

Ridker PM (2003). Clinical applications of C-reactive protein for cardiovascular disease detection and prevention. *Circulation* 107:363–369.

Ridker PM, Brown NJ, Vaughan DE, Harrison DG, Mehta JL (2004). Established and emerging plasma biomarkers in the prediction of first atherothrombotic events. *Circulation* 109 (Suppl IV):IV-6–IV-19.

Rifkind BM (1998). Clinical trials of reducing low-density lipoprotein concentrations. *Endocrinol Metab Clin North Am* 27:585–595.

Rimm EB, Stampfer MJ, Ascherio A, Giovannucci E, Colditz GA, Willett WC (1993). Vitamin E consumption and the risk of coronary heart disease in men. *N Engl J Med* 328:1450–1456.

Ross R (1993). The pathogenesis of atherosclerosis: a perspective for 1990s. *Nature* 362:801–809.

Ross R (1999). Atherosclerosis – An inflammatory disease. *N Engl J Med* 340:115–126.

Saito Y, Yoshida Y, Nishio K, Hayakawa M, Niki E (2004). Characterization of cellular uptake and distribution of vitamin E. *Ann N Y Acad Sci* 1031:368–375.

Scanu AM, Fless GM (1990). Lipoprotein (a): heterogeneity and biological relevance. *J Clin Invest* 86:1709–1715.

Schaffer S, Muller WE, Eckert GP (2005). Tocotrienols: constitutional effects in aging and disease. *J Nutr*, 135:151–154.

Schneider C (2005). Chemistry and biology of vitamin E. *Mol Nutr Food Res* 49:7–30.

Sen CK, Khanna S, Roy S (2006). Tocotrienols: vitamin E beyond tocopherols. *Life Sci* 78(18):2088–2098.

Sen CK, Khanna S, Roy S (2007). Tocotrienols in health and disease: The other half of the natural vitamin E family. *Mol Aspects Med* 28:692–728.

Sen CK, Khanna S, Roy S, Packer LJ (2000). Molecular basis of vitamin E action. *J Biol Chem* 275:13049–13055.

Serbinova E, Kagan V, Han D, Packer L (1991). Free radical recycling and intramembrane mobility in the antioxidant properties of alpha-tocopherol and alpha-tocotrienol. *Free Radic Biol Med* 10:263–275.

Serbinova EA, Packer L (1994). Antioxidant properties of alpha-tocopherol and alpha-tocotrienol. *Methods Enzymol* 234:354–366.

Setiadi DH, Chass GA, Torday LL, Varro A, Papp JG (2002). Vitamin E models. Conformational analysis and stereochemistry of tetralin, chroman, thiochroman and selenochroman. *J Mol Struct* (Theochem) 594: 161–172.

Sever N, Song BL, Yabe D, Goldstein JL, Brown MS, DeBose-Boyd RA. (2003). Insig-dependent ubiquitination and degradation of mammalian 3-hydroxy-3-methylglutaryl-CoA reductase stimulated by sterols and geranylgeraniol. *J Biol Chem* 278:52479–52490.

Shringarpure R, Teoh C, Khaliulin I, Das DD, Davies KJA, Schwalb H. Oxidized and ubiquitinated proteins may predict recovery of postischemic cardiac function: essential role of the proteasome. *Antioxid Redox Signal* 7(5–6):538–546.

Sniderman A, Shapiro S, Marpole D, Skinner B, Teng B, Kwiterovich PO (1980). Association of coronary atherosclerosis with hyperbetalipoproteinemia increased protein but normal cholesterol levels in human plasma low-density (beta) lipoproteins. *Proc Natl Acad Sci USA* 77:604–608.

Song BL, Debose-Boyd RA (2006). Insig-dependent ubiquitination and degradation of 3hydroxy-3-methylglutaryl coenzyme A reductase stimulated by d- and c-tocotrienols. *J Biol Chem* 281:25054–25061.

Srinath RK, Salim Y (1998). Emerging Epidemic of cardiovascular disease in developing countries. *Circulation* 97:596–601.

Stampfer MJ, Hennekens CH, Manson JE, Colditz GA, Rosner B, Willett WC (1993). Vitamin E consumption and the risk of coronary disease in women. *N Engl J Med* 328(20):1444–1449.

Steinberg D (2002). Atherogenesis in perspective: hypercholesterolemia and inflammation as partners in crime. *Nat Med* 8:1211–1217.

Steinberg D, Parthasarathy S, Carew TE, Khoo JC, Witztum JL (1989). Beyond cholesterol: modification of low density lipoprotein that increases its atherogenicity. *N Engl J Med* 320:915–924.

Suarna C, Hood RL, Dean RT, Stocker R (1993). Comparative antioxidant activity of tocotrienols and other natural lipid-soluble antioxidants in a homogeneous system and in rat and human lipoproteins. *Biochim Biophys Acta* 24:163–170.

Suzuki YJ, Tsuchiya M, Wassall SR, Choo YM, Govil G, Kagan VE, Packe L (1993). Structural and dynamic membrane properties of alpha-tocopherol and alpha- tocotrienol: implication to the molecular mechanism of their antioxidant potency. *Biochemistry* 32:10692–10699.

Tan B (2010). Tocotrienols: the new vitamin E. *Spacedocnet*, March 10, 2010.

Temple NJ (2000). Antioxidants and disease: more questions than answers. *Nutr Res* 20:449–459.

Theriault A, Chao J-T, Gapor A (2002). Tocotrienol is the most effective vitamin E for reducing endothelial expression of adhesion molecules and adhesion to monocytes. *Atherosclerosis* 160:21–30.

Theriault A, Chao JT, Wang Q, Gapor A, Adeli K (1999). Tocotrienols: A review of its therapeutic potential. *Clin Biochem* 32(5):309–319.

Tomeo AC, Geller M, Watkins TR, Gapor A, Bierenbaum ML (1995). Antioxidant effects of tocotrienols in patients with hyperlipidemia and carotid stenosis. *Lipids* 30:1179–1183.

Upston JM, Witting PK, Brown AJ, Stocker R, Keaney JF Jr (2001). Effect of vitamin E on aortic lipid oxidation and intimal proliferation after arterial injury in cholesterol-fed rabbits. *Free Radic Biol Med* 31(10):1245–1253.

Valentin HE, Qi Q (2005). Biotechnological production and application of vitamin E: current state and prospects. *Appl Microbiol Biotechnol* 68:436–444.

Vivekananthan DP, Pen MS, Sapp SK, Hsu A, Topol EJ (2003). Use of antioxidant vitamins for the prevention of vascular disease: Meta-analysis of randomized trials. *Lancet* 361(9374):2017–2023.

Wilson PWF, Dagostino RB, Levy D, Belanger AM, Silbershatz H, Kannel WB (1998). Prediction of coronary heart disease using risk factor categories. *Circulation* 97:1837–1847.

Wu SJ, Liu PL, Lean-Teik N (2008). c-Tocotrienol-rich fraction of palm oil exhibits anti-inflammatory property by suppressing the expression of inflammatory mediators in human monocytic cells. *Mol Nutr Food Res* 52:921–929.

Yoshida Y, Hayakawa M, Habuchi Y, Itoh N, Niki E (2007). Evaluation of lipophilic antioxidant efficacy in vivo by the biomarkers hydroxyoctadecadienoic acid and isoprostane. *Lipids* 42:463–472.

Zieliński H (2002). Low molecular weight antioxidants in the cereal grains. *Pol J Food Nutr Sci* 11/52:3–9.

13 Tocotrienols
Viable Options for Managing Metabolic Diseases

Chi-Wai Wong

CONTENTS

13.1 INTRODUCTION

Diabetes, dyslipidemia, and hypercholesterolemia are major risk factors for cardiovascular disease and stroke. These metabolic diseases are affecting an increasing number of people in not only developed but also developing countries. The World Health Organization estimates that more than 220 million people worldwide currently have diabetes with more than 80% of diabetes-associated deaths occurring disproportionately in low- and middle-income countries (http://www.who.int/mediacentre/factsheets/fs312/en/index.html). In this decade, China is estimated to lose $558 billion in foregone national income due to heart disease, stroke, and diabetes. The importance of understanding the etiology of metabolic diseases cannot be understated for administrating appropriate treatments and developing preventive strategies.

13.2 OXIDATIVE STRESS, INSULIN RESISTANCE, AND DIABETES

Diabetes is characterized by hyperglycemia or elevated blood glucose level. Unmanaged hyperglycemia causes damage to nerves and blood vessels, leading to diabetic complications such as neuropathy, retinopathy, and nephropathy. Normally, pancreatic beta-islet cells secrete more insulin in response to a raise in blood glucose level. As a hormone, insulin signals to responsive cells including those of the liver, muscle, and fat depot to absorb and store glucose in the form of glycogen or triglyceride in these tissues, thereby lowering blood glucose level. Type I diabetes results from a loss of insulin-producing pancreatic beta-islet cells, often due to attacks by autoimmune antibodies (Waldron-Lynch and Herold, 2011). On the other hand, more than 90% of diabetics are type II, which is primarily due to insulin resistance, that is, a loss of insulin responsiveness, in target tissues (Petersen and Shulman, 2006).

The inability to properly respond to insulin or insulin resistance is thought to be a precursor to developing diabetes. Insulin binds to insulin receptor (IR), a transmembrane receptor tyrosine kinase, and triggers a signaling cascade to downstream effectors to affect glucose uptake, glycogen synthesis, and other metabolic pathways (Petersen and Shulman, 2006). Insulin receptor substrates (IRS) are important mediators that are phosphorylated at tyrosine residues by IR. IR-mediated tyrosine phosphorylation of IRS recruits other signaling molecules such as phosphatidylinositol 3-kinases (PI3Ks) to form a signaling complex. In turn, the PI3K pathway is activated to transmit the signal downstream to effectors including glucose transporters and glycogen synthase to affect glucose uptake and glycogen synthesis. On the other hand, phosphorylation of IRS at serine residues by other kinases affects the ability of IR to tyrosine phosphorylate IRS. In particular, phosphorylation by stress-activated kinases such as JNK and p38MAPK suppresses the ability of IR to phosphorylate IRS; thus, stress, in particular oxidative stress, has a negative impact on insulin signaling and is one of the causes of insulin resistance (Evans et al., 2002). Other conditions such as chronic inflammation are also known to contribute to insulin resistance partly through cross-talking with stress-activated kinases.

Sustained oxidative stress is an important contributor of insulin resistance; therefore, understanding the sources of oxidative stress becomes a priority for preventing diabetes (Whaley-Connell et al., 2011). Oxidative stress is a result of an imbalance between the production and detoxification of reactive oxygen species (ROS). ROS can be produced by a number of enzymes including those in the mitochondrial electron transport chain. Activated oxygen produced in mitochondria during oxidative phosphorylation is a major source of ROS. It is believed that excessive nutrition or obesity provides too much fuel for mitochondrial oxidative phosphorylation and elevates the level of ROS. An antioxidant system, comprised of detoxifying enzymes such as superoxide dismutase, catalase, and glutathione peroxidase, is normally in place to keep the amount of ROS in check. However, this defense system may be overwhelmed by excessive nutrition or chronic inflammation, triggering oxidative stress-activated kinases and contributing to insulin resistance.

13.3   VITAMIN E: TOCOPHEROLS

As an essential nutrient, vitamin E has been studied for its anticancer, antioxidant, and anti-inflammatory actions (Schneider, 2005). Based on these properties, vitamin E is popularly believed to be chemopreventive and antiaging as well as expected to alleviate symptoms due to oxidative stress or chronic inflammation. Two structurally distinct classes of chemicals, namely, tocopherols and tocotrienols, comprise vitamin E. α-tocopherol is the commonly available form found in health supplements; thus, most clinical studies are conducted using α-tocopherol as the major form of vitamin E. Disappointingly, long-term clinical studies concluded that vitamin E is not chemopreventive or cardioprotective. Specifically, no significant effect on the incidences of myocardial infarction, stroke, and total cancer (breast, lung, and colon cancers) were observed in the Women's Health Study (Lee et al., 2005). Additional analyses of the Women's Health Study also showed no significant reductions in the risk of developing diabetes (Liu et al., 2006) and rheumatoid arthritis (Karlson et al., 2008). In fact, vitamin E was associated with a higher risk of heart failure and hospitalization for heart failure in the initial Heart Outcomes Prevention Evaluation (HOPE) and the extended HOPE-The Ongoing Outcomes (HOPE-TOO) trials (Lonn et al., 2005). This cardiovascular risk was further confirmed in the GISSI-Prevenzione trial showing that vitamin E treatment was associated with a significant 50% increase of congestive heart failure in patients with left ventricular dysfunction (Marchioli et al., 2006). These adverse effects are perhaps reasons behind a statistically significant relationship between vitamin E dosage and all-cause mortality (Miller et al., 2005). Collectively, these studies suggest that vitamin E in the form of α-tocopherol is not effective in reducing the risks of a multitude of diseases.

13.4   VITAMIN E: TOCOTRIENOLS

α-, β-, γ-, and δ-tocotrienol are different forms of vitamin E that are naturally found in rice barn, wheat germ, barley, saw palmetto, palm fruits, and annatto. Tocotrienols differ from tocopherols by possessing three double bonds in the phytyl side chain. Studies on tocotrienols reveal not only their antioxidant activities but also several intriguing aspects, particularly in regard to metabolic pathways, that are different from tocopherols.

13.4.1   TOCOTRIENOLS AS CHOLESTEROL- AND TRIGLYCERIDE-SUPPRESSING AGENTS

Excessive amount of serum cholesterol particularly in the form of low-density-lipoprotein cholesterol (LDL-C) is a major contributor to atherosclerosis development. A rate-limiting enzyme in cholesterol synthesis is 3-hydroxy-3-methyl-glutaryl-coenzyme A (HMG-CoA) reductase. While the most commercially successful class of cholesterol-lowering drug statins act as direct inhibitors of HMG-CoA reductase, tocotrienols suppress the activity of HMG-CoA reductase at posttranscriptional levels (Parker et al., 1993; Pearce et al., 1992, 1994). The mechanism of action is thought to involve ubiquitin-mediated degradation of HMG-CoA reductase (Song et al., 2006). The ability of tocotrienols to suppress the activity of HMG-CoA reductase appears to contribute to their anti-atherosclerosis effects in animal models (Black et al., 2000; Ismail et al., 2000). However, strong clinical evidence supporting that tocotrienols are effective in lowering serum cholesterol levels in humans and preventing atherosclerosis development is still missing. Intriguingly, tocotrienols had been shown in borderline-high cholesterol patients to lower serum triglycerides with concomitant reductions in triglyceride-rich very-low-density lipoprotein and chylomicrons (Zaiden et al., 2010). In addition, in type II diabetic patients, tocotrienols reduced serum triglycerides, total cholesterol, and LDL-C levels (Baliarsingh et al., 2005). Data from these small-scale trials imply that tocotrienols are effective in modifying unfavorable parameters associated with metabolic diseases in human.

13.4.2   TOCOTRIENOLS AS ANTIDIABETIC AGENTS

Investigations into whether tocotrienols can also function as antidiabetic agents are primarily based on animal models. Streptozotocin (STZ) is a chemical that is particularly toxic to the insulin-producing pancreatic beta-islet cells. It is frequently used in medical research to produce animal models for type I diabetes. In an STZ-induced diabetic rat model, tocotrienol rich fraction (TRF) from palm oil reduced serum glucose and glycated hemoglobin concentrations in addition to lowering serum total cholesterol, LDL-C, and triglyceride levels (Budin et al., 2009). Similarly, a rice bran oil diet containing γ-tocotrienol improved insulin sensitivity as well as lowered serum triglyceride, LDL-C, and hepatic triglyceride levels in type II diabetes rats induced by STZ and nicotinamide (Chen et al., 2006; Chou et al., 2009). Besides strengthening the lipid lowering effects observed in previously mentioned clinical trials, these studies further suggest that tocotrienols may be effective in enhancing insulin sensitivity. In fact, there are additional tantalizing pieces of evidence to suggest that tocotrienols alleviate symptoms of diabetic complication such as nephropathy and neuropathy. Assessed by biochemical markers of renal function in urine and oxidative stress markers in kidney tissue, both TRF from palm oil and rice bran oil significantly improved renal function in type I diabetic rats (Siddiqui et al., 2010). Furthermore, diabetic rats develop neuropathy shown by marked hyperalgesia and allodynia associated with enhanced nitrosative stress, and release of inflammatory mediators. Tocotrienols significantly attenuated behavioral, biochemical, and molecular changes associated with diabetic neuropathy (Kuhad et al., 2009). Although these studies generally support the notion that tocotrienols are antidiabetic, how tocotrienols function at the molecular level to enhance insulin sensitivity is still not known.

13.4.3 TOCOTRIENOLS AS SELECTIVE PEROXISOME PROLIFERATORS-ACTIVATED RECEPTOR MODULATORS

Since chronic inflammation contributes to diabetes, tocotrienols may function as anti-inflammatory agents to prevent the development of diabetes. Nuclear factor kappa-light-chain-enhancer of activated B cells (NF-κB) protein complex is intimately involved in cellular inflammatory responses to oxidative stress such as ROS, pro-inflammatory cytokines such as tumor necrosis factor alpha (TNFα), and bacterial or viral agents such as lipopolysaccharide (LPS). Activation of NF-κB is in part mediated through phosphorylation and degradation of an inhibitor complex IκB by an IκB kinase. NF-κB controls the transcription of genes including inducible nitric oxide synthase (iNOS) and cyclooxygenase-2 (COX2) that respectively catalyze the production of nitric oxide and prostaglandins serving as secondary signals. γ-tocotrienol had been found to abolish TNFα- and LPS-induced NF-κB activation (Ahn et al., 2007). Specifically, γ-tocotrienol blocked TNFα-induced phosphorylation and degradation of IκB through inhibiting IκB kinase activation; thus, leading to a suppression of phosphorylation and nuclear translocation of NF-κB (Ahn et al., 2007). TRF of palm oil also suppressed the inductions of iNOS and COX2 expression by LPS-activated NF-κB (Shu-Jing Wu, 2008). Among the different isoforms within TRF, δ-tocotrienol appeared to be the most effective (Yam et al., 2009). Importantly, α-tocopherol was not effective, indicating that being an antioxidant *per se* is not sufficient to suppress NF-κB activation.

Since tocotrienols suppress NF-κB activation, it is possible that tocotrienols utilize mechanisms close to other natural or synthetic chemicals that modulate NF-κB activity. Intriguingly, a set of insulin sensitizers, drugs that are proven to improve insulin signaling and clinically used to treat type II diabetes, collectively referred to as thiazolidinediones share similar anti-inflammatory properties by suppressing NF-κB activity. Among these thiazolidinediones, rosiglitazone and pioglitazone are still being marketed while troglitazone was withdrawn from the market due to idiosyncratic liver toxicity. These thiazolidinediones function as ligands for peroxisome proliferator–activated receptors (PPARs), in particular, PPARγ.

Three distinctive genes encode PPARα, PPARγ, and PPARδ isotypes that belong to the nuclear hormone receptor superfamily of ligand-regulated transcription factors (Desvergne et al., 1999). For example, PPARγ contains an N-terminal ligand-independent transcriptional domain, a centrally located DNA binding domain (DBD), a variable hinge region, and a C-terminally located ligand binding domain (LBD) that is responsible for recognizing and binding to a variety of structurally distinctive ligands such as thiazolidinediones. PPARs play essential roles during the development of diabetes and atherosclerosis through regulating energy metabolism and inflammation. Endogenous ligands for PPARs such as unsaturated fatty acid, prostaglandins, and lysophosphatidic acid are key physiological regulators of metabolic pathways and inflammatory responses (Forman et al., 1995; Gupta et al., 2000; Keller et al., 1993; Kliewer et al., 1995; Yu et al., 1995). Besides, genetic mutations of PPARγ are associated with insulin resistance and diabetes in human (Stumvoll and Haring, 2002). Additionally, manipulating PPAR expression levels in rodents suggested that PPARs participate in regulating insulin sensitivity and atherosclerosis development (Jones et al., 2005; Lee et al., 2006; Wang et al., 2003). Importantly, synthetic PPARα ligands such as fibrates and PPARγ ligands such as thiazolidinediones are prescription drugs for dyslipidemia and diabetes (Staels and Fruchart, 2005), whereas synthetic ligands for PPARδ are currently under development for metabolic diseases (Oliver et al., 2001).

The actions of tocotrienols in many respects mirror ligands that modulate the activities of PPARs. First of all, both preliminary clinical and animal model studies suggest that tocotrienols not only function as insulin sensitizers to alleviate the symptoms of diabetes but also as agents that reduce serum lipids levels (Baliarsingh et al., 2005; Budin et al., 2009; Chen et al., 2006; Zaiden et al., 2010). These aspects are reminiscent of PPARγ ligands thiazolidinediones and PPARα ligands fibrates. Second, tocotrienols are anti-inflammatory similar to thiazolidinediones and fibrates by suppressing the activation of NF-κB (Ahn et al., 2007; Shu-Jing Wu, 2008; Yam et al., 2009). Third, both thiazolidinediones and TRF had been demonstrated in animal models to be cardioprotective by reducing the extent of myocardial infarction induced by global ischemia followed by reperfusion (Das et al., 2008; Lekli et al., 2010). Finally, the chromanol ring of tocotrienol is commonly found in troglitazone, a ligand of PPARγ. These coincidents imply that tocotrienols may bind to PPARs and function as selective modulators to exert their anti-inflammatory and insulin-sensitizing effects.

The hypothesis that tocotrienols are PPAR modulators was tested recently by my group (Fang et al., 2010; Li et al., 2010). We examined whether TRF of palm oil modulated the activities of PPARs by reporter-based assays under the control of PPARs and found that TRF dose-dependently and potently activated the activity of PPARα while modestly activated the activities of PPARγ and PPARδ (Fang et al., 2010; Li et al., 2010). We further found that purified α-, γ-, and δ-tocotrienol dose-dependently and potently enhanced the activity of PPARα while δ-tocotrienol modestly enhanced the activities of PPARγ and PPARδ, recapitulating the pan-agonistic activities of TRF. Since PPARs recruit cofactors such as PPARγ coactivator-1α (PGC-1α) through its LXXLL motifs in a ligand-dependent manner for activation (Puigserver et al., 1998), we also examined the abilities of tocotrienols to enhance this interaction. We employed a cell-free *in vitro* system to confirm if α-, γ-, and δ-tocotrienol can bind to the LBD of PPARα and recruit LXXLL peptides derived from PGC-1α. We found that purified PPARα-LBD was indeed induced dose-dependently to interact with LXXLL peptides by α-, γ-, and δ-tocotrienol (Fang et al., 2010). Collectively, these results suggest that α-, γ-, and δ-tocotrienol are direct agonists for PPARs with a preference for PPARα.

Besides these *in vitro* and cell-based results, we additionally examined if TRF of palm oil can function as PPAR modulators to improve glucose disposal and insulin sensitivity in diabetic *Db/Db* mice. Oral glucose tolerance test (OGTT) and insulin tolerance test (ITT) were used to assess the glucose and insulin sensitivities of *Db/Db* mice. We found that TRF was able to lower the fasting blood glucose level and reduce the areas under the curve in both OGTT and ITT (Fang et al., 2010), indicating improvements in both glucose and insulin sensitivities. Importantly, we found in a major insulin-responsive tissue responsible for metabolizing the majority of glucose, that is, the skeletal muscle, that the mRNA expression patterns of key metabolic regulatory genes were altered. Specifically, TRF treatment enhanced the expression levels of glucose transporter 4 (Glut4), which is primarily responsible for insulin-stimulated glucose uptake in skeletal muscle (Ishiki et al., 2005), under both fasting and fed states (Fang et al., 2010). Similarly, we found that the expression level of carnitine palmitoyl transferase 2 (CPT2), which is responsible for initiating long-chain fatty acid β-oxidation in mitochondria (Brady et al., 1993), was induced by TRF in the fed state (Fang et al., 2010). On the other hand, we found that the expression level of uncoupling protein 3 (UCP3), which is responsible for fine tuning mitochondrial membrane potential and promoting β-oxidation (Bezaire et al., 2007), was significantly enhanced in the fed state (Fang et al., 2010). Of note, the transcriptional regulations of Glut4, CPT2, and UCP3 in the muscle had been demonstrated to be regulated in part by PPARs (Dressel et al., 2003; Muoio et al., 2002; Ye et al., 2001). These data collectively suggest that TRF altered expression levels of PPAR-target genes associated with glucose uptake and β-oxidation to promote energy utilization.

PPARs have also been implicated to play essential roles during the development of atherosclerosis and synthetic ligands of these receptors have anti-atherogenic activities in rodent models of atherosclerosis. Specifically, synthetic ligands of PPARs prevent the developments of atherosclerosis in apolipoprotein E-null (*ApoE$^{-/-}$*) and low density lipoprotein receptor-null (*LDLR$^{-/-}$*) animals. In particular, the mechanism of action of PPARγ is thought to be mediated at least in part through enhancing the expression of liver X receptor alpha (LXRα) in macrophages (Chawla et al., 2001). The induced LXR in turn promotes the expressions of ATP-binding cassette (ABC) transporter family including subfamily A member 1 (ABCA1) and subfamily G member 1 (ABCG1) as well as apolipoprotein C-I (ApoC-I) and C-II (ApoC-II) (Mak et al., 2002; Oliver et al., 2001). These transporters and lipoproteins help promote the efflux of cholesterol from macrophages to the liver to be converted into bile acids or exported as high density lipoproteins. Therefore, we further addressed if TRF can attenuate the extent of atherosclerosis in $ApoE^{-/-}$ mice. We found that TRF induced the expression of cholesterol transporters, apolipoproteins, and LXRα in $ApoE^{-/-}$ mice, but TRF did not act as an agonist for LXRs (Li et al., 2010). Since PPARs are upstream of LXRα in promoting reverse cholesterol transport, it is reasonable to speculate that TRF may induce the expression of LXRα and apolipoproteins through PPARs. Importantly, TRF treatment reduced the amount of fatty streak lesion in proximal aorta, strongly indicating that TRF can attenuate the development of atherosclerosis (Li et al., 2010). These two studies collectively indicated that tocotrienols function as selective PPAR modulators (SPPARMs) to prevent diabetes and atherosclerosis development.

Other apparent health beneficial effects of tocotrienols can also be explained by considering tocotrienols as SPPARMs. Interleukin-6 (IL-6) is an important cytokine that is associated with suppressing insulin signaling. Signal transducers and activators of transcription (STATs) are activated by IL-6. An activated STAT3 induces the expression of suppressor of cytokine signaling 3 (SOCS3) as a negative feedback mechanism. SOCS3 is also a negative regulator of insulin signaling by blocking IRS phosphorylation by IR. Intriguingly, a synthetic PPARδ ligand suppresses IL-6-mediated activation of STAT3 (Kino et al., 2007). Having demonstrated that PPARδ is preferentially activated by δ-tocotrienol, it is conceivable that δ-tocotrienol enhances insulin signaling by acting through PPARδ to interfere with STAT3 activation by IL-6, thereby blocking the induction of SOCS3, the negative regulator of insulin signaling (Serrano-Marco et al., 2011). This mechanism may also be relevant in the context of cancer as tocotrienols also interfere with STAT3 in cancer cells (Kannappan et al., 2010; Rajendran et al., 2011). Additionally, this synthetic PPARδ ligand synergizes with exercise training to increase oxidative myofibers and running endurance in adult mice (Narkar et al., 2008). Coincidentally, TRF has similar capability (Lee et al., 2009). Moreover, other synthetic PPARδ ligands elevated high-density lipoprotein cholesterol (HDL-C) in animal models. As a PPARδ modulator, perhaps it is not surprising to find that TRF also elevated HDL-C level in an animal model (Budin et al., 2009). These links are further suggestive of tocotrienols functioning as SPPARMs to exert their health beneficial effects.

13.4.4 TOCOTRIENOLS AS VIABLE OPTIONS FOR MANAGING METABOLIC DISEASES

Diabetes and cardiovascular diseases are major health risks. Countless efforts have been spent on developing better treatments for these diseases. PPARγ ligands like rosiglitazone and pioglitazone are currently used for management of diabetes while PPARα ligands like gemfibrozil and bezafibrate are prescribed for dyslipidemia. However, side effects ranging from edema, weight gain, to compromised heart function contribute to the debate regarding the risks and benefits of using PPARγ synthetic ligands for diabetes (Nissen et al., 2007). Importantly, a dual PPARα and PPARγ agonist actually increased cardiovascular risk and was terminated from marketing even after getting regulatory approval (Nissen et al., 2005). Since tocotrienol supplements have not been associated with adverse cardiovascular events but in fact reduce cardiovascular risk factors in small clinical trials, our results also raise an intriguing question whether these natural PPAR ligands may be better medicines for management of metabolic syndrome compared to synthetic PPAR ligands. Additionally, our results call into question whether the vitamin E supplement taken by millions of people daily in the form of α-tocopherol is the right form of vitamin E that confers the greatest beneficial effect.

REFERENCES

Ahn, KS, Sethi, G, Krishnan, K, Aggarwal, BB (2007) {Gamma}-tocotrienol inhibits nuclear factor-{kappa}B signaling pathway through inhibition of receptor-interacting protein and TAK1 leading to suppression of antiapoptotic gene products and potentiation of apoptosis. *J Biol Chem* 282(1): 809–820.

Baliarsingh, S, Beg, ZH, Ahmad, J (2005) The therapeutic impacts of tocotrienols in type 2 diabetic patients with hyperlipidemia. *Atherosclerosis* 182(2): 367–374.

Bezaire, V, Seifert, EL, Harper, ME (2007) Uncoupling protein-3: clues in an ongoing mitochondrial mystery. *FASEB J* 21(2): 312–324.

Black, TM, Wang, P, Maeda, N, Coleman, RA (2000) Palm tocotrienols protect ApoE +/– mice from diet-induced atheroma formation. *J Nutr* 130(10): 2420–2426.

Brady, PS, Ramsay, RR, Brady, LJ (1993) Regulation of the long-chain carnitine acyltransferases. *FASEB J* 7(11): 1039–1044.

Budin, SB, Othman, F, Louis, SR, Bakar, MA, Das, S, Mohamed, J (2009) The effects of palm oil tocotrienol-rich fraction supplementation on biochemical parameters, oxidative stress and the vascular wall of strep-tozotocin-induced diabetic rats. *Clinics (Sao Paulo)* 64(3): 235–244.

Chawla, A, Boisvert, WA, Lee, C-H, Laffitte, BA, Barak, Y, Joseph, SB, Liao, D, Nagy, L, Edwards, PA, Curtiss, LK, Evans, RM, Tontonoz, P (2001) A PPAR[gamma]-LXR-ABCA1 pathway in macrophages is involved in cholesterol efflux and atherogenesis. *Molecular Cell* 7(1): 161–171.

Chen, C-W, Cheng, H-H (2006) A rice bran oil diet increases LDL-receptor and HMG-CoA reductase mRNA expressions and insulin sensitivity in rats with streptozotocin/nicotinamide-induced type 2 diabetes. *J Nutr* 136(6): 1472–1476.

Chou, TW, Ma, CY, Cheng, HH, Chen, YY, Lai, MH (2009) A rice bran oil diet improves lipid abnormalities and suppress hyperinsulinemic responses in rats with streptozotocin/nicotinamide-induced type 2 diabetes. *J Clin Biochem Nutr* 45(1): 29–36.

Das, S, Lekli, I, Das, M, Szabo, G, Varadi, J, Juhasz, B, Bak, I, Nesaretam, K, Tosaki, A, Powell, SR, Das, DK (2008) Cardioprotection with palm oil tocotrienols: Comparison of different isomers. *Am J Physiol Heart Circ Physiol* 294(2): H970–H978.

Desvergne, B, Wahli, W (1999) Peroxisome proliferator-activated receptors: nuclear control of metabolism. *Endocr Rev* 20(5): 649–688. DOI: 10.1210/er.20.5.649.

Dressel, U, Allen, TL, Pippal, JB, Rohde, PR, Lau, P, Muscat, GEO (2003) The peroxisome proliferator-acti-vated receptor {beta}/{delta} agonist, GW501516, regulates the expression of genes involved in lipid catabolism and energy uncoupling in skeletal muscle cells. *Mol Endocrinol* 17(12): 2477–2493. DOI: 10.1210/me.2003-0151.

Evans, JL, Goldfine, ID, Maddux, BA, Grodsky, GM (2002) Oxidative stress and stress-activated signaling pathways: a unifying hypothesis of type 2 diabetes. *Endocr Rev* 23(5): 599–622.

Fang, F, Kang, Z, Wong, C (2010) Vitamin E tocotrienols improve insulin sensitivity through activating peroxi-some proliferator-activated receptors. *Mol Nutr Food Res* 54(3): 345–352.

Forman, BM, Tontonoz, P, Chen, J, Brun, RP, Spiegelman, BM, Evans, RM (1995) 15-deoxy-[delta]12,14-prostaglandin J2 is a ligand for the adipocyte determination factor PPAR[gamma]. *Cell* 83(5): 803–812.

Gupta, RA, Tan, J, Krause, WF, Geraci, MW, Willson, TM, Dey, SK, DuBois, RN (2000) Prostacyclin-mediated activation of peroxisome proliferator-activated receptor delta in colorectal cancer. *Proc Natl Acad Sci USA* 97(24): 13275–13280. DOI: 10.1073/pnas.97.24.13275.

Ishiki, M, Klip, A (2005) Minireview: recent developments in the regulation of glucose transporter-4 traffic: new signals, locations, and partners. *Endocrinology* 146(12): 5071–5078.

Ismail, NM, Ghafar, NA, Jaarin, K, Khine, JH, Top, GM (2000) Vitamin E and factors affecting atherosclerosis in rabbits fed a cholesterol-rich diet. *Int J Food Sci Nutr* 51(0): 79–94.

Jones, JR, Barrick, C, Kim, K-A, Lindner, J, Blondeau, B, Fujimoto, Y, Shiota, M, Kesterson, RA, Kahn, BB, Magnuson, MA (2005) Deletion of PPAR{gamma} in adipose tissues of mice protects against high fat diet-induced obesity and insulin resistance. *Proc Natl Acad Sci USA* 102(17): 6207–6212. DOI: 10.1073/pnas.0306743102.

Kannappan, R, Yadav, VR, Aggarwal, BB (2010) {Gamma}-tocotrienol but not {gamma}-tocopherol blocks STAT3 cell signaling pathway through induction of protein-tyrosine phosphatase SHP-1 and sensitizes tumor cells to chemotherapeutic agents. *J Biol Chem* 285(43): 33520–33528.

Karlson, EW, Shadick, NA, Cook, NR, Buring, JE, Lee, IM (2008) Vitamin E in the primary prevention of rheumatoid arthritis: the Women's Health Study. *Arthritis Rheum* 59(11): 1589–1595.

Keller, H, Dreyer, C, Medin, J, Mahfoudi, A, Ozato, K, Wahli, W (1993) Fatty acids and retinoids control lipid metabolism through activation of peroxisome proliferator-activated receptor-retinoid X receptor heterodimers. *Proc Natl Acad Sci USA* 90(6): 2160–2164.

Kino, T, Rice, KC, Chrousos, GP (2007) The PPARdelta agonist GW501516 suppresses interleukin-6-mediated hepatocyte acute phase reaction via STAT3 inhibition. *Eur J Clin Invest* 37(5): 425–433.

Kliewer, SA, Lenhard, JM, Willson, TM, Patel, I, Morris, DC, Lehmann, JM (1995) A prostaglandin J2 metab-olite binds peroxisome proliferator-activated receptor [gamma] and promotes adipocyte differentiation. *Cell* 83(5): 813–819.

Kuhad, A, Chopra, K (2009) Tocotrienol attenuates oxidative-nitrosative stress and inflammatory cascade in experimental model of diabetic neuropathy. *Neuropharmacology* 57(4): 456–462.

Lee, IM, Cook, NR, Gaziano, JM, Gordon, D, Ridker, PM, Manson, JE, Hennekens, CH, Buring, JE (2005) Vitamin E in the primary prevention of cardiovascular disease and cancer: The Women's Health Study: A randomized controlled trial. *JAMA* 294(1): 56–65.

Lee, SP, Mar, GY, Ng, LT (2009) Effects of tocotrienol-rich fraction on exercise endurance capacity and oxidative stress in forced swimming rats. *Eur J Appl Physiol* 107(5): 587–595.

Lee, C-H, Olson, P, Hevener, A, Mehl, I, Chong, L-W, Olefsky, JM, Gonzalez, FJ, Ham, J, Kang, H, Peters, JM, Evans, RM (2006) PPAR{delta} regulates glucose metabolism and insulin sensitivity. *Proc Natl Acad Sci USA* 103(9): 3444–3449. DOI: 10.1073/pnas.0511253103.

Lekli, I, Ray, D, Mukherjee, S, Gurusamy, N, Ahsan, MK, Juhasz, B, Bak, I et al. (2010) Co-ordinated autophagy with resveratrol and gamma-tocotrienol confers synergetic cardioprotection. *J Cell Mol Med* 14(10): 2506–2518.

Li, F, Tan, W, Kang, Z, Wong, CW (2010) Tocotrienol enriched palm oil prevents atherosclerosis through modulating the activities of peroxisome proliferators-activated receptors. *Atherosclerosis* 211(1): 278–282.

Liu, S, Lee, IM, Song, Y, Van Denburgh, M, Cook, NR, Manson, JE, Buring, JE (2006) Vitamin E and risk of type 2 diabetes in the women's health study randomized controlled trial. *Diabetes* 55(10): 2856–2862.

Lonn, E, Bosch, J, Yusuf, S, Sheridan, P, Pogue, J, Arnold, JM, Ross, C et al. (2005) Effects of long-term vitamin E supplementation on cardiovascular events and cancer: a randomized controlled trial. *JAMA* 293(11): 1338–1347.

Mak, PA, Laffitte, BA, Desrumaux, C, Joseph, SB, Curtiss, LK, Mangelsdorf, DJ, Tontonoz, P, Edwards, PA (2002) Regulated expression of the apolipoprotein E/C-I/C-IV/C-II gene cluster in murine and human macrophages. A CRITICAL ROLE FOR NUCLEAR LIVER X RECEPTORS alpha AND beta 10.1074/jbc.M202993200. *J Biol Chem* 277(35): 31900–31908.

Marchioli, R, Levantesi, G, Macchia, A, Marfisi, RM, Nicolosi, GL, Tavazzi, L, Tognoni, G, Valagussa, F (2006) Vitamin E increases the risk of developing heart failure after myocardial infarction: results from the GISSI-Prevenzione trial. *J Cardiovasc Med (Hagerstown)* 7(5): 347–350.

Miller, ER, 3rd, Pastor-Barriuso, R, Dalal, D, Riemersma, RA, Appel, LJ, Guallar, E (2005) Meta-analysis: High-dosage vitamin E supplementation may increase all-cause mortality. *Ann Intern Med* 142(1): 37–46.

Muoio, DM, Way, JM, Tanner, CJ, Winegar, DA, Kliewer, SA, Houmard, JA, Kraus, WE, Dohm, GL (2002) Peroxisome proliferator-activated receptor-{alpha} regulates fatty acid utilization in primary human skeletal muscle cells. *Diabetes* 51(4): 901–909.

Narkar, VA, Downes, M, Yu, RT, Embler, E, Wang, YX, Banayo, E, Mihaylova, MM, Nelson, MC, Zou, Y, Juguilon, H, Kang, H, Shaw, RJ, Evans, RM (2008) AMPK and PPARdelta agonists are exercise mimetics. *Cell* 134(3): 405–415.

Nissen, SE, Wolski, K (2007) Effect of rosiglitazone on the risk of myocardial infarction and death from cardiovascular causes. *N Engl J Med* 356(24): 2457–2471.

Nissen, SE, Wolski, K, Topol, EJ (2005) Effect of muraglitazar on death and major adverse cardiovascular events in patients with type 2 diabetes mellitus. *JAMA* 294(20): 2581–2586.

Oliver, WR Jr, Shenk, JL, Snaith, MR, Russell, CS, Plunket, KD, Bodkin, NL, Lewis, MC et al. (2001) A selective peroxisome proliferator-activated receptor delta agonist promotes reverse cholesterol transport. *Proc Natl Acad Sci USA* 98(9): 5306–5311.

Parker, R, Pearce, B, Clark, R, Gordon, D, Wright, J (1993) Tocotrienols regulate cholesterol production in mammalian cells by post-transcriptional suppression of 3-hydroxy-3-methylglutaryl-coenzyme A reductase. *J Biol Chem* 268(15): 11230–11238.

Pearce, BC, Parker, RA, Deason, ME, Dischino, DD, Gillespie, E, Qureshi, AA, Wright, JJK, Volk, K (1994) Inhibitors of cholesterol biosynthesis. 2. Hypocholesterolemic and antioxidant activities of benzopyran and tetrahydronaphthalene analogs of the tocotrienols. *J Med Chem* 37(4): 526–541.

Pearce, BC, Parker, RA, Deason, ME, Qureshi, AA, Wright, JJK (1992) Hypocholesterolemic activity of synthetic and natural tocotrienols. *J Med Chem* 35(20): 3595–3606.

Petersen, KF, Shulman, GI (2006) Etiology of insulin resistance. *Am J Med* 119(5 Suppl 1): S10–S16.

Puigserver, P, Wu, Z, Park, CW, Graves, R, Wright, M, Spiegelman, BM (1998) A cold-inducible coactivator of nuclear receptors linked to adaptive thermogenesis. *Cell* 92(6): 829–839.

Rajendran, P, Li, F, Manu, KA, Shanmugam, MK, Loo, SY, Kumar, AP, Sethi, G (2011) Gamma-tocotrienol is a novel inhibitor of constitutive and inducible STAT3 signalling pathway in human hepatocellular carcinoma: potential role as an antiproliferative, pro-apoptotic and chemosensitizing agent. *Br J Pharmacol* 163(2): 283–298.

Schneider, C (2005) Chemistry and biology of vitamin E. *Mol Nutr Food Res* 49(1): 7–30.

Serrano-Marco, L, Rodriguez-Calvo, R, El Kochairi, I, Palomer, X, Michalik, L, Wahli, W, Vazquez-Carrera, M (2011) Activation of peroxisome proliferator-activated receptor-{beta}/-{delta} (PPAR-{beta}/-{delta}) ameliorates insulin signaling and reduces SOCS3 levels by inhibiting STAT3 in interleukin-6-stimulated adipocytes. *Diabetes* 60(7): 1990–1999.

Shu-Jing Wu, P-LL, Lean-Teik Ng (2008) Tocotrienol-rich fraction of palm oil exhibits anti-inflammatory property by suppressing the expression of inflammatory mediators in human monocytic cells. *Mol Nutr Food Res* 52(8): 921–929.

Siddiqui, S, Rashid Khan, M, Siddiqui, WA (2010) Comparative hypoglycemic and nephroprotective effects of tocotrienol rich fraction (TRF) from palm oil and rice bran oil against hyperglycemia induced nephropathy in type 1 diabetic rats. *Chem Biol Interact* 188(3): 651–658.

Song, BL, DeBose-Boyd, RA (2006) Insig-dependent ubiquitination and degradation of 3-hydroxy-3-methylglutaryl coenzyme a reductase stimulated by delta- and gamma-tocotrienols. *J Biol Chem* 281(35): 25054–25061.

Staels, B, Fruchart, J-C (2005) Therapeutic roles of peroxisome proliferator-activated receptor agonists. *Diabetes* 54(8): 2460–2470.

Stumvoll, M, Haring, H (2002) The peroxisome proliferator-activated receptor-{gamma}2 pro12Ala polymorphism. *Diabetes* 51(8): 2341–2347.

Waldron-Lynch, F, Herold, KC (2011) Immunomodulatory therapy to preserve pancreatic beta-cell function in type 1 diabetes. *Nat Rev Drug Discov* 10(6): 439–452.

Wang YX, Lee CH, Tiep S, Yu RT, Ham J, Kang H, RM., E (2003) Peroxisome-proliferator-activated receptor delta activates fat metabolism to prevent obesity. *Cell* 113(2): 159–170.

Whaley-Connell, A, McCullough, PA, Sowers, JR (2011) The role of oxidative stress in the metabolic syndrome. *Rev Cardiovasc Med* 12(1): 21–29.

Yam, ML, Abdul Hafid, SR, Cheng, HM, Nesaretnam, K (2009) Tocotrienols suppress proinflammatory markers and cyclooxygenase-2 expression in RAW264.7 macrophages. *Lipids* 44(9): 787–797.

Ye, J-M, Doyle, PJ, Iglesias, MA, Watson, DG, Cooney, GJ, Kraegen, EW (2001) Peroxisome Proliferator–Activated Receptor (PPAR)-{alpha} activation lowers muscle lipids and improves insulin sensitivity in high fat–fed rats: comparison with PPAR-{gamma} activation. *Diabetes* 50(2): 411–417.

Yu, K, Bayona, W, Kallen, CB, Harding, HP, Ravera, CP, McMahon, G, Brown, M, Lazar, MA (1995) Differential activation of peroxisome proliferator-activated receptors by eicosanoids. *J Biol Chem* 270(41): 23975–23983.

Zaiden, N, Yap, WN, Ong, S, Xu, CH, Teo, VH, Chang, CP, Zhang, XW, Nesaretnam, K, Shiba, S, Yap, YL (2010) Gamma delta tocotrienols reduce hepatic triglyceride synthesis and VLDL secretion. *J Atheroscler Thromb* 17(10): 1019–1032.

14 Tocotrienols as Possible Treatments for Obesity

Wong Weng-Yew and Lindsay Brown

CONTENTS

14.1 DEFINING THE EXTENT OF THE OBESITY PROBLEM

Obesity is excessive fat storage, usually defined in humans by the ratio of body mass to height^2 (body mass index or BMI). In European populations, overweight is defined as BMI values >25 and obesity as values >30. In Asian populations, these cutoffs are usually decreased to 23 for overweight and 27 for obesity, since, at a given BMI, Asians have an increased percentage of body fat compared to Europeans (Deurenberg-Yap et al., 2000; WHO Expert Consultation, 2004). The incidence of obesity is increasing worldwide. The World Health Organization (WHO) estimates that more than 1 billion adults worldwide are overweight; of these, at least 300 million are obese (Ahima and Flier, 2000). In Australia, the proportion of overweight and obese adults increased from 41% in 1995 to 49% in 2004–2005 and about 61% in 2007–2008. In 2008, 42.2% of adult males were overweight and 25.4% were obese while the comparable figures for females were 31.1% and 23.7%, respectively (Australian Institute of Health and Welfare, 2008, 2010; Australian Bureau of Statistics, 2011a). This mirrors changes in other developed countries. In 2007–2008, the prevalence of obesity was 32.2% among adult men and 35.5% among adult women in the United States (Flegal et al., 2010). In the United Kingdom, the prevalence of obesity increased markedly from 13.2% of men in 1993 to 26.2% in 2010 and from 16.4% of women in 1993 to 26.2% in 2010 while the proportion of overweight was stable at 40% for men and 30% for women (The NHS Information Centre, Lifestyles Statistics, 2012)). In Sweden, this figure increased from 35% in 1980 to 52% in 2007 in adult men and from 27% to 36% in adult women (Johansson, 2010). The problem is less marked in developing countries but these societies are also showing an increasing incidence of overweight and obesity. In the decade from 1996 to 2006, the prevalence of overweight adults in Malaysia increased from 20.7% to 29.1% with an even larger proportional increase in obesity from 5.5% to 14.0% (Khambalia and Seen, 2010). In China, the prevalence of overweight and obesity (BMI ≥ 25.0 kg/m^2) among adults aged 18 years or older increased from 14.6% in 1992 to 21.8% in 2002, and the prevalence among adults aged from 18 to 44 years almost tripled (Wang et al., 2006). In populations from industrial areas in India, 30.9% of men and 32.8% of women showed abdominal obesity in 2002–2003 (Reddy et al., 2006).

Chronic diseases associated with obesity include diabetes, cardiovascular disease, liver disease, kidney disease, arthritis, and osteoporosis. Diabetes affects about 6.6% of the Australian population, with the incidence increasing with age (Australian Institute of Health and Welfare, 2010). Of the people who were registered on the National Diabetic Register in Australia between 2000 and 2007, around 69% were diagnosed with type 2 diabetes and 15% with type 1 diabetes. The remaining 16% are gestational diabetes and others. At diagnosis, 65% of the registrants were aged 45 years or over and 10% were aged <25 years (Australian Institute of Health and Welfare, 2010). Hypertension is the most common cardiovascular abnormality in Australia. Between 1999 and 2000, it was estimated that almost 30% of Australians aged 25 years and over had the disorder, or about 3.7 million Australians, with similar incidence in males and females. The proportion of those with high blood pressure increased with age in both males and females (Australian Institute of Health and Welfare, 2011a). The most common damage to the liver is fatty liver disease, considered as the liver component of metabolic syndrome, occurring in 20%–30% of adult populations in Europe and the United States, with men having approximately double the incidence of women (Aleffi et al., 2005). Obesity has been implicated as a possible risk factor for microalbuminuria with BMI positively associated with progression of IgA glomerulone-phritis (Ejerblad et al., 2006). In the Framingham Offspring cohort, BMI was positively correlated to a glomerular filtration rate in the fifth or lower percentile after long-term follow-up (Fox et al., 2004). Similarly, follow-up among participants in health screening programs in the United States (Hsu et al., 2006) and Japan (Iseki et al., 2004) demonstrated a positive relationship between BMI and risk for end-stage renal failure. Obesity is a potential risk factor for the onset and deterioration of musculoskeletal conditions of the hip, knee, ankle, foot, and shoulder. Osteoarthritis is the major cause of disability and chronic pain in Australia, placing a large burden on the community, and is more common in females than males. About 3.85 million Australians (17.1% of the male population and 19.9% of the female population) are affected by arthritis (Arthritis Queensland, 2011). Almost 700,000 Australians (3% of the population, 82% females) have been diagnosed with osteoporosis (Australian Institute of Health and Welfare, 2010) but about 2.2 million people were affected in 2006 and this is expected to increase to 3 million by 2021 (Access Economics, 2001). Osteoporosis is most common in older age groups, with <1% of people aged <25 years having osteoporosis, compared with 16% of people aged 65 years or over (Australian Bureau of Statistics, 2011b). Further, the risk of osteoporosis is increased by obesity, contrary to the common view that overweight people have higher bone density (Zhao et al., 2007).

Obesity represents a major cost to the community. In 2008 alone, the overall cost of obesity to Australian society and governments was estimated to be $58.2 billion, with the total direct financial cost of obesity for the Australian community estimated to be $8.3 billion or almost $400 for every Australian of any age (Colagiuri et al., 2010). Cardiovascular disease incurs the highest health-care cost in Australia, with direct costs of $5.94 billion in 2004–2005 or 11% of overall recurrent health system expenditure (Australian Institute of Health and Welfare, 2010). The total health sector cost for providing renal replacement therapy services from 2004 to 2010 was estimated to be between $4.26 and $4.52 billion. The costs of treating end-stage kidney disease from 2009 to 2020 were estimated to be around $12 billion to the Australian Government (Cass et al., 2010). Arthritis is esti-mated to incur around $23.9 billion each year in medical and indirect costs in Australia (Arthritis Queensland, 2011). In 2004–2005, the total direct health expenditure for osteoporosis was $304 million (Australian Institute of Health and Welfare, 2011b).

An increased BMI has long been associated with increased mortality. Large cohort studies with European patients have evaluated the increased risk as BMI increases (Flegal et al., 2005; Prospective Studies Collaboration, 2009). Median survival is reduced by 2–4 years at 30–35 kg/m^2 and by 8–10 years at 40–45 kg/m^2 (Prospective Studies Collaboration, 2009). In a similarly large study in Asian populations, underweight was associated with a substantially increased risk of death but the excess risk of death associated with a high BMI was seen among Chinese, Koreans, and Japanese only and not among Indians and Bangladeshis, possibly showing a relationship between lifestyle, education, and access to health care (Zheng et al., 2011). In the East Asia cohort, the lowest risk of death was seen among persons with a BMI in the range of 22.6–27.5. The risk was elevated among persons with higher or lower BMI values by a factor of up to 1.5 among those with a BMI of >35.0 and by a factor of 2.8 among those with a BMI of 15.0 or less (Zheng et al., 2011).

Animal models in obesity research are widely used to study the pathogenesis of obesity in early stages and the effects of drug or food interventions. Studies are usually performed on male rats and mice. There are many rodent models for obesity, such as WNIN/Ob strain (Kiran et al., 2007), the Otsuka Long-Evans Tokushima Fatty (OLETF) rats with the absence of CCK(1) receptors (Schroeder et al., 2010), Spontaneous Hypertensive/NIH Corpulent (SHR/N-cp) rat (Atgié et al., 2009), human GH (hGH) transgenic rats (Furuhata et al., 2002), *ob/ob* mice (Ingalls et al., 1996), and obese (*fa/fa*) Zucker rats (Ruth et al., 2008), yet few of these are diet-induced. To be realistic, rodent models of obesity should closely mimic the range of signs seen in the human disease and preferably these signs should be induced by diet as in humans. Models such as high fat, high carbohydrate-induced obese rats mimic the changes observed in diet-induced obese humans including obesity, diabetes, hypertension, and cardiovascular changes with liver, pancreatic, and kidney dysfunction (Panchal and Brown, 2011; Panchal et al., 2011).

Dietary changes have been perceived as the first-line intervention in obesity and its related metabolic disorders. Targeting selected components of foods as medications, defined as treatment with functional foods or nutrapharmacology, could provide protection against obesity and metabolic disorders (Ness and Powles, 1997; Srinath and Katan, 2004; Sirtori et al., 2009). Functional or medicinal foods and phytonutrients are widely accepted for maintaining well-being, enhancing health, and modulating immune function to prevent specific diseases (D'Ambrosio, 2007; Zhao, 2007). Several reviews have discussed treatment options for obesity including spices (Iyer et al., 2009), functional foods (Riccardi et al., 2005), and plant extracts (Vermaak et al., 2011). We have shown that food components such as anthocyanins from purple carrots (*Daucus carota* L. ssp. *sativus* var. *atrorubens* Alef.) (Poudyal et al., 2010), rutin from onions (Panchal et al., 2011), and Coffee (Panchal et al., 2012) reduced obesity, hypertension, fatty liver, and inflammation in rats fed a high carbohydrate, high fat diet. Epigallocatechin-3-gallate (EGCG) from green tea (*Camellia sinensis*) and curcumin from turmeric (*Curcuma longa*) produced antiobesity responses in animals and humans (Vermaak et al., 2011).

Obesity is now widely accepted as a chronic, low-grade inflammatory state (Iyer et al., 2010). Inflammation is the sum of the short-term physiological responses to cell and tissue injury and is crucial for the initiation of tissue repair. This response turns pathological when prolonged. In metabolic diseases, such as obesity and diabetes, the prolonged response is triggered by nutrients and metabolic surplus, utilizing a similar set of molecules and signaling pathways as in inflammation (Hotamisligil, 2006; Gregor and Hotamisligil, 2011). Unlike inflammation as an injury repair mechanism, the chronic inflammation in metabolic disease limits endogenous nutrient output and exogenous nutrient intake by activating multiple redundant mechanisms in response to an increase in nutrients (Hotamisligil, 2006).

There is now strong evidence that insulin resistance and inflammation are intertwined (Iyer et al., 2010; Iyer and Brown, 2010). Insulin resistance is associated with increased pro-inflammatory proteins in the circulation and metabolic tissues (Van Gaal et al., 2006). Although systemic inflammation is not always accompanied by impaired insulin action and obesity, the traditional immune/inflammatory and lipid-derived mediators could play a role in causing or aggravating insulin resistance and contributing to its establishment in a feed-forward mechanism (Pedersen and Febbraio, 2010). Surplus or excess fat from the plasma disturbs primary metabolism of fats by altering synthesis and action of metabolic hormones. Excess fat also gets deposited in the liver, heart, muscle, and pancreatic beta cells, causing lipotoxicity or initiation of specialized extracellular and intracellular signaling through lipid-derived mediators that lead to systemic inflammation and insulin resistance (Li et al., 2010).

Chronic excessive free fatty acid deposition in organs may activate NFκB pathways resulting in inflammation, formation of reactive oxygen species, and lipid-induced beta-cell apoptosis leading to beta-cell failure, type II diabetes, and insulin resistance (Unger and Zhou, 2001; Cusi, 2010). The NFκB is a family of transcription factors that plays a central role in regulating genes critical for inflammation and immunity. Suppression of the NFκB pathway will eventually lead to a lower expression of pro-inflammatory enzymes and cytokines (Yam et al., 2009). Tocotrienols blocked the activation of NFκB (Ahn et al., 2007; Aggarwal et al., 2010; Kaileh and Sen, 2010; Shirode and Sylvester, 2010). Human myeloid KBM-5 cells incubated with 25 μM γ-tocotrienol for 24 h did not activate NFκB, and TNF-α-induced NFκB activation was almost maximally abolished at 12 h in contrast to the lack of response to α-tocopherol (Ahn et al., 2007). In addition, combined treatment with subeffective doses of γ-tocotrienol (0.25 μM) and the cyclooxygenase 2 inhibitor, celecoxib (2.5 μM), resulted in a synergistic effect to downregulate NFκB, with reduced prostaglandin E2 (PGE2) synthesis and decreased cyclooxygenase 2, phospho-Akt, and phospho-NFκB concentrations (Shirode and Sylvester, 2010). The tocotrienol-rich fraction and α-, δ-, and γ-tocotrienols inhibited the release of interleukin-6 and nitric oxide, pro-inflammatory cytokines involved in acute and chronic inflammation, in lipopolysaccharide-stimulated RAW264.7 macrophages; γ-tocotrienol was the most effective homologue in most assays, possibly by NFκB inhibition (Yam et al., 2009).

14.2 VITAMIN E: TOCOPHEROLS AND TOCOTRIENOLS

Vitamin E consists of two groups of closely related compounds, the tocopherols and tocotrienols. They share a common chromanol ring with the tocopherols having a saturated phytyl side chain, differing from the geranylgeranyl side chain with three double bonds in the tocotrienols (Figure 14.1). Each group has α-, β-, γ-, and δ-homologues.

Vitamin E has been an active research area for nearly a century since the first report as a micronutrient essential for reproduction in rats (Evans and Bishop, 1922), but this research focused on α-tocopherol, since this compound was more abundant in plasma (Yap et al., 2001; Fairus et al., 2006). Despite *in vitro* and *in vivo* studies demonstrating positive antioxidant and anti-atherogenic effects with tocopherols, large clinical studies have not demonstrated benefits of tocopherols in the primary and secondary prevention of cardiovascular disease, with supplementation possibly associated with increases in total mortality, heart failure, and hemorrhagic stroke (Saremi and Arora, 2010). These neutral or negative clinical results with tocopherols warrant reconsideration of the efficacy of the tocotrienols, as new evidence has shown unique functions of these compounds (Nesaretnam

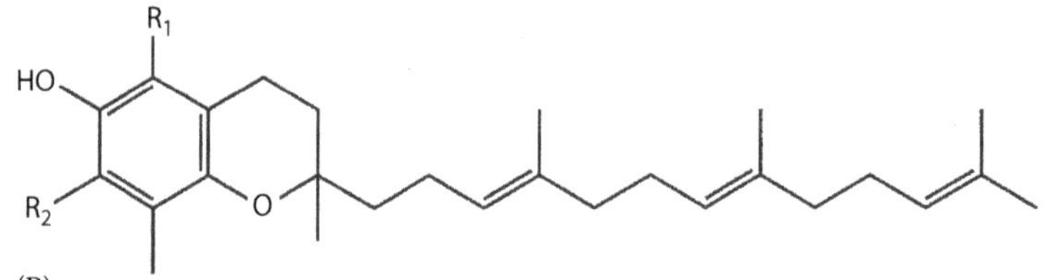

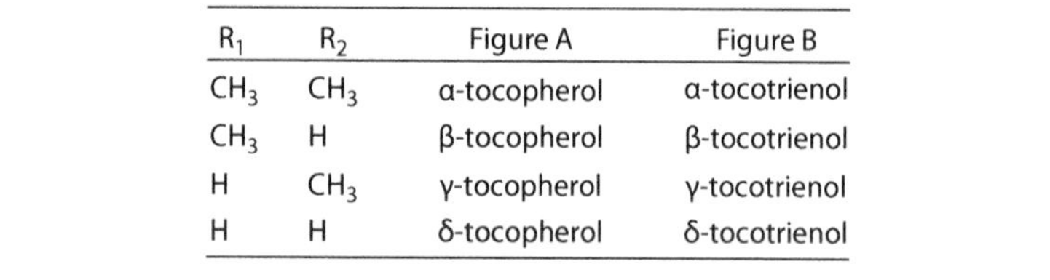

R$_1$	R$_2$	Figure A	Figure B
CH$_3$	CH$_3$	α-tocopherol	α-tocotrienol
CH$_3$	H	β-tocopherol	β-tocotrienol
H	CH$_3$	γ-tocopherol	γ-tocotrienol
H	H	δ-tocopherol	δ-tocotrienol

FIGURE 14.1 Chemical structures of naturally occuring tocopherols and tocotrienols.

et al., 2007b; Aggarwal et al., 2010). Tocotrienols possess neuroprotective, anticancer, and cholesterol-lowering properties that are often not exhibited by tocopherols (Sen et al., 2006; Aggarwal et al., 2010). α-Tocotrienol, but not α-tocopherol, prevents neurodegeneration at nanomolar concentrations, relevant considering the low plasma concentrations (Sen et al., 2007). This suggests that the molecular and therapeutic targets of the tocotrienols are distinct from those of the tocopherols (Aggarwal et al., 2010).

Conventionally, being members of the vitamin E family, tocotrienols are widely recognized for their antioxidant effects (Serbinova et al., 1991; Suzuki et al., 1993; Kamal-Eldin and Appelqvist, 1996; Kamat et al., 1997). Tocotrienols show responses additional to their antioxidant effects including anti-inflammatory, antiproliferative, antidiabetic, and cholesterol-lowering effects *in vitro* and *in vivo* (Watkins et al., 1993; McIntyre et al., 2000; Qureshi et al., 2001; Wan Nazaimoon and Khalid, 2002; Baliarsingh et al., 2005; Yam et al., 2009; Aggarwal et al., 2010; Nesaretnam et al., 2010; Yap et al., 2010; Zaiden et al., 2010). In addition, tocotrienols exhibited anti-angiogenic responses in animal models, suggesting potential in combating angiogenic disorders such as cancer and arthritis via the modulation of abnormal blood vessel formation (Carmeliet and Jain, 2000; Nakagawa et al., 2007; Miyazawa et al., 2009; Wong et al., 2009; Cao, 2010). These anti-angiogenic responses may be appropriate in the treatment of obesity.

14.3 ANGIOGENESIS AS A TARGET IN OBESITY

The vascular system is comparable to a closed plumbing system with the circulating fluid being blood, transferring various supplies that are essential for the growth of our body as well as ridding it of waste products. Proteins, vitamins, minerals, ions, and waste products are transported through this complicated vascular network. Angiogenesis is the process that is responsible for generating blood vessels in the body. It is a physiological process involving the formation of new blood vessels from existing vessels in the body.

Angiogenesis is a complex process that relies on the coordination of many different activities in cell types such as endothelial cells, pericytes, and fibroblasts, with immune mediators that express several kinds of cytokines and growth factors. These chemical mediators then modulate sequential steps involved in angiogenesis such as proteolysis, proliferation, migration, adhesion, and vessel stabilization. Hypoxia induces angiogenesis as a reparative mechanism (Bouïs et al., 2006). One of the key players in cellular hypoxia response is hypoxia-inducible factor-1α (HIF-1α). During the development of organs or when blood vessels are clogged, supply of nutrients and oxygen diminishes and this causes the body to generate new blood vessels to overcome this decrease in nutrients and oxygen. Angiogenesis is tightly controlled and regulated by a series of "on" and "off" switches. The "on" switch involves positive regulators or angiogenesis-stimulating factors such as vascular endothelial growth factor (VEGF), basic fibroblast growth factor (bFGF), transforming growth factor-β (TGF-β), interleukin-8 (IL-8), and angiopoietin-1 (Ang1) (Claffey et al., 1996; Bussolino et al., 1997; Goldman et al., 1998). The "off" switches include angiogenesis inhibitors such as angiostatin, endostatin, and interleukin-12 (IL-12) (Hayes et al., 1999). HIF-1α acts on the VEGF promoter to upregulate angiogenic gene expression (Lal et al., 2001).

In disease states, the tight balance between stimulation and inhibition is shifted, leading to unregulated angiogenesis. The excess production of pro-angiogenic factors signals to the body to generate more blood vessels (Carmeliet, 2003; Fan et al., 2006). This can have a major impact on health as angiogenesis contributes to pathological processes including tumor growth, rheumatoid arthritis, diabetic retinopathy, psoriasis, obesity, and metabolic disorders (Folkman, 1971, 1995; Hoeben et al., 2004; Lijnen, 2008; Cao, 2010). Angiogenesis is especially important for the growth of tumors as the delivery of blood-borne nutrients to the tumor cells is essential for their survival (Hanathan, 1996) and for the spread of metastatic tumor cells (Skobe et al., 1997). This discovery led to the targeting of tumor angiogenesis as a promising potential therapeutic approach for cancer treatment (Muehlbauer, 2003). This concept may also be valid in the treatment of obesity as lipids are transported to and from adipocytes by the blood.

14.4 STARVING THE ADIPOCYTES AS A CONCEPT: ANTIANGIOGENESIS WITH TOCOTRIENOLS

Angiogenesis involves several steps, including endothelial cell proliferation, migration, differentiation, and tube formation, thus providing potential targets for therapeutic intervention. Tocotrienols show anti-angiogenic properties in cancer (Nakagawa et al., 2007; Shibata et al., 2008; Miyazawa et al., 2009; Wong et al., 2009; Selvaduray et al., 2011). *In vitro* studies showed that tocotrienols inhibited the proliferation, migration, and tube formation of human umbilical vein and bovine aortic endothelial cells; δ-tocotrienol was the most potent inhibitor with potency decreasing in the order of δ->β->γ->α-tocotrienol (Miyazawa et al., 2004; Wong et al., 2009). α-Tocopherol produced no responses, suggesting that tocotrienols, but not α-tocopherol, have considerable potential as angiogenic inhibitors (Miyazawa et al., 2004; Wong et al., 2009).

The anti-angiogenic effects of tocotrienols have been shown in dorsal air sac and chick embryo chorioallantoic membrane (CAM) assays. These assays assess the formation of vessels in a biological system together with biochemical interventions (Miyazawa et al., 2009; Ribatti et al., 2001). In the dorsal air sac assay, increased neovascularization was suppressed in mice implanted with tumor cells (human colon carcinoma, DLD-1) by dietary supplementation of 10 mg/day of tocotrienol-rich fraction (equivalent to 4.4 mg/day tocotrienol mixtures) compared with control (Nakagawa et al., 2007). In CAM assay, direct inhibition of blood vessels with 200 μg/mL tocotrienol-rich fraction (Wong et al., 2009) was observed compared with control. δ-Tocotrienol (500–1000 μg/egg) inhibited new blood vessel formation on the growing CAM, while δ-Tocotrienol at 1000 μg produced a larger avascular zone (50% of tocotrienol-treated group), while α-tocopherol did not inhibit vascularization in CAM (Nakagawa et al., 2007), indicating the selective *in vivo* anti-angiogenic effects of tocotrienols.

VEGF is one of the earliest signals to stimulate tumor angiogenesis. The binding of VEGF to its receptors is important for the activation of phosphatidylinositol-3 kinase (PI3K)/PDK/Akt signaling in endothelial cells, leading to increased proliferation, survival, permeability, and migration of cells (Hoeben et al., 2004). Suppression of angiogenesis by tocotrienol-rich fraction was mediated through reduction in serum concentrations of VEGF, corresponding with a reduction in tumor size in BALB/c mice treated with 1 mg/mL/d tocotrienol-rich fraction (Wong et al., 2009) and decreased expression of VEGF and the mRNA of its receptors; VEGF-R1 (fms-like tyrosine kinase, Flt-1) and VEGF-R2 (kinase-insert-domain-containing receptor, KDR/Flk-2), in tumors excised from BALB/c mice (Selvaduray et al., 2011). PI3K is a lipid signaling kinase that activates PDK, leading to activation of Akt, which in turn phosphorylates intracellular substrates associated with cell proliferation and apoptosis (Toker, 2000). Tocotrienols induced anti-angiogenic responses via suppression of growth factor-dependent activation of PI3K/PDK/Akt signaling in neoplastic mammary cells (Samant and Sylvester, 2006; Nakagawa et al., 2007). δ-Tocotrienol suppressed the phosphorylation of phosphoinositide-dependent protein kinase (PDK) and Akt (Nakagawa et al., 2007). Further, it increased the phosphorylation of apoptosis signal-regulating kinase and p38 in fibroblast growth factor–treated human umbilical vein endothelial cells (HUVEC), indicating that the anti-angiogenic effects of tocotrienols are associated with changes in growth factor-dependent PI3K/PDK/Akt signaling as well as induction of apoptosis in endothelial cells (Nakagawa et al., 2007). Tocotrienols also suppressed the FGF receptor tyrosine phosphorylation (Nakagawa et al., 2007). Since antiangiogenesis has been recognized as an appropriate strategy in combating cancer (Kim et al., 1993), it may also be applicable in metabolic diseases.

The central feature of metabolic disorders is an increase in abdominal adipose tissue (Soares, 2009). Adipose tissue is much more than an energy storage depot as it is a complex and dynamic organ, including lipid-filled adipocytes, endothelial cells, pericytes, fibroblasts, preadipocytes, mast cells, and immune cells such as resident macrophages and T cells (Lee et al., 2010). Adipocytes and immune cells within adipose tissue release many bioactive molecules, known as adipokines and pro-inflammatory cytokines, to initiate vascular dysfunction, atherosclerosis, and impaired glucose metabolism (Haffner, 2006; Van Gaal et al., 2006). Adipose growth is regulated by angiogenesis; the vasculature responds by increasing blood vessel density to supply the growing adipose tissue with nutrients and oxygen (Lijnen, 2008). Adipose tissue angiogenesis has been described as a cause of metabolic disorders since modulators of angiogenesis can regulate the expansion and metabolism of fat mass (Lijnen, 2008; Cao, 2010).

14.5 ADIPOSE TISSUE VASCULATURE

Angiogenesis is essential for adipose tissue. Unlike most other tissues, adipose tissue continuously undergoes expansion and regression throughout adult life. The expansion requires the parallel growth of its capillary network for the supply of oxygen, nutrients, plasma rich in growth factors and cytokines, stem cells required for differentiation, monocytes, and neutrophils to infiltrate the tissue (Crossno et al., 2006; Hotamisligil, 2006; Cao, 2007, 2010; Powell, 2007; Christiaens and Lijnen, 2010). Therefore, adipogenesis is tightly associated with angiogenesis.

Adipose tissue has a well-defined vascular system with capillaries surrounding every adipocyte. Its development is characterized by the appearance of a number of fat cell clusters, also known as the "primitive organs." These are vascular structures in the adipose tissue with few or no fat cells. Formation of primitive fat organs occurs at perivascular sites during embryo development (Hausman and Richardson, 1982). Human preadipocytes and capillary endothelial cells express $\alpha_v\beta_3$ integrin and plasminogen activator inhibitor 1 (PAI-1), regulating and coordinating the migration of preadipocytes with capillary endothelial cell development at the same locus (Crandall et al., 2000). PPAR-γ mediated both preadipocyte differentiation and angiogenesis; inhibition of PPAR-γ impaired development of both (Panigrahy et al., 2002; Fukumura et al., 2003; Cao, 2007). In addition, inhibition of VEGF receptor signals prevents angiogenesis and preadipocyte differentiation, suggesting VEGF acts on endothelial cells to regulate preadipocyte differentiation (Fukumura et al., 2003).

The development of white adipose tissue (WAT) requires constant remodeling of the vasculature system, primarily of primitive capillary networks. The expansion of WAT, both adipocyte hyperplasia and hypertrophy, can be supported by neovascularization for the former and dilation as well as remodeling of existing capillaries for the latter (Lijnen, 2008). The main function of brown adipose tissue (BAT) is energy metabolism. Thus, its expansion and function rely on an efficient blood perfusion to supply nutrients and oxygen and to export heat. BAT hyperplasia is critically dependent on angiogenesis, as it requires rapid activation of mitosis in fat precursor cells and endothelial cells to develop capillaries (Bukowiecki et al., 1980).

14.6 ANGIOGENIC FACTORS

Apart from the direct crosstalk between endothelial cells and adipocytes, several conditions stimulate angiogenesis during obesity, such as hypoxia and chronic inflammation (Soares, 2009). These conditions result in the expression of transcription factors, hormones, cytokines, and growth factors, which trigger the formation of blood vessels, such as HIF-1α, VEGF, bFGF, and the matrix metalloproteinases (MMPs) (Cao, 2007; Soares, 2009).

Hypoxia plays an important role in angiogenesis of obesity. As adipose tissue expands, the demand for oxygen increases, resulting in a hypoxic condition. As a response to hypoxia, adipose tissues produce HIF-1α-induced angiogenic factors such as VEGF, leptin, tumor necrosis factor-α (TNF-α), and PAI-1, which regulate angiogenesis and vasculogenesis (Carmeliet and Jain, 2000). The tip region of adult epididymal adipose tissue was hypoxic and released high concentrations of VEGF, VEGFRs, MMP, and stromal cell-derived factor-1, which collectively attracted the accumulation of bone marrow-derived lymphatic endothelium hyaluronan receptor-positive macrophages (Cho et al., 2007).

It has been speculated that lipid mediators localized in the circulation and adipose tissue may bind to immune receptors such as class A G protein-coupled receptors and Toll-like receptors (TLRs), and induce low-grade tissue inflammation (Iyer and Brown, 2010). Chronic inflammation with concomitant cytokine and growth factors release is another primary stimulus for angiogenesis as it induces expression of angiogenic factors. Monocytes, macrophages, platelets, mast cells, and other leukocytes release a myriad of angiogenic factors including VEGF, bFGF, platelet-derived growth factor (PDGF), TNF-α, TGF-β, IL-8, Ang1, hepatocyte growth factor (HGF), insulin-like growth factor-1 (IGF-1), and monocyte chemoattractant protein-1 (MCP-1) (Carmeliet and Jain, 2000). Angiogenesis further contributes to inflammation by providing oxygen and nutrients for metabolic requirements in inflammatory sites, besides enabling extravasation of immune cells (Costa et al., 2007; Soares, 2009).

Adipose tissue is no longer considered to be an inert tissue functioning solely as an energy depot, as it is a complex and dynamic organ that secretes hormones and cytokines for both normal and abnormal tissue functions. To adapt adipose tissue to changes in size and metabolic rate, the adipose tissue vascular network is tightly regulated by angiogenic factors such as VEGF, bFGF, IL-8, Ang1, TNF-α, and PDGF (Carmeliet, 2003; Cao, 2007; Lijnen, 2008). Apart from the classical ones, several adipokines, including leptin, resistin, and visfatin, modulate angiogenic and vascular survival activities (Sierra-Honigmann et al., 1998; Tilg and Moschen, 2006; Cao, 2010). The classical angiogenic factors and angiogenic adipokines could synergistically induce angiogenesis. For example, leptin upregulated the expression of VEGF-A and synergistically induced angiogenesis (Cao et al., 2001; Aleffi et al., 2005).

Leptin is a pleiotropic molecule that regulates food intake and metabolic and endocrine responses and plays a regulatory role in hematopoiesis, inflammation, and immunity (Ahima and Flier, 2000; Fantuzzi and Faggioni, 2000). Elevated leptin concentrations correlated with obesity, hyperinsulinemia, and insulin resistance; conditions found in most patients with type 2 diabetes (Zimmet et al., 1999). Leptin produced in adipocytes is secreted into the bloodstream, but it may also act locally upon endothelial cells in a paracrine fashion, causing increased fatty acid oxidation and an angiogenic response that maintains an appropriate balance between blood supply and fat depot size (Sierra-Honigmann et al., 1998). Further, *in vitro* leptin (10–40 ng/mL) induced proliferation of HUVEC and elevation of MMP-2, MMP-9, tissue inhibitors of metalloproteinases (TIMP-1), and TIMP-2 expression in a concentration-dependent manner, apart from eliciting a comparable angiogenic activity with VEGF in rat corneal tissue (Park et al., 2001). It was suggested that leptin induced angiogenesis by upregulating the expression of HIF-1α, which regulated angiogenic gene expression via the PI3K/PDK/AKT (Aleffi et al., 2005).

The MMPs belong to a family of over 25 neutral endopeptidases. They cleave all of the extracellular matrix (ECM) components and several non-ECM proteins, namely, adhesion molecules, cytokines, protease inhibitors, and other pro-MMPs (Gomez et al., 1997; Lijnen, 2008). MMPs are involved in the development of adipose tissue. The mRNAs of some MMPs (MMP-3, -11, -12, -13, -14) mRNA were upregulated, while others (MMP-7, -9, -16, -24) were downregulated in obese mice (Maquoi et al., 2002). Most of these modulations were specific to the gonadal fat (Lijnen, 2008). The binding of VEGF to its receptors is important for the activation of PI3K/PDK/Akt signaling in endothelial cells, leading to increased proliferation, survival, permeability, and migration of cells (Hoeben et al., 2004).

VEGF, through stimulation of proliferation and migration of endothelial cells, accounts for much of the angiogenic activity of adipose tissue (Hausman and Richardson, 2004). Administration of a VEGFR-2 blocking antibody to mice reduced angiogenesis and tissue growth and also inhibited preadipocyte differentiation (Fukumura et al., 2003). These findings revealed a reciprocal regulation of adipogenesis and angiogenesis and suggested that blockade of VEGF signaling could inhibit adipose tissue formation (Fukumura et al., 2003). Oral administration of PTK787 (Vatalanib), an inhibitor of vascular endothelial growth factor receptor (VEGFR) tyrosine kinases, for 4 weeks to C57Bl/6 mice fed a high fat diet, reduced total body weight and subcutaneous and gonadal adipose tissue mass (Lijnen et al., 2007).

14.7 ANTI-ANGIOGENIC TREATMENT IN OBESITY: THE POSSIBLE ROLE OF TOCOTRIENOLS

Tocotrienols reduce tumor mass via the attenuation of angiogenesis, preventing tumors from getting blood supplies needed for survival and metastasis. To do so, tocotrienols reduce VEGF secretion and expression, regulate the PI3K/PDK/AKT pathway, hence retarding increases in the tumor vascular network (Nakagawa et al., 2007; Shibata et al., 2008; Wong et al., 2009; Selvaduray et al., 2011). This raises the question of whether tocotrienols reduce angiogenesis in non-neoplastic tissues such as adipose tissue.

The original hypothesis that angiogenesis could be a target for obesity therapy was based on the idea that the expansion and growth of WAT is dependent on angiogenesis (Cao, 2007). Therefore, as has been proven for tumor growth, inhibition of adipose tissue angiogenesis should inhibit WAT growth and ultimately impair development of obesity. Indeed, adipose tissue growth in mice can be impaired with angiogenesis inhibitors such as TNP-470 (a synthetic analog of fumagillin that selectively inhibits endothelial cell growth by suppression of methionine aminopeptidase) (Rupnick et al., 2002) and endogenous angiogenic inhibitors such as angiostatin and endostatin (Cao, 2010). Treatment with TNP-470 20 mg/kg for 16 weeks to mice fed with high fat diet reduced total body fat by 63% compared with controls (Kusaka et al., 1991). A study with 3T3-F442A preadipocytes injected into severe combined immunodeficient (SCID) mice induced angiogenesis and adipocyte differentiation (Mandrup et al., 1997). Adipogenesis and *de novo* adipose tissue formation in this model can be impaired by inhibition of PPAR-γ or VEGFR-2 (Fukumura et al., 2003) and by administration of a placental growth factor (PlGF, a member of VEGF family) neutralizing monoclonal antibody (Lijnen et al., 2006). Further, the use of an anti-VEGF antibody inhibited angiogenesis, as well as the formation of adipo/angiogenic cell clusters indicating that coupling of adipogenesis and angiogenesis is essential for differentiation of adipocytes in obesity, confirming that VEGF is a key mediator (Nishimura et al., 2007; Lijnen, 2008).

Tumors and obesity use similar mechanisms to induce angiogenesis. Both pathologies require blood vessels to survive and VEGF plays a significant role to establish vessels in these sites. VEGF binds to VEGF-R, activating the PI3K/PDK/Akt pathway that leads to differentiation of endothelial cells, migration, and thus vessel formation. These targets serve as good sites for tocotrienols to exert anti-angiogenic effects, preventing vessel sprouting to these tissues, as shown in tumors (Nakagawa et al., 2007; Shibata et al., 2008; Wong et al., 2009; Selvaduray et al., 2011). Tumor formation and adipose tissue development are stimulated by hypoxia resulting in HIF-1α binding to HRE, hence expression of angiogenic factors ensue. Tocotrienols prevented the expression of HIF-1α in tumors (Shibata et al., 2008) and this may likely work in obesity. Tocotrienols suppressed the insulin-induced mRNA expression of adipocyte-specific genes, PPAR-γ, which mediates preadipocyte differentiation and regulates angiogenesis. Inhibition of PPAR-γ impaired development of both (Panigrahy et al., 2002; Fukumura et al., 2003; Cao, 2007). Chronic inflammation with concomitant cytokine and growth factors release is another primary stimulus for angiogenesis as it induces expression of angiogenic factors. Tocotrienols reduce the release of pro-inflammatory cytokines (Yam et al., 2009). Taken together, tocotrienols may be a plausible anti-angiogenic agent for the treatment of obesity, since new evidence has shown unique functions of this compound (Nesaretnam et al., 2007b; Aggarwal et al., 2010). Further, *in vivo* studies indicated that tocotrienols accumulated in adipose tissues (Khanna et al., 2005; Nesaretnam et al., 2007a). There are therefore solid reasons why tocotrienols, not tocopherols, should be tested as possible antiobesity agents. Positive results would expand the armamentarium of compounds useful in obesity and obesity-related conditions.

REFERENCES

Access Economics 2001. The burden of brittle bones; costing osteoporosis in Australia. Canberra, Australian Capital Territory, Australia. www.boneandjointdecade.org/ViewDocument.aspx?ContId=534 (accessed on 4.5.2012).

Aggarwal, B. B., C. Sundaram, S. Prasad, and R. Kannappan 2010. Tocotrienols, the vitamin E of the 21st century: Its potential against cancer and other chronic diseases. *Biochem Pharmacol.* 80, 1613–1631.

Ahima, R. S. and J. S. Flier 2000. Leptin. *Annu Rev Physiol* 62, 413–437.

Ahn, K. S., G. Sethi, K. Krishnan, and B. B. Aggarwal 2007. γ-Tocotrienol inhibits nuclear factor-κB signaling pathway through inhibition of receptor-interacting protein and TAK1 leading to suppression of antiapoptotic gene products and potentiation of apoptosis. *J Biol Chem* 282, 809–820.

Aleffi, S., I. Petrai, C. Bertolani et al. 2005. Upregulation of proinflammatory and proangiogenic cytokines by leptin in human hepatic stellate cells. *Hepatology* 42, 1339–1348.

Arthritis Queensland. 2011. www.arthritis.org.au/page/Arthritis/Arthritis_statistics [accessed 4 May 2012].

Atgié, C., A. Hadi-Sassi, L. Bukowiecki, and P. Mauriège 2009. High lipolytic activity and dyslipidemia in a Spontaneous Hypertensive/NIH Corpulent (SHR/N-*cp*) rat: A genetic model of obesity and type 2 diabetes mellitus. *J Physiol Biochem* 65, 33–41.

Australian Bureau of Statistics 2011a—Overweight and obesity in adults in Australia: A snapshot, 2007–2008. Cat. no. 4842.0.55.001. http://www.ausstats.abs.gov.au

Australian Bureau of Statistics 2011b. http://www.aihw.gov.au. —Arthritis and osteoporosis in Australia: A snapshot, 2007–2008. Cat. no. 4843.0.55.001. http://www.ausstats.abs.gov.au

Australian Institute of Health and Welfare 2008. *Australian Institute of Health and Welfare 2008. Diabetes: Australian Facts 2008.* Diabetes series no. 8. Cat. no. CVD 40. Canberra: AIHW. http://www.aihw.gov.au

Australian Institute of Health and Welfare 2011a. *Australian Institute of Health and Welfare 2011. Cardiovascular Disease: Australian Facts 2011.* Cardiovascular disease series. Cat. no. CVD 53. Canberra: AIHW. http://www.aihw.gov.au

Australian Institute of Health and Welfare 2011b. *A Snapshot of Osteoporosis in Australia 2011.* Arthritis series no. 15. Cat. no. PHE 137. Canberra: AIHW. http://www.aihw.gov.au

Australia's Health 2010 Australia's Health 2010, Australian Institute of Health and Welfare Canberra Cat. no. AUS 122.

Baliarsingh, S., Z. H. Beg, and J. Ahmad 2005. The therapeutic impacts of tocotrienols in type 2 diabetic patients with hyperlipidemia. *Atherosclerosis* 182, 367–374.

Bouïs, D., Y. Kusumanto, C. Meijer, N. H. Mulder, and G. A. P. Hospers 2006. A review on pro- and anti-angiogenic factors as targets of clinical intervention. *Pharmacol Res* 53, 89–103.

Bukowiecki, L., J. Lupien, N. Follea et al. 1980. Mechanism of enhanced lipolysis in adipose tissue of exercise-trained rats. *Am J Physiol* 239, E422–E429.

Bussolino, F., A. Mantovani, and G. Percisco 1997. Molecular mechanisms of blood vessel formation. *Trends Biochem Sci* 22, 251–256.

Cao, Y. 2007. Angiogenesis modulates adipogenesis and obesity. *J Clin Invest* 117, 2362–2368.

Cao, Y. 2010. Adipose tissue angiogenesis as a therapeutic target for obesity and metabolic diseases. *Nat Rev Drug Discov* 9, 107–115.

Cao, R., E. Brakenhielm, C. Wahlestedt, J. Thyberg, and Y. Cao 2001. Leptin induces vascular permeability and synergistically stimulates angiogenesis with FGF-2 and VEGF. *Proc Natl Acad Sci USA* 98, 6390–6395.

Carmeliet, P. 2003. Angiogenesis in health and disease. *Nat Med* 9, 653–660.

Carmeliet, P. and R. K. Jain 2000. Angiogenesis in cancer and other diseases. *Nature* 407, 249–257.

Cass, A., S. Chadban, J. Craig et al. 2010. The economic impact of end-stage kidney disease in Australia: Projection to 2020. ISBN 978-1-74249-201-8; Cat. no. PHE 150; 64 pp. http://www.kidney.org.au/HealthProfessionals/CKDinAustralia/tabid/622/Default.aspx [accessed 4 May 2012].

Cho, C.-H., Y. H. Koh, J. Han et al. 2007. Angiogenic role of LYVE-1–positive macrophages in adipose tissue. *Circ Res* 100, e47–e57.

Christiaens, V. and H. R. Lijnen 2010. Angiogenesis and development of adipose tissue. *Mol Cell Endocrinol* 318, 2–9.

Claffey, K. P., L. F. Brown, L. F. Aguila et al. 1996. Expression of vascular permeability factor/vascular endothelial growth factor by melanoma cells increases tumour growth, angiogenesis, and experimental metastasis. *Cancer Res* 56, 172–181.

Colagiuri, S., C. M. Lee, R. Colagiuri et al. 2010. The cost of overweight and obesity in Australia. *Med J Aust* 192, 260–264.

Costa, C., J. Incio, and R. Soares 2007. Angiogenesis and chronic inflammation: Cause or consequence? *Angiogenesis* 10, 149–166.

Crandall, D. L., D. E. Busler, B. Mchendry-Rinde, T. M. Groeling, and J. G. Kral 2000. Autocrine regulation of human preadipocyte migration by plasminogen activator inhibitor-1. *J Clin Endocrinol Metab* 85, 2609–2614.

Crossno, J. T., S. M. Majka, T. Grazia, R. G. Gill, and D. J. Klemm 2006. Rosiglitazone promotes development of a novel adipocyte population from bone marrow–derived circulating progenitor cells. *J Clin Invest* 116, 3220–3228.

Cusi, K. 2010. The role of adipose tissue and lipotoxicity in the pathogenesis of type 2 diabetes. *Curr Diab Rep* 10, 306–315.

D'ambrosio, S. M. 2007. Phytonutrients: A more natural approach toward cancer prevention. *Semin Cancer Biol* 17, 345–346.

Deurenberg-Yap, M., G. Schmidt, W. A. Van Staveren, and P. Deurenberg 2000. The paradox of low body mass index and high body fat percentage among Chinese, Malays and Indians in Singapore. *Int J Obes Relat Metab Disord* 24, 1011–1017.

Diwan, V., H. Poudyal, and L. Brown 2011. Piperine attenuates cardiovascular, liver and metabolic changes in high carbohydrate, high fat-fed rats. *Cell Biochem Biophys* In press.

Ejerblad, E., C. M. Fored, P. Lindblad et al. 2006. Obesity and risk for chronic renal failure. *J Am Soc Nephrol* 17, 1695–1702.

Evans, H. M. and K. S. Bishop 1922. On the existence of a hitherto unrecognized dietary factor essential for reproduction. *Science* 56, 650–651.

Fairus, S., R. M. Nor, H. M. Cheng, and K. Sundram 2006. Postprandial metabolic fate of tocotrienol-rich vitamin E differs significantly from that of alpha-tocopherol. *Am J Clin Nutr* 84, 835–842.

Fan, T.-P., J.-C. Yeh, K. W. Leung, P. Y. K. Yue, and R. N. S. Wong 2006. Angiogenesis: from plants to blood vessels. *Trends Pharmacol Sci* 27, 297–309.

Fantuzzi, G. and R. Faggioni 2000. Leptin in the regulation of immunity, inflammation, and hematopoiesis. *J Leukoc Biol* 68, 437–446.

Flegal, K. M., M. D. Carroll, C. L. Ogden, and L. R. Curtin 2010. Prevalence and trends in obesity among US adults, 1999–2008. *JAMA* 303, 235–241.

Flegal, K. M., B. I. Graubard, D. F. Williamson, and M. H. Gail 2005. Excess deaths associated with underweight, overweight, and obesity. *JAMA* 293, 1861–1867.

Folkman, J. 1971. Tumor angiogenesis: Therapeutic implications. *N Engl J Med* 285, 1182–1186.

Folkman, J. 1995. Angiogenesis in cancer, vascular, rheumatoid, and other disease. *Nat Med* 1, 27–31.

Fox, C. S., M. G. Larson, E. P. Leip et al. 2004. Predictors of new-onset kidney disease in a community-based population. *JAMA* 291, 844–850.

Fukumura, D., A. Ushiyama, D. G. Duda et al. 2003. Paracrine regulation of angiogenesis and adipocyte differentiation during in vivo adipogenesis. *Circ Res* 93, 88–97.

Furuhata, Y., K. Hirabayashi, T. Yonezawa, M. Takahashi, and M. Nishihara 2002. Effects of pair-feeding and growth hormone treatment on obese transgenic rats. *Eur J Endocrinol* 146, 245–249.

Goldman, C. K., R. L. Kendall, G. Cabrera et al. 1998. Paracrine expression of a native soluble vascular endothelial growth factor receptor inhibits tumor growth, metastasis and mortality rate. *Proc Natl Acad Sci USA* 95, 8795–8800.

Gomez, D. E., D. F. Alonso, H. Yoshiji, and U. P. Thorgeirsson 1997. Tissue inhibitors of metalloproteinases: Structure, regulation and biological functions. *Eur J Cell Biol* 74, 111–122.

Gregor, M. F. and G. S. Hotamisligil 2011. Inflammatory mechanisms in obesity. *Annu Rev Immunol* 29, 415–445.

Haffner, S. M. 2006. The metabolic syndrome: Inflammation, diabetes mellitus, and cardiovascular disease. *Am J Cardiol* 97, 3–11.

Hanathan, D. and J. Folkman (1996). 1996. Patterns and imaging mechanism of the angiogenic switch during tumorigenesis. *Cell* 86, 353–364.

Hausman, G. J. and L. R. Richardson 1982. Histochemical and ultrastructural analysis of developing adipocytes in the fetal pig. *Acta Anat (Basel)* 114, 228–247.

Hausman, G. J. and L. R. Richardson 2004. Adipose tissue angiogenesis. *J Anim Sci* 82, 925–934.

Hayes, A. J., L. Y. Li, and M. E. Lippman 1999 Antivascular therapy: A new approach to cancer treatment. *BMJ* 318, 853–856.

Hoeben, A., B. Landuyt, M. S. Highley et al. 2004. Vascular endothelial growth factor and angiogenesis. *Pharmacol Rev* 56, 549–580.

Hotamisligil, G. S. 2006. Inflammation and metabolic disorders. *Nature* 444, 860–867.

Hsu, C.-y., C. E. McCollough, C. Iribarren, J. Darbinian, and A. S. Go 2006. Body mass index and risk for endstage renal disease. *Ann Intern Med* 144, 21–28.

Ingalls, A. M., M. M. Dickie, and G. D. Snell 1996. Obese, a new mutation in the house mouse. *Obes Res* 41, 101.

Iseki, K., Y. Ikemiya, K. Kinjo et al. 2004. Body mass index and the risk of development of end-stage renal disease in a screened cohort. *Kidney Int* 65, 1870–1876.

Iyer, A. and L. Brown 2010. Lipid mediators and inflammation in glucose intolerance and insulin resistance. *Drug Discov Today Dis Mech* 7, e191–e197.

Iyer, A., D. P. Fairlie, J. B. Prins, B. D. Hammock, and L. Brown 2010. Inflammatory lipid mediators in adipocyte function and obesity. *Nat Rev Endocrinol* 6, 71–82.

Iyer, A., S. Panchal, H. Poudyal, and L. Brown 2009. Potential health benefits of Indian spices in the symptoms of the metabolic syndrome: A review. *Indian J Biochem Biophys* 46, 467–481.

Johansson, G. 2010. Overweight and obesity in Sweden. A five year follow-up, 2004–2008. *Scand J Public Health* 38, 803–809.

Kaileh, M. and R. Sen 2010. Role of NFκB in the anti-inflammatory effects of tocotrienols. *J Am Coll Nutr* 29, 334–339.

Kamal-Eldin, A. and L.-Å. Appelqvist 1996. The chemistry and antioxidant properties of tocopherols and tocotrienols. *Lipids* 31, 671–701.

Kamat, J. P., H. D. Sarma, T. P. Devasagayam, K. Nesaretnam, and Y. Basiron 1997. Tocotrienols from palm oil as effective inhibitors of protein oxidation and lipid peroxidation in rat liver microsomes. *Mol Cell Biochem* 170, 131–137.

Khambalia, A. Z. and L. S. Seen 2010. Trends in overweight and obese adults in Malaysia (1996–2009): A systematic review. *Obes Rev* 11, 403–412.

Khanna, S., V. Patel, C. Rink, S. Roy, and C. K. Sen 2005. Delivery of orally supplemented α-tocotrienol to vital organs of rats and tocopherol-transport protein deficient mice. *Free Radic Biol Med* 39, 1310–1319.

Kim, K. J., B. Li, J. Winer et al. 1993. Inhibition of vascular endothelial growth factor-induced angiogenesis suppresses tumour growth *in vivo*. *Nature* 362, 841–844.

Kiran, K., B. Vijaya, R. Vishnuvardhan, and N. Giridharan 2007. DNA fingerprinting and phylogenetic analysis of WNIN rat strain and its obese mutants using microsatellite markers. *Biochem Genet* 45, 77–91.

Kusaka, M., K. Sudo, T. Fujita et al. 1991. Potent anti-angiogenic action of AGM-1470: Comparison to the fumagillin parent. *Biochem Biophys Res Commun* 174, 1070–1076.

Lal, A., H. Peters, B. St Croix et al. 2001. Transcriptional response to hypoxia in human tumors. *J Natl Cancer Inst* 93, 1337–1343.

Lee, M. J., Y. Y. Wu, and S. K. Fried 2010. Adipose tissue remodeling in pathophysiology of obesity. *Curr Opin Clin Nutr Metab Care* 13, 371–376.

Li, L. O., E. L. Klett, and R. A. Coleman 2010. Acyl-CoA synthesis, lipid metabolism and lipotoxicity. *Biochim Biophys Acta* 1801, 246–251.

Lijnen, H. R. 2008. Angiogenesis and obesity. *Cardiovasc Res* 78, 286–293.

Lijnen, H. R., V. Christiaens, I. Scroyen et al. 2006. Impaired adipose tissue development in mice with inactivation of placental growth factor function. *Diabetes* 55, 2698–2704.

Lijnen, H. R., B. Van Hoef, D. Kemp, and D. Collen 2007. Inhibition of vascular endothelial growth factor receptor tyrosine kinases impairs adipose tissue development in mouse models of obesity. *Biochim Biophys Acta* 1770, 1369–1373.

Mandrup, S., T. M. Loftus, O. A. MacDougald, F. P. Kuhajda, and M. D. Lane 1997. Obese gene expression at in vivo levels by fat pads derived from s.c. implanted 3T3-F442A preadipocytes. *Proc Natl Acad Sci USA* 94, 4300–4305.

Maquoi, E., C. Munaut, A. Colige, D. Collen, and H. R. Lijnen 2002. Modulation of adipose tissue expression of murine matrix metalloproteinases and their tissue inhibitors with obesity. *Diabetes* 51, 1093–1101.

McIntyre, B. S., K. P. Briski, A. Gapor, and P. W. Sylvester 2000. Antiproliferative and apoptotic effects of tocopherols and tocotrienols on preneoplastic and neoplastic mouse mammary epithelial cells. *Proc Soc Exp Biol Med* 224, 292–301.

Miyazawa, T., A. Shibata, P. Sookwong et al. 2009. Antiangiogenic and anticancer potential of unsaturated vitamin E (tocotrienol). *J Nutr Biochem* 20, 79–86.

Miyazawa, T., T. Tsuzuki, K. Nakagawa, and M. Igarashi 2004. Antiangiogenic potency of vitamin E. *Ann N Y Acad Sci* 1031, 401–404.

Muehlbauer, P. M. 2003. Anti-angiogenesis in cancer therapy. *Semin Oncol Nurs* 19, 180–192.

Nakagawa, K., A. Shibata, S. Yamashita et al. 2007. In vivo angiogenesis is suppressed by unsaturated vitamin E, tocotrienol. *J Nutr* 137, 1938–1943.

Nesaretnam, K., P. A. Gomez, K. R. Selvaduray, and G. A. Razak 2007a. Tocotrienol levels in adipose tissue of benign and malignant breast lumps in patients in Malaysia. *Asia Pac J Clin Nutr* 16, 498–504.

Nesaretnam, K., D. Mahalingam, A. K. Radhakrishnan, and R. Premier 2010. Supplementation of tocotrienol-rich fraction increases interferon-gamma production in ovalbumin-immunized mice. *Eur J Lipid Sci Technol* 112, 531–536.

Nesaretnam, K., W. Y. Wong, and M. B. Wahid 2007b. Tocotrienols and cancer: Beyond antioxidant activity. *Eur J Lipid Sci Technol* 109, 445–452.

Ness, A. R. and J. W. Powles 1997. Fruit and vegetables, and cardiovascular disease: A review. *Int J Epidemiol* 26, 1–13.

Nishimura, S., I. Manabe, M. Nagasaki et al. 2007. Adipogenesis in obesity requires close interplay between differentiating adipocytes, stromal cells and blood vessels. *Diabetes* 56, 1517–1526.

Panchal, S. K. and L. Brown 2011. Rodent models for metabolic syndrome research. *J Biomed Biotechnol.* 2011, 351982.

Panchal, S. K., H. Poudyal, A. Iyer et al. 2011. High-carbohydrate high-fat diet–induced metabolic syndrome and cardiovascular remodeling in rats. *J Cardiovasc Pharmacol* 57, 51–64.

Panchal, S. K., H. Poudyal, J. Waanders, and L. Brown 2012. Coffee extract attenuates changes in cardiovascular and hepatic structure and function without decreasing obesity in high-carbohydrate, high-fat diet-fed male rats. *J Nutr.* 142, 690–697.

Panigrahy, D., S. Singer, L. Q. Shen et al. 2002. PPARγ ligands inhibit primary tumor growth and metastasis by inhibiting angiogenesis. *J Clin Invest* 110, 923–932.

Park, H. Y., H. M. Kwon, H. J. Lim et al. 2001 Potential role of leptin in angiogenesis: Leptin induces endothelial cell proliferation and expression of matrix metalloproteinases in vivo and in vitro. *Exp Mol Med* 33, 95–102.

Pedersen, B. K. and M. A. Febbraio 2010. Diabetes: treatment of diabetes mellitus: New tricks by an old player. *Nat Rev Endocrinol* 6, 482–483.

Poudyal, H., S. Panchal, and L. Brown 2010. Comparison of purple carrot juice and β-carotene in a high-carbohydrate, high-fat diet-fed rat model of the metabolic syndrome. *Br J Nutr* 104, 1322–1332.

Powell, K. 2007. Obesity: the two faces of fat. *Nature* 447, 525–527.

Prospective Studies Collaboration 2009. Body-mass index and cause-specific mortality in 900000 adults: Collaborative analyses of 57 prospective studies. *Lancet* 373, 1083–1096.

Qureshi, A. A., S. A. Sami, W. A. Salser, and F. A. Khan 2001. Synergistic effect of tocotrienol-rich fraction (TRF25) of rice bran and lovastatin on lipid parameters in hypercholesterolemic humans. *J Nutr Biochem* 12, 318–329.

Reddy, K., D. Prabhakaran, V. Chaturvedi et al. 2006. Methods for establishing a surveillance system for cardiovascular diseases in Indian industrial populations. *Bull World Health Organ* 84, 461–469.

Ribatti, D., B. Nico, A. Vacca et al. 2001. Chorioallantoic membrane capillary bed: A useful target for studying angiogenesis and antiangiogenesis in vivo. *Anat Rec* 264, 317–324.

Riccardi, G., B. Capaldo, and O. Vaccaro 2005. Functional foods in the management of obesity and type 2 diabetes. *Curr Opin Clin Nutr Metab Care* 8, 630–635.

Rupnick, M. A., D. Panigrahy, C. Y. Zhang et al. 2002. Adipose tissue mass can be regulated through the vasculature. *Proc Natl Acad Sci USA* 99, 10730–10735.

Ruth, M. R., C. G. Taylor, P. Zahradka, and C. J. Field 2008. Abnormal immune responses in *fa/fa* Zucker rats and effects of feeding conjugated linoleic acid. *Obesity* 16, 1770–1779.

Samant, G. V. and P. W. Sylvester 2006. γ-Tocotrienol inhibits ErbB3-dependent PI3K/Akt mitogenic signalling in neoplastic mammary epithelial cells. *Cell Prolif* 39, 563–574.

Saremi, A. and R. Arora 2010. Vitamin E and cardiovascular disease. *Am J Ther* 17, e56–e65.

Schroeder, M., T. H. Moran, and A. Weller 2010. Attenuation of obesity by early-life food restriction in genetically hyperphagic male OLETF rats: Peripheral mechanisms. *Horm Behav* 57, 455–462.

Selvaduray, K. R., A. K. Radhakrishnan, M. K. Kutty, and K. Nesaretnam 2011. Palm tocotrienols decrease levels of pro-angiogenic markers in human umbilical vein endothelial cells (HUVEC) and murine mammary cancer cells. *Genes Nutr*, 7, 53–61.

Sen, C. K., S. Khanna, and S. Roy 2006. Tocotrienols: Vitamin E beyond tocopherols. *Life Sci* 78, 2088–2098.

Sen, C. K., S. Khanna, and S. Roy 2007. Tocotrienols in health and disease: the other half of the natural vitamin E family. *Mol Aspects Med* 28, 692–728.

Serbinova, E., V. Kagan, D. Han, and L. Packer 1991. Free radical recycling and intramembrane mobility in the antioxidant properties of alpha-tocopherol and alpha-tocotrienol. *Free Radic Biol Med* 10, 263–275.

Shibata, A., K. Nakagawa, P. Sookwong et al. 2008. Tocotrienol inhibits secretion of angiogenic factors from human colorectal adenocarcinoma cells by suppressing hypoxia-inducible factor-1α. *J Nutr* 138, 2136–2142.

Shirode, A. B. and P. W. Sylvester 2010. Synergistic anticancer effects of combined γ-tocotrienol and celecoxib treatment are associated with suppression in Akt and NFkB signaling. *Biomed Pharmacother* 64, 327–332.

Sierra-Honigmann, M. R., A. K. Nath, C. Murakami et al. 1998. Biological action of leptin as an angiogenic factor. *Science* 281, 1683–1686.

Sirtori, C. R., C. Galli, J. W. Anderson, E. Sirtori, and A. Arnoldi 2009. Functional foods for dyslipidaemia and cardiovascular risk prevention. *Nutr Res Rev* 22, 244–261.

Skobe, M., P. Rockwell, N. Goldstein, S. Vosseler, and N. E. Fusenig 1997. Halting angiogenesis suppresses carcinoma cell invasion. *Nat Med* 3, 1222–1227.

Soares, R. 2009. Angiogenesis in the metabolic syndrome. In: Soares, R. and Costa, C. (eds.) *Oxidative Stress, Inflammation and Angiogenesis in the Metabolic Syndrome*. Springer: Houten, the Netherlands.

Srinath, R. K. and M. B. Katan 2004. Diet, nutrition and the prevention of hypertension and cardiovascular diseases. *Public Health Nutr* 7, 167–186.

Suzuki, Y. J., M. Tsuchiya, S. R. Wassall et al. 1993. Structural and dynamic membrane properties of α-tocopherol and α-tocotrienol: Implication to the molecular mechanism of their antioxidant potency. *Biochemistry* 32, 10692–10699.

The NHS Information Centre, L. S. 2012. Statistics on obesity, physical activity and diet: England, 2012. http://www.ic.nhs.uk/statistics-and-data-collections/health-and-lifestyles/obesity/statistics-on-obesity-physical-activity-and-diet-england-2012 [accessed 4 May 2012].

Tilg, H. and A. R. Moschen 2006. Adipocytokines: Mediators linking adipose tissue, inflammation and immunity. *Nat Rev Immunol* 6, 772–783.

Toker, A. 2000. Protein kinases as mediators of phosphoinositide 3-kinase signaling. *Mol Pharmacol.* 57, 652–658.

Unger, R. H. and Y. T. Zhou 2001. Lipotoxicity of beta-cells in obesity and in other causes of fatty acid spillover. *Diabetes* 50, S118–S121.

Van Gaal, L. F., I. L. Mertens, and C. E. De Block 2006. Mechanisms linking obesity with cardiovascular disease. *Nature* 444, 875–880.

Vermaak, I., A. M. Viljoen, and J. H. Hamman 2011. Natural products in anti-obesity therapy. *Nat Prod Rep* 28, 1493–1533.

Wan Nazaimoon, W. M. and B. A. Khalid 2002. Tocotrienols-rich diet decreases advanced glycosylation end-products in non-diabetic rats and improves glycemic control in streptozotocin-induced diabetic rats. *Malaysian J Pathol* 24, 77–82.

Wang, Y., J. Mi, X. Y. Shan, Q. J. Wang, and K. Y. Ge 2006. Is China facing an obesity epidemic and the consequences? The trends in obesity and chronic disease in China. *Int J Obes* 31, 177–188.

Watkins, L., P. Lenz, A. Gapor et al. 1993. Gamma-tocotrienol as a hypocholesterolemic and antioxidant agent in rats fed atherogenic diets. *Lipids* 28, 1113–1118.

Who Expert Consultation 2004. Appropriate body-mass index for Asian populations and its implications for policy and intervention strategies. *Lancet* 363, 157–163.

Wong, W. Y., K. R. Selvaduray, H. M. Cheng, and K. Nesaretnam 2009. Suppression of tumor growth by palm tocotrienols via the attenuation of angiogenesis. *Nutr Cancer* 61, 367–373.

Yam, M. L., S. Abdul Hafid, H. M. Cheng, and K. Nesaretnam 2009. Tocotrienols suppress proinflammatory markers and cyclooxygenase-2 expression in RAW264.7 macrophages. *Lipids* 44, 787–797.

Yap, S. P., K. H. Yuen, and J. W. Wong 2001. Pharmacokinetics and bioavailability of alpha-, gamma- and delta-tocotrienols under different food status. *J Pharm Pharmacol* 53, 67–71.

Yap, W. N., N. Zaiden, S. Y. Luk et al. 2010. In vivo evidence of γ-tocotrienol as a chemosensitizer in the treatment of hormone-refractory prostate cancer. *Pharmacology* 85, 248–258.

Zaiden, N., W. N. Yap, S. Ong et al. 2010. Gamma delta tocotrienols reduce hepatic triglyceride synthesis and VLDL secretion. *J Atheroscler Thromb* 17, 1019–1032.

Zhao, J. 2007. Nutraceuticals, nutritional therapy, phytonutrients, and phytotherapy for improvement of human health: A perspective on plant biotechnology application. *Recent Pat Biotechnol* 1, 75–97.

Zhao, L.-J., Y.-J. Liu, P.-Y. Liu et al. 2007. Relationship of obesity with osteoporosis. *J Clin Endocrinol Metab* 92, 1640–1646.

Zheng, W., D. F. Mclerran, B. Rolland et al. 2011. Association between body-mass index and risk of death in more than 1 million Asians. *N Engl J Med* 364, 719–729.

Zimmet, P., E. J. Boyko, G. R. Collier, and M. De Courten 1999. Etiology of the metabolic syndrome: potential role of insulin resistance, leptin resistance, and other players. *Ann N Y Acad Sci* 892, 25–44.

15 Tocotrienols, Inflammation, and Cancer
How Are They Linked?

*Sahdeo Prasad, Bokyung Sung, Sridevi Patchva,
Subash C. Gupta, and Bharat B. Aggarwal*

CONTENTS

15.1 INTRODUCTION

In 1900, the top three causes of death in the United States were pneumonia/influenza, tuberculosis, and diarrhea/enteritis. Since the 1940s, however, most deaths in the United States have resulted from heart disease and cancer (NCHS 1900, 1948). Cancer is the second most common cause of death in the United States, after heart disease. Since 1950, the incidence of heart diseases has sharply decreased, but cancer incidence has not declined. It has been estimated that in the year 2011, about 1,596,670 new cancer cases will be diagnosed and about 571,950 Americans are expected to die of cancer, or more than 1500 people a day. In the United States, cancer accounts for nearly one of every four deaths. According to the International Agency for Research on Cancer (IARC), by the year 2030, almost 21.4 million new cases of this disease will be diagnosed annually and >13.2 million people will die of cancer each year, almost double the number who died of the disease in 2008. Therefore, it is necessary to better understand the prognosis, diagnosis, and treatment of cancer.

Cancer was first described in an ancient Egyptian textbook on trauma surgery that dates back to about 1600 BC. However, the term "cancer" was first used by the Greek physician Hippocrates (460–370 BC), who used the terms "*carcinos*" and "*carcinoma*" to describe "non-ulcer forming" and "ulcer-forming tumors." Cancer cells arise from normal cells. Usually, normal cells, which are the building blocks of living beings, multiply and die as needed by the body. However, cancer occurs when the growth of cells in the body is out of control and cells divide and multiply rapidly. Cancer cells acquire this property by gain of function mutations in oncogenes and loss of function mutations in tumor suppressor genes (Hanahan and Weinberg, 2011). However, only 5%–10% of cancers are caused by mutations; the majority (90%–95%) of cancers are attributed to environmental factors and lifestyle (Anand et al., 2008).

The common environmental and lifestyle factors that account for 90%–95% of cancer risk include tobacco, diet and obesity, infections, radiation, stress, lack of physical activity, and environmental pollutants (Anand et al., 2008). The underlying mechanisms by which these risk factors induce cancer are becoming increasingly evident. One process that seems to be common to all these risk factors is their ability to induce inflammation (Aggarwal et al., 2009; Chinenov and Kerppola, 2001; Mantovani et al., 2008). Inflammation is a process by which the body reacts to the insults incurred by internal or external stimuli. The clinical and fundamental signs of inflammation include redness, swelling, heat, pain, and loss of function. Inflammation can be classified as acute or chronic. Acute inflammation is an immediate response of the body and is required to ward off harmful pathogens. However, when inflammation persists for a longer time, progressive change in the type of cells at the site of damage occurs and leads to chronic inflammation. Research over the past several years has indicated that chronic inflammation is a major culprit for most chronic diseases including cancer (Aggarwal et al., 2006b; Karin and Greten, 2005; Li et al., 2005; Prasad et al., 2010). Implications of all these indicate that anti-inflammatory agents might have potential for the prevention and treatment of cancer.

In recent decades, numerous anti-inflammatory agents including synthetic drugs and antibodies have been developed. Although cancer is caused by dysregulation of multiple inflammatory pathways, most of the synthetic drugs are based on the modulation of more specifically a single target and therefore are less likely to be effective. In addition, these drugs produce numerous side effects and cannot be consumed chronically. Therefore, there is an urgent need for the identification of agents that are multitargeted, cost-effective, and immediately available. In this regard, agents derived from natural sources called nutraceuticals seem to fulfill most of these criteria (Jensen, 2006; Jensen and Roubenoff, 2008). Tocotrienol (T3) is one such nutraceutical that is present in palm oil, rice bran oil, red annatto, coconut, wheat germ oil, barley, cocoa, oat, grape seed oil, hazelnut, maize, olive oil, flax seed oil, poppy seed oil, safflower oil, buckthorn berry, and rye (Figure 15.1A).

In this chapter, we discuss in detail the modulation of inflammatory transcription factors by tocotrienol. We focus on the modulation of both pro-inflammatory (activator protein-1 [AP-1], signal transducer and activator of transcription 3[STAT3], nuclear factor-κB [NF-κB], hypoxia-inducible factor-1 [HIF-1], Wnt/β-catenin) and anti-inflammatory (nuclear factor erythroid 2-related factor [NRF2] and peroxisome-proliferator-activated receptors [PPARs]) transcription factors by this nutraceutical.

15.2 TOCOTRIENOL: HISTORY, SOURCE, AND STRUCTURE

Tocotrienol is one of the two derivatives of vitamin E. The other derivative of vitamin E is tocopherol. Both tocotrienol and tocopherol are composed of four isomers: alpha, beta, gamma, and delta. The tocopherols are the saturated forms of vitamin E, whereas the tocotrienols are unsaturated and possess an isoprenoid side chain. Tocopherols are much more common and more studied than tocotrienols. However, current studies have shown that tocotrienols are more effective in reducing the risk of several diseases and disorders, including heart strokes, high cholesterol, diabetes, and cancers such as pancreatic, breast, skin, and prostate cancer.

Tocotrienols were first discovered in 1964 by Pennock and Whittle while separating tocotrienols from rubber (Whittle et al., 1966). However, the importance and health benefits of tocotrienol did not become evident for another 2 decades. In the 1980s, its effect on lowering of cholesterol was noted by Qureshi (Qureshi et al., 1986), and in the 1990s, tocotrienols were found to be effective against various cancers (Pearce et al., 1992). Since then, researchers have worked to discover the

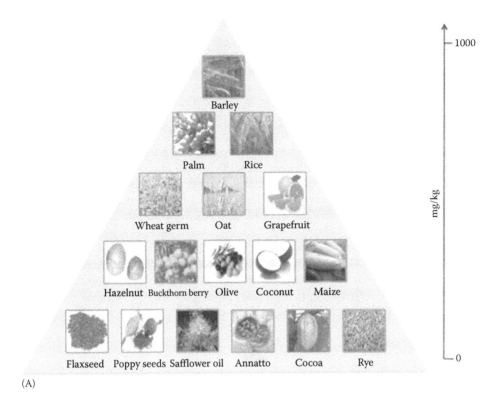

(A)

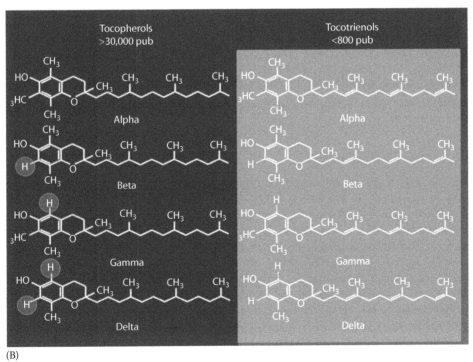

(B)

FIGURE 15.1 (A) Natural sources of tocotrienols. The upward arrow indicates increasing concentration of tocotrienol in different sources. (B) Chemical structure of tocopherol and tocotrienol.

mechanism of action of tocotrienols against cancer and other diseases. Because of the health benefits shown by tocotrienols, Barrie Tan invented techniques for their isolation from palm, rice, and annatto and patented these techniques between 1992 and 2002.

In nature, tocotrienols are present in very low levels, whereas commercially they are extracted from palm, rice, and annatto. Other natural sources of tocotrienols are rice bran oil, coconut oil, cocoa butter, barley, and wheat germ (Packer et al., 2001). Among these, barley and palm oil are the richest source of tocotrienols, containing 910 and 738 mg/kg, respectively. Other sources such as rice bran contain 465 mg/kg, wheat germ 189 mg/kg, barley 910 mg/kg, oat 210 mg/kg, coconut oil 25 mg/kg, and cocoa butter 2 mg/kg (www.tocotrienol.org). Various isomers of tocotrienols have been detected in very low quantities in human milk (Kobayashi et al., 1975) as well. Tocotrienol can also be synthesized through chemical reactions. Chemically synthesized tocotrienols are available in racemic mixtures of isomers D and L (right and left), forms that are lateral inversions of one another. Moreover, researchers are working to synthesize pure isomers of either the D- or L-tocotrienol isomers.

Tocopherols consist of a chromanol ring and a 15-carbon tail. The presence of three *trans* double bonds in the tail distinguishes tocotrienols from tocopherols (Figure 15.1B). Tocotrienols are also distinguished by having a 20-carbon-geranylgeranyl tail attached to the benzene ring, in contrast to the 20-carbon-phytyl tail (including pyranol ring) in tocopherols. The isomeric forms of tocotrienol are distinguished by the number and location of methyl groups on the chromanol rings: α-tocotrienol is 5,7,8-trimethyl, β-tocotrienol is 5,8-dimethyl, γ-tocotrienol is 7,8-dimethyl, and δ-tocotrienol is 8-monomethyl.

15.3   ROLE OF TOCOTRIENOLS IN INFLAMMATORY PATHWAYS

Most oncogenes and tumor suppressor genes are transcription factors, which control the expression of genes and regulate numerous signaling pathways. Dysregulation of transcription factors results in changes in gene expression, protein–protein interactions, and posttranslational modifications, leading to dysregulation of gene products that are involved in both inflammation and cancer (Chaturvedi et al., 2011). In this section, our focus is on selected transcription factors: NF-κB, AP-1, STAT3, Wnt/β-catenin, HIF-1, NRF2, and PPARγ. We discuss how tocotrienol can modulate these inflammatory transcription factors and thereby play a positive role in the prevention and treatment of cancer (Table 15.1).

15.3.1   Nuclear Factor-Kappa B

NF-κB is one of the major pro-inflammatory transcription factors with potential to modulate more than 500 genes (Gupta et al., 2010a,b). It was first discovered by Sen and Baltimore in 1986 in the nucleus of the B cell as an enhancer of the κ immunoglobulin chain (Sen and Baltimore, 1986). In unstimulated cells, NF-κB is located in the cytosol in an inactive form. NF-κB is activated in response to several stimuli, such as stress, pathogens, TNF-α, IL-1, and environmental and lifestyle factors (Ahn et al., 2007a). When these inducers bind to their respective receptors, signaling impinges on a common molecular target, the inhibitor of κB (IκB) kinase (IKK) complex, leading to phosphorylation, polyubiquitination, and subsequent degradation of inhibitory subunit (IκBα), thereby allowing active NF-κB to translocate to the nucleus where NF-κB exerts its function as a transcriptional regulator (Figure 15.2). NF-κB can regulate numerous gene products linked with survival, proliferation, invasion, and angiogenesis of tumor cells. The intimate relationship between NF-κB and cancer has already been extensively reviewed (Aggarwal et al., 2006b; Karin and Greten, 2005; Li et al., 2005; Prasad et al., 2010). Here, we describe whether tocotrienols modulate the NF-κB signaling pathway.

The role of tocotrienols in modulating NF-κB signaling pathway has been studied by us as well as by other groups. Theriault et al. (2002) have shown that α-T3 has potential to inhibit TNF-α-induced

TABLE 15.1
Effect of Tocotrienols on Inflammation-Related Pathways

NF-κB
- Inhibits NF-κB activation and thereby reduces cellular adhesion molecule expression and monocytic cell adherence (Theriault et al., 2002)
- Inhibits the NF-κB signaling pathway through inhibition of RIP and TAK1 in human chronic myeloid leukemia cells (Ahn et al., 2007b)
- Inhibits tumor growth and enhances antitumor properties of gemcitabine in an orthotopic mouse model of human pancreatic cancer by downregulating NF-κB and its regulated gene products (Kunnumakkara et al., 2010)
- Inhibits tumor growth in murine breast cancer cells and shows synergistic anticancer effects with celecoxib by reducing phospho-NF-κB levels (Shirode and Sylvester, 2010)
- Inhibits the nuclear translocation of NF-κB p65 protein in human colon carcinoma HT-29 cells (Xu et al., 2009)
- Inhibits NF-κB expression in human monocytic cells (Wu et al., 2008)
- Inhibits NF-κB activity in breast cancer cells (Shah and Sylvester, 2005; Sylvester et al., 2005)

AP-1:
- Suppresses concanavalin A–induced AP-1-dependent gene expression (Wilankar et al., 2011)

STAT3
- Inhibits both the constitutive and inducible activation of STAT3 through the upregulation of SHP-1 in HCC and multiple myeloma (Kannappan et al., 2010; Rajendran et al., 2011)
- Inhibits STAT3 activity in murine breast cancer cells in combination with tyrosine kinase inhibitor (Bachawal et al., 2010)
- Inhibits STAT3 and reduces chemoresistance of mesothelioma cells (Kashiwagi et al., 2009)

Wnt/β-Catenin
- Reduces β-catenin expression and inhibits angiogenesis in HUVECs (Li et al., 2011)
- Reduces the expression of β-catenin and Wnt-1 proteins in human colon carcinoma cells (Zhang et al., 2011)

HIF-1α
- Suppresses HIF-1α in human colorectal adenocarcinoma cells (Shibata et al., 2008)
- Reduces HIF-1α protein accumulation by inhibiting p-ERK1/2 in human gastric adenocarcinoma cells (Bi et al., 2010)

NRF2
- Activates NRF2-mediated oxidative stress response in human breast cancer cells (Patacsil et al., 2011)

PPAR-γ
- α- and γ-tocotrienol activate PPARα, while δ-tocotrienol activates PPARα, PPARγ, and PPARδ (Fang et al., 2010)
- Increases PPAR-γ-activating ligand 15-S-hydroxyeicosatetraenoicacid by increasing the levels of 15-lipoxygenase-2 enzyme in prostate cancer cells (Campbell et al., 2011)
- Upregulates PPAR-γ in human colon cancer cells (Stone et al., 2004)

STAT, signal transducers and activators of transcription; HCC, hepatocellular carcinoma; NF-κB, nuclear factor-κB; STZ, streptozotocin, NRF2, NF-E2-related factor 2; AP-1, activator protein-1; PPAR, peroxisome-proliferator-activated receptor; HIF, hypoxia-inducible factors; ERK, extracellular-signal-regulated kinases.

monocyte adhesion through inhibition of NF-κB pathway. Among the four isotypes of T3, γ-T3 has been well studied with respect to its suppressive ability on the NF-κB signaling pathway. We found that γ-T3, but not γ-tocopherol, has the potential to completely abolish TNF-induced NF-κB activation in human leukemia cells. Mechanistically, γ-T3 inhibited NF-κB activation through suppression of phosphorylation and degradation of IκBα, inhibition of IKK activation, and suppression of phosphorylation and nuclear translocation of p65. Further, inhibition in NF-κB activation was correlated with downregulation in NF-κB-dependent-gene products linked with antiapoptosis (IAP1, IAP2, Bcl-xL, Bcl-2, cFLIP, XIAP, Bfl-1/A1, TRAF1, and survivin), proliferation (cyclin D1,

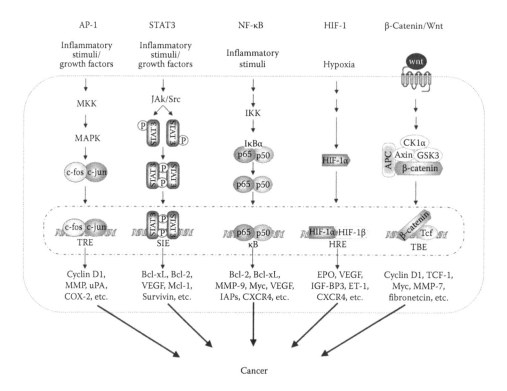

FIGURE 15.2 Regulation of selected pro-inflammatory transcription factors and their association with cancer. AP-1, activator protein-1; APC, adenomatous polyposis coli; Bcl-2, B-cell lymphoma-2; Bcl-xL, B-cell lymphoma-extra large; CK1, casein kinase 1; COX-2, cyclooxygenase-2; c-Myc, cellular v-myc myelocytomatosis viral oncogene homolog (avian); CXCR4, C-X-C chemokine receptor type 4; EPO, erythropoietin; ET-1, endothelin-1; GSK3, glycogen synthase kinase 3; HIF-1, hypoxia-inducible factor-1; HRE, hypoxia-responsive element; IAPs, inhibitor of apoptosis proteins; IGF-BP3, insulin-like growth factor binding protein 3; IKK, IκB kinase; IκBα, inhibitor of κB; Jak, Janus kinase; MAPK, mitogen-activated protein kinase; Mcl-1, myeloid cell leukemia-1; MKK, MAPK kinases; MMP, matrix metalloproteinase; NF-κB, nuclear factor-kappa B; P, phosphorylation; STAT3, signal transducer and activator of transcription 3; TBE, Tcf/β-catenin binding element; Tcf, T-cell factor; TRE, 12-O-tetradecanoylphorbol-13-acetate (TPA)-responsive element; uPA, urokinase-type plasminogen activator; VEGF, vascular endothelial growth factor.

COX2, and c-Myc), invasion (MMP-9 and ICAM-1), and angiogenesis (vascular endothelial growth factor) (Ahn et al., 2007b). In another orthotropic murine model of human pancreatic cancer, γ-T3 (400 mg/kg body weight) was shown to inhibit tumor growth and to sensitize tumors to gemcitabine by suppressing NF-κB-mediated inflammatory pathways (Kunnumakkara et al., 2010). Similarly, Campbell et al. (2011) also reported that the γ- and δ-isoforms of T3 inhibited the growth of prostate cancer cells more effectively compared with the γ- and δ-forms of tocopherol. The group demonstrated that the growth inhibitory effect of γ-T3 was mediated through inhibition of the NF-κB pathway (Campbell et al., 2011). Ha et al. (2011) also reported that α-T3 but not α-tocopherol has potential to inhibit osteoclastogenesis. Further, α-T3 but not α-tocopherol inhibited the expression of receptor activator of NF-κB ligand (RANKL) and c-Fos through inhibition of NF-κB activation (Ha et al., 2011).

Tocotrienols have been demonstrated to possess antiproliferative effects through modulation of NF-κB pathway in prostate and melanoma cancer cells as well. One study found that γ-T3 is one of the most potent tocotrienols in inducing apoptosis and inhibiting proliferation of prostate and melanoma cancer cells (Chang et al., 2009; Yap et al., 2008). Similarly, δ-T3 was shown to inhibit cell growth, cell migration, tumor cell invasiveness, and to induce apoptosis in human non-small-cell lung cancer cells through downregulation of NF-κB (Ji et al., 2011). Some other cancer types where tocotrienols have been shown to inhibit cancer cell development through modulation of NF-κB pathway are listed in Table 15.1.

15.3.2 ACTIVATOR PROTEIN-1

AP-1, which is involved in mediating cellular responses and pro-inflammatory stimuli, was first identified as a transcription factor that binds to an essential *cis*-element of the human metallothionein promoter (Lee et al., 1987). AP-1 activity can be regulated by a plethora of physiological stimuli and environmental factors, including pro-inflammatory cytokines, growth factors, and oxidative stress. AP-1 exists as a dimeric transcription factor comprising of basic leucine zipper family members including Jun (c-Jun, JunB, and JunD), Fos (c-Fos, FosB, Fra1, and Fra2), ATF (ATF2, B-ATF, JDP1, and JDP2), and Maf (MafA, MafB, c-Maf, and MafG/F/K) protein families (Eferl and Wagner, 2003; Shaulian and Karin, 2002). The AP-1 dimer complex can recognize the 12-*O*-tetradecanoylphorbol-13-acetate (TPA, also called PMA) response elements (TREs) or cyclic adenosine monophosphate (AMP) response elements within the promoter region of target genes (Chinenov and Kerppola, 2001) (Figure 15.2).

AP-1 is considered to be one of the key players in tumorigenesis through regulation of inflammation. This transcription factor has been shown to play a critical role in the osteoclastogenesis activated by RANKL (Kong et al., 1999; Zenz et al., 2008). The role of AP-1 in tumor promotion was first discovered by Bernstein and Colburn (Bernstein and Colburn, 1989), who reported that transformation-resistant JB6 cells failed to activate AP-1 in response to tumor promoters such as TPA and EGF, whereas the AP-1 response was intact in transformation-sensitive JB6 cells. Elevated AP-1 activity has been detected in a variety of cancers and tumor cell lines, suggesting a role for AP-1 in tumor progression (Young et al., 2003). Thus, AP-1 is a good target for both prevention and treatment of inflammatory diseases.

Numerous reports indicated that tocopherols inhibit the activation of AP-1 in cancer cells (Crispen et al., 2007; Kuchide et al., 2003; Mukhopadhyay et al., 2009; Qian et al., 1997). However, very little is known about the effect of T3 on AP-1. Recently, γ-T3 was found to suppress concanavalin A (ConA)-induced AP-1 activation in mice lymphocytes (Wilankar et al., 2011). Further, a comparison of immunomodulatory potential of γ-T3 with α-T3 revealed that γ-T3 was more potent in suppressing ConA-mediated proliferation of T cells.

15.3.3 SIGNAL TRANSDUCER AND ACTIVATOR OF TRANSCRIPTION

STAT3 is a member of the family of STAT transcription factors that is normally present in the cytoplasm of most cells. In response to certain inflammatory stimuli (e.g., IL-6) and growth factors (e.g., EGF), STAT3 undergoes phosphorylation at Tyr^{705}, homodimerization, nuclear translocation, DNA binding, and gene transcription. Several protein kinases including Janus-activated kinase 1, 2, and 3 and Src are involved in the STAT3 phosphorylation. STAT3 also undergoes dephosphorylation by specific phosphatases such as SHP-1. STAT3 is involved in the regulation of genes associated with tumor development (Aggarwal et al., 2006a, 2009) (Figure 15.2).

Emerging evidence suggests that STAT3 plays a crucial role in the inflammatory microenvironment, in both initiation and progression of cancer (Catlett-Falcone et al., 1999; Grivennikov et al., 2009; Kortylewski et al., 2009; Kujawski et al., 2008; Mantovani et al., 2008). The elevated STAT3 activity has been detected in a wide variety of cancers, including head and neck, breast, colorectal, ovarian, pancreatic, renal, leukemia, lymphoma, and multiple myeloma (Aggarwal et al., 2009). Rebouissou et al. (2009) showed that STAT3 is linked to inflammation and tumorigenesis, which is initiated by genetic alterations in tumor hepatocytes.

Several studies have indicated that γ-T3 inhibits STAT3 activation and induces apoptosis in various cancer types (Bachawal et al., 2010; Kannappan et al., 2010; Rajendran et al., 2011). A report from our group showed that γ-T3 has potential to inhibit the phosphorylation, nuclear translocation, and DNA binding of STAT3 in human multiple myeloma cells (Kannappan et al., 2010). This suppression of STAT3 activity by γ-T3 was correlated with inhibition of Src kinase and JAK1 and JAK2 kinases. The suppression of STAT3 by γ-T3 further lead to inhibition of the expression of STAT3-regulated antiapoptotic (Bcl-2, Bcl-xL, and Mcl-1), proliferative (cyclin D1), and angiogenic (VEGF) gene products (Bachawal et al., 2010; Kannappan et al., 2010; Rajendran et al., 2011). γ-T3, in combination with the receptor tyrosine kinase inhibitors has been shown to inhibit tumor cell growth through the modulation of STAT3 activity (Bachawal et al., 2010). Recently, Rajendran et al. (2011) reported that γ-T3 induced apoptosis in hepatocellular carcinoma by inactivating STAT3 and downregulating STAT3-regulated gene expression linked to tumorigenesis. In addition to natural γ-T3, a redox-silent analogue of α-T3, 6-*O*-carboxypropyl-α-T3 (T3E), has been shown to suppress STAT3 activation in chemoresistant H28 mesothelioma cells (Kashiwagi et al., 2009).

15.3.4 WNT/β-CATENIN

The Wnt pathway plays a critical role in the development of multicellular organisms; however, abnormal Wnt signaling has been associated with many human diseases including cancer. The *wnt1* gene (originally called "*Int-1*") in mice was first identified in 1982 by Nusse and Varmus as a preferential integration site for the mouse mammary tumor virus in breast tumors (Nusse and Varmus, 1982). Since that discovery, 19 Wnt ligands have been identified in mammals that are known to activate β-catenin-dependent (canonical) and β-catenin-independent (noncanonical) signaling pathways on binding to the Frizzled-LRP coreceptor complex. When Wnt ligands bind to their receptors—that is, proteins of the Frizzled family—the result is the inactivation of a complex of cytoplasmic proteins (including adenomatous polyposis coli [APC] and axin). This inactivation promotes the degradation of β-catenin, leading to its cytoplasmic accumulation and nuclear localization. In the nucleus, β-catenin interacts with T-cell factor/lymphoid enhancer factors (TCF/LEFs) to regulate the expression of target gene products (Figure 15.2). Thus, given the critical and pleiotropic roles of Wnt signaling, it is not surprising that perturbations/mutations in Wnt signaling have been implicated in a variety of human diseases, including cancer (Clevers, 2006).

The nuclear accumulation of β-catenin, a hallmark of activated Wnt signaling, has been clearly observed in cancer cells (Bienz and Clevers, 2003). Hyperactive β-catenin turns on a genetic program sufficient to initiate the development of a multitude of different tumor types, primarily those of gastrointestinal origin. Loss-of-function mutations in the components of the β-catenin degradation complex have been observed in many human cancers. For instance, >70% of colorectal cancers have been shown to bear mutations in *APC*, by which it fails to degrade β-catenin. Similarly, inactivating mutations in the axin scaffold protein have been implicated in hepatocellular carcinomas (Giles et al., 2003).

Tocotrienols have been reported to regulate the β-catenin/Wnt signaling pathway. γ-T3 has been shown to regulate Wnt signaling by decreasing β-catenin expression in human umbilical vein endothelial cells (HUVECs). This suppression was associated with inhibition of proliferation, migration, and tube formation of HUVEC cells (Li et al., 2011). Similarly, δ-T3 was found to induce cell death in human colon carcinoma SW620 cells, which was associated with the suppression of the Wnt signaling pathway (Zhang et al., 2011). δ-T3 also downregulated the expression of β-catenin and Wnt-1 protein that lead to suppression of downstream target proteins of the Wnt signaling pathway such as cyclin D1, c-myc, c-jun, and MMP-7 in the human colorectal cancer cells. These observations indicate that the ability of T3 to modulate the β-catenin/Wnt signaling pathway may provide a potential way to prevent and treat cancer.

15.3.5 Hypoxia Inducible Factor-1

HIF-1 is involved in the transcription of genes encoding proteins that mediate adaptive responses to reduced oxygen availability. This transcription factor consists of an O_2-regulated HIF-1α and a constitutively expressed HIF-1β subunit (Wang et al., 1995).

A growing body of evidence suggests that the upregulation of HIF has a crucial role in the progression of a broad range of human malignancies (Giaccia et al., 2003; Maxwell et al., 2001; Semenza, 2003). For instance, accumulation of HIF-1α has been associated with poor survival of patients with a variety of cancers, including cervical, breast, ovarian, endometrial, and oropharyngeal squamous cell carcinoma (Bertout et al., 2008). HIF can directly upregulate a number of angiogenic factors, including VEGF, VEGF receptors, plasminogen activator inhibitor-1, angiopoietins (ANG-1 and -2), platelet-derived growth factor B, the TIE-2 receptor, and MMPs (Hickey and Simon, 2006). As a transcription factor, HIF-1 can also induce the expression of gene products encoding the glycolytic enzymes phosphoglycerate kinase-1 and lactate dehydrogenase A, which provide energy for cancer cells under hypoxic conditions (Firth et al., 1994). Indeed, HIF-1 has been shown to be a potent inducer of metastatic genes including chemokine receptor 4, its ligands, and lysyl oxidase in a broad range of tumors (Arya et al., 2007), as well as E-cadherin, a key factor governing metastatic probability in the majority of epithelial cancers (Hanahan and Weinberg, 2011).

The δ-isomer of tocotrienol has been reported to inhibit hypoxia-induced inflammation by inhibiting COX-2 and IL-8 in human colorectal cancer cells and hepatoma cells. δ-T3 has been shown to suppress HIF-1α expression, which in turn leads to inhibition of angiogenesis in human colorectal cancer cells (Shibata et al., 2008). When T3 isomers were compared for their effect on VEGF secretion, the inhibitory effect was ranked as δ- > β- > γ- > α-T3. γ-T3 has been shown to significantly inhibit both basal and cobalt (II) chloride-induced HIF-1α protein accumulation and VEGF expression in the human gastric adenocarcinoma cells (Bi et al., 2010). This effect is mediated through the inhibition of hypoxia-mediated activation of ERK1/2 and subsequently a decrease of HIF-1α accumulation, which leads to downregulation of gene expression and secretion of VEGF.

Similarly, an ether derivative of α-T3, 6-O-carboxypropyl-α-tocotrienol (T3E) has been shown to exert an effect on HIF-2α. This redox-silent analogue of α-T3 has been shown to decrease hypoxia-induced HIF-2α protein levels in lung cancer cells (Kashiwagi et al., 2008). HIF-2α is known to be strongly associated with adaptation of cancer cells during prolonged hypoxia (Lin et al., 2011). Moreover, the inhibition of HIF-2α by α-T3 reduced invasion capacity through downregulation of transcription of plasminogen activator-1 in lung cancer cells. Overall, these results suggest that inhibition of HIF by T3 could have potential in the treatment of cancers.

15.3.6 Nuclear Factor Erythroid 2–Related Factor

The transcription factor NRF2 is normally retained in the cytoplasm by binding with its negative regulator Keap1 (Dinkova-Kostova et al., 2002). Once NRF2 dissociates from Keap1, it translocates to the nucleus, heterodimerizes with small Maf, and binds to ARE, resulting in the expression of a responsive gene (Itoh et al., 1999) (Figure 15.3). NRF2 regulates the expression of approximately 100 cytoprotective genes, including glutathione S-transferases (GSTs), heme oxygenase-1 (HO-1), NAD(P)H:quinoneoxidoreductase 1 (NQO1), and peroxiredoxin 1. NRF2 also plays a major role as a central regulator of the adaptive response to oxidative stress. When exposed to xenobiotics or chemicals that generate intracellular oxidative stress, $nrf2^{-/-}$ mice display increased tissue damage and prolonged inflammation; high amounts of DNA, lipid, and protein oxidation; and an increased incidence of cancer (Aoki et al., 2001; Ramos-Gomez et al., 2001, 2003). Thus, agents with potential to activate NRF2 are considered to be promising chemopreventive agents, and some of these are now undergoing human trials for cancer chemoprevention.

Tocotrienols and tocopherols are known for their antioxidative effects. However, tocopherols have been studied quite extensively for their antioxidative properties and limited information is

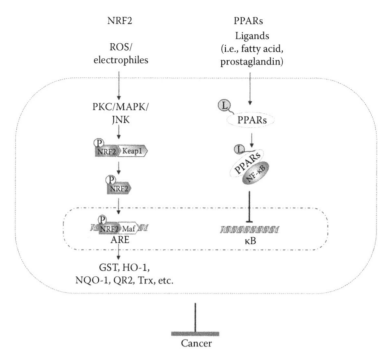

FIGURE 15.3 Anti-inflammatory signaling pathways (NRF2 and PPARs) that suppress tumorigenesis. ARE, antioxidant response element; GST, glutathione-S-transferase; HO-1, heme oxygenase-1; JNK, c-Jun N terminal kinases; Keap1, Kelch-like erythroid cell-derived protein with CNC homology (ECH)-associated protein 1; L, ligands; MAPK, mitogen-activated protein kinase; NQO-1, NAD(P)H:quinone oxidoreductase 1; NRF2, nuclear factor erythroid 2-related factor 2; P, phosphorylation; PKC, protein kinase C; PPARγ, peroxisome proliferator-activated receptor gamma; ROS, reactive oxygen species.

available on T3s. Recently, Hsieh et al. (2010) reported that T3s could suppress cell proliferation and could modulate antioxidant enzyme expression in human breast cancer cells. The authors also showed that δ-T3 was more active than α- or γ-T3 in upregulating the antioxidant glutathione peroxidase; however, these three T3s had comparable activity in inducing thioredoxin in the estrogen receptor–negative human breast cancer cell line MDA-MB-231. Interestingly, in estrogen receptor–positive MCF-7 cells, expressions of quinone reductase 2 and thioredoxin were increased by γ- and δ-T3, whereas quinone reductase 1 was unaffected by any T3s. In MDA-MB-231 cells, T3s upregulated the expression of NRF2 with a corresponding decrease in Keap1. In contrast, no significant change in either NRF2 or Keap1 was found in MCF-7 cells. The authors suggested that the action of T3s in activating NRF2 might have therapeutic potential against cancer.

15.3.7 PEROXISOME-PROLIFERATOR-ACTIVATED RECEPTOR-γ

PPARs, members of the nuclear receptor superfamily, are best understood as regulators of lipid metabolism (Figure 15.3). PPARs are also known to directly downregulate the expression of pro-inflammatory gene products in a ligand-dependent manner by antagonizing the activity of pro-inflammatory transcription factors such as NF-κB and AP-1 (Jiang et al., 1998; Marx et al., 1998; Ricote et al., 1998). PPARs are involved in the regulation of cellular differentiation, development, metabolism, and tumorigenesis as well (Belfiore et al., 2009). There are three forms of PPAR: α, β/δ, and γ (Ricote and Glass, 2007). Among PPARs, PPARγ (also known as the glitazone receptor) is one of the nuclear receptor proteins that acts as a transcription factor and controls the expression of different genes. PPARγ is normally present in diverse systems such as adipocytes, skeletal muscle cells, osteoclasts, osteoblasts, and several immune-type cells. Interestingly, somatic mutations in PPARγ have been found in sporadic colorectal carcinomas (Kinzler and Vogelstein, 1996). These findings suggest an important role for PPARγ as a tumor suppressor. However, under certain circumstances, PPARγ ligands may stimulate cancer formation as well (Koeffler, 2003).

Numerous lines of evidence have indicated that tocotrienols can activate PPARs. In one study, both α- and γ-T3 were found to activate PPARα, whereas δ-T3 activated PPARα, PPARγ, and PPARδ (Fang et al., 2010). T3s also enhanced the interaction of the ligand-binding domain of PPARα with the receptor-interacting motif of coactivator-1α (Fang et al., 2010). Recently, Campbell et al. found that γ-T3 has potential to inhibit growth of prostate cancer cells in a PPAR-γ-dependent mechanism. The group also observed that γ-T3 treatment increased the level of the 15-lipoxygenase-2 enzyme, which is responsible for the conversion of arachidonic acid to the PPAR-γ-activating ligand 15-S-hydroxyeicosatrienoic acid (Campbell et al., 2011). Implications of these observations indicate that modulating the activities of PPARs by tocotrienols may have therapeutic potential for the prevention and treatment of cancer.

15.4 CONCLUSIONS

It is clear from the previous discussion that chronic inflammation is tightly linked with cancer. Tocotrienols can suppress inflammatory pathways and thus may help in the prevention and treatment of cancer. Tocotrienols can modulate multiple transcription factors that are involved in tumor development. The recommendations made by the U.S. National Cancer Institute are that a chemopreventive agent should be nontoxic to normal and healthy people, should have high efficacy against multiple sites, should be orally bioavailable, should have a known mechanism of action, should be easily accessible, and should be acceptable to most of the human population. Tocotrienols appear to meet most of these requirements. However, the use of tocotrienol for cancer prevention and treatment in the clinic awaits the answer of several unresolved questions, including those about bioavailability and safety. Future studies in this direction will hopefully bring this fascinating nutraceutical to the forefront of cancer therapeutics for human use.

ACKNOWLEDGMENTS

We thank Michael Worley of the Department of Scientific Publications for carefully editing this chapter and providing valuable comments. Dr. Aggarwal is the Ransom Horne Jr., Professor of Cancer Research. This work was supported by Malaysian Palm Oil Board, Kaula Lumpur, Malaysia.

REFERENCES

Aggarwal BB, Kunnumakkara AB, Harikumar KB, Gupta SR, Tharakan ST, Koca C, Dey S and Sung B (2009) Signal transducer and activator of transcription-3, inflammation, and cancer: How intimate is the relationship? *Ann N Y Acad Sci* 1171:59–76.

Aggarwal BB, Sethi G, Ahn KS, Sandur SK, Pandey MK, Kunnumakkara AB, Sung B and Ichikawa H (2006a) Targeting signal-transducer-and-activator-of-transcription-3 for prevention and therapy of cancer: Modern target but ancient solution. *Ann N Y Acad Sci* 1091:151–169.

Aggarwal BB, Shishodia S, Sandur SK, Pandey MK and Sethi G (2006b) Inflammation and cancer: How hot is the link? *Biochem Pharmacol* 72(11):1605–1621.

Ahn KS, Sethi G and Aggarwal BB (2007a) Nuclear factor-kappa B: From clone to clinic. *Curr Mol Med* 7(7):619–637.

Ahn KS, Sethi G, Krishnan K and Aggarwal BB (2007b) Gamma-tocotrienol inhibits nuclear factor-kappaB signaling pathway through inhibition of receptor-interacting protein and TAK1 leading to suppression of antiapoptotic gene products and potentiation of apoptosis. *J Biol Chem* 282(1):809–820.

Anand P, Kunnumakkara AB, Sundaram C, Harikumar KB, Tharakan ST, Lai OS, Sung B and Aggarwal BB (2008) Cancer is a preventable disease that requires major lifestyle changes. *Pharm Res* 25(9):2097–2116.

Aoki Y, Sato H, Nishimura N, Takahashi S, Itoh K and Yamamoto M (2001) Accelerated DNA adduct formation in the lung of the Nrf2 knockout mouse exposed to diesel exhaust. *Toxicol Appl Pharmacol* 173(3):154–160.

Arya M, Ahmed H, Silhi N, Williamson M and Patel HR (2007) Clinical importance and therapeutic implications of the pivotal CXCL12-CXCR4 (chemokine ligand-receptor) interaction in cancer cell migration. *Tumour Biol* 28(3):123–131.

Bachawal SV, Wali VB and Sylvester PW (2010) Combined gamma-tocotrienol and erlotinib/gefitinib treatment suppresses Stat and Akt signaling in murine mammary tumor cells. *Anticancer Res* 30(2):429–437.

Belfiore A, Genua M and Malaguarnera R (2009) PPAR-gamma agonists and their effects on IGF-I receptor signaling: implications for cancer. *PPAR Res* 2009:830501.

Bernstein LR and Colburn NH (1989) AP1/jun function is differentially induced in promotion-sensitive and resistant JB6 cells. *Science* 244(4904):566–569.

Bertout JA, Patel SA and Simon MC (2008) The impact of O2 availability on human cancer. *Nat Rev Cancer* 8(12):967–975.

Bi S, Liu JR, Li Y, Wang Q, Liu HK, Yan YG, Chen BQ and Sun WG (2010) gamma-Tocotrienol modulates the paracrine secretion of VEGF induced by cobalt(II) chloride via ERK signaling pathway in gastric adenocarcinoma SGC-7901 cell line. *Toxicology* 274(1–3):27–33.

Bienz M and Clevers H (2003) Armadillo/beta-catenin signals in the nucleus—Proof beyond a reasonable doubt? *Nat Cell Biol* 5(3):179–182.

Campbell SE, Rudder B, Phillips RB, Whaley SG, Stimmel JB, Leesnitzer LM, Lightner J, Dessus-Babus S, Duffourc M, Stone WL, Menter DG, Newman RA, Yang P, Aggarwal BB and Krishnan K (2011) gamma-Tocotrienol induces growth arrest through a novel pathway with TGFbeta2 in prostate cancer. *Free Radic Biol Med* 50(10):1344–1354.

Catlett-Falcone R, Landowski TH, Oshiro MM, Turkson J, Levitzki A, Savino R, Ciliberto G et al. (1999) Constitutive activation of Stat3 signaling confers resistance to apoptosis in human U266 myeloma cells. *Immunity* 10(1):105–115.

Chang PN, Yap WN, Lee DT, Ling MT, Wong YC and Yap YL (2009) Evidence of gamma-tocotrienol as an apoptosis-inducing, invasion-suppressing, and chemotherapy drug-sensitizing agent in human melanoma cells. *Nutr Cancer* 61(3):357–366.

Chaturvedi MM, Sung B, Yadav VR, Kannappan R and Aggarwal BB (2011) NF-kappaB addiction and its role in cancer: 'One size does not fit all'. *Oncogene* 30(14):1615–1630.

Chinenov Y and Kerppola TK (2001) Close encounters of many kinds: Fos-Jun interactions that mediate transcription regulatory specificity. *Oncogene* 20(19):2438–2452.

Clevers H (2006) Wnt/beta-catenin signaling in development and disease. *Cell* 127(3):469–480.

Crispen PL, Uzzo RG, Golovine K, Makhov P, Pollack A, Horwitz EM, Greenberg RE and Kolenko VM (2007) Vitamin E succinate inhibits NF-kappaB and prevents the development of a metastatic phenotype in prostate cancer cells: implications for chemoprevention. *Prostate* 67(6):582–590.

Dinkova-Kostova AT, Holtzclaw WD, Cole RN, Itoh K, Wakabayashi N, Katoh Y, Yamamoto M and Talalay P (2002) Direct evidence that sulfhydryl groups of Keap1 are the sensors regulating induction of phase 2 enzymes that protect against carcinogens and oxidants. *Proc Natl Acad Sci USA* 99(18):11908–11913.

Eferl R and Wagner EF (2003) AP-1: A double-edged sword in tumorigenesis. *Nat Rev Cancer* 3(11):859–868.

Fang F, Kang Z and Wong C (2010) Vitamin E tocotrienols improve insulin sensitivity through activating peroxisome proliferator-activated receptors. *Mol Nutr Food Res* 54(3):345–352.

Firth JD, Ebert BL, Pugh CW and Ratcliffe PJ (1994) Oxygen-regulated control elements in the phosphoglycerate kinase 1 and lactate dehydrogenase A genes: Similarities with the erythropoietin 3' enhancer. *Proc Natl Acad Sci USA* 91(14):6496–6500.

Giaccia A, Siim BG and Johnson RS (2003) HIF-1 as a target for drug development. *Nat Rev Drug Discov* 2(10):803–811.

Giles RH, van Es JH and Clevers H (2003) Caught up in a Wnt storm: Wnt signaling in cancer. *Biochim Biophys Acta* 1653(1):1–24.

Grivennikov S, Karin E, Terzic J, Mucida D, Yu GY, Vallabhapurapu S, Scheller J et al. (2009) IL-6 and Stat3 are required for survival of intestinal epithelial cells and development of colitis-associated cancer. *Cancer Cell* 15(2):103–113.

Gupta SC, Kim JH, Prasad S and Aggarwal BB (2010a) Regulation of survival, proliferation, invasion, angiogenesis, and metastasis of tumor cells through modulation of inflammatory pathways by nutraceuticals. *Cancer Metastasis Rev* 29(3):405–434.

Gupta SC, Sundaram C, Reuter S and Aggarwal BB (2010b) Inhibiting NF-kappaB activation by small molecules as a therapeutic strategy. *Biochim Biophys Acta* 1799(10–12):775–787.

Ha H, Lee JH, Kim HN and Lee ZH (2011) alpha-Tocotrienol inhibits osteoclastic bone resorption by suppressing RANKL expression and signaling and bone resorbing activity. *Biochem Biophys Res Commun* 406(4):546–551.

Hanahan D and Weinberg RA (2011) Hallmarks of cancer: the next generation. *Cell* 100(1):57–70.

Hickey MM and Simon MC (2006) Regulation of angiogenesis by hypoxia and hypoxia-inducible factors. *Curr Top Dev Biol* 76:217–257.

Hsieh TC, Elangovan S and Wu JM (2010) Differential suppression of proliferation in MCF-7 and MDA-MB-231 breast cancer cells exposed to alpha-, gamma- and delta-tocotrienols is accompanied by altered expression of oxidative stress modulatory enzymes. *Anticancer Res* 30(10):4169–4176.

Itoh K, Wakabayashi N, Katoh Y, Ishii T, Igarashi K, Engel JD and Yamamoto M (1999) Keap1 represses nuclear activation of antioxidant responsive elements by Nrf2 through binding to the amino-terminal Neh2 domain. *Genes Dev* 13(1):76–86.

Jensen GL (2006) Inflammation as the key interface of the medical and nutrition universes: A provocative examination of the future of clinical nutrition and medicine. *JPEN J Parenter Enteral Nutr* 30(5):453–463.

Jensen GL and Roubenoff R (2008) Introduction: Nutrition and inflammation: Research Makes The Connection–Intersociety Research Workshop, Chicago, February 8–9, 2008. *JPEN J Parenter Enteral Nutr* 32(6):625.

Ji X WZ, Geamanu A, Sarkar FH, Gupta SV (2011) Inhibition of cell growth and induction of apoptosis in non- small cell lung cancer cells by delta- tocotrienol is associated with Notch- 1 down- regulation. *J Cell Biochem* 112(10):2773–2783.

Jiang C, Ting AT and Seed B (1998) PPAR-gamma agonists inhibit production of monocyte inflammatory cytokines. *Nature* 391(6662):82–86.

Kannappan R, Yadav VR and Aggarwal BB (2010) gamma-Tocotrienol but not gamma-tocopherol blocks STAT3 cell signaling pathway through induction of protein-tyrosine phosphatase SHP-1 and sensitizes tumor cells to chemotherapeutic agents. *J Biol Chem* 285(43):33520–33528.

Karin M and Greten FR (2005) NF-kappaB: Linking inflammation and immunity to cancer development and progression. *Nat Rev Immunol* 5(10):749–759.

Kashiwagi K, Harada K, Yano Y, Kumadaki I, Hagiwara K, Takebayashi J, Kido W, Virgona N and Yano T (2008) A redox-silent analogue of tocotrienol inhibits hypoxic adaptation of lung cancer cells. *Biochem Biophys Res Commun* 365(4):875–881.

Kashiwagi K, Virgona N, Harada K, Kido W, Yano Y, Ando A, Hagiwara K and Yano T (2009) A redox-silent analogue of tocotrienol acts as a potential cytotoxic agent against human mesothelioma cells. *Life Sci* 84(19–20):650–656.

Kinzler KW and Vogelstein B (1996) Lessons from hereditary colorectal cancer. *Cell* 87(2):159–170.

Kobayashi H, Kanno C, Yamauchi K and Tsugo T (1975) Identification of alpha-, beta-, gamma-, and delta-tocopherols and their contents in human milk. *Biochim Biophys Acta* 380(2):282–290.

Koeffler HP (2003) Peroxisome proliferator-activated receptor gamma and cancers. *Clin Cancer Res* 9(1):1–9.

Kong YY, Feige U, Sarosi I, Bolon B, Tafuri A, Morony S, Capparelli C et al. (1999) Activated T cells regulate bone loss and joint destruction in adjuvant arthritis through osteoprotegerin ligand. *Nature* 402(6759):304–309.

Kortylewski M, Xin H, Kujawski M, Lee H, Liu Y, Harris T, Drake C, Pardoll D and Yu H (2009) Regulation of the IL-23 and IL-12 balance by Stat3 signaling in the tumor microenvironment. *Cancer Cell* 15(2):114–123.

Kuchide M, Tokuda H, Takayasu J, Enjo F, Ishikawa T, Ichiishi E, Naito Y, Yoshida N, Yoshikawa T and Nishino H (2003) Cancer chemopreventive effects of oral feeding alpha-tocopherol on ultraviolet light B induced photocarcinogenesis of hairless mouse. *Cancer Lett* 196(2):169–177.

Kujawski M, Kortylewski M, Lee H, Herrmann A, Kay H and Yu H (2008) Stat3 mediates myeloid cell-dependent tumor angiogenesis in mice. *J Clin Invest* 118(10):3367–3377.

Kunnumakkara AB, Sung B, Ravindran J, Diagaradjane P, Deorukhkar A, Dey S, Koca C et al. (2010) {Gamma}-tocotrienol inhibits pancreatic tumors and sensitizes them to gemcitabine treatment by modulating the inflammatory microenvironment. *Cancer Res* 70(21):8695–8705.

Lee W, Haslinger A, Karin M and Tjian R (1987) Activation of transcription by two factors that bind promoter and enhancer sequences of the human metallothionein gene and SV40. *Nature* 325(6102):368–372.

Li Y, Sun WG, Liu HK, Qi GY, Wang Q, Sun XR, Chen BQ and Liu JR (2011) gamma-Tocotrienol inhibits angiogenesis of human umbilical vein endothelia cell induced by cancer cell. *J Nutr Biochem* 22(12):1127–1136.

Li Q, Withoff S and Verma IM (2005) Inflammation-associated cancer: NF-kappaB is the lynchpin. *Trends Immunol* 26(6):318–325.

Lin Q, Cong X and Yun Z (2011) Differential hypoxic regulation of hypoxia-inducible factors 1alpha and 2alpha. *Mol Cancer Res* 9(6):757–765.

Mantovani A, Allavena P, Sica A and Balkwill F (2008) Cancer-related inflammation. *Nature* 454(7203):436–444.

Marx N, Schonbeck U, Lazar MA, Libby P and Plutzky J (1998) Peroxisome proliferator-activated receptor gamma activators inhibit gene expression and migration in human vascular smooth muscle cells. *Circ Res* 83(11):1097–1103.

Maxwell PH, Pugh CW and Ratcliffe PJ (2001) Activation of the HIF pathway in cancer. *Curr Opin Genet Dev* 11(3):293–299.

Mukhopadhyay S, Mukherjee S, Stone WL, Smith M and Das SK (2009) Role of MAPK/AP-1 signaling pathway in the protection of CEES-induced lung injury by antioxidant liposome. *Toxicology* 261(3):143–151.

NCHS (1900) National center for health statistics, National office of vital statistics.67.

NCHS (1948) National Center for health statistics, National office of vital statistics.55.

Nusse R and Varmus HE (1982) Many tumors induced by the mouse mammary tumor virus contain a provirus integrated in the same region of the host genome. *Cell* 31(1):99–109.

Packer L, Weber SU and Rimbach G (2001) Molecular aspects of alpha-tocotrienol antioxidant action and cell signalling. *J Nutr* 131(2):369S–373S.

Patacsil D TAT, Cho YS, Suy S, Saenz F, Malyukova I, Ressom H, Collins SP, Clarke R, Kumar D (2011) Gamma- tocotrienol induced apoptosis is associated with unfolded response in human breast cancer cells. *J Nutr Biochem* 23(1):93–100.

Pearce BC, Parker RA, Deason ME, Qureshi AA and Wright JJ (1992) Hypocholesterolemic activity of synthetic and natural tocotrienols. *J Med Chem* 35(20):3595–3606.

Prasad S, Ravindran J and Aggarwal BB (2010) NF-kappaB and cancer: How intimate is this relationship. *Mol Cell Biochem* 336(1–2):25–37.

Qian M, Kralova J, Yu W, Bose HR, Jr., Dvorak M, Sanders BG and Kline K (1997) c-Jun involvement in vitamin E succinate induced apoptosis of reticuloendotheliosis virus transformed avian lymphoid cells. *Oncogene* 15(2):223–230.

Qureshi AA, Burger WC, Peterson DM and Elson CE (1986) The structure of an inhibitor of cholesterol biosynthesis isolated from barley. *J Biol Chem* 261(23):10544–10550.

Rajendran P, Li F, Manu KA, Shanmugam MK, Loo SY, Kumar AP and Sethi G (2011) gamma-Tocotrienol is a novel inhibitor of constitutive and inducible STAT3 signalling pathway in human hepatocellular carcinoma: potential role as an antiproliferative, pro-apoptotic and chemosensitizing agent. *Br J Pharmacol* 163(2):283–298.

Ramos-Gomez M, Dolan PM, Itoh K, Yamamoto M and Kensler TW (2003) Interactive effects of nrf2 genotype and oltipraz on benzo[a]pyrene-DNA adducts and tumor yield in mice. *Carcinogenesis* 24(3):461–467.

Ramos-Gomez M, Kwak MK, Dolan PM, Itoh K, Yamamoto M, Talalay P and Kensler TW (2001) Sensitivity to carcinogenesis is increased and chemoprotective efficacy of enzyme inducers is lost in nrf2 transcription factor-deficient mice. *Proc Natl Acad Sci USA* 98(6):3410–3415.

Rebouissou S, Amessou M, Couchy G, Poussin K, Imbeaud S, Pilati C, Izard T, Balabaud C, Bioulac-Sage P and Zucman-Rossi J (2009) Frequent in-frame somatic deletions activate gp130 in inflammatory hepatocellular tumours. *Nature* 457(7226):200–204.

Ricote M and Glass CK (2007) PPARs and molecular mechanisms of transrepression. *Biochim Biophys Acta* 1771(8):926–935.

Ricote M, Li AC, Willson TM, Kelly CJ and Glass CK (1998) The peroxisome proliferator-activated receptor-gamma is a negative regulator of macrophage activation. *Nature* 391(6662):79–82.

Semenza GL (2003) Targeting HIF-1 for cancer therapy. *Nat Rev Cancer* 3(10):721–732.

Sen R and Baltimore D (1986) Multiple nuclear factors interact with the immunoglobulin enhancer sequences. *Cell* 46(5):705–716.

Shah SJ and Sylvester PW (2005) Gamma-tocotrienol inhibits neoplastic mammary epithelial cell proliferation by decreasing Akt and nuclear factor kappaB activity. *Exp Biol Med (Maywood)* 230(4):235–241.

Shaulian E and Karin M (2002) AP-1 as a regulator of cell life and death. *Nat Cell Biol* 4(5):E131–E136.

Shibata A, Nakagawa K, Sookwong P, Tsuduki T, Tomita S, Shirakawa H, Komai M and Miyazawa T (2008) Tocotrienol inhibits secretion of angiogenic factors from human colorectal adenocarcinoma cells by suppressing hypoxia-inducible factor-1alpha. *J Nutr* 138(11):2136–2142.

Shirode AB and Sylvester PW (2010) Synergistic anticancer effects of combined gamma-tocotrienol and celecoxib treatment are associated with suppression in Akt and NFkappaB signaling. *Biomed Pharmacother* 64(5):327–332.

Stone WL, Krishnan K, Campbell SE, Qui M, Whaley SG and Yang H (2004) Tocopherols and the treatment of colon cancer. *Ann N Y Acad Sci* 1031:223–233.

Sylvester PW, Shah SJ and Samant GV (2005) Intracellular signaling mechanisms mediating the antiproliferative and apoptotic effects of gamma-tocotrienol in neoplastic mammary epithelial cells. *J Plant Physiol* 162(7):803–810.

Theriault A, Chao JT and Gapor A (2002) Tocotrienol is the most effective vitamin E for reducing endothelial expression of adhesion molecules and adhesion to monocytes. *Atherosclerosis* 160(1):21–30.

Wang GL, Jiang BH, Rue EA and Semenza GL (1995) Hypoxia-inducible factor 1 is a basic-helix-loop-helix-PAS heterodimer regulated by cellular O2 tension. *Proc Natl Acad Sci USA* 92(12):5510–5514.

Whittle KJ, Dunphy PJ and Pennock JF (1966) The isolation and properties of delta-tocotrienol from Hevea latex. *Biochem J* 100(1):138–145.

Wilankar C, Sharma D, Checker R, Khan NM, Patwardhan R, Patil A, Sandur SK and Devasagayam TP (2011) Role of immunoregulatory transcription factors in differential immunomodulatory effects of tocotrienols. *Free Radic Biol Med* 51(1):129–143.

Wu SJ, Liu PL and Ng LT (2008) Tocotrienol-rich fraction of palm oil exhibits anti-inflammatory property by suppressing the expression of inflammatory mediators in human monocytic cells. *Mol Nutr Food Res* 52(8):921–929.

Xu WL, Liu JR, Liu HK, Qi GY, Sun XR, Sun WG and Chen BQ (2009) Inhibition of proliferation and induction of apoptosis by gamma-tocotrienol in human colon carcinoma HT-29 cells. *Nutrition* 25(5):555–566.

Yap WN, Chang PN, Han HY, Lee DT, Ling MT, Wong YC and Yap YL (2008) Gamma-tocotrienol suppresses prostate cancer cell proliferation and invasion through multiple-signalling pathways. *Br J Cancer* 99(11):1832–1841.

Young MR, Yang HS and Colburn NH (2003) Promising molecular targets for cancer prevention: AP-1, NF-kappa B and Pdcd4. *Trends Mol Med* 9(1):36–41.

Zenz R, Eferl R, Scheinecker C, Redlich K, Smolen J, Schonthaler HB, Kenner L, Tschachler E and Wagner EF (2008) Activator protein 1 (Fos/Jun) functions in inflammatory bone and skin disease. *Arthritis Res Ther* 10(1):201.

Zhang JS, Li DM, He N, Liu YH, Wang CH, Jiang SQ, Chen BQ and Liu JR (2011) A paraptosis-like cell death induced by delta-tocotrienol in human colon carcinoma SW620 cells is associated with the suppression of the Wnt signaling pathway. *Toxicology* 285(1–2):8–17.

16 1-Modulating NF-κB Activity by Tocotrienols

Mary Kaileh and Ranjan Sen

CONTENTS

16.1 INTRODUCTION

The NF-κB family of transcription factors is composed of homo- and heterodimers of REL homology domain (RHD)-containing polypeptides. The RHD is a 300-amino-acid domain that mediates protein–protein interactions as well as DNA binding. Mammals contain five RHD-containing proteins NF-κB1, NF-κB2, REL, RELA, and RELB. The RHDs of REL family members are located at the N-termini of these proteins. NF-κB1 and NF-κB2, the longest polypeptides (105 and 100 kD, respectively), are further processed to generate p50 and p52 proteins that are composed mostly of the RHD itself (Basak et al. 2007). p50 forms homodimers and heterodimerizes primarily with RELA (p65) and REL; p52 also forms homodimers but heterodimerizes primarily with RELB. Thus, despite substantial homology between these proteins, p50 and p52 serve different cellular functions. The other three REL family members (REL, RELA, and RELB) contain C-terminal extensions beyond the RHD that act as transcription activation domains. REL and RELA can form homodimers and REL/RELA heterodimers in addition to p50-containing heterodimers. RELB is believed not to homodimerize and forms heterodimers largely with p52 (Bonizzi and Karin 2004). REL, RELA, and RELB polypeptides do not undergo proteolytic processing but can be posttranslationally modified by phosphorylation and acetylation (Chen and Greene 2003; Neumann and Naumann 2007). These modifications have been shown to alter their transcriptional properties. It is obvious that "NF-κB" constitutes a family of DNA binding proteins, thus analysis of NF-κB-dependent gene transcription must account for which family member(s) is being used to activate genes of interest.

NF-κB is a family of inducible transcription factors, which means that they are activated in response to cell stimulation. NF-κB-dependent transcription can be divided into classical and alternate NF-κB responses. The classical response is mediated primarily by REL- and RELA-containing homo- and heterodimeric transcription factors (Hayden and Ghosh 2008). These factors are present in inactivated cells in a non-DNA binding state due to association with a family of inhibitory proteins known as IκBs. In response to cell stimulation, IκB proteins are phosphorylated by IκB kinase 2 (IKK2) marking them for proteasome-mediated degradation. Upon degradation of IκB, REL and RELA-containing NF-κB translocate to the nucleus to activate gene transcription

(Sen and Smale 2010). This form of activation has two important characteristics. First, because the DNA-binding transcription factor is present in cells prior to stimulation, this form of activation does not require new protein synthesis. Thus, it is rapid. Second, one of the targets of RELA-containing NF-κB is the *Nfkbia* (IκBα) gene. *De novo* transcription of *Nfkbia* leads to production of IκBα protein, which can reassociate with DNA-binding NF-κB and functionally sequester it (Ghosh and Karin 2002). This process makes classical NF-κB activation transient and is also responsible for the observation of NF-κB "superinduction" when activation is carried out in the presence of inhibitors of protein synthesis.

Activation of the alternate pathway requires stabilization of basally translated NF-κB-inducing kinase (NIK), which activates the IκB kinase 1 (IKK1) (Qing et al. 2005). IKK1 phosphorylates NF-κB2 leading to its processing to p52, thereby producing p52/RELB complexes to activate gene transcription (Bonizzi and Karin 2004). The requirement for the stabilization of NIK to activate this pathway means that it is slower. Moreover, since p52/RELB heterodimers do not activate transcription of any known inhibitor of this transcription factor, the alternate pathway is not subject to feedback inhibition like the classical pathway. This implies that once induced p52/RELB can continuously activate gene transcription. However, this circumstance would reduce the effectiveness of NF-κB as an inducible transcription factor. Therefore, it is likely that there are means to terminate alternate pathway activation. However, as of now this remains an open and interesting question in NF-κB biology.

Cellular stimuli can activate the classical pathway, the alternate pathway, or both pathways. The best characterized activators of the classical pathway are the cytokines TNFα and interleukin-1 (IL-1); conversely, lymphotoxin β and the B cell survival cytokine BAFF primarily activate the alternate pathway. The TNF receptor superfamily member CD40 that is essential for effective humoral responses effectively activates both classical and alternate pathways (Zarnegar et al. 2004; Elgueta et al. 2009; Rickert et al. 2011). While there are receptors that primarily activate one or the other NF-κB pathway, it is quite likely that *in vivo* both pathways may often be activated simultaneously via two different receptors. This becomes particularly important in optimizing cross-talk between the two pathways. The question of cross-talk emerges from the demonstration that both *Nfkb2* and *Relb* genes are transcriptional targets of the classical pathway (Lombardi et al. 1995; Bren et al. 2001; Basak et al. 2008). Thus, one can envisage the following plausible scenario. Activation of the alternate pathway leads to NF-κB2 processing and p52/RELB-dependent transcription. Sooner or later, the cellular pool of NF-κB2 runs out, thereby functionally terminating further activation of the alternate pathway. However, if the classical pathway has been simultaneously activated, then NF-κB-dependent *Nfkb2* and *Relb* transcription and consequent protein production will maintain a continuous pool of NF-κB2/RELB dimers to serve as the substrate for the alternate pathway. We have previously shown this form of effective cross-talk in spleen B lymphocytes stimulated via the B cell antigen receptor (an activator of classical NF-κB) and the BAFF receptor (an activator of alternate NF-κB) (Stadanlick et al. 2008).

Tom Gilmore and colleagues maintain a website that lists putative NF-κB target genes. These genes can be broadly categorized as (1) anti-apoptotic genes (such as Bclx, A1, and GADD45β), (2) cytokine and chemokine genes (such as IL-1, 2, 6, TNFα, CCL3, and CCL4), (3) cell cycle regulators (such as c-myc and cyclin D2), and (4) cell adhesion molecules (such as ICAM and VCAM). There are several other putative target genes that do not fall into these categories. The importance of NF-κB as a regulator of inflammation stems not only from the nature of genes induced but also from the fact that some NF-κB target genes are themselves inducers of NF-κB. The most prominent of these are TNFα and IL-1. Thus, once a stimulus induces NF-κB to activate TNFα, the cytokine can itself feedback on the cells (or the cellular microenvironment) to induce NF-κB. This has the potential to establish a self-sustaining, or self-amplifying, loop that persistently activates inflammatory gene expression. Additional perspectives on NF-κB biology and NF-κB-dependent gene expression can be found in several recent reviews and monographs (Sen and Smale 2010; Staudt and Karin 2010; Shih et al. 2011).

16.2   TOCOTRIENOLS AND NF-κB

Tocotrienols belong to the vitamin E family and mediate broad biological activities such as antioxidant, anti-inflammatory, antitumor, and anti-angiogenic effects. The chemical structures of tocotrienols are made up of an aromatic chromanol ring and an isoprenoid chain containing multiple unsaturated C-C bonds (Sen et al. 2007). Depending on the number and position of methyl substitutions on the chromanol ring, tocotrienols are further subdivided into four isomers (α, β, γ, and δ). The higher degrees of unsaturation in combination with a hypomethylated chroman ring in tocotrienols have suggested that they are more potent antioxidants compared to tocopherols. The richest sources of tocotrienols are palm oil, rice bran, and annatto oils (Sen et al. 2006). We have recently reviewed the effects of tocotrienols on NF-κB induction and function (Kaileh and Sen 2010). Here, we incorporate additional studies that have been published since then to provide an up-to-date perspective on the relationship of this important family of compounds to a critical transcription factor.

16.2.1   T3 MODULATION OF INDUCIBLE NF-κB

The normal function of NF-κB is as an inducible transcription factor that responds to extracellular stimuli. Thus, one important situation in which to consider the effects of tocotrienols is on inducible NF-κB function. One of the earliest studies to do this showed that TNFα-induced activation of cell adhesion molecules VCAM-1 and ICAM-1 was significantly reduced by pretreatment of human umbilical vein endothelial cells (HUVECs) with α-tocotrienol (αT3) for 20 h (Theriault et al. 2002). αT3 reduced the adherence of monocytic THP-1 cells to TNFα-treated HUVECs, probably because of attenuated expression of these adhesion molecules. Theriault et al. found that cell adhesion induced by IL-1 and phorbol ester (PMA) was also reduced by αT3. Interestingly, all three inducing agents are well-known activators of NF-κB, and, indeed, NF-κB induction by TNFα was reduced, but not eliminated, by αT3 in this study. The use of primary untransformed endothelial cells and the implications for the use of tocotrienols as means of intervention in atherosclerosis made this a notable pioneering study.

Ahn et al. (2007) carried out the most comprehensive analysis to date of the effects of tocotrienol on NF-κB induction (Ahn et al. 2007). In this study, γT3 blocked TNFα-induced NF-κB activation in several human tumor cell lines. For the effect to be observed the cells were incubated with γT3 for 12 h prior to activation. Reduced NF-κB induction was mediated by reduced phosphorylation and degradation of IκBα. The proposed mechanism by which NF-κB was inhibited involved reduced phosphorylation of Akt. This was similar to the work of Sylvester and colleagues, who showed that constitutive Akt phosphorylation was inhibited by γT3 in mammary epithelial cells. Ahn et al. suggested that the repression of NF-κB by γT3 may be mediated by Akt in these cells because Akt has been suggested to be an inducer of NF-κB (Ozes et al. 1999; Romashkova and Makarov 1999). Reduced NF-κB induction in the presence of γT3 correlated with lack of anti-apoptotic protein expression and increased cell death. In a more recent study, Shin-Kang et al. demonstrated that γT3 and δT3 inhibit the activation of Akt by downregulating ErbB2 expression in pancreatic cancer cells (Shin-Kang et al. 2011). As ErbB2 has been proposed to be upstream of NF-κB, the authors suggested that the downregulation of ErbB2 may have a role in inhibiting NF-κB in these cells. The relative contribution of ErB2 or Akt in these circumstances remains to be evaluated.

Inhibition of lipopolysaccharide-induced NF-κB activation has been examined in several studies using a human monocytic cell line (THP1) (Wu et al. 2008), murine macrophage cell line RAW264.7, and peritoneal macrophages (Meyskens et al. 1999; McNulty et al. 2001; Yam et al. 2009). All studies reached similar conclusions. In THP-1 cells, tocotrienol-rich fraction (TRF) blocked TNFα and IL-1β secretion, as well as cytosolic cyclo-oxygenase 2 (COX2) and inducible nitric oxide synthase (iNOS) production. Yam et al. compared the effects of TRF and individual

T3 isomers on cytokine secretion, and iNOS and COX1 and 2 expressions in the LPS-activated RAW264.7 cells. They found that δT3 was the most effective isomer in most assays. In a similar study, Qureshi et al. compared the effects of α-tocopherol (αT) and three isomers of T3 (α, γ, and δ) on the secretion of TNFα in LPS-stimulated RAW264.7 cells and in peritoneal macrophages derived from BALB/c mice. All three T3 isomers inhibited the secretion of TNFα, but the maximal inhibition was obtained with δT3. They also showed that δT3 blocked LPS-induced TNFα, IL-1β, IL-6, and iNOS gene expression (Qureshi et al. 2010). Furthermore, these authors demonstrated that LPS-induced activation of NF-κB and its target genes, TNFα and iNOS, was suppressed by δT3 in RAW264.7 cells and in the peritoneal macrophages. Interestingly, these authors found that IκBα was phosphorylated normally, but not degraded in cells treated with δT3. These observations led them to propose that δT3 works as a proteasome inhibitor (Qureshi et al. 2011a). In a recent study on the effect of δT3 on macrophage responsiveness in young and old mice, animals were fed with δT3 supplemented diet, followed by *ex vivo* stimulation of macrophages with LPS. LPS-induced NO secretion and iNOS expression was suppressed in macrophages from δT3-fed mice. The effect was accentuated in macrophages from older mice, in part due to higher levels of LPS-induced iNOS expression in these animals. TNFα induction by LPS was also suppressed in macrophages from δT3-fed mice (Qureshi et al. 2011b).

Wilankar et al. carried out the first study on the immunomodulatory activity of tocotrienols on murine splenic CD4[+] T cells. In this study, γT3 blocked Con-A-induced T-cell proliferation *in vitro* and blocked anti-CD3/CD28-induced T-cell proliferation *in vitro* and *in vivo*. Stimulation of T cells with either Con-A or anti-CD3/CD28 for 24 h induced IL-2, 4, 6, and INFγ secretion, while cotreatment of these cells with γT3 suppressed the secretion of these cytokines. These authors also showed that pretreatment of T cells with γT3 for 12 h completely inhibited Con-A-induced activation of NF-κB (Wilankar et al. 2011). Although some of the aforementioned studies did not directly examine the effect of TRF and T3s on NF-κB activity *per se*, the examined genes such as TNFα, COX2, IL-6, and iNOS are NF-κB targets; therefore, the biological effects reported were likely mediated by this transcription factor. Furthermore, the differential effects seen with TRF and different T3 isomers highlight the importance of using all of these compounds in future studies of the NF-κB/T3 connection.

16.2.2 T3 Modulation of Constitutive NF-κB

Although NF-κB's most prominent function is to regulate inducible gene transcription in response to activating stimuli, there are circumstances where NF-κB also regulates constitutive gene transcription in the absence of overt cell stimulation. The earliest example of constitutive NF-κB activity was described in B lymphocytes, but constitutive NF-κB has been implicated in many cancers, including hepatic carcinomas, mammary epithelial carcinomas, human melanomas, and B lymphomas (Meyskens et al. 1999; Landesman-Bollag et al. 2001; McNulty et al. 2001; Shaffer et al. 2006; Vainer et al. 2008; Lenz and Staudt 2010). Thus, it is important to examine the response of cells that constitutively express nuclear NF-κB to tocotrienols. Indeed, this has been an area of considerable activity since we previously summarized the state of the NF-κB/tocotrienol connection. Tocotrienols have been shown to reduce constitutive NF-κB activity in a mammary epithelial cell line (Shah and Sylvester 2005), prostate cancer cell line (Yap et al. 2008), multiple myeloma cell line (Ahn et al. 2007), colon carcinoma cell line (Xu et al. 2009), breast cancer cell line (Yap et al. 2010), pancreatic cancer cell line (Kunnumakkara et al. 2010; Husain et al. 2011), human melanoma cell line (Chang et al. 2009), lung cancer cell line (Ji et al. 2011), in tumor tissues of mice xenografted with a pancreatic cancer cell line (Husain et al. 2011), and in an orthotopic pancreatic tumor model in nude mice (Kunnumakkara et al. 2010). Despite the use of different kinds of assays to measure NF-κB induction, which makes it difficult to directly compare these studies, the diversity of tumor lines that respond to T3 indicates that tocotrienols may prove effective in reducing tumor growth. Several recent studies showing constitutive NF-κB inhibition by tocotrienols in pancreatic cancer cells are grounds for particular optimism because these cells are often particularly refractory to common forms of chemotherapy (Bilimoria et al. 2007).

Some of these studies are briefly considered below. Ji et al. showed that treatment of the non-small-cell lung cancer cells, A549 and H1299, with δT3 for 72h results in reduced NF-κB/DNA binding and inhibits the NF-κB target genes Bcl-x$_L$, VEGF, and MMP9 (Ji et al. 2011). They showed that δT3 inhibited cell growth and induced apoptosis through the inhibition of Notch-1 and NF-κB. Yap et al. demonstrated that γT3 suppressed constitutive NF-κB activity in breast cancer cells, MDA-231, by inhibiting the IκB kinase. They also showed that γT3 downregulates the NF-κB target gene Bcl-2 and leads to apoptosis of these cells (Yap et al. 2010). Selvaduray et al. studied the anti-angiogenic effect of TRF, γT3, and δT3 on HUVEC and on 4T1 mouse mammary cancer cells. HUVEC cells treated with TRF, γT3, and δT3 showed reduced levels of the pro-angiogenic cytokines IL-8 and IL-6. Similar treatment of 4T1 cells showed reduced levels of IL-8 and VEGF (Selvaduray et al. 2011). Finally, in a study that examined the effects of tocotrienols *in vivo*, Qureshi et al. showed that supplementation of control diet with δT3 for 4 weeks results in reduced serum levels of TNFα and nitric oxide (NO) in female chickens (Qureshi et al. 2011c).

16.2.3 SYNERGY OF T3 WITH OTHER CHEMOTHERAPEUTIC AGENTS

Cumulatively, all the studies described in the aforementioned sections showed that γT3 and δT3 appear to be the most potent inhibitors of NF-κB and NF-κB-dependent gene expression. However, it is worthwhile to test the efficacy of each isomer and TRF in future studies because their activity may be different in different cell types or pathologic states. Second, the effects of T3 isomers in most of the studies required long-term (several days) treatment of cells prior to analysis. This is unlike the effects of NF-κB-blocking antioxidants. We previously suggested that this extended time course of tocotrienol effects on NF-κB may mediate an indirect mode of function (Kaileh and Sen 2010). That is, tocotrienols alter cell physiology over several days of treatment, and this altered cell physiology leads to NF-κB downregulation. If this hypothesis is true, we had proposed that these effects of tocotrienols could be enhanced by secondary treatments. One example comes from the work of Shirode et al., who showed that γT3 synergizes with the cyclo-oxygenase inhibitor, celecoxib, to downregulate NF-κB and induce apoptosis of mammary epithelial cells (Shirode and Sylvester 2010, 2011). More recently, Kunnumakkara et al. also observed similar results, where γT3 potentiates the antitumor activity of gemcitabine, a nucleoside analog used as a standard treatment for pancreatic cancer, by inhibiting constitutively active NF-κB and its regulated genes such as Bcl2, COX2, and VEGF in human pancreatic cancer cells (Kunnumakkara et al. 2010). These authors also showed that in an orthotopic nude mouse model of human pancreatic cancer, oral administration of tocotrienol in combination with gemcitabine for 28 days enhanced the antitumor properties of gemcitabine by inhibiting constitutively active NF-κB. Similarly, Husain et al. demonstrated that δT3 enhances gemcitabine inhibition of cell proliferation and induction of apoptosis in part due to the inactivation of NF-κB and its downstream genes *in vitro* in pancreatic cancer cells and *in vivo* in a pancreatic tumor model in SCID nude mice (Husain et al. 2011). Finally, Chang and Yap showed that γT3 synergizes with docetaxel to inhibit NF-κB activation and to induce apoptosis in the human amelanotic cells C32 (Chang et al. 2009). These studies demonstrate the validity of continuing to search for compounds that enhance NF-κB suppression by tocotrienols.

We previously emphasized the need for continued systematic analyses of tocotrienol effects, particularly in the context of mouse models of inflammatory disease. This was based on the observations of Wu and Ng who reported that treatment of HeLa (human cervical carcinoma) cells with αT3 or γT3 resulted in increased IL-6 production by the cells prior to undergoing apoptosis (Wu and Ng 2010). A similar observation was made by Wilankar et al., who found that short-term γT3 treatment of CD4$^+$ T cells led to higher levels of NF-κB. Since IL-6 is a well-known NF-κB target gene, these observations imply that NF-κB activity was upregulated by these treatments.

These results underscore the possibility of context-specific effects that may need to be taken into consideration. One way to reconcile the disparate observations is that IL-6 upregulation by α- and γT3 may have occurred at a posttranscriptional step, such as stabilization of the IL-6 mRNA, which would be NF-κB-independent. Effects of T3 isomers on posttranscriptional gene regulation are completely unexplored at present, and may explain differential effects on different NF-κB target genes.

16.3 CONCLUSIONS AND FUTURE DIRECTIONS

Overall, most studies to date demonstrate that tocotrienols reduce NF-κB induction and, thereby, NF-κB-dependent gene transcription. The specific effects vary from cell type to cell type. However, since these studies are carried out with transformed cell lines, some of the variations may also be due to the nature of the transforming events. While the importance of suppressing NF-κB in tumors and thereby reducing tumor growth is of unquestionable importance, in our opinion studies of the effects of tocotrienols on NF-κB function in untransformed cells are also necessary. Such information would be important to minimize adverse effects of the lack of NF-κB induction, such as diminution of immune response to pathogens. Finally, the mechanism by which tocotrienols suppress NF-κB is of utmost importance. Even if the effects are indirect, it will be useful to identify alterations in cell physiology that ultimately affect NF-κB induction in tocotrienol-treated cells. Understanding the changes that make tocotrienol-exposed cells unresponsive to NF-κB activation will permit the design of rational intervention strategies that maximize the therapeutic efficacy of tocotrienols.

ACKNOWLEDGMENT

The contributors are supported by the Intramural Research Program of the National Institute on Aging (Baltimore, MD).

REFERENCES

Ahn, K. S., G. Sethi et al. (2007). Gamma-tocotrienol inhibits nuclear factor-kappaB signaling pathway through inhibition of receptor-interacting protein and TAK1 leading to suppression of antiapoptotic gene products and potentiation of apoptosis. *J Biol Chem* 282(1): 809–820.

Basak, S., H. Kim et al. (2007). A fourth IkappaB protein within the NF-kappaB signaling module. *Cell* 128(2): 369–381.

Basak, S., V. F. Shih et al. (2008). Generation and activation of multiple dimeric transcription factors within the NF-kappaB signaling system. *Mol Cell Biol* 28(10): 3139–3150.

Bilimoria, K. Y., D. J. Bentrem et al. (2007). Validation of the 6th edition AJCC pancreatic cancer staging system: Report from the national cancer database. *Cancer* 110(4): 738–744.

Bonizzi, G. and M. Karin (2004). The two NF-kappaB activation pathways and their role in innate and adaptive immunity. *Trends Immunol* 25(6): 280–288.

Bren, G. D., N. J. Solan et al. (2001). Transcription of the RelB gene is regulated by NF-kappaB. *Oncogene* 20(53): 7722–7733.

Chang, P. N., W. N. Yap et al. (2009). Evidence of gamma-tocotrienol as an apoptosis-inducing, invasion-suppressing, and chemotherapy drug-sensitizing agent in human melanoma cells. *Nutr Cancer* 61(3): 357–366.

Chen, L. F. and W. C. Greene (2003). Regulation of distinct biological activities of the NF-kappaB transcription factor complex by acetylation. *J Mol Med (Berl)* 81(9): 549–557.

Elgueta, R., M. J. Benson et al. (2009). Molecular mechanism and function of CD40/CD40L engagement in the immune system. *Immunol Rev* 229(1): 152–172.

Ghosh, S. and M. Karin (2002). Missing pieces in the NF-kappaB puzzle. *Cell* 109 Suppl: S81–S96.

Hayden, M. S. and S. Ghosh (2008). Shared principles in NF-kappaB signaling. *Cell* 132(3): 344–362.

Husain, K., R. A. Francois et al. (2011). Vitamin E delta-tocotrienol augments the antitumor activity of gemcitabine and suppresses constitutive NF-kappaB activation in pancreatic cancer. *Mol Cancer Ther* 10(12): 2363–2372.

Ji, X., Z. Wang et al. (2011). Inhibition of cell growth and induction of apoptosis in non-small cell lung cancer cells by delta-tocotrienol is associated with notch-1 down-regulation. *J Cell Biochem* 112(10): 2773–2783.

Kaileh, M. and R. Sen (2010). Role of NF-kappaB in the anti-inflammatory effects of tocotrienols. *J Am Coll Nutr* 29(3 Suppl): 334S–339S.

Kunnumakkara, A. B., B. Sung et al. (2010). {Gamma}-tocotrienol inhibits pancreatic tumors and sensitizes them to gemcitabine treatment by modulating the inflammatory microenvironment. *Cancer Res* 70(21): 8695–8705.

Landesman-Bollag, E., D. H. Song et al. (2001). Protein kinase CK2: Signaling and tumorigenesis in the mammary gland. *Mol Cell Biochem* 227(1–2): 153–165.

Lenz, G. and L. M. Staudt (2010). Aggressive lymphomas. *N Engl J Med* 362(15): 1417–1429.

Lombardi, L., P. Ciana et al. (1995). Structural and functional characterization of the promoter regions of the NFKB2 gene. *Nucleic Acids Res* 23(12): 2328–2336.

McNulty, S. E., N. B. Tohidian et al. (2001). RelA, p50 and inhibitor of kappa B alpha are elevated in human metastatic melanoma cells and respond aberrantly to ultraviolet light B. *Pigment Cell Res* 14(6): 456–465.

Meyskens, F. L. Jr., J. A. Buckmeier et al. (1999). Activation of nuclear factor-kappa B in human metastatic melanomacells and the effect of oxidative stress. *Clin Cancer Res* 5(5): 1197–1202.

Neumann, M. and M. Naumann (2007). Beyond IkappaBs: Alternative regulation of NF-kappaB activity. *FASEB J* 21(11): 2642–2654.

Ozes, O. N., L. D. Mayo et al. (1999). NF-kappaB activation by tumour necrosis factor requires the Akt serine-threonine kinase. *Nature* 401(6748): 82–85.

Qing, G., Z. Qu et al. (2005). Stabilization of basally translated NF-kappaB-inducing kinase (NIK) protein functions as a molecular switch of processing of NF-kappaB2 p100. *J Biol Chem* 280(49): 40578–40582.

Qureshi, A. A., J. C. Reis et al. (2010). Tocotrienols inhibit lipopolysaccharide-induced pro-inflammatory cytokines in macrophages of female mice. *Lipids Health Dis* 9: 143.

Qureshi, A. A., J. C. Reis et al. (2011c). delta-Tocotrienol and quercetin reduce serum levels of nitric oxide and lipid parameters in female chickens. *Lipids Health Dis* 10: 39.

Qureshi, A. A., X. Tan et al. (2011b). Inhibition of nitric oxide in LPS-stimulated macrophages of young and senescent mice by delta-tocotrienol and quercetin. *Lipids Health Dis* 10(1): 239.

Qureshi, A. A., X. Tan et al. (2011a). Suppression of nitric oxide induction and pro-inflammatory cytokines by novel proteasome inhibitors in various experimental models. *Lipids Health Dis* 10: 177.

Rickert, R. C., J. Jellusova et al. (2011). Signaling by the tumor necrosis factor receptor superfamily in B-cell biology and disease. *Immunol Rev* 244(1): 115–133.

Romashkova, J. A. and S. S. Makarov (1999). NF-kappaB is a target of AKT in anti-apoptotic PDGF signalling. *Nature* 401(6748): 86–90.

Selvaduray, K. R., A. K. Radhakrishnan et al. (2012). Palm tocotrienols decrease levels of pro-angiogenic markers in human umbilical vein endothelial cells (HUVEC) and murine mammary cancer cells. *Genes Nutr* 7(1): 53–61.

Sen, C. K., S. Khanna et al. (2006). Tocotrienols: Vitamin E beyond tocopherols. *Life Sci* 78(18): 2088–2098.

Sen, C. K., S. Khanna et al. (2007). Tocotrienols: The emerging face of natural vitamin E. *Vitam Horm* 76: 203–261.

Sen, R. and S. T. Smale (2010). Selectivity of the NF-{kappa}B response. *Cold Spring Harb Perspect Biol* 2(4): a000257.

Shaffer, A. L., G. Wright et al. (2006). A library of gene expression signatures to illuminate normal and pathological lymphoid biology. *Immunol Rev* 210: 67–85.

Shah, S. J. and P. W. Sylvester (2005). Gamma-tocotrienol inhibits neoplastic mammary epithelial cell proliferation by decreasing Akt and nuclear factor kappaB activity. *Exp Biol Med (Maywood)* 230(4): 235–241.

Shih, V. F., R. Tsui et al. (2011). A single NFkappaB system for both canonical and non-canonical signaling. *Cell Res* 21(1): 86–102.

Shin-Kang, S., V. P. Ramsauer et al. (2011). Tocotrienols inhibit AKT and ERK activation and suppress pancreatic cancer cell proliferation by suppressing the ErbB2 pathway. *Free Radic Biol Med* 51(6): 1164–1174.

Shirode, A. B. and P. W. Sylvester (2010). Synergistic anticancer effects of combined gamma-tocotrienol and celecoxib treatment are associated with suppression in Akt and NFkappaB signaling. *Biomed Pharmacother* 64(5):327–332.

Shirode, A. B. and P. W. Sylvester (2011). Mechanisms mediating the synergistic anticancer effects of combined gamma-tocotrienol and celecoxib treatment. *J Bioanal Biomed* 3: 1–7.

Stadanlick, J. E., M. Kaileh et al. (2008). Tonic B cell antigen receptor signals supply an NF-kappaB substrate for prosurvival BLyS signaling. *Nat Immunol* 9(12): 1379–1387.

Staudt, L. M., Karin M, ed. (2010). *Cold Spring Harbor Perspectives in Biology*. New York: Cold Spring Harbor Laboratory Press.

Theriault, A., J. T. Chao et al. (2002). Tocotrienol is the most effective vitamin E for reducing endothelial expression of adhesion molecules and adhesion to monocytes. *Atherosclerosis* 160(1): 21–30.

Vainer, G. W., E. Pikarsky et al. (2008). Contradictory functions of NF-kappaB in liver physiology and cancer. *Cancer Lett* 267(2): 182–188.

Wilankar, C., D. Sharma et al. (2011). Role of immunoregulatory transcription factors in differential immuno-modulatory effects of tocotrienols. *Free Radic Biol Med* 51(1): 129–143.

Wu, S. J., P. L. Liu et al. (2008). Tocotrienol-rich fraction of palm oil exhibits anti-inflammatory property by suppressing the expression of inflammatory mediators in human monocytic cells. *Mol Nutr Food Res* 52(8): 921–929.

Wu, S. J. and L. T. Ng (2010). Tocotrienols inhibited growth and induced apoptosis in human HeLa cells through the cell cycle signaling pathway. *Integr Cancer Ther* 9(1): 66–72.

Xu, W. L., J. R. Liu et al. (2009). Inhibition of proliferation and induction of apoptosis by gamma-tocotrienol in human colon carcinoma HT-29 cells. *Nutrition* 25(5): 555–566.

Yam, M. L., S. R. Abdul Hafid et al. (2009). Tocotrienols suppress proinflammatory markers and cyclooxygenase-2 expression in RAW264.7 macrophages. *Lipids* 44(9): 787–797.

Yap, W. N., P. N. Chang et al. (2008). Gamma-tocotrienol suppresses prostate cancer cell proliferation and invasion through multiple-signalling pathways. *Br J Cancer* 99(11): 1832–1841.

Yap, W. N., N. Zaiden et al. (2010). Id1, inhibitor of differentiation, is a key protein mediating anti-tumor responses of gamma-tocotrienol in breast cancer cells. *Cancer Lett* 291(2): 187–199.

Zarnegar, B., J. Q. He et al. (2004). Unique CD40-mediated biological program in B cell activation requires both type 1 and type 2 NF-kappaB activation pathways. *Proc Natl Acad Sci U S A* 101(21): 8108–8113.

17 Antioxidant Action of Tocotrienols

Etsuo Niki

CONTENTS

17.1 INTRODUCTION

Do we need eight homologues and does each homologue exert specific function? This is one of the major questions on vitamin E. Among the eight compounds in the vitamin E family, α-tocopherol is by far the major type found in humans with smaller amounts of γ-tocopherol. The physiological concentrations of tocotrienols (T3s) are much lower than tocopherols (Ts). Thus, a question arises: Do we need T3, and why do some plants such as palm, rice, and annatto beans contain high T3s?

The role and function of T3 have received much attention recently (Miyazawa et al. 2009; Aggarwal et al. 2010; Colombo 2010; Sen et al. 2010; Frank et al. 2011; Nesaretnam and Meganathan 2011). Some studies have reported more potent antioxidant activity of T3 than T. Moreover, biological functions such as cholesterol lowering, antiatherogenic, anticancer, anti-inflammatory, antiallergic, antiangiogenic, antithrombotic, and antiasthmatic effects by modulation of signaling pathways, not related to antioxidant activity, have been reported. Nearly 100 molecular targets for T3s have been reported (Aggarwal et al. 2010). It is important to demonstrate whether T3s really exert more potent antioxidant capacity than Ts and whether or not the specific non-antioxidant functions of T3s, which Ts do not share, are important *in vivo*.

17.2 ACTIVITY OF TOCOTRIENOLS AND TOCOPHEROLS FOR RADICAL SCAVENGING

The important physiological function of vitamin E is to act as a radical scavenging antioxidant. It has been established that vitamin E inhibits lipid peroxidation *in vivo* as well as *in vitro* by scavenging lipid peroxyl radicals that act as chain-carrying species (Niki 2009). Lipid peroxidation is mediated by free radicals and enzymes such as lipoxygenase and cytochrome P450. Vitamin E suppresses the formation of lipid peroxidation products such as *trans, trans*-hydroperoxyoctadecadienoates that are specific for free-radical-mediated oxidation and used as a specific biomarker for free radical lipid peroxidation. Both T3 and T scavenge oxygen radicals by donating phenolic hydrogen at the sixth position of the chroman ring. The reactivity of phenolic hydrogen is determined by the bond dissociation energy or ionization potential.

It has been clearly shown that the reactivities of T3s and Ts toward oxygen radicals decrease in the order $\alpha > \beta$, $\gamma > \delta$ and that the corresponding T3 and T exert the same reactivity (Yoshida et al. 2003). The reactivities of antioxidants toward free radicals can be measured by several methods (Niki 2010). The reactivities of α-, β-, γ-, and δ-T3 and T were measured from their effect on the rate of consumption of pyrogallol red used as a reference probe. The hydrodynamic voltammogram also showed that the half-wave potential of α-T3 and α-T is the same and smaller than that of γ-T3 and γ-T, which is also the same. Furthermore, it was shown that the corresponding T and T3 were consumed at the same rate and also that they suppressed the oxidation of methyl linoleate and β-linoleoyl-γ-palmitoyl phosphatidylcholine in homogeneous solution and in phosphatidylcholine liposomal membranes in aqueous dispersions, respectively, mediated by free radicals. These results clearly confirm that the reactivities of T3s and Ts toward oxygen radicals decrease in the order $\alpha > \beta$, $\gamma > \delta$ and that the corresponding T3 and T exert the same reactivity On the other hand, it was reported that α-T3 possessed 40–60 times higher antioxidant activity than α-T against Fe(II) + ascorbate and Fe(II) + nicotinamide adenine dinucleotide phosphate (NADPH)-induced lipid peroxidation in rat liver microsomal membranes (Serbinova et al. 1991), but in this experiment, the rate of lipid oxidation was not measured. It may be noteworthy that both α-T and α-T3 reduced cupric ion Cu(II) to cuprous ion Cu(I) with concomitant formation of α-T-quinone and α-T3-quinone, respectively, but that β-, γ-, and δ-T and T3 did not (Yoshida et al. 2003). Therefore, α-T and α-T3 may act as a prooxidant under certain conditions in the presence of transition metal ion.

17.3   ACTION OF TOCOTRIENOL AND TOCOPHEROL IN THE MEMBRANES

T has a saturated phytyl side chain, while T3 has an unsaturated isoprenoid side chain with three double bonds at 3′, 7′, and 11′ position, respectively. Although these different side chains do not affect the chemical reactivities of T and T3 toward radicals, they exert physical effects such as fluidity in the membrane and mobility between the membranes (Atkinson et al. 2008). The electron paramagnetic resonance (EPR) studies using spin labels having stable nitroxide radical at the different position of stearic acid revealed that T increased membrane rigidity slightly more significantly than the corresponding T3 (Suzuki et al. 1993; Yoshida et al. 2003). As described earlier, Serbinova et al. observed higher antioxidant capacity of α-T3 than α-T and ascribed this difference to its higher recycling efficiency from chromanoxyl radicals, its more uniform distribution in membrane bilayer, and its stronger disordering of membrane lipids, which makes interaction of chromanols with lipid radicals more efficient than α-T (Serbinova et al. 1991).

The effects of side chains on the rate of incorporation into the membranes were found more significant, that is, T3 is incorporated into and transferred between the membranes more rapidly than T (Yoshida 2003). This may be ascribed to a shorter chain of T3 than T. It has been shown that the shorter the side chain length of chromanols, the faster the rate of incorporation into the membranes (Niki et al. 1988). This difference is important in the cell culture system as described in the following.

17.4   PROTECTIVE EFFECT OF TOCOTRIENOLS AND TOCOPHEROLS AGAINST OXIDATIVE STRESS IN CULTURED CELLS

Cell culture systems have been used often to investigate the action of T and T3, since they are more relevant to biological systems than the simple test tube. The protective effects of T3 against various oxidative stresses have been studied extensively and documented (Noguchi et al. 2008). It was reported that nanomolar amounts of α-T3, but not α-T, blocked glutamate-induced death by suppressing glutamate-induced early activation of c-Src kinase (Sen et al. 2000), oxidation by 12-lipoxygenase (Khanna et al. 2003), and by inhibiting phospholipase A2 activation (Khanna et al. 2010). Several other studies also have observed a more potent protective effect of T3 than T against oxidative stress in cultured cells (Osakada et al. 2004; Fukui et al. 2011). However, it should be emphasized that the apparent protective effects depend on the rate of antioxidant incorporation into the cells. T3s are incorporated into cultured cells much faster than the corresponding Ts, which

TABLE 17.1

Protective Effect of Vitamin E Homologues against Glutamate-Induced Neuronal Cell Death (%)

T or T3	Cotreatment		Pretreatment	
	0.25 µM	2.5 µM	0.25 µM	2.5 µM
α-T	24	42	31	103
α-T3	98	92	98	107
β-T	25	75	51	81
β-T3	62	63	82	81
γ-T	25	51	45	73
γ-T3	69	87	58	96
δ-T	23	59	52	66
δ-T3	78	83	76	83

Source: Saito, Y. et al., *Free Radic. Biol. Med.*, 49, 1542, 2010.

results in higher apparent activity of T3 than T (Saito et al. 2003, 2010; Numakawa et al. 2006). The treatment of immature primary cortical neurons with glutamate induces the depletion of glutathione, the generation of reactive oxygen species (ROS), and free-radical-mediated lipid peroxidation. All eight vitamin E homologues protected neuronal cells from glutamate toxicity by scavenging ROS and suppressing lipid peroxidation. Four types of T3s exhibited higher apparent cytoprotective activity than the corresponding Ts, but when the intracellular concentrations are considered, T3 and T exerted essentially the same capacity (Saito et al. 2010). As shown in Table 17.1, the preincubation of Ts increases the apparent protective effect of Ts more significantly than T3s (Saito et al. 2010).

A more potent effect of T3 than T was reported in reducing endothelial expression of adhesion molecules (Theriault et al. 2002). Similar effects were observed for the inhibition of cell adhesion to endothelial cells (Noguchi et al. 2003) and also surface expression of adhesion molecules (Naito et al. 2005), that is, α-T3 exerted higher apparent activity than α-T, but the activity was the same when intracellular concentrations were adjusted.

These results suggest that the intracellular concentrations of antioxidants should be measured, by which the protective effects of antioxidants should be assessed, rather than by the concentration added to the cell culture system. It should also be noted that the amount of lipophilic antioxidants such as T3 and T should be chosen carefully considering the concentration of lipids in the cell culture. Often, T3 and T higher than 10 µM are added to the culture medium, but this may be too high considering the amount of lipids in the cell culture and physiological molar ratio of vitamin E to lipids, which is about 1–500 or 1000. The concentration of lipids in the cell culture is usually below 100 µM, and hence T and T3 below 1 µM is enough (Table 17.1). It may be noted that T and T3 are distributed similarly within the nuclear, mitochondrial, microsomal, and cytosolic fractions of the cells, whose distribution was directly proportional to lipid distribution (Saito et al. 2004). It is disappointing that these issues are not considered in many studies and the protective effects are discussed without measuring the intracellular concentrations of antioxidants.

17.5 ANTIOXIDANT ACTION OF TOCOTRIENOLS *IN VIVO*

Several reports show the antioxidant effect of T3 *in vivo*. Ultraviolet B (UVB) irradiation shortens the life span of *Caenorhabditis elegans*. Treatment of *C. elegans* with T3-rich fraction (TRF) from palm oil, containing 22% α-T, 24% α-T3, 37% γ-T3, and 12% δ-T3, was found to reduce the accumulation of protein carbonyl, a biomarker of oxidative stress, and also recovered the mean life span to that of unirradiated groups (Adachi and Ishii 2000). α-Tocopheryl quinone is an oxidation product of α-T. In contrast to γ-tocopheryl quinine, which may exert cytotoxicity, α-tocopheryl quinone is not cytotoxic but acts as a potent antioxidant after reduction to hydroquinone (Shi et al. 1999). α-Tocotrienol quinone is a metabolite of α-T3 and has been reported to act as a cellular protectant against oxidative stress and aging (Shrader et al. 2011).

It has been known that α-T is effective in reducing the ischemia-induced brain damage and α-T3 was also effective in decreasing the size of cerebral infarcts induced by middle cerebral artery occlusion (Mishima et al. 2003). It was also found that α-T3 reduced malondialdehyde (MDA), a biomarker of lipid peroxidation, and prevented intracerebroventricular streptozotocin-induced cognitive impairment in rat (Tiwari et al. 2009). The preventive effect of T3 against carbon tetrachloride-induced liver damage was also reported (Yachi et al. 2010). This is a well-established model of oxidative stress *in vivo*. It was found that TRF containing 37.8% α-T3, 4.0% β-T3, 45.5% γ-T3, and 10.7% δ-T3 significantly reduced triacylglycerols and alanine aminotransferase (ALT) in the liver. The reduction of hepatic triglyceride synthesis by T3 was also reported (Zaiden et al. 2010). As described earlier, several studies showed that T3 protected neuronal cells from oxidative stress in cell culture systems. It was reported that α-T3 supplementation protected mice and rats from stroke-dependent brain tissue damage, which was attributed to lowering of c-Src activation and 12-lipoxygenase phosphorylation (Khanna et al. 2005). A more potent protective effect of T3 than T was observed in the rats exposed to experimental restraint stress (Azlina et al. 2005). The oral administration of γ-T3 was found to suppress ultraviolet B (UVB)-induced changes in skin thickness, COX-2 expression, and hyperplasia, but α-T did not (Shibata et al. 2010). T3 reduced the MDA level in gastric tissues and blocked the stress-induced changes in the gastric acidity and gastrin level. Further, dietary supplementation with T3s was found to enhance immune function in mice, suggesting a beneficial effect of T3 in improving the age-related decline in T-cell function (Ren et al. 2010).

Several human studies on T3 have been carried out, but the reported results are not consistent (Aggarwal et al. 2010). Some studies observed lowering of plasma cholesterol by T3, but others did not. In one study, it was examined if the daily supplements of placebo or α-, γ-, or δ-tocotrienyl acetates would alter serum cholesterol or low density lipoprotein (LDL) oxidative resistance in hypercholesterolemic subjects in a double-blind, placebo-controlled study (O'Byrne et al. 2000). Subjects were randomly assigned to receive placebo ($n = 13$), α-($n = 13$), γ-($n = 12$), or δ-($n = 13$) tocotrienyl acetate supplements (250 mg/day). Following supplementation in the respective groups, plasma concentrations were α-T3 $0.98 \pm 0.80\,\mu M$, γ-T3 $0.54 \pm 0.45\,\mu M$, and δ-T3 $0.09 \pm 0.07\,\mu M$. Tocotrienyl acetate supplements did not lower cholesterol in hypercholesterolemic subjects. α-T3 increased *in vitro* LDL oxidative resistance, but the effect of tocotrienyl acetate supplementation on the plasma level of lipid peroxidation was not measured.

In a more recent study, the effects of TRF supplementation on lipid profile and oxidative status were assessed. The subjects were given a capsule per day containing 70.4, 4.8, 57.6, 33.6, and 48 mg α-T3, β-T3, γ-T3, δ-T3, and α-T for 6 months (Chin et al. 2011). It was found that plasma level of α-T was increased, whereas change in T3s were small, high density lipoprotein (HDL) cholesterol was increased, protein carbonyl was decreased, but that the levels of advanced glycation end products (AGE) and MDA did not change significantly.

An inherent problem with T3 is its low bioavailability (Chow 1975) because of its low affinity to α-tocopherol transfer protein and fast metabolism. Vitamin E is distributed into circulation from the liver by α-tocopherol transfer protein, which determines the concentrations in biological fluids and tissues. The relative affinity of α-T3 to α-tocopherol transfer protein is only 12% of α-T (Hosomi et al. 1997). Furthermore, T3s are metabolized much faster than their T counterparts by cytochrome P450 4F2 (CYP4F2), which catalyzes the ω-hydroxylation of the side chain of T3 and T to give the final metabolite 2-carboxyethyl-6-hydroxychroman (CEHC) (Sontag and Parker 2007).

TABLE 17.2
Tissue Levels of α-Tocopherol and α-Tocotrienol in Rat Eyes after Topical Administration[a]

	Eye Tissue α-T/α-T3				
	Cornea	Crystalline Lens	Iris	Neural Retina	Eye Cup
Administration					
None	4.42/nd	0.47/nd	32.19/nd	43.05/0.06	18.57/0.36
α-T	4.58/0.02	0.56/0.01	28.85/0.01	35.28/0.05	20.38/0.04
α-T3	3.45/2.42	0.54/0.13	36.12/3.86	44.39/2.61	17.56/4.54
Net increase					
α-T/α-T3	0.16/2.42	0.09/0.13	–/3.86	–/2.55	1.81/4.18

Source: Tanito, M. et al., *Lipids*, 39, 469, 2004.
nd, not detected.
[a] In nmol/g tissue. α-T or α-T3 (5 μL, 2.2 mg) was applied to each eye once a day for four consecutive days. $n = 4$ (8 eyes).

CEHCs having phenolic hydrogen are capable of acting as a radical scavenging antioxidant. Therefore, it is difficult to raise the concentrations of T3 in extracellular fluids and tissues, although T3 concentrations may be increased in some peripheral organs such as adipose tissue and skin (Ikeda et al. 2001; Kawakami et al. 2007). However, topical administration of T3 to skin or eye, for example, may be useful to increase its local concentration. In fact, it was found that α-T3 was increased more significantly than α-T in ocular tissues after topical ophthalmic administration (Table 17.2) (Tanito et al. 2004).

It has been observed that α-T suppresses the uptake and distribution of T3 in extracellular fluids and tissues. It was recently pointed out that α-T supplementation is undesirable, since it does more harm than good and that, since α-T acts as an antagonist, T3-rich materials free from α-T may be preferable (Gee 2011). This is apparently a premature statement. Many inconsistent results and statements have been reported. Sound and solid experimental design and interpretation of results are essential for proper understanding of the action and function of T3.

17.6 CONCLUSION

The following conclusions may be noted:

1. Both T3 and T act as radical scavenging antioxidant *in vitro* and *in vivo*. The reactivities of corresponding T3 and T toward free radicals are substantially the same, and the reactivities decrease in the order of α- > β- and γ- > δ-T3 and T.
2. α-T3 and α-T reduce ferric and cupric ion, Fe(III) and Cu(II), to the lower valency state, Fe(II) and Cu(I), respectively, but β-, γ-, and δ-T3 and T do not.
3. The inherent drawback of T3 is the low bioavailability because of low affinity to α-tocopherol transfer protein and fast metabolism. However, T3s are more rapidly incorporated into cells than Ts and topical administration may be useful.
4. The significance of non-antioxidant functions of T3, especially in humans, such as gene regulation and signaling, which are outside the scope of this chapter, should be elucidated in future studies.

REFERENCES

Adachi, H. and Ishii, N. 2000. Effects of tocotrienols on life span and protein carbonylation in *Caenorhabditis elegans*. *J. Gerontol. A Biol. Sci. Med. Sci.* 55: 280–285.

Aggarwal, B. B., Sundaram, C., Prasad, S., and Kannappan, R. 2010. Tocotrienols, the vitamin E of the 21st century: Its potential against cancer and other chronic diseases. *Biochem. Pharmacol.* 80: 1613–1631.

Atkinson, J, Epand, R. F., and Epand, R. M. 2008. Tocopherols and tocotrienols in membranes: A critical review. *Free Radic. Biol. Med.* 44: 739–764.

Azlina, M. F., Nafeeza, M. I., and Khalid, B. A. 2005. A comparison between tocopherol and tocotrienol on gastric parameters in rats exposed to stress. *Asia Pac. J. Clin. Nutr.* 14: 358–365.

Chin, S. F., Ibahim, J., Makpol, S. et al. 2011. Tocotrienol rich fraction supplementation improved lipid profile and oxidative status in healthy older adults: A randomized controlled study. *Nutr. Metab (Lond).* 8: 42.

Chow, C. K. 1975. Distribution of tocopherols in human plasma and red blood cells. *Am. J. Clin. Nutr.* 28: 756–760.

Colombo, M. L. 2010. An update on vitamin E, tocopherol and tocotrienol-perspectives. *Molecules* 15: 2103–2113.

Frank, J., Chin, X. W., Shrader, C., Eckert, G. P., and Rimbach, G. 2012. Do tocotrienol have potential as neuroprotective dietary factors? *Ageing Res. Rev.* 11: 163–180.

Fukui, K., Takatsu, H., Koike, T., and Urano, S. 2011. Hydrogen peroxide induces neurite degeneration: Prevention by tocotrienols. *Free Radic. Res.* 45: 681–691.

Gee, P. T. 2011. Unleashing the untold and misunderstood observations on vitamin E. *Genes Nutr.* 6: 5–16.

Hosomi, A., Arita, M., Sato, Y. et al. 1997. Affinity for alpha-tocopherol transfer protein as a determinant of the biological activities of vitamin E analogs. *FEBS Lett.* 409: 105–108.

Ikeda, S., Toyoshima, K., and Yamshita, K. 2001. Dietary sesame seeds elevate α- and γ-tocotrienol concentrations in skin and adipose tissue of rats fed the tocotrienol-rich fraction extracted from palm oil. *J. Nutr.* 131: 2892–2897.

Kawakami, Y., Tuszuki, T., Nakagawa, K., and Miyazawa, T. 2007. Distribution of tocotrienols in rats fed a rice bran tocotrienol concentrate. *Biosci. Biotechnol. Biochem.* 71: 464–471.

Khanna, S., Parinandi, N. L., and Kotha, S. R. 2010. Nanomolar vitamin E alpha-tocotrienol inhibits glutamate-induced activation of phospholipase A2 and causes neuroprotection. *J. Neurochem.* 112: 1249–1260.

Khanna, S., Roy, S., Ryu, H. et al. 2003. Molecular basis of vitamin E action: tocotrienol modulates 12-lipoxygenase, a key mediator of glutamate-induced neurodegeneration. *J. Biol. Chem.* 278: 43508–43515.

Khanna, S., Roy, S., Slivka, A. et al. 2005. Neuroprotective properties of the natural vitamin E α-tocotrienol. *Stroke.* 36: e144–e152.

Mishima, K., Tanaka, T., Pu, F. et al. 2003. Vitamin E isoforms α-tocopherol and γ-tocopherol prevent cerebral infarction in mice. *Neurosci. Lett.* 337: 56–60.

Miyazawa, T., Shibata, A., Sookwong, P. et al. 2009. Antiangiogenic and anticancer potential of unsaturated vitamin E (tocotrienol). *J. Nutr. Biochem.* 20: 79–86.

Naito, Y., Shimozawa, M., Kuroda, M. et al. 2005. Tocotrienols reduce 25-hydroxycholesterol-induced monocyte-endothelial cell interaction by inhibiting the surface expression of adhesion molecules. *Atherosclerosis* 180: 19–25.

Nesaretnam, K. and Meganathan, P. 2011. Tocotrienols: inflammation and cancer. *Ann. N. Y. Acad. Sci.* 1229:18–22.

Niki, E. 2009. Lipid peroxidation: Physiological levels and dual biological effects. *Free Radic. Biol Med.* 47: 469–484.

Niki, E. 2010. Assessment of antioxidant capacity in vitro and in vivo. *Free Radic. Biol. Med.* 49: 503–515.

Niki, E., Komuro, E., Takahashi, M et al. 1988. Oxidative hemolysis of erythrocytes and its inhibition by free radical scavengers. *J. Biol. Chem.* 263:19809–19814.

Noguchi, N., Hanyu, R., Nonaka, A., Okimoto, Y., and Kodama, T. 2003. Inhibition of THP-1 cell adhesion to endothelial cells by alpha-tocopherol and alpha-tocotrienol is dependent on intracellular concentration of the antioxidants. *Free Radic. Biol. Med.* 34: 1614–1620.

Noguchi, N., Saito, Y., and Niki, E. 2008. Uptake, distribution and protective action of tocotrienols in cultured cells. Watson, R. and Preedy V. R. (eds). In: *Tocotrienols: Vitamin E Beyond Tocopherols*, pp. 159–170. Boca Raton, FL: CRC Press.

Numakawa, Y., Numakawa, T., Matsumoto T. et al. 2006. Vitamin E protected cultured cortical neurons from oxidative stress-induced cell death through the activation of mitogen-activated protein kinase and phosphatidylinositol 3-kinase. *J. Neurochem.* 97: 1191–1202.

O'Byrne, D., Grundy, S., Packer, L. et al. 2000. Studies of LDL oxidation following alpha-, gamma-, or delta-tocotrienyl acetate supplementation of hypercholesterolemic humans. *Free Radic. Biol. Med.* 29: 834–845.

Osakada, F., Hashino, A., Kume, T., Katsuki, H., Kaneko, S., and Akaike, A. 2004. α-Tocotrienol provides the most potent neuroprotection among vitamin E analogs on cultured striatal neurons. *Neuropharmacol.* 47: 904–915.

Ren, Z., Pae, M., Dao, M. C. et al. 2010. Dietary supplementation with tocotrienols enhances immune function in C57BL/6 mice. *J. Nutr.* 140: 1335–1341.

Saito, Y., Nishio, K., Akazawa-Ogawa, Y. et al. 2010. Cytoprotective effects of vitamin E homologues against glutamate-induced cell death in immature primary cortical neuron cultures: Tocopherols and tocotrienols exert similar effects by antioxidant function. *Free Radic. Biol. Med.* 49: 1542–1549.

Saito, Y., Yoshida, Y., Akazawa, T., Takahashi, K., and Niki, E. 2003. Cell death caused by selenium deficiency and protective effect of antioxidants. *J. Biol. Chem.* 278: 39428–39434.

Saito, Y., Yoshida, Y., Nishio, K., Hayakawa, M., and Niki, E. 2004. Characterization of cellular uptake and distribution of vitamin E. *Ann. N. Y. Acad. Sci.* 1031: 368–375.

Sen, C.K., Khanna, S., Roy, S., and Packer, L. 2000. Molecular basis of vitamin E action. Tocotrienol potently inhibits glutamate-induced pp60(c-Src) kinase activation and death of HT4 neuronal cells. *J. Biol. Chem.* 275: 13049–13055.

Sen, C. K., Rink, C., and Khanna, S. 2010. Palm oil-derived vitamin E alpha-tocotrienol in brain health and disease. *J. Am. Coll. Nutr.* 29: 314S–323S.

Serbinova, E., Kagan, V., Han, D., and Packer, L. 1991. Free radical recycling and intramembrane mobility in the antioxidant properties of alpha-tocopherol and alpha-tocotrienol. *Free Radic. Biol. Med.* 10: 263–275.

Shibata, A., Nakagawa, K., Kawakami, Y., Tsuzuki, T., and Miyazawa, T. 2010. Suppression of gamma-tocotrienol on UVB induced inflammation in HaCaT keratinocytes and HR-1 hairless mice via inflammatory mediators multiple signaling. *J. Agric. Food Chem.* 58: 7013–7020.

Shrader W. D., Amagata, A., Barnes, A. et al. 2011. A-Tocotorienol quinine modulates oxidative stress response and the biochemistry of aging. *Bioorg. Med. Chem. Lett.* 21: 3693–3698.

Shi, H., Noguchi, N., and Niki, E. 1999. Comparative study on dynamics of antioxidative action of a-tocopheryl quinone, ubiquinol, and a-tocopherol against lipid peroxidation. *Free Radic. Biol. Med.* 27: 334–346.

Sontag, T. J. and Parker, R. S. 2007. Influence of major structural features of tocopherols and tocotrienols on their omega-oxidation by tocopherol-omega-hydroxylase. *J. Lipid Res.* 48: 1090–1098.

Suzuki, Y. J., Tsuchiya, M., Wassall, S. R. et al. 1993. Structural and dynamic membrane properties of α-tocopherol and α-tocotrienol: Implication to the molecular mechanisms of their antioxidant potency. *Biochemistry.* 32: 10692–10699.

Tanito, M., Itoh, N., Yoshida, Y. et al. 2004. Distribution of tocopherols and tocotrienols to rat ocular tissues after topical ophthalmic administration. *Lipids* 39: 469–474.

Theriault, A., Chao, J. T., and Gapor, A. 2002. Tocotorienol is the most effective vitamin E for reducing endothelial expression of adhesion molecules and adhesion to monocytes. *Atherosclerosis* 160: 21–30.

Tiwari, V., Kuhad, A., Bishnoi, M., and Chopra, K. 2009. Chronic treatment with tocotrienol, an isoform of vitamin E, prevents intracerebroventricular streptozotocin-induced cognitive impairment and oxidative-nitrosative stress in rats. *Pharmacol. Biochem. Behav.* 93: 183–189.

Yachi, R., Igarashi, O., and Kiyose, C. 2010. Protective effects of vitamin E analogs against carbon tetrachloride-induced fatty liver in rats. *J. Clin. Biochem. Nutr.* 47: 148–154.

Yoshida, Y., Niki, E., and Noguchi, N. 2003. Comparative study on the action of tocopherols and tocotrienols as antioxidant: chemical and physical effects. *Chem. Phys. Lipids.* 123: 63–75.

Zaiden, N., Yap, W. N., Ong, S. et al. 2010. Gamma delta tocotrienols reduce hepatic triglyceride synthesis and VLDL secretion. *J. Atheroscler. Thromb.* 17: 1019–1032.

18 Tocotrienol in Human Pancreatic Cancer

Mokenge P. Malafa and Kazim Husain

CONTENTS

18.1 INTRODUCTION

Pancreatic cancer is a major disease responsible for the death of hundreds of thousands of men and women. Worldwide, there are about 230,000 new cases of pancreatic cancer yearly, and about 225,000 patients will die from this disease (Kamangar et al. 2006). Pancreatic cancer is a rapidly fatal disease with a median survival rate of 4–6 months. The death/incidence ratio of pancreatic cancer, >0.95, is the highest of all malignancies thus making it the most lethal cancer (Jemal et al. 2006). In the United States, it is the fourth leading cause of cancer-related deaths (Jemal et al. 2010). Despite the use of surgery, radiation therapy, and various types of chemotherapy, progress in reducing the death rate for pancreatic cancer overall has remained unchanged for decades (Ko and Tempero 2005; Hochster et al. 2006). Even when diagnosed at its earliest stages and therefore amenable to complete surgical resection, long-term survival is rare with >70% of the patients succumbing to recurrent or metastatic disease (Han et al. 2006). In metastatic pancreatic cancer, standard chemotherapy with either gemcitabine or 5-fluorouracil results in response rate on the order of 10%–20%, but responses last only a few months, and time to disease progression is only 4–6 months. Therefore, existing therapies fail in a large number of patients and the need for agents that can prevent the disease or enhance current therapy is a high priority.

There has been intense interest in the role of nutrition in the etiology and prevention of cancer (Taylor and Greenwald 2005). In the past 30 years, there have been hundreds of observational studies of diet and cancer, and the vast majority show that individuals who consume more fruit, vegetables, and cereal grains have lower cancer risk (Steinmetz and Potter 1991; Cotugna et al. 1992). Of the six prospective studies that have examined fruit, vegetable, and cereal grain intake and the risk of pancreatic cancer, four have demonstrated an inverse association (Mills et al. 1988;

Shibata et al. 1994; Stolzenberg-Solomon et al. 2002; Chan et al. 2005), while two have not shown any clear association (Zheng et al. 1993; Coughlin et al. 2000). In contrast, at least 11 case–control studies and 1 cohort study have reported inverse associations for risk of pancreatic cancer (Gold et al. 1985; Norell et al. 1986; Falk et al. 1988; Olsen et al. 1989; La Vecchia et al. 1990; Baghurst et al. 1991; Bueno de Mesquita et al. 1991; Lyon et al. 1993; Ji et al. 1995; Silverman et al. 1998; Stolzenberg-Solomon et al. 1999; Nkondjock et al. 2005a,b). These results suggest that increasing vegetable, fruit, and cereal consumption may provide protection against developing pancreatic cancer.

Natural vitamin E, an essential nutrient for the body, was named as tocopherol in 1924 and chemically synthesized in 1938 (Sen et al. 2007). Vitamin E is made up of eight different isoforms consisting of alpha-(α-), beta-(β-), gamma-(γ-), and delta-(δ)-tocopherols (T) and α-, β-, γ-, and δ-tocotrienols (T3) (Figure 18.1). The tocopherols are saturated forms of vitamin E, whereas the tocotrienols are unsaturated and contain an isoprenoid side chain. Tocopherols consist of a chromanol ring and a 15-carbon tail. The name tocotrienol was first suggested by Bunyan et al. (1961), and the tocotrienols were described in *Nature* in the 1960s (Whittle et al. 1966). The isomeric forms of tocotrienol are distinguished by the number and location of methyl groups on the chromanol rings: α-tocotrienol is 5,7,8-trimethyl, β-tocotrienol is 5,8-dimethyl, γ-tocotrienol is 7,8-dimethyl, and δ-tocotrienol is 8-monomethyl. Tocotrienols are present only in a small fraction of plants, whereas tocopherols are rich in most plants. The natural sources of tocotrienols are red annatto, palm oil, rice bran oil, grape seed oil, maize, wheat germ oil, hazel nut, olive oil, buckthorn berry, rye, oat, barley, flax seed oil, poppy seed oil, and sunflower oil (Aggarwal et al. 2010). Rice bran, palm, and annatto oils are some of the richest sources of tocotrienols. Several studies have suggested that tocotrienols are better antioxidants than tocopherols both *in vitro* as well as *in vivo* (Komiyama et al. 1989; Suarna et al. 1993). Animal and human studies suggest that natural vitamin E tocotrienols are safe and nontoxic at higher doses (Qureshi et al. 1986, 2002; Parker et al. 1993; Yap et al. 2001; Husain et al. 2009b). The biological significance of tocotrienols was clearly delineated in the 1980s, when its ability to lower cholesterol was reported (Qureshi et al. 1986). Later anticancer effects of tocotrienols were discovered (Komiyama et al. 1989; Sundram et al. 1989). Structure–activity studies of the proapoptotic effects of vitamin E compounds in cancer cells have clearly documented the importance of the unsaturated isoprenoid tail of the vitamin E compounds in their antitumor bioactivity

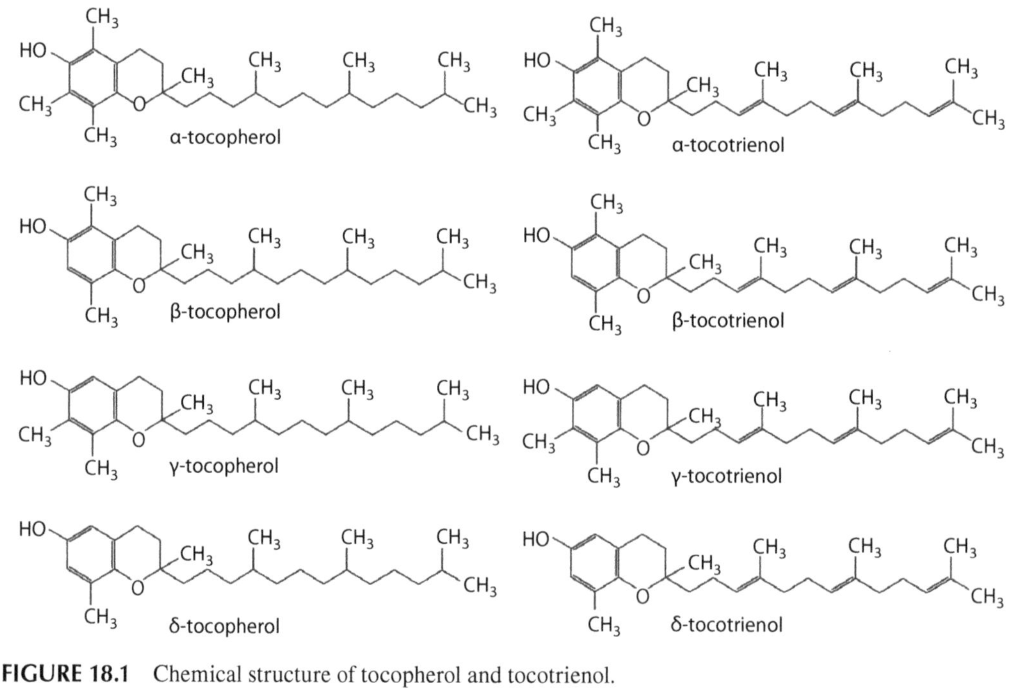

FIGURE 18.1   Chemical structure of tocopherol and tocotrienol.

(Birringer et al. 2003). Furthermore, these studies also demonstrate that decreasing the number of methyl substitutions on the chromanol ring, is associated with increasing antitumor potency in tocotrienol compounds (Inokuchi et al. 2003; Miyazawa et al. 2004). Thus, δ-tocotrienol should be the most potent natural tocotrienol against cancer cells. We have confirmed this observation in pancreatic cancer *in vitro* as well as *in vivo*. However, the molecular mechanisms pertaining to the anticancer activities of tocotrienols are still under investigation. The focus of this chapter is on the mechanisms of anticancer activities and molecular targets of different isoforms of tocotrienol specifically in pancreatic cancer both *in vitro* as well as *in vivo*, including a current clinical trial.

18.2 ANTICANCER/ANTITUMOR ACTIVITY OF TOCOTRIENOLS

Isoprenoids are well known to elicit potent anticancer activity (Mo and Elson 1999; Birringer et al. 2003), and tocotrienols contain an isoprenoid side chain in their chemical structure while tocopherols do not. Hence, tocotrienols possess potent anticancer activity both *in vitro* as well as *in vivo*.

18.2.1 *In Vitro* Studies

Tocotrienols have been shown to inhibit the growth and proliferation and induce cell death/apoptosis in a wide variety of tumor cells. Table 18.1 summarizes the *in vitro* anticancer activities of tocotrienols. Breast cancer has been most extensively studied in cell culture to validate the efficacy of tocotrienols. Initial studies were carried out using the tocotrienol-rich fraction (TRF), which contains the mixture of α-, β-, γ-, and δ-tocotrienols as well as some α-tocopherol. TRF has been shown to inhibit the cell proliferation and growth of MDA-MB-435, MDA-MB-231, ZR-75-1, and MCF-7 estrogen receptor-negative as well as -positive human breast cancer cells, whereas α-tocopherol was ineffective even at higher concentrations (Nesaretnam et al. 1995, 1998, 2000; Guthrie et al. 1997; Mo and Elson 1999). In a study, it was observed that normal mammary epithelial cells isolated from mice and treated with TRF inhibited the cell growth, whereas α-tocopherol had no effect (McIntyre et al. 2000b). The effect of TRF on preneoplastic, neoplastic, and highly malignant mouse mammary epithelial cells over a 5 day culture significantly inhibited the growth of the cells and demonstrated higher sensitivity of malignant cells than pre-neoplastic cells to the antiproliferative effects of TRF (McIntyre et al. 2000a). Studies with individual tocotrienols (α, β, γ, and δ) on breast cancer cells showed differential antiproliferative activity. γ- and δ-Tocotrienol were the most effective isomers in the inhibition of human breast cancer cells (Guthrie et al. 1997; Yu et al. 1999). Studies on the influence of tocotrienols on mitogenic signaling pathways have also been conducted. The antiproliferative effects of tocotrienols in pre-neoplastic mammary epithelial cells did not show any decrease in the EGF receptor mitogenic responsiveness but inhibited the early postreceptor events involved in cAMP production upstream due to EGF-dependent MAPK and PI3Kinase/Akt mitogenic signaling (Sylvester et al. 2002). The antitumor activity of tocotrienols has also been reported due to induction of programmed cell death (apoptosis) in breast cancer cells. Preneoplastic, neoplastic, and highly malignant mouse mammary epithelial cells treated with TRF undergo cell death due to induction of apoptosis, and the sensitivity of malignant cells to the apoptotic effects of TRF (McIntyre et al. 2000a) was higher than pre-neoplastic cells. Treatment with TRF and γ-tocotrienol but not α-tocopherol induced apoptosis in highly malignant mouse mammary epithelial cells (Shah et al. 2003). γ- and δ-Tocotrienols significantly inhibited cell proliferation and malignant transformation in both estrogen-responsive MCF-7 cells and estrogen-nonresponsive MDA-MB-231 cells, but α-tocopherol had no effect at doses up to 10 μM (Hsieh et al. 2010). The apoptosis-inducing properties of tocotrienols and tocopherols were compared in estrogen-responsive MCF-7 cells and estrogen-nonresponsive MDA-MB-435 cells. The estrogen-responsive MCF-7 cells were found to be more sensitive than estrogen-nonresponsive MDA-MB-435 cells to tocotrienol (γ and δ)-induced apoptosis (Yu et al. 1999). The molecular mechanisms by which tocotrienols selectively kill breast cancer cells have been explored. Treatment with TRF and γ-tocotrienol increased intracellular activity and levels of cleaved

TABLE 18.1
In Vitro **Studies with Tocotrienols for Anticancer Activity**

Cancer Type	References
Breast cancer	
Inhibition of cell proliferation of pre-neoplastic mammary epithelial cells	Sylvester et al. (2002), McIntyre et al. (2000)
Inhibition of estrogen receptor-negative and receptor-positive cell proliferation	Ayoub et al. (2011), Comitato et al. (2010), Guthrie et al. (1997), Hsieh et al. (2010), Mo and Elson (1999), Nesaretnam et al. (1995, 1998, 2000), Park et al. (2010), Pierpaoli et al. (2010), Samant et al. (2010), Selvaduray et al. (2010), Yap et al. (2010), Yu et al. (1999)
Inhibition of proliferation by cell cycle arrest	Samant et al. (2010), Elangovan et al. (2008), Wali et al. (2009)
Inhibition of anchorage-independent growth	Park et al. (2010), Hsieh et al. (2010)
Induction of apoptosis	McIntyre et al. (2000), Samant et al. (2010), Park et al. (2010), Pierpaoli et al. (2010), Shah et al. (2003), Shah and Sylvester (2004), Takahashi and Loo (2004), Wali et al. (2009), Yu et al. (1999)
Induction of apoptosis through TGF-β-Fas-JNK signaling	Shun et al. (2004)
Induction of apoptosis through PDK-1/Akt/GSK3/(FLIP) pathway	Shah and Sylvester (2004, 2005a,b)
Downregulation of API5 and upregulation of the MIG6 gene	Ramdas et al. (2011)
Prostate cancer	
Inhibition of cell growth	Srivastava and Gupta (2006), Yap et al. (2010)
Induction of apoptosis	Yap et al. (2008), Jiang et al. (2011)
Downregulation of TGFβ receptor I, SMAD-2, p38, and NF-κB signaling	Campbell et al. (2011)
Colon cancer	
Inhibition of cell growth	Agarwal et al. (2004), Xu et al. (2009), Kannappan et al. (2010)
Induction of cell death/apoptosis	Zhang et al. (2011), Xu et al. (2009), Kannappan et al. (2010)
Hepatic cancer	
Inhibition of cell growth	Sakai et al. (2004), Har and Keong (2005), Wada et al. (2005), Hiura et al. (2009)
Induction of apoptosis	Hiura et al. (2009), Sakai et al. (2006)
Downregulation of STAT3 pathway	Rajendran et al. (2011)
Gastric cancer	
Inhibition of cell growth	Li et al. (2011)
Induction of apoptosis	Sun et al. (2008, 2009), Liu et al. (2010)
Skin cancer	
Inhibition of cell growth	Mo and Elson (1999), Chang et al. (2009), Fernandes et al. (2010)
Induction of apoptosis	De Mesquita et al. (2011), Chang et al. (2009)
Lung cancer	
Inhibition of cell growth	Nakashima et al. (2010), Kashiwagi et al. (2008), Yu et al. (2005)
Induction of apoptosis	Ji et al. (2011)
Hematological cancer	
Inhibition of cell growth	Kannappan et al. (2010)
Induction of apoptosis	Inoue et al. (2011), Fu et al. (2009)

caspase-8 and caspase-3, but not caspase-9. Furthermore, treatment with specific caspase-8 and caspase-3 inhibitor, but not caspase-9 inhibitor, blocked tocotrienol-induced apoptosis in highly malignant mouse mammary epithelial cells. These findings suggest that tocotrienol-induced apoptosis in highly malignant mouse mammary epithelial cells is mediated by activation of the extrinsic caspase-8 signaling pathway and is independent of intrinsic caspase-9 activation (Shah et al. 2003). However, tocotrienol-induced caspase-8 activation was not associated with death receptor apoptotic signaling (Shah and Sylvester 2004). In contrast, γ- and δ-tocotrienol reduced cell viability and induced apoptosis possibly via the mitochondrial pathway, as well as the expression of senescent-like growth arrest markers such as p53, p21, p16, and downregulated HER-2/neu in breast tumor cells overexpressing this oncogene (Pierpaoli et al. 2010). γ-Tocotrienol inhibited ErbB3-receptor tyrosine phosphorylation and subsequent reduction in PI3K/PDK-1/Akt mitogenic signaling in malignant mouse mammary epithelial cells (Samant and Sylvester 2006). Treatment of MDA-MB-231 with γ-tocotrienol resulted in membrane blebbing, formation of apoptotic bodies, chromatin condensation/fragmentation, and phosphatidylserine externalization, the hallmark of apoptosis (Takahashi and Loo 2004). In γ-tocotrienol treated human breast cancer cells, the functional capacity of the mitochondrial membrane was impaired followed by the release of mitochondrial cytochrome C (Takahashi and Loo 2004). δ-Tocotrienol induced transforming growth factor (TGF-β) receptor II expression and activated the TGF-β-, Fas-, and c-Jun NH (2)-terminal kinase (JNK)-signaling pathways in breast cancer cells (Shun et al. 2004), while γ-tocotrienol downregulated the intracellular levels of (PI3Kinase)-dependent kinase 1 (phospho-PDK-1), phospho-Akt/ phospho-GSK3, and FLICE-inhibitory protein (FLIP), an antiapoptotic protein that inhibits caspase-8 activation and nuclear factor-kappa B (NF-κB) activation in highly malignant mouse mammary epithelial cells (Shah and Sylvester 2004, 2005a,b). γ-Tocotrienol induced apoptosis which was associated with a corresponding increase in poly (ADP) ribosyl polymerase (PARP) cleavage and activation of protein kinase-like endoplasmic reticulum (ER) kinase/eukaryotic translational initiation factor/activating transcription factor 4 (PERK/eIF2alpha/ATF-4) pathway, a marker of ER stress response, increase in C/EBP homologous protein (CHOP) levels, a key component of ER stress mediated apoptosis that increases expression of tribbles 3 (TRB3), and also reduced full-length caspase-12 levels, an indication of caspase-12 cleavage and activation in highly malignant mouse mammary epithelial cells (Wali et al. 2009). Cell culture studies (Park et al. 2010) showed that γ-tocotrienol inhibited colony formation of a mouse mammary cancer cell line and human breast cancer cell lines. The antiproliferative effects of tocotrienols were highly correlated with an increase in apoptosis. Tocotrienol isomers (α-, γ-, and δ-tocotrienol) and TRF inhibited the growth of the 4T1 murine mammary cancer cells, caused induction of the interleukin (IL) 24 messenger ribonucleic acid (mRNA) levels, and decreased IL-8 and vascular endothelial growth factor (VEGF) mRNA levels, indicating potent antiangiogenic and antitumor effects (Selvaduray et al. 2010). Treatment of human MDA-MB-231 and MCF-7 cells with γ-tocotrienol induced cleavages of PARP as well as caspase-8, -9, and -3. Additional analyses showed that γ-tocotrienol activated JNK and p38 MAPK, and upregulated death receptor 5 (DR5) as well as C/EBP homologous protein (CHOP), an ER stress marker. Ahn et al. (2007) reported that γ-tocotrienol treatment significantly downregulated the NF-κB activity and suppressed the NF-κB-regulated gene products associated with antiapoptotic activity such as IAPI, Bcl-xL, Bcl2, cFLIP, XIAP, and survivin in cancer cells. δ-Tocotrienol inhibited cell proliferation in a model estrogen receptor-negative human breast cancer cell line MDA-MB-231, which was mediated by the loss of cyclin D1 and associated suppression of site-specific Rb phosphorylation (Elangovan et al. 2008). Samant et al. (2010) have shown that antiproliferative effects of γ-tocotrienol were associated with reduction in cell cycle progression from G(1) to S (as evidenced by increased p27 levels) and a corresponding decrease in cyclin D1, CDK2, CDK4, CDK6, and phosphorylated Rb levels in highly malignant mouse mammary epithelial cells. γ-Tocotrienol-induced breast cancer cell death was associated with the suppression of inhibitor of differentiation protein (Id1) and NF-κB through modulation of their upstream regulators (Src, Smad1/5/8, Fak, and LOX) (Yap et al. 2010b). In another study, γ- and δ-tocotrienol increased the ERbeta translocation into the nucleus, which in turn activated estrogen-responsive genes (MIC-1, EGR-1, and cathepsin D), DNA fragmentation, and caspase-3 activation in breast cancer cells (Comitato et al. 2009). In an MCF-7 breast cancer cell expressing both ERalpha and ERbeta, TRF treatment increases ERbeta nuclear translocation, and significantly inhibits ERalpha expression as well as complete destruction of the protein from the nucleus (Comitato et al. 2010). γ-Tocotrienol suppressed MCF-7 cell proliferation, which was associated with loss of cyclin D1 and inhibition of specific Rb phosphorylation (pRb-p at Thr821) (Hsieh et al. 2010). A recent study showed that TRF and isomers of tocotrienols (α, γ, and δ) cause the downregulation of the API5 gene, upregulation of the MIG6 gene, and the differential expression of other genes involved in the regulation of immune response, tumor growth and metastatic suppression, apoptotic signaling, transcription, and protein biosynthesis in MCF-7 cells (Ramdas et al. 2011). γ-Tocotrienol induced apoptosis in MDA-MB 231 and MCF-7 breast cancer cells (PARP cleavage and caspase-7 activation). Gene expression analysis of MCF-7 cells treated with γ-tocotrienol revealed alterations in NRF-2-mediated oxidative stress response, TGF-β signaling, endoplasmic reticulum (ER) stress response (activation of PERK and pIRE1α pathway), and activating transcription factor 3 (ATF3) gene (Patacsil et al. 2011). Recently, studies on the mechanism of tocotrienol binding to estrogen receptor (ER) and signaling indicated a high affinity of specific forms of tocotrienols for ERβ, but not for ERα, increased ERβ translocation into the nucleus, which in turn activates the expression of estrogen-responsive genes (MIC-1, EGR-1, and Cathepsin D) in breast cancer cells only expressing ERβ cells (MDA-MB-231) and in cells expressing both ER isoforms (MCF-7). The binding of tocotrienol to ERβ was associated with caspase-3 activation, DNA fragmentation, and apoptosis (Nesaretnam et al. 2011). The production of IL-8 and IL-6 (pro-angiogenic cytokines) was lowest in δ-tocotrienol-treated human umbilical vein endothelial cells (HUVECs) followed by γ-tocotrienol and TRF. There was a significant reduction in IL-8 and VEGF production in 4T1 cells treated with TRF or δ-tocotrienol (Selvaduray et al. 2011). Treatment with γ-tocotrienol or Met inhibitor significantly inhibited HGF-dependent +SA cell replication, inhibited HGF-induced Met autophosphorylation, but had no effect on total Met levels. Combined treatment with γ-tocotrienol and Met inhibitor reduced both the total Met levels and HGF-induced Met autophosphorylation health benefits in prevention and/or treatment of breast cancer in women with deregulated HGF/Met signaling (Ayoub et al. 2011).

The growth inhibitory and apoptotic effects of TRF were tested in normal human prostate epithelial cells (PrEC), virally transformed normal human prostate epithelial cells (PZ-HPV-7), and human prostate cancer cells (LNCaP, DU145, and PC-3). Other studies have demonstrated that TRF selectively inhibited the growth of cancer cells (but not normal cells), malignant transformation, caused G0/G1 phase cell cycle arrest and sub-G1 accumulation, and induced apoptosis (Srivastava and Gupta 2006). γ-Tocotrienol was the most potent in induction of apoptosis as evidenced by activation of procaspases and the presence of sub-G(1) cell population. Cell death was associated with suppression of NF-κB, EGF-R, and Id family proteins (Id1 and Id3), induction of JNK-signaling pathway, suppression of mesenchymal markers, and the restoration of E-cadherin and gamma-catenin expression, which was associated with suppression of cell invasion capability of prostate Ca cells (Yap et al. 2008). Yap et al. (2010) demonstrated that γ-tocotrienol downregulated the expression of prostate CSC markers (CD133/CD44) and suppressed the spheroid formation ability of the androgen-independent prostate cancer cell lines (PC-3 and DU145). Both γ and δ isoforms of tocotrienol were more effective in the inhibition of the growth of prostate cancer cell lines (PC-3 and LNCaP) compared with the γ and δ forms of tocopherol. In addition, the latent precursor and the mature forms of TGFβ2 are downregulated after treatment with γ-tocotrienol, with concomitant disruptions in TGFβ receptor I, SMAD-2, p38, and NF-κB signaling (Campbell et al. 2011). A recent study showed that γ-tocotrienol promoted apoptosis, necrosis, and autophagy in human prostate PC-3 and LNCaP cancer cells, which was associated with marked increase of intracellular dihydroceramide and dihydrosphingosine (sphingolipid intermediates), but had no effect on ceramide or sphingosine (Jiang et al. 2011).

Consistent with the aforementioned breast and prostate cancer cell growth inhibition and apoptosis induction, tocotrienols inhibited the growth of hepatoma cells (dRLh-84), but not normal cells, of rats and mice and induced apoptosis (Sakai et al. 2004; Har and Keong 2005). The tocotrienol-induced apoptosis in hepatoma cells was mediated by caspase-8 and caspase-3 activation. γ-Tocotrienol treatment inhibited the proliferation of human hepatoma Hep3B cells, induced apoptosis by increasing the PARP cleavage, caspase-8, caspase-9, and caspase-3 activation, and upregulation of pro-apoptotic protein Bax and fragment of Bid (Sakai et al. 2006). δ-Tocotrienol was more potent in the inhibition of growth, S-phase cell cycle arrest, and induction of apoptosis in human hepatocellular carcinoma HepG2 cells (Wada et al. 2005). The evaluation of the antitumor activities of γ-tocotrienol and δ-tocotrienol in murine hepatoma MH134 cells was shown *in vitro* and *in vivo*. We found that δ-tocotrienol inhibited the growth of MH134 cells more strongly than γ-tocotrienol by inducing apoptosis (Hiura et al. 2009). A recent study showed that γ-tocotrienol inhibited both the constitutive and inducible activation of STAT3 with minimum effect on STAT5, inhibited the activation of Src, JAK1, and JAK2 implicated in STAT3 activation, induced the expression of the tyrosine phosphatase SHP-1, and downregulated the expression of STAT3-regulated gene products (cyclin D1, Bcl-2, Bcl-xL, survivin, Mcl-1, VEGF) in hepatocellular cancer cells (Rajendran et al. 2011).

With regard to gastric cancer, γ-tocotrienol induced apoptosis in a human gastric adenocarcinoma SGC-7901 cell line through downregulation of the ERK signaling pathway. Furthermore, γ-tocotrienol-induced apoptosis was accompanied by downregulation of Bcl-2, upregulation of Bax, activation of caspase-3, and subsequent PARP cleavage. γ-Tocotrienol also downregulated the activation of the Raf-ERK signaling pathway and downregulated c-Myc by decreasing the expressions of Raf-1 and p-ERK1/2 proteins (Sun et al. 2008). In a subsequent study, Sun et al. (2009) demonstrated that γ-tocotrienol's antitumor effect in SGC-7901 cells was associated with DNA damage, cell cycle arrest at G(0)/G(1) phase, activation of caspase-9 and caspase-3, and increased PARP cleavage, suggesting a mitochondria-dependent apoptosis pathway. Using a similar human gastric adenocarcinoma SGC-7901 cell line (Liu et al. 2010) showed that γ-tocotrienol inhibited cell migration and cell invasion through downregulation of the mRNA expressions of MMP-2 and MMP-9 and upregulation of tissue inhibitor of metalloproteinase-1 (TIMP-1) and TIMP-2, suggesting γ-tocotrienol-mediated antitumor metastasis activity. Similarly, a recent study demonstrated that γ-tocotrienol suppressed proliferation, migration, and tube formation of HUVECs induced by SGC-7901 cells. Moreover, the inhibitory effects of γ-tocotrienol on HUVECs were correlated with induction of apoptosis and arrest of cell cycle at the G(0)/G(1) phase, and inhibition of angiogenesis by downregulation of β-catenin, cyclin D1, CD44, phospho-VEGFR-2, and MMP-9 (Li et al. 2011).

The anticancer activity of TRF has also been evaluated in colon carcinoma RKO cells. TRF inhibited both anchorage-dependent and anchorage-independent growth of RKO cells. In addition, TRF induced CDK inhibitor p21 levels and increased Bax/Bcl2 ratio, which was associated with cytochrome c release from mitochondria, induction of APAF-1, activation of caspase-9, and finally activation of caspase-3 (Agarwal et al. 2004). In another study, γ-tocotrienol inhibited cell growth and arrested HT-29 cells in G(0)/G(1) phase and induced apoptosis, which was accompanied by downregulation of Bcl-2, upregulation of Bax, and activation of caspase-3, reduced NF-κB p65 protein and its nuclear translocation (Xu et al. 2009). Furthermore, γ-tocotrienol significantly downregulated the expression of antiapoptotic proteins (c-IAP2 and Bcl-xL), induced the expression of the TRAIL receptors and death receptors (DR-4 and DR-5) in human colon cancer (HCT-116) cells, and sensitized the cancer cells to TRAIL-induced apoptosis. Upregulation of DRs by γ-tocotrienol required the production of reactive oxygen species (ROS), activation of extracellular signal-regulated kinase 1 (ERK1), expression of p53, and Bax (Kannappan et al. 2010). A recent study showed that δ-tocotrienol inhibited proliferation of SW620 cells and induced paraptosis-like death, which was correlated with the vacuolation from swelling and fusion of mitochondria and/or the ER. δ-Tocotrienol reduced the expression of β-catenin and Wnt-1 proteins, decreased cyclin D1, c-jun, and MMP-7 protein levels, indicating that δ-tocotrienol induced paraptosis-like cell death, which was associated with the suppression of the Wnt signaling pathway (Zhang et al. 2011).

The growth-inhibitory activity of tocotrienols has been reported in murine melanoma B16F10 cells (Mo and Elson 1999). Studies have shown that δ-tocotrienol was most effective in the inhibition of melanoma cell proliferation. Chang et al. (2009), on the other hand, showed that the inhibitory effect of γ-tocotrienol was most potent in human melanoma cell lines.

γ-Tocotrienol-induced apoptosis was evidenced by activation of procaspases and the accumulation of sub-G1 cell population. Examination of the prosurvival genes revealed that γ-tocotrienol-induced cell death was associated with suppression of NF-κB, EGF-R, and Id family proteins. γ-Tocotrienol treatment also resulted in induction of JNK signaling pathway, suppression of mesenchymal markers, and the restoration of E-cadherin and γ-catenin expression, which was associated with suppression of cell invasion capability. However, recent studies have shown that δ-tocotrienol inhibited cell proliferation, cell cycle arrest at the G1-phase, reduced expression of CDK4, induced caspase-3 activation, as well as apoptosis in human A2058 and A375 melanoma cells (Fernandes et al. 2010; de Mesquita et al. 2011).

The antioxidant or redox silencing of α-tocotrienol rendered it to be toxic to human lung adenocarcinoma A549 cells (Yu et al. 2005) and suppressed hypoxia adaptation of A549 cells by the inhibition in hypoxia-induced activation of Src signaling (Kashiwagi et al. 2008). Nakashima et al. (2010) have reported that TRF treatment caused reduction in the viability of mesothelioma H28 cells, and this effect was enhanced by the combination treatment with cisplatin. The cytotoxic effect was closely related to the inhibition of phosphatidylinositol 3-kinase (PI3K)-AKT signaling. A recent study showed that treatment with δ-tocotrienol resulted in inhibition of cell growth, cell migration, tumor cell invasiveness, and induction of apoptosis in non-small cell lung cancer cells. Real-time RT-PCR and western blot analysis showed that antitumor activity by δ-tocotrienol was associated with a decrease in Notch-1, Hes-1, survivin, MMP-9, VEGF, and Bcl-xL expression. In addition, there was a decrease in NF-κB-DNA binding activity. These results suggest a downregulation of Notch-1 via inhibition of NF-κB signaling pathways by δ-tocotrienol (Ji et al. 2011).

The anticancer activity of tocotrienols has also been tested in hematological malignancies. α-, δ-, and γ-tocotrienol induced apoptosis in human hematological cancer cell lines HL-60, NB-4, Raji, and SY-5Y cells (Inoue et al. 2011). γ-Tocotrienol demonstrated more effective induction than the other derivatives in HL-60 cells. Induction of apoptosis was related to activation of the caspase cascade, cytochrome c release, Bid cleavage, and mitochondrial membrane depolarization. Furthermore, γ-tocotrienol showed cytotoxicity for leukemic cells from various patients regardless of lymphoblastic, myeloblastic, or relapsed leukemia, but the cytotoxic effect was weak in normal mononuclear cells.

The entrapment of TRF in transferrin-bearing vesicles led to a 3-fold higher TRF uptake and more than 100-fold improved cytotoxicity in A431 (epidermoid carcinoma), T98G (glioblastoma), and A2780 (ovarian carcinoma) cell lines compared to TRF solution (Fu et al. 2009). Recently, Kannappan et al. (2010) have shown that γ-tocotrienol, but not γ-tocopherol, inhibited constitutive activation of STAT3 as well as STAT3 DNA binding, which was correlated with inhibition of Src kinase and JAK1 and JAK2 kinases in multiple myeloma U266 cells. Furthermore, γ-tocotrienol induced the expression of the tyrosine phosphatase SHP-1, and downregulated the expression of STAT3-regulated antiapoptotic (Bcl-2, Bcl-xL, and Mcl-1), proliferative (cyclin D1), and angiogenic (VEGF) gene products. This, in turn, correlated with suppression of proliferation, the accumulation of cells in sub-G (1) phase of the cell cycle, and induction of apoptosis.

18.2.2 *In Vivo* Studies

The antitumor activity of tocotrienols in animal models of cancer was reported for the first time in 1989 and is summarized in Table 18.2. α- and γ-tocotrienol at doses of 5–40 mg/kg/day resulted in reduction of sarcoma 180, Ehrlich carcinoma, and invasive mammary carcinoma. The antitumor activity of γ-tocotrienol was higher than that of α-tocotrienol (Komiyama et al. 1989). Another study in the same year reported that dietary feeding of palm oil rich in tocotrienols for 5 months inhibited tumor formation in rats treated with a single dose of 5 mg of mammary chemical carcinogen 7,12-dimethylbenz (a) anthracene (DMBA) intragastrically (Sundram et al. 1989). Tocotrienols and tocopherols were studied for chemoprevention in a mammary chemical carcinogenesis rat model, and it was reported that tocotrienol-treated animals showed enhanced tumor latency

TABLE 18.2
In Vivo **Studies with Tocotrienols for Antitumor Activity**

Cancer Type	References
Breast cancer	
Inhibition of tumor growth in animals	Komiyama et al. (1989), Sundaram et al. (1989), Nesaretnam et al. (2004) Selvaduray et al. (2010, 2011), Iqbal et al. (2003), Gould et al. (1991)
Prostate cancer	
Inhibition of tumor growth in animals	Kumar et al. (2006), Jiang et al. (2011), Berve et al. (2010)
Hepatic cancer	
Inhibition of tumor growth in animals	Ngah et al. (1991), Rahmat et al. (1993), Makpol et al. (1997), Iqbal et al. (2003), Hiura et al. (2009)
Skin cancer	
Inhibition of tumor growth in animals	Yamada et al. (2008), Kausar et al. (2003)

compared to tocopherol (Gould et al. 1991). Feeding of TRF (10 mg/kg/day) for 6 months to DMBA-treated rats attenuated the severity and extent of malignant transformation in the mammary glands (Iqbal et al. 2003). Feeding of TRF (1 mg/day) for 20 weeks to athymic nude mice bearing MCF-7 tumor xenografts delayed the onset, incidence, and size of the tumors. The tumors tissues were subjected to cDNA array analysis. Data showed that 10 genes were downregulated and 20 genes were upregulated. Further, interferon-inducible transmembrane protein 1 and CD59 genes were significantly upregulated, whereas c-myc gene was significantly downregulated (Nesaretnam et al. 2004). Dietary delivery of γ-tocotrienol suppressed tumor growth in a syngeneic implantation mouse mammary cancer model (Nesaretnam et al. 2004). Tumor incidence and tumor load in TRF-supplemented BALB/c mice bearing 4T1 murine mammary cancer cells were decreased by 57.1% and 93.6%, respectively, and IL-24 mRNA levels in tumor tissues increased twofold, suggesting the inhibition of tumor growth and angiogenesis (Selvaduray et al. 2010). Decreased expression of VEGF and its receptors—VEGF-R1 (fms-like tyrosine kinase, Flt-1) and VEGF-R2 (kinase-insert-domain-containing receptor, KDR/Flk-2)—in tumor tissues excised from mice supplemented with TRF was observed. There was also decreased expression of VEGF-R2 in lung tissues of mice supplemented with TRF (Selvaduray et al. 2011).

In a prostate tumor model, PC3 cells were injected into BALB/c mice, treated with γ-tocotrienol (400 mg/kg, sc), and irradiated with 12 Gy. The results showed that the tumor size decreased to 40%, and the efficacy of radiotherapy was enhanced with γ-tocotrienol (Kumar et al. 2006). A recent study showed that mixed-tocotrienol feeding decreased incidence of tumor formation along with a significant reduction in the average wet weight of the genitourinary apparatus in transgenic adenocarcinoma mouse prostate (TRAMP) mice. Furthermore, mixed tocotrienols significantly reduced the levels of high-grade neoplastic lesions, which was associated with increased expression of proapoptotic proteins BAD, Bcl2, and cleaved caspase-3, p21 and p27, whereas the expression of cyclins A and E were decreased (Barve et al. 2010). In a recent study, γ-tocotrienol inhibited LNCaP xenograft tumor growth by 53% compared to 33% by γ-tocopherol in nude mice (Jiang et al. 2011).

Treatment with TRF for 6 months in rats bearing hepatocarcinoma induced by diethylnitrosamine (DEN)/2-acetylaminofluorene (AAF) significantly reduced the chemical carcinogenicity (Ngah et al. 1991; Rahmat et al. 1993; Makpol et al. 1997; Iqbal et al. 2003). In C3H/HeN, mice implanted with MH134 and fed γ-tocotrienol and δ-tocotrienol, tumor growth was significantly delayed. Both tocotrienols were detected in the tumor, but not in normal tissues, suggesting that tocotrienol accumulation is critical for the antitumor activities of the compound (Hiura et al. 2009).

The feeding of an experimental diet containing γ-tocotrienol and α-tocopherol to C57BL mice implanted with melanoma B16F10 cells reduced the tumor growth by 36% and 50%, respectively, suggesting that both tocotrienol and tocopherol are effective against melanoma tumors. Topical application of palm oil 1 h prior to application of 12-O-tetradecanoyl-phorbol-13-acetate (TPA) resulted in a significant protection against skin tumor promotion in mice. The animals pretreated with palm oil showed a decrease in both tumor incidence and tumor yield as compared to the TPA (alone)-treated group. Palm oil application also reduced the development of malignant tumors (Kausar et al. 2003). Dietary TRF fed to mice for 6 weeks reduced the extent of UVB (sunburn) and incidence of tumor (Yamada et al. 2008).

18.2.3 CLINICAL TRIALS

During a 5 year study using TRF, 8 patients died of breast cancer, whereas in 36 patients, a local or systemic recurrence developed. Five year breast cancer-specific survival rate was 98.3% in the intervention group and 95% in the control group, whereas the 5 year disease-free survival rate was 86.7% and 83.3%, respectively. Risk of mortality due to breast cancer was 60% lower in the intervention group versus the controls after adjustment for age, ethnicity, stage, and lymph node status, but this was not statistically significant. Adjuvant TRF therapy was not associated with breast cancer recurrence (Nesaretnam et al. 2010).

18.3 ANTITUMOR ACTIVITY OF TOCOTRIENOLS IN HUMAN PANCREATIC CANCER

Although antitumor activity of TRF and tocotrienols *in vitro*, *in vivo*, and in clinical trials has been reported mostly in breast cancer, *in vitro* and *in vivo* antitumor activity of TRF and tocotrienols has also been documented in prostate, gastric, colon, melanoma, and hepatic cancer. During the last 5 years, antitumor activity of tocotrienols in pancreatic cancer has been thoroughly studied and reported specifically from our laboratory. Since loss of viability and induction of apoptosis are two major mechanisms by which chemotherapeutic agents kill cancer cells, we conceptualized that tocotrienols might inhibit the growth and induce apoptosis in human pancreatic cancer cells.

18.3.1 IN VITRO STUDIES

Table 18.3 summarizes studies of the effect of tocotrienols in pancreatic cancer *in vitro*. The first report appeared in 2007, demonstrating that when a transformed phenotype of pancreatic satellite

TABLE 18.3
Antitumor Activity of Tocotrienol in Pancreatic Cancer

Study Type	References
In vitro	
Inhibition of anchorage-dependent growth	Husain et al. (2008, 2009a, 2010, 2011), Hussein and Mo (2009), Kannappan et al. (2010), Kunnumakkara et al. (2010), Shin-Kang et al. (2011)
Inhibition of anchorage-independent growth	Husain et al. (2008, 2009a, 2010, 2011)
Induction of apoptosis	Vaquero et al. 2007, Husain et al. (2008, 2009a, 2010, 2011) Kannappan et al. (2010), Kunnumakkara et al. (2010), Shin-Kang et al. (2011)
Induction of apoptosis through inhibition of NF-κB pathway	Husain et al. (2010, 2011) Kunnumakkara et al. (2010)
Induction of apoptosis through death receptor pathway	Kannappan et al. (2010)
In vivo	
Inhibition of tumor growth in animals	Husain et al. (2009a, 2010, 2011) Kannappan et al. (2010), Kunnumakkara et al. (2010)

cells (PSCs) was exposed to tocotrienols, autophagic and apoptotic signaling was induced (Vaquero et al. 2007). At the annual American Association for Cancer Research (AACR) meeting in 2008, 2009, and 2010 we reported the differential antitumor activity of tocotrienols in pancreatic cancer cells (Husain et al. 2008, 2009a, 2010). Tocotrienols had variable inhibitory effects on human pancreatic cancer cells AsPc-1 and MiaPaCa-2. δ-, γ-, β-, and α-tocotrienol inhibited cell viability by 60%, 54%, 40%, and 0%, respectively, at 50 μM concentration for 72 h. The IC_{50} values were 40 ± 7, 45 ± 5, 60 ± 6, and >100 μM for δ-, γ-, β-, and α-tocotrienol, respectively. The relative potency of the tocotrienols in inhibiting anchorage-independent growth was δ-tocotrienol (65%), γ-tocotrienol (30%), β-tocotrienol (13%), and α-tocotrienol (2%). Tocotrienols also had variable apoptosis-inducing effects on human pancreatic cancer MiaPaCa-2 cells. The relative potency of the tocotrienols in inducing apoptosis (cell death ELISA) was δ-tocotrienol (14-fold), γ-tocotrienol (7-fold), β-tocotrienol (2.5-fold), and α-tocotrienol (0-fold) at 50 μM concentrations after 72 h. δ-, γ-, and β-tocotrienol also significantly increased caspase-8 and caspase-3 activity, as well as PARP1 cleavage. These data clearly show that δ-tocotrienol is the most active antitumor agent against human pancreatic cancer. Later, Hussein and Mo (2009) also demonstrated that δ-tocotrienol significantly inhibited cell proliferation and induced apoptosis and G1-phase cell cycle arrest in human pancreatic cancer cells MIA PaCa-2, PANC-1, and BxPC-3. Subsequently, Husain et al. (2011) have shown that δ-tocotrienol augmented gemcitabine activity in pancreatic cancer cells (AsPc-1 and MiaPaCa-2) through suppression of NF-κB activity and the expression of NF-κB transcriptional targets [Bcl-xL, X-linked inhibitor of apoptosis (XIAP)]. Kannappan et al. (2010) reported that γ-tocotrienol, but not tocopherol, induced the expression of the TRAIL receptors death receptor DR-4 and DR5 in pancreatic cancer MIA PaCa-2 and PANC-1 cells, and suggested that γ-tocotrienol may sensitize tumor cells to TRAIL by upregulating death receptors through the ROS/ERK/p53 pathway and by downregulating cell survival proteins (c-IAP2 and Bcl-xL). γ-Tocotrienol inhibited the proliferation of pancreatic cancer cell lines (BxPC-3, MIA PaCa-2, and PANC-1) and potentiated gemcitabine-induced apoptosis. These effects correlated with an inhibition of NF-κB activation by γ-tocotrienol and a suppression of key cellular regulators including cyclin D1, c-Myc, cyclooxygenase-2 (COX-2), Bcl-2, cellular inhibitor of apoptosis protein, survivin, VEGF, and ICAM-1 (Kunnumakkara et al. 2010). Shin-Kang et al. (2011), using both γ- and δ-tocotrienols, have shown potent antiproliferative activity and cell death in pancreatic cancer cells (Panc-28, MIA PaCa-2, Panc-1, and BxPC-3). γ- and δ-tocotrienol treatment of cells inhibited the activation of ERK MAP kinase, RSK (ribosomal protein S6 kinase) and AKT, leading to downregulation of p-GSK-3β accompanied by nuclear translocation of Foxo3. These effects were mediated by the downregulation of Her2/ErbB2 at the messenger level. Recently, we have shown that γ- and δ-tocotrienols inhibit NF-κB activity and the survival of human pancreatic cancer cells (AsPc-1 and MiaPaCa-2) (Husain et al. 2011). Importantly, the bioactivity of the four tocotrienols (α-, β-, δ-, and γ-tocotrienol) was directly related to their ability to suppress NF-κB activity. The most bioactive tocotrienol for pancreatic cancer, δ-tocotrienol, significantly enhanced the efficacy of gemcitabine to inhibit pancreatic cancer cell growth and survival. Moreover, augmentation of gemcitabine's antitumor activity by δ-tocotrienol in pancreatic cancer cells was associated with significant suppression of NF-κB activity and the expression of NF-κB transcriptional targets Bcl-xL, XIAP, and survivin. Our study represents the first comprehensive pre-clinical evaluation of the activity of natural vitamin E compounds in pancreatic cancer.

18.3.2 *In Vivo Studies*

Table 18.3 summarizes the studies of tocotrienol's effect in pancreatic cancer *in vivo*. We have shown that oral administration of 100 mg/kg/day of δ-tocotrienol to mice resulted in levels that were 10 times higher in pancreas than in pancreatic tumor or liver tissue (Husain et al. 2009b). Subsequently, we used human pancreatic cancer (AsPc-1) cells xenografted in mice to test the comparative efficacy of tocotrienols *in vivo*. We found that δ-, γ-, and β-tocotrienol feeding (200 mg/kg × 2/day) for 4 weeks significantly inhibited the growth of pancreatic tumor in mice (Husain et al. 2008, 2009a, 2010, 2011). *In vivo* data validate the *in vitro* data that δ-tocotrienol is most active in the regression of tumor growth in mice. We further investigated whether the effects of combining δ-tocotrienol and gemcitabine on tumor growth in mice were associated with inhibition of NF-κB activation. δ-Tocotrienol augmented the antitumor activity of gemcitabine in pancreatic tumors, which was associated with significant suppression of NF-κB activity and NF-κB-regulated antiapoptotic proteins (Bcl-xL, survivin, and XIAP). In an orthotopic nude mouse model of human pancreatic cancer, oral administration of γ-tocotrienol (400 mg/kg/day) inhibited tumor growth and enhanced the antitumor properties of gemcitabine (Kunnumakkara et al. 2010). Immunohistochemical analysis indicated a correlation between tumor growth inhibition and reduced expression of Ki-67, COX-2, matrix metalloproteinase-9 (MMP-9), NF-κB p65, and VEGF in the tissue. Combination of gemcitabine and tocotrienol has been shown to downregulate NF-κB activity along with the NF-κB-regulated gene products (cyclin D1, c-Myc, VEGF, MMP-9, and CXCR4). Kannappan et al. (2010) have also shown that γ-tocotrienol at a dose of 400 mg/kg/day for 4 weeks inhibited STAT3 activation (phosphorylation) in tumor tissues of mice orthotopically injected with MiaPaCa-2 cells.

18.3.3 CLINICAL TRIALS

The clinical experience with TRF and tocotrienols is mainly in the chemoprevention of cardio-vascular diseases (Qureshi et al. 1986, 2002; Parker et al. 1993; Yap et al. 2001). The clinical trial data have established a favorable pharmacodynamic effect of δ-tocotrienol at 100–800 mg/day. δ-Tocotrienol has a terminal elimination half-life of 6–8 h (Yap et al. 2001). On the basis of the pharmacokinetic profile of δ-tocotrienol, steady state is reached in 2–3 weeks using twice-a-day dosing. No toxicities were observed with up to 800 mg/day dosing and with chronic administration of δ-tocotrienol of several months duration. Pre-surgical trials of potential chemoprevention agents have been particularly useful in prostate and breast cancer (Singletary et al. 2000; Lieberman 2001). Only a single clinical trial has been reported using TRF in breast cancer patients (Nesaretnam et al. 2010). Moreover, a phase I dose-escalating study evaluating the effect of pure δ-tocotrienol toward individuals with pancreatic cancer is currently underway at the Moffitt Cancer Center, and is the first tocotrienol study that is being clinically evaluated in humans toward pancreatic cancer. Clinical data show that δ-tocotrienol is well tolerated at doses up to 800 mg daily without toxic-ity. Treatment of patients with δ-tocotrienol at doses >200 mg daily induces expression of p27 and increases apoptosis in pancreatic tumors. This study demonstrates the feasibility of employing a pre-surgical trial design for determination of biologically effective doses to modulate signaling pathways in pancreatic cancer.

18.4 POTENTIAL MOLECULAR TARGETS, SIGNALING, AND BIOMARKER OF TOCOTRIENOLS IN PANCREATIC CANCER

Several mechanisms by which tocotrienols exert their anticancer effects in pancreatic can-cer have been reported. The growth-inhibitory activity of tocotrienols is mediated through modulation of growth factors such as VEGF and HER2/ErbB2 (Kunnumakkara et al. 2010; Shin-Kang et al. 2011) in pancreatic cancer. Inhibition of mitogen-activated protein kinases (MAPK) ERK, phosphorylation of PI3K/Akt/GSK-3β pathway, cyclin-dependent kinases (CDK2/CDK4/CDK6) and their inhibitors (p21, p27, and p53), and cyclin D1 are also related to the anti-proliferative effects of tocotrienols in pancreatic cancer (Hussein and Mo 2009; Kannappan et al. 2010; Kunnumakkara et al. 2010; Shin-Kang et al. 2011). Tocotrienols also inhibit the cell survival proteins [Bcl-2, Bcl-xL, c-FLIP, survivin, Cox-2, XIAP, IAP-1] in pancreatic cancer (Kunnumakkara et al. 2010; Husain et al. 2011; Shin-Kang et al. 2011). Tocotrienols can induce apoptosis through activation of intrinsic and extrinsic pathways. The intrinsic pathway involves induction of Bax, cleavage of Bid, and activation of caspase-9 leading to activation of caspase-3 and PARP1 cleavage (Kannappan et al. 2010; Kunnumakkara et al. 2010; Shin-Kang et al. 2011). The extrinsic pathway involves induction of death receptors, caspase-8 activation leading to caspase-3 activation, and PARP1 cleavage (Kannappan et al. 2010; Kunnumakkara et al. 2010; Husain et al. 2011; Shin-Kang et al. 2011). Tocotrienols also induce apoptosis through DNA fragmentation and p53 upregulation (Kannappan et al. 2010). Studies have also shown that tocotrienols exhibit potent anti-inflammatory activity. Tocotrienols inhibit transcription factor NF-κB pathway and STAT3 signaling pathways in pancreatic cancer (Kannappan et al. 2010; Kunnumakkara et al. 2010; Husain et al. 2011; Shin-Kang et al. 2011). These findings clearly indicate that antitumor activity of tocotrienols is implicated in multiple cancer signaling pathways of pancreatic cancer.

18.5   NEW PERSPECTIVES AND FUTURE DIRECTIONS

Tocotrienols have been shown to induce apoptosis and inhibit tumor growth in many human cancer models including pancreatic cancer. However, the specific molecular target gene/receptor/enzyme/ transcription factor to which tocotrienols bind directly and initiate antitumor effects is unknown. Earlier studies have shown the unspecific direct molecular targets of tocotrienols such as drug metabolizing enzymes (GST P1-1), steroids and xenobiotic receptor (SXR), and HMG-CoA reductase (Parker et al. 1993; van Haaften et al. 2002; Zhou et al. 2004). Therefore, research on tocotrienol's direct binding target, which elicits antitumor activity, is warranted. We have recently identified some direct binding partners of tocotrienols using affinity column chromatography and mass spectrometry in human pancreatic cancer cells, which are in the process of validation and characterization. Moreover, the efficacy of tocotrienol as an antitumor agent has been evaluated in orthotopic pancreatic cancer nude mouse models (Husain et al. 2009a, 2010, 2011; Kunnumakkara et al. 2010). Therefore, the genetic mouse model of pancreatic cancer such as Kras^{G12D} and Kras^{G12D} + p53, which recapitulate the main characteristics of pancreatic cancer development on the histopathologic and genetic level, must be evaluated for chemoprevention and treatment. To conclude, given the impressive pre-clinical data, δ-tocotrienol warrants evaluation in phase I and II clinical trials as well as combination with standard radiation/chemotherapy regimen in patients with advanced pancreatic cancer.

18.6   CONCLUSION

Natural vitamin E includes eight chemically distinct molecules: α-, β-, γ-, and δ-tocopherol and α-, β-, γ-, and δ-tocotrienol. The biological significance of tocotrienol as a cholesterol-lowering agent was delineated in the 1980s. Later, anticancer effects of tocotrienols were discovered. Antiproliferative and apoptosis-inducing effects of tocotrienols (γ and δ) have been reported *in vitro* as well as *in vivo*, specifically in breast, prostate, hepatic, gastric, colon, melanoma, pancreatic, and lung cancer as well as in some hematological malignancies. In pancreatic cancer, both γ- and δ-tocotrienol inhibited anchorage-dependent and anchorage-independent growth, and induced apoptosis in most of the human pancreatic cancer cells (AsPc-1, BxPC-3, MiaPaCa-2, Panc-1, and Panc-28) and in tumor tissues of the orthotopic mouse model. The antiproliferative and apoptotic effects of tocotrienols were mediated through inhibition of NF-κB signaling and NF-κB-regulated gene products (cyclin D1, c-Myc, Cox-2, VEGF, MMP-9, CXCR4, c-IAP2, Bcl2, Bcl-xL, XIAP, and survivin), downregulation of MAPK, ERK, RSK (ribosomal protein S6 kinase), AKT/p-GSK-3β pathway, and STAT3 phosphorylation. However, the pancreatic antitumor activity of δ-tocotrienol was greatest among the vitamin E isomers. The lack of specific direct binding targets of δ-tocotrienol, which elicits its antitumor activity, facilitates the active research in this area. Moreover, with impressive pre-clinical data, δ-tocotrienol warrants evaluation in phase I and II clinical trials as well as combination with standard radiation/chemotherapy regimen in patients with advanced pancreatic cancer.

REFERENCES

Agarwal, M. K., M. L. Agarwal et al. (2004). Tocotrienol-rich fraction of palm oil activates p53, modulates Bax/Bcl2 ratio and induces apoptosis independent of cell cycle association. *Cell Cycle* 3(2): 205–211.

Aggarwal, B. B., C. Sundaram et al. (2010). Tocotrienols, the vitamin E of the 21st century: Its potential against cancer and other chronic diseases. *Biochemical Pharmacology* 80(11): 1613–1631.

Ahn, K. S., G. Sethi et al. (2007). Gamma-tocotrienol inhibits nuclear factor-kappaB signaling pathway through inhibition of receptor-interacting protein and TAK1 leading to suppression of antiapoptotic gene products and potentiation of apoptosis. *Journal of Biological Chemistry* 282(1): 809–820.

Ayoub, N. M., S. V. Bachawal et al. (2011). Gamma-tocotrienol inhibits HGF-dependent mitogenesis and Met activation in highly malignant mammary tumour cells. *Cell Proliferation* 44(6): 516–526.

Baghurst, P. A., A. J. McMichael et al. (1991). A case-control study of diet and cancer of the pancreas. *American Journal of Epidemiology* 134(2): 167–179.

Barve, A., T. O. Khor et al. (2010). Mixed tocotrienols inhibit prostate carcinogenesis in TRAMP mice. *Nutrition and Cancer* 62(6): 789–794.

Birringer, M., J. H. EyTina et al. (2003). Vitamin E analogues as inducers of apoptosis: Structure-function relation. *British Journal of Cancer* 88(12): 1948–1955.

Bueno de Mesquita, H. B., P. Maisonneuve et al. (1991). Intake of foods and nutrients and cancer of the exocrine pancreas: A population-based case-control study in the Netherlands. *International Journal of Cancer* 48(4): 540–549.

Bunyan, J., H. D. McHale et al. (1961). Biological potencies of epsilon- and zeta-1-tocopherol and 5-methyltocol. *British Journal of Nutrition* 15: 253–257.

Campbell, S. E., B. Rudder et al. (2011). Gamma-tocotrienol induces growth arrest through a novel pathway with TGFbeta2 in prostate cancer. *Free Radical Biology & Medicine* 50(10): 1344–1354.

Chan, J. M., F. Wang et al. (2005). Vegetable and fruit intake and pancreatic cancer in a population-based case-control study in the San Francisco bay area. *Cancer Epidemiology, Biomarkers & Prevention* 14(9): 2093–2097.

Chang, P. N., W. N. Yap et al. (2009). Evidence of gamma-tocotrienol as an apoptosis-inducing, invasion-suppressing, and chemotherapy drug-sensitizing agent in human melanoma cells. *Nutrition and Cancer* 61(3): 357–366.

Comitato, R., G. Leoni et al. (2010). Tocotrienols activity in MCF-7 breast cancer cells: Involvement of ERbeta signal transduction. *Molecular Nutrition & Food Research* 54(5): 669–678.

Comitato, R., K. Nesaretnam et al. (2009). A novel mechanism of natural vitamin E tocotrienol activity: Involvement of ERbeta signal transduction. *American Journal of Physiology, Endocrinology and Metabolism* 297(2): E427–E437.

Cotugna, N., A. F. Subar et al. (1992). Nutrition and cancer prevention knowledge, beliefs, attitudes, and practices: The 1987 National Health Interview Survey. *Journal of the American Dietetic Association* 92(8): 963–968.

Coughlin, S. S., E. E. Calle et al. (2000). Predictors of pancreatic cancer mortality among a large cohort of United States adults. *Cancer Causes & Control: CCC* 11(10): 915–923.

Elangovan, S., T. C. Hsieh et al. (2008). Growth inhibition of human MDA-mB-231 breast cancer cells by delta-tocotrienol is associated with loss of cyclin D1/CDK4 expression and accompanying changes in the state of phosphorylation of the retinoblastoma tumor suppressor gene product. *Anticancer Research* 28(5A): 2641–2647.

Falk, R. T., L. W. Pickle et al. (1988). Life-style risk factors for pancreatic cancer in Louisiana: A case-control study. *American Journal of Epidemiology* 128(2): 324–336.

Fernandes, N. V., P. K. Guntipalli et al. (2010). D-delta-Tocotrienol-mediated cell cycle arrest and apoptosis in human melanoma cells. *Anticancer Research* 30(12): 4937–4944.

Fu, J. Y., D. R. Blatchford et al. (2009). Tumor regression after systemic administration of tocotrienol entrapped in tumor-targeted vesicles. *Journal of Controlled Release* 140(2): 95–99.

Gold, E. B., L. Gordis et al. (1985). Diet and other risk factors for cancer of the pancreas. *Cancer* 55(2): 460–467.

Gould, M. N., J. D. Haag et al. (1991). A comparison of tocopherol and tocotrienol for the chemoprevention of chemically induced rat mammary tumors. *American Journal of Clinical Nutrition* 53(4 Suppl): 1068S–1070S.

Guthrie, N., A. Gapor et al. (1997). Inhibition of proliferation of estrogen receptor-negative MDA-MB-435 and -positive MCF-7 human breast cancer cells by palm oil tocotrienols and tamoxifen, alone and in combination. *Journal of Nutrition* 127(3): 544S–548S.

van Haaften, R. I., G. R. Haenen et al. (2002). Tocotrienols inhibit human glutathione S-transferase P1-1. *IUBMB Life* 54(2): 81–84.

Han, S. S., J. Y. Jang et al. (2006). Analysis of long-term survivors after surgical resection for pancreatic cancer. *Pancreas* 32(3): 271–275.

Har, C. H. and C. K. Keong (2005). Effects of tocotrienols on cell viability and apoptosis in normal murine liver cells (BNL CL.2) and liver cancer cells (BNL 1ME A.7R.1), in vitro. *Asia Pacific Journal of Clinical Nutrition* 14(4): 374–380.

Hiura, Y., H. Tachibana et al. (2009). Specific accumulation of gamma- and delta-tocotrienols in tumor and their antitumor effect in vivo. *Journal of Nutritional Biochemistry* 20(8): 607–613.

Hochster, H. S., D. G. Haller et al. (2006). Consensus report of the international society of gastrointestinal oncology on therapeutic progress in advanced pancreatic cancer. *Cancer* 107(4): 676–685.

Hsieh, T. C., S. Elangovan et al. (2010). Differential suppression of proliferation in MCF-7 and MDA-MB-231 breast cancer cells exposed to alpha-, gamma- and delta-tocotrienols is accompanied by altered expression of oxidative stress modulatory enzymes. *Anticancer Research* 30(10): 4169–4176.

Husain, K., R. Francois et al. (2008). Abstract #3826: Delta-tocotrienol is the most bioactive natural tocotrienol in the prevention of pancreatic cancer transformation. *2008 Annual Meeting of the American Association for Cancer Research*, San Diego, CA. p 3826.

Husain, K., R. Francois et al. (2009a). Abstract #964: Comparative evaluation of natural tocotreinols as antitumor compounds for pancreatic cancer. *2009 Annual Meeting of the American Association for Cancer Research*, Denver, CO. p 964.

Husain, K., R. A. Francois et al. (2009b). Vitamin E delta-tocotrienol levels in tumor and pancreatic tissue of mice after oral administration. *Pharmacology* 83(3): 157–163.

Husain, K., R. A. Francois et al. (2011). Vitamin E {delta}-tocotrienol augments the anti-tumor activity of gemcitabine and suppresses constitutive NF-{kappa}B activation in pancreatic cancer. *Molecular Cancer Therapeutics* 10(12): 2363–2372.

Husain, K., M. Perez et al. (2010). Abstract #5416: Delta-tocotrienol potentiates antitumor activity of gemcitabine in pancreatic cancer through inhibition of nuclear factor-κB. *2010 Annual Meeting of the American Association for Cancer Research*, Washington, DC. p 5416.

Hussein, D. and H. Mo (2009). D-delta-Tocotrienol-mediated suppression of the proliferation of human PANC-1, MIA PaCa-2, and BxPC-3 pancreatic carcinoma cells. *Pancreas* 38(4): e124–e136.

Inokuchi, H., H. Hirokane et al. (2003). Anti-angiogenic activity of tocotrienol. *Bioscience, Biotechnology, and Biochemistry* 67(7): 1623–1627.

Inoue, A., K. Takitani et al. (2011). Induction of apoptosis by gamma-tocotrienol in human cancer cell lines and leukemic blasts from patients: Dependency on bid, cytochrome c, and caspase pathway. *Nutrition and Cancer* 63(5): 763–770.

Iqbal, J., M. Minhajuddin et al. (2003). Suppression of 7,12-dimethylbenz[alpha]anthracene-induced carcinogenesis and hypercholesterolaemia in rats by tocotrienol-rich fraction isolated from rice bran oil. *European Journal of Cancer Prevention* 12(6): 447–453.

Jemal, A., R. Siegel et al. (2006). Cancer statistics, 2006. *CA: A Cancer Journal for Clinicians* 56(2): 106–130.

Jemal, A., R. Siegel et al. (2010). Cancer statistics, 2010. *CA: A Cancer Journal for Clinicians* 60(5): 277–300.

Ji, B. T., W. H. Chow et al. (1995). Dietary factors and the risk of pancreatic cancer: A case-control study in Shanghai China. *Cancer Epidemiology, Biomarkers & Prevention* 4(8): 885–893.

Ji, X., Z. Wang et al. (2011). Inhibition of cell growth and induction of apoptosis in non-small cell lung cancer cells by delta-tocotrienol is associated with notch-1 down-regulation. *Journal of Cellular Biochemistry* 112(10): 2773–2783.

Jiang, Q., X. Rao et al. (2011). Gamma-tocotrienol induces apoptosis and autophagy in prostate cancer cells by increasing intracellular dihydrosphingosine and dihydroceramide. *International Journal of Cancer* 130(3): 685–693.

Kamangar, F., G. M. Dores et al. (2006). Patterns of cancer incidence, mortality, and prevalence across five continents: Defining priorities to reduce cancer disparities in different geographic regions of the world. *Journal of Clinical Oncology* 24(14): 2137–2150.

Kannappan, R., V. R. Yadav et al. (2010). gamma-Tocotrienol but not gamma-tocopherol blocks STAT3 cell signaling pathway through induction of protein-tyrosine phosphatase SHP-1 and sensitizes tumor cells to chemotherapeutic agents. *Journal of Biological Chemistry* 285(43): 33520–33528.

Kashiwagi, K., K. Harada et al. (2008). A redox-silent analogue of tocotrienol inhibits hypoxic adaptation of lung cancer cells. *Biochemical and Biophysical Research Communications* 365(4): 875–881.

Kausar, H., G. Bhasin et al. (2003). Palm oil alleviates 12-O-tetradecanoyl-phorbol-13-acetate-induced tumor promotion response in murine skin. *Cancer Letters* 192(2): 151–160.

Ko, A. H. and M. A. Tempero (2005). Treatment of metastatic pancreatic cancer. *Journal of the National Comprehensive Cancer Network* 3(5): 627–636.

Komiyama, K., K. Iizuka et al. (1989). Studies on the biological activity of tocotrienols. *Chemical and Pharmaceutical Bulletin* 37(5): 1369–1371.

Kumar, K. S., M. Raghavan et al. (2006). Preferential radiation sensitization of prostate cancer in nude mice by nutraceutical antioxidant gamma-tocotrienol. *Life Sciences* 78(18): 2099–2104.

Kunnumakkara, A. B., B. Sung et al. (2010). {Gamma}-tocotrienol inhibits pancreatic tumors and sensitizes them to gemcitabine treatment by modulating the inflammatory microenvironment. *Cancer Research* 70(21): 8695–8705.

La Vecchia, C., E. Negri et al. (1990). Medical history, diet and pancreatic cancer. *Oncology* 47(6): 463–466.

Li, Y., W. G. Sun et al. (2011). Gamma-tocotrienol inhibits angiogenesis of human umbilical vein endothelial cell induced by cancer cell. *Journal of Nutritional Biochemistry* 22(12): 1127–1136.

Lieberman, R. (2001). Prostate cancer chemoprevention: Strategies for designing efficient clinical trials. *Urology* 57(4 Suppl 1): 224–229.

Liu, H. K., Q. Wang et al. (2010). Inhibitory effects of gamma-tocotrienol on invasion and metastasis of human gastric adenocarcinoma SGC-7901 cells. *Journal of Nutritional Biochemistry* 21(3): 206–213.

Lyon, J. L., M. L. Slattery et al. (1993). Dietary intake as a risk factor for cancer of the exocrine pancreas. *Cancer Epidemiology, Biomarkers & Prevention* 2(6): 513–518.

Makpol, S., N. A. Shamaan et al. (1997). Different starting times of alpha-tocopherol and gamma-tocotrienol supplementation and tumor marker enzyme activities in the rat chemically induced with cancer. *General Pharmacology* 28(4): 589–592.

de Mesquita, M. L., R. M. Araujo et al. (2011). Cytotoxicity of delta-tocotrienols from *Kielmeyera coriacea* against cancer cell lines. *Bioorganic & Medicinal Chemistry* 19(1): 623–630.

McIntyre, B. S., K. P. Briski et al. (2000a). Antiproliferative and apoptotic effects of tocopherols and tocotrienols on preneoplastic and neoplastic mouse mammary epithelial cells. *Proceedings of the Society for Experimental Biology and Medicine* 224(4): 292–301.

McIntyre, B. S., K. P. Briski et al. (2000b). Antiproliferative and apoptotic effects of tocopherols and tocotrienols on normal mouse mammary epithelial cells. *Lipids* 35(2): 171–180.

Mills, P. K., W. L. Beeson et al. (1988). Dietary habits and past medical history as related to fatal pancreas cancer risk among Adventists. *Cancer* 61(12): 2578–2585.

Miyazawa, T., H. Inokuchi et al. (2004). Anti-angiogenic potential of tocotrienol in vitro. *Biochemistry* 69(1): 67–69.

Mo, H. and C. E. Elson (1999). Apoptosis and cell-cycle arrest in human and murine tumor cells are initiated by isoprenoids. *Journal of Nutrition* 129(4): 804–813.

Nakashima, K., N. Virgona et al. (2010). The tocotrienol-rich fraction from rice bran enhances cisplatin-induced cytotoxicity in human mesothelioma H28 cells. *Phytotherapy Research* 24(9): 1317–1321.

Nesaretnam, K., R. Ambra et al. (2004). Tocotrienol-rich fraction from palm oil affects gene expression in tumors resulting from MCF-7 cell inoculation in athymic mice. *Lipids* 39(5): 459–467.

Nesaretnam, K., S. Dorasamy et al. (2000). Tocotrienols inhibit growth of ZR-75-1 breast cancer cells. *International Journal of Food Sciences and Nutrition* 51 Suppl: S95–S103.

Nesaretnam, K., N. Guthrie et al. (1995). Effect of tocotrienols on the growth of a human breast cancer cell line in culture. *Lipids* 30(12): 1139–1143.

Nesaretnam, K., P. Meganathan et al. (2011). Tocotrienols and breast cancer: The evidence to date. *Genes & Nutrition* 7(1): 3–9.

Nesaretnam, K., K. R. Selvaduray et al. (2010). Effectiveness of tocotrienol-rich fraction combined with tamoxifen in the management of women with early breast cancer: A pilot clinical trial. *Breast Cancer Research: BCR* 12(5): R81.

Nesaretnam, K., R. Stephen et al. (1998). Tocotrienols inhibit the growth of human breast cancer cells irrespective of estrogen receptor status. *Lipids* 33(5): 461–469.

Ngah, W. Z., Z. Jarien et al. (1991). Effect of tocotrienols on hepatocarcinogenesis induced by 2-acetylamino-fluorene in rats. *American Journal of Clinical Nutrition* 53(4 Suppl): 1076S–1081S.

Nkondjock, A., P. Ghadirian et al. (2005a). Dietary intake of lycopene is associated with reduced pancreatic cancer risk. *Journal of Nutrition* 135(3): 592–597.

Nkondjock, A., D. Krewski et al. (2005b). Dietary patterns and risk of pancreatic cancer. *International Journal of Cancer* 114(5): 817–823.

Norell, S. E., A. Ahlbom et al. (1986). Diet and pancreatic cancer: A case-control study. *American Journal of Epidemiology* 124(6): 894–902.

Olsen, G. W., J. S. Mandel et al. (1989). A case-control study of pancreatic cancer and cigarettes, alcohol, coffee and diet. *American Journal of Public Health* 79(8): 1016–1019.

Park, S. K., B. G. Sanders et al. (2010). Tocotrienols induce apoptosis in breast cancer cell lines via an endoplasmic reticulum stress-dependent increase in extrinsic death receptor signaling. *Breast Cancer Research and Treatment* 124(2): 361–375.

Parker, R. A., B. C. Pearce et al. (1993). Tocotrienols regulate cholesterol production in mammalian cells by post-transcriptional suppression of 3-hydroxy-3-methylglutaryl-coenzyme A reductase. *Journal of Biological Chemistry* 268(15): 11230–11238.

Patacsil, D., A. T. Tran et al. (2011). Gamma-tocotrienol induced apoptosis is associated with unfolded protein response in human breast cancer cells. *Journal of Nutritional Biochemistry* 23(1): 93–100.

Pierpaoli, E., V. Viola et al. (2010). Gamma- and delta-tocotrienols exert a more potent anticancer effect than alpha-tocopheryl succinate on breast cancer cell lines irrespective of HER-2/neu expression. *Life Sciences* 86(17–18): 668–675.

Qureshi, A. A., W. C. Burger et al. (1986). The structure of an inhibitor of cholesterol biosynthesis isolated from barley. *Journal of Biological Chemistry* 261(23): 10544–10550.

Qureshi, A. A., S. A. Sami et al. (2002). Dose-dependent suppression of serum cholesterol by tocotrienol-rich fraction (TRF25) of rice bran in hypercholesterolemic humans. *Atherosclerosis* 161(1): 199–207.

Rahmat, A., W. Z. Ngah et al. (1993). Long-term administration of tocotrienols and tumor-marker enzyme activities during hepatocarcinogenesis in rats. *Nutrition* 9(3): 229–232.

Rajendran, P., F. Li et al. (2011). Gamma-Tocotrienol is a novel inhibitor of constitutive and inducible STAT3 signalling pathway in human hepatocellular carcinoma: Potential role as an antiproliferative, pro-apoptotic and chemosensitizing agent. *British Journal of Pharmacology* 163(2): 283–298.

Ramdas, P., M. Rajihuzzaman et al. (2011). Tocotrienol-treated MCF-7 human breast cancer cells show down-regulation of API5 and up-regulation of MIG6 genes. *Cancer Genomics & Proteomics* 8(1): 19–31.

Sakai, M., M. Okabe et al. (2004). Induction of apoptosis by tocotrienol in rat hepatoma dRLh-84 cells. *Anticancer Research* 24(3a): 1683–1688.

Sakai, M., M. Okabe et al. (2006). Apoptosis induction by gamma-tocotrienol in human hepatoma Hep3B cells. *Journal of Nutritional Biochemistry* 17(10): 672–676.

Samant, G. V. and P. W. Sylvester (2006). gamma-Tocotrienol inhibits ErbB3-dependent PI3K/Akt mitogenic signalling in neoplastic mammary epithelial cells. *Cell Proliferation* 39(6): 563–574.

Samant, G. V., V. B. Wali et al. (2010). Anti-proliferative effects of gamma-tocotrienol on mammary tumour cells are associated with suppression of cell cycle progression. *Cell Proliferation* 43(1): 77–83.

Selvaduray, K. R., A. K. Radhakrishnan et al. (2010). Palm tocotrienols inhibit proliferation of murine mammary cancer cells and induce expression of interleukin-24 mRNA. *Journal of Interferon & Cytokine Research* 30(12): 909–916.

Selvaduray, K. R., A. K. Radhakrishnan et al. (2011). Palm tocotrienols decrease levels of pro-angiogenic markers in human umbilical vein endothelial cells (HUVEC) and murine mammary cancer cells. *Genes & Nutrition* 7(1): 53–61.

Sen, C. K., S. Khanna et al. (2007). Tocotrienols: The emerging face of natural vitamin E. *Vitamins and Hormones* 76: 203–261.

Shah, S., A. Gapor et al. (2003). Role of caspase-8 activation in mediating vitamin E-induced apoptosis in murine mammary cancer cells. *Nutrition and Cancer* 45(2): 236–246.

Shah, S. and P. W. Sylvester (2004). Tocotrienol-induced caspase-8 activation is unrelated to death receptor apoptotic signaling in neoplastic mammary epithelial cells. *Experimental Biology and Medicine* 229(8): 745–755.

Shah, S. J. and P. W. Sylvester (2005a). Gamma-tocotrienol inhibits neoplastic mammary epithelial cell proliferation by decreasing Akt and nuclear factor kappaB activity. *Experimental Biology and Medicine* 230(4): 235–241.

Shah, S. J. and P. W. Sylvester (2005b). Tocotrienol-induced cytotoxicity is unrelated to mitochondrial stress apoptotic signaling in neoplastic mammary epithelial cells. *Biochemistry and Cell Biology* 83(1): 86–95.

Shibata, A., T. M. Mack et al. (1994). A prospective study of pancreatic cancer in the elderly. *International Journal of Cancer* 58(1): 46–49.

Shin-Kang, S., V. P. Ramsauer et al. (2011). Tocotrienols inhibit AKT and ERK activation and suppress pancreatic cancer cell proliferation by suppressing the ErbB2 pathway. *Free Radical Biology & Medicine* 51(6): 1164–1174.

Shun, M. C., W. Yu et al. (2004). Pro-apoptotic mechanisms of action of a novel vitamin E analog (alpha-TEA) and a naturally occurring form of vitamin E (delta-tocotrienol) in MDA-MB-435 human breast cancer cells. *Nutrition and Cancer* 48(1): 95–105.

Silverman, D. T., C. A. Swanson et al. (1998). Dietary and nutritional factors and pancreatic cancer: A case-control study based on direct interviews. *Journal of the National Cancer Institute* 90(22): 1710–1719.

Singletary, E., R. Lieberman et al. (2000). Novel translational model for breast cancer chemoprevention study: Accrual to a presurgical intervention with tamoxifen and N-[4-hydroxyphenyl] retinamide. *Cancer Epidemiology, Biomarkers & Prevention* 9(10): 1087–1090.

Srivastava, J. K. and S. Gupta (2006). Tocotrienol-rich fraction of palm oil induces cell cycle arrest and apoptosis selectively in human prostate cancer cells. *Biochemical and Biophysical Research Communications* 346(2): 447–453.

Steinmetz, K. A. and J. D. Potter (1991). Vegetables, fruit, and cancer. I. Epidemiology. *Cancer Causes & Control: CCC* 2(5): 325–357.

Stolzenberg-Solomon, R. Z., D. Albanes et al. (1999). Pancreatic cancer risk and nutrition-related methyl-group availability indicators in male smokers. *Journal of the National Cancer Institute* 91(6): 535–541.

Stolzenberg-Solomon, R. Z., P. Pietinen et al. (2002). A prospective study of medical conditions, anthropometry, physical activity, and pancreatic cancer in male smokers (Finland). *Cancer Causes & Control: CCC* 13(5): 417–426.

Suarna, C., R. L. Hood et al. (1993). Comparative antioxidant activity of tocotrienols and other natural lipid-soluble antioxidants in a homogeneous system, and in rat and human lipoproteins. *Biochimica et Biophysica Acta* 1166(2–3): 163–170.

Sun, W., Q. Wang et al. (2008). Gamma-tocotrienol-induced apoptosis in human gastric cancer SGC-7901 cells is associated with a suppression in mitogen-activated protein kinase signalling. *British Journal of Nutrition* 99(6): 1247–1254.

Sun, W., W. Xu et al. (2009). gamma-Tocotrienol induces mitochondria-mediated apoptosis in human gastric adenocarcinoma SGC-7901 cells. *Journal of Nutritional Biochemistry* 20(4): 276–284.

Sundram, K., H. T. Khor et al. (1989). Effect of dietary palm oils on mammary carcinogenesis in female rats induced by 7,12-dimethylbenz(a)anthracene. *Cancer Research* 49(6): 1447–1451.

Sylvester, P. W., A. Nachnani et al. (2002). Role of GTP-binding proteins in reversing the antiproliferative effects of tocotrienols in preneoplastic mammary epithelial cells. *Asia Pacific Journal of Clinical Nutrition* 11(Suppl 7): S452–459.

Takahashi, K. and G. Loo (2004). Disruption of mitochondria during tocotrienol-induced apoptosis in MDA-MB-231 human breast cancer cells. *Biochemical Pharmacology* 67(2): 315–324.

Taylor, P. R. and P. Greenwald (2005). Nutritional interventions in cancer prevention. *Journal of Clinical Oncology* 23(2): 333–345.

Vaquero, E. C., M. Rickmann et al. (2007). Tocotrienols: Balancing the mitochondrial crosstalk between apoptosis and autophagy. *Autophagy* 3(6): 652–654.

Wada, S., Y. Satomi et al. (2005). Tumor suppressive effects of tocotrienol in vivo and in vitro. *Cancer Letters* 229(2): 181–191.

Wali, V. B., S. V. Bachawal et al. (2009). Endoplasmic reticulum stress mediates gamma-tocotrienol-induced apoptosis in mammary tumor cells. *Apoptosis* 14(11): 1366–1377.

Whittle, K. J., P. J. Dunphy et al. (1966). The isolation and properties of delta-tocotrienol from Hevea latex. *Biochemical Journal* 100(1): 138–145.

Xu, W. L., J. R. Liu et al. (2009). Inhibition of proliferation and induction of apoptosis by gamma-tocotrienol in human colon carcinoma HT-29 cells. *Nutrition* 25(5): 555–566.

Yamada, Y., M. Obayashi et al. (2008). Dietary tocotrienol reduces UVB-induced skin damage and sesamin enhances tocotrienol effects in hairless mice. *Journal of Nutritional Science and Vitaminology* 54(2): 117–123.

Yap, W. N., P. N. Chang et al. (2008). Gamma-tocotrienol suppresses prostate cancer cell proliferation and invasion through multiple-signalling pathways. *British Journal of Cancer* 99(11): 1832–1841.

Yap, S. P., K. H. Yuen et al. (2001). Pharmacokinetics and bioavailability of alpha-, gamma- and delta-tocotrienols under different food status. *Journal of Pharmacy and Pharmacology* 53(1): 67–71.

Yap, W. N., N. Zaiden et al. (2010a). In vivo evidence of gamma-tocotrienol as a chemosensitizer in the treatment of hormone-refractory prostate cancer. *Pharmacology* 85(4): 248–258.

Yap, W. N., N. Zaiden et al. (2010b). Id1, inhibitor of differentiation, is a key protein mediating anti-tumor responses of gamma-tocotrienol in breast cancer cells. *Cancer Letters* 291(2): 187–199.

Yu, F. L., A. Gapor et al. (2005). Evidence for the preventive effect of the polyunsaturated phytol side chain in tocotrienols on 17beta-estradiol epoxidation. *Cancer Detection and Prevention* 29(4): 383–388.

Yu, W., M. Simmons-Menchaca et al. (1999). Induction of apoptosis in human breast cancer cells by tocopherols and tocotrienols. *Nutrition and Cancer* 33(1): 26–32.

Zhang, J. S., D. M. Li et al. (2011). A paraptosis-like cell death induced by delta-tocotrienol in human colon carcinoma SW620 cells is associated with the suppression of the Wnt signaling pathway. *Toxicology* 285(1–2): 8–17.

Zheng, W., J. K. McLaughlin et al. (1993). A cohort study of smoking, alcohol consumption, and dietary factors for pancreatic cancer (United States). *Cancer Causes & Control: CCC* 4(5): 477–482.

Zhou, C., M. M. Tabb et al. (2004). Tocotrienols activate the steroid and xenobiotic receptor, SXR, and selectively regulate expression of its target genes. *Drug Metabolism and Disposition: The Biological Fate of Chemicals* 32(10): 1075–1082.

19 Tocotrienols in the Treatment of Dyslipidemia

Mark Houston

CONTENTS

19.1 INTRODUCTION

Vitamin E is the generic name of a mixture of lipid-soluble phenols, tocopherols, and tocotrienols, possessing general structural features: an aromatic chromanol head and a 16-carbon hydrocarbon tail (Serbinova et al. 1991). The amount of methyl substituents in the chromanol nucleus gives rise to alpha, beta, gamma, and delta isomers (Serbinova et al. 1991). Tocotrienols are a naturally occurring derivative of tocopherols in the vitamin E family (Serbinova et al. 1991). Tocopherols have four isomers: alpha, beta, gamma, and delta (Serbinova et al. 1991). Tocotrienols have the same four isomers but differ in the number of double bonds in the side chains (Serbinova et al. 1991). The tocotrienols have more potent antioxidant activity than tocopherols (Serbinova et al. 1991). Tocotrienol and tocopherol concentrates are often referred to as "tocotrienol-rich fractions" or TRFs, and are obtained primarily from rice bran or palm oil and contain about 30%–50% tocopherols (Khor et al. 1995). Tocotrienols naturally occur in coconut oil, cocoa butter, barley, the annatto plant, and wheat germ in addition to rice bran and palm oil. The annatto plant has the highest concentration of gamma- and delta-tocotrienol isomers. If the TRFs contain >20% tocopherol, the cholesterol-lowering effect is diminished (Qureshi et al. 1986; Qureshi 1996; Hosomi and Arita 1997). Tocotrienols are more effective in reducing low-density lipoprotein (LDL) and total cholesterol if the concentration of tocotrienols is high and the tocopherol concentration is low (Qureshi et al. 1986; Qureshi 1996; Hosomi and Arita 1997). The relative potency of the tocotrienols varies, with the delta isomer being the best at reducing LDL, total cholesterol, and triglycerides (Serbinova et al. 1991; O'Byrne et al. 2000; Song and DeBose-Boyd 2006). This review covers the mechanism of action, animal studies, and clinical human trials of tocotrienols as effective natural compounds to treat dyslipidemia. Specific clinical recommendations are made on optimal dosing and combinations of tocotrienols with other natural agents for dyslipidemia as well as with statins.

19.2 MECHANISM OF ACTION AND STRUCTURE–FUNCTION RELATIONSHIP

The tocotrienols demonstrate one of the most important structure–function relationships in natural medicine. Tocotrienols are composed of a chroman ring with a variable number of methyl groups and a long phytyl side chain with three double bonds (Serbinova et al. 1991). As the number of methyl groups decreases on the chroman ring from the alpha (trimethyl) to the delta isomer (monomethyl), the lipid-lowering potency increases (Serbinova et al. 1991; Qureshi et al. 2002). The gamma isomer is about 30× more potent in lipid-lowering capability as compared to the alpha isomer (Serbinova et al. 1991; Qureshi et al. 2002). The location of the double bonds and the structure of tocotrienols is very close to that of farnesyl (farnesylated benzopyran analogs), which is the compound preceding the formation of squalene in cholesterol synthesis (Parker et al. 1993). Farnesyl is also the compound converted to ubiquinone (coenzyme Q-10) via the formation of all-*trans*-geranylgeranyl pyrophosphate, as well as to various prenylated proteins and dolicols. Tocotrienols increase the conversion of farnesyl to farnesol, which reduces the conversion of farnesyl to squalene and then to cholesterol (Parker et al. 1993). This also increases endogenous levels of ubiquinone in mitochondria. In addition, the farnesol signals two post-transcriptional pathways suppressing 3-hydroxy-3-methylglutaryl-coenzyme A (HMG-CoA) reductase activity by increasing the controlled degradation of the reductase protein and reducing the efficiency of translation of HMG-CoA reductase mRNA (Parker et al. 1993; Correll et al. 1994; Khor et al. 1995). This prevents upregulation of the HMG-CoA enzyme in response to statin therapy and further reduces LDL cholesterol when tocotrienols are used in combination with statin therapy in humans.

The 2.4× increase in degradation of the reductase enzyme reduces the T 1/2 from 3.73–1.59 h. There is a 57%–76% decreased efficiency of translation of the reductase mRNA and a 23%–76% decrease in reductase protein mass levels. In addition, the LDL receptor protein is augmented, increasing the number of LDL receptors and LDL removal as well as stimulation of apolipoprotein B degradation clearance (Pearce et al. 1992, 1994; Parker et al. 1993). There is a dose-dependent cholesterol reduction associated with tocotrienols. As the dose of tocotrienols increases, additional conversion to alpha-tocopherol may occur, which will limit the antilipid effects (Qureshi et al. 2002). If the alpha-tocopherol concentration is >20%, it will inhibit the tocotrienol lipid-lowering effects (Qureshi et al. 1986, 1996; Hosomi and Arita 1997). Alpha-tocopherol may compete for binding with the alpha-tocopherol transfer protein (TTP), and thus interfere with the transport of tocotrienols in the circulation (Hosomi and Arita 1997). In addition, alpha-tocopherol attenuates the inhibitory effects of tocotrienols on HMG-CoA reductase and actually induces enzymatic activity (Qureshi et al. 1996, 2002). This increase in HMG-CoA reductase activity with alpha-tocopherol may be one of the reasons that moderate to high dose alpha-tocopherol—as has been used exclusively in clinical trials—has not consistently reduced cardiovascular events in human prospective clinical trials. It is estimated that about 40% of the plasma tocotrienols are carried in LDL (O'Byrne et al. 2000).

Recent studies have demonstrated specific differences between the gamma- and delta-tocotrienol mechanism of action on lipid reduction (Song and DeBose-Boyd 2006). The degradation as well as the complex multivalent feedback regulation of the HMG-CoA reductase enzyme results from sterol-induced binding of the reductase to the endoplasmic reticulum (ER) membrane proteins called Insigs (Song and DeBose-Boyd 2006). Delta-tocotrienol stimulates ubiquitination and degradation of HMG-CoA reductase and blocks processing of sterol regulatory element binding proteins (SREBPs), another sterol-mediated action of Insigs (Song and DeBose-Boyd 2006). Gamma-tocotrienol is more selective in enhancing reductase ubiquitination and degradation than blocking SREBP processing (Song and DeBose-Boyd 2006). This may provide additional lipid-lowering effect when used in conjunction with statins (Song and DeBose-Boyd 2006). However, the efficacy of gamma-tocotrienol may be limited by a rapid rate of metabolism, which appears to be mediated by the induction of CYP3A4 through the action of the pregnane X receptor (PXR), a nuclear receptor that plays a major role in xenobiotic detoxification (Song and DeBose-Boyd 2006). The absorption of tocotrienols is greater when they are given with a meal than when they are given to subjects in a fasting state (Yap et al. 2001).

19.3 ANIMAL STUDIES

Tocotrienols provide significant lipid-lowering effects in experimental animals (Qureshi et al. 1991a, 2001; Teoh et al. 1994; Iqbal et al. 2003; Minhajuddin et al. 2005; Yu et al. 2006). In a study of 5 week old female chickens, there was a dose–response reduction in total and LDL cholesterol of

22%–52% ($p < 0.05$), respectively, with supplemental TRF (TRF of palm oil) (Yu et al. 2006). The alpha-tocotrienol fraction reduced total cholesterol and LDL cholesterol by 17% and 33%, respectively. However, the more potent gamma- and delta fractions reduced total and LDL cholesterol by 32% and 66%, respectively. Triglycerides were also significantly reduced, but high-density lipoprotein (HDL) was unchanged. In experimentally induced hyperlipidemic rats, a TRF isolate from rice bran oil produced a dose-dependent reduction in total cholesterol of 48%, LDL cholesterol of 60%, and triglycerides of 42%, with no change in HDL cholesterol but an improvement in oxidative stress parameters at doses of 8 mg TRF/kg/day (Minhajuddin et al. 2005).

Feeding TRF to rats resulted in a significant decline of 30% in total cholesterol and 67% in LDL cholesterol (Iqbal et al. 2003). In a swine study, administration of TRF with tocotrienols significantly reduced total cholesterol 32%–38%, LDL 35%–43%, apolipoprotein B 22%–35%, triglycerides 15%–19%, platelet factor 4 by 12%–24%, thromboxane B2 by 11%–18%, and glucose by 22%–25% (Qureshi et al. 1991, 2001).

In rabbits fed a gamma-tocotrienol complex of 80% with 20% alpha- and beta-tocotrienols, there was a significant reduction in lipid levels, as well as reduction in lipid streaks and atheroma in the aorta (Teoh et al. 1994).

19.4 HUMAN STUDIES

Most prospective studies have demonstrated significant lipid-lowering effects of tocotrienols in humans (Qureshi et al. 1991, 1995; Tomeo et al. 1995; O'Byrne et al. 2000). Those studies that were negative generally have methodological flaws that may account for the discrepant results (Mensink et al. 1999; Mustad et al. 2002). A double-blind, 8 week, crossover study in 25 subjects compared the effects of TRF palm oil at 200 mg of palmvitee capsules per day versus 300 mg of corn oil per day on serum lipids in hypercholesterolemic humans (Qureshi et al. 1991). Total cholesterol fell 15%, LDL 8%, Apo B 10%, thromboxane 25%, PF4 16%, and glucose 12% (all values $p < 0.05$). The HDL and triglyceride levels were not significantly changed. However, there was significant variation in the response rate as indicated by a large standard deviation in the lipid results of those subjects receiving the tocotrienol complex. Some of this may be accounted for by the lack of control of cholesterol and fat intake in the subjects. Another explanation would be that efficacy of tocotrienols would be limited to those subjects who have an inherent overproduction of cholesterol. Finally, alpha-tocopherol at concentrations over 20% inhibits the effectiveness of the tocotrienol lipid-lowering effect. Tocotrienols may be less effective in those subjects with ad lib intake of cholesterol and fats due to the downregulation of the HMG-CoA reductase enzyme. Those receiving 200 mg of 100% gamma-tocotrienol formulation had a much greater reduction in total cholesterol of 31%, LDL of 27%, and triglycerides of 15%, indicating a greater potency of this subfraction. The effects on lipids persisted for 2–6 weeks following discontinuation of the tocotrienols.

Qureshi et al. (1995) evaluated 36 subjects with dyslipidemia treated for 8 weeks with an AHA Step 1 dietary regimen, followed by administration of palmvitee capsules or 200 mg of gamma-tocotrienol for an additional 4 weeks. The palmvitee capsules contained 40 mg of alpha-tocopherol, 48 mg of alpha-tocotrienol, 112 mg of gamma-tocotrienol, and 60 mg of delta-tocotrienol. The total cholesterol level was reduced by 10% ($p < 0.05$), LDL 13% ($p < 0.05$), apolipoprotein B 7% ($p < 0.05$), thromboxane B2 ($p < 0.05$), and glucose 15% ($p < 0.05$) in the palmvitee group. The total cholesterol fell 13% ($p < 0.05$), LDL fell 15% ($p < 0.05$), and apolipoprotein B fell 8% ($p < 0.05$) in the gamma-tocotrienol group ($p < 0.05$). There were no significant changes in triglycerides, HDL, or apolipoprotein A1 in either group.

Tomeo et al. (1995) demonstrated regression for carotid artery stenosis with duplex ultrasonography in 7 of 25 subjects with known cerebrovascular disease treated over 18 months with a mixture of alpha-tocopherol and gamma-tocotrienols. There was a reduction in platelet peroxidation in this group, but there were no significant changes in serum lipids. None of the subjects in the control group showed regression, and 10 of 25 showed progression.

Mensink et al. (1999) evaluated 20 men in a randomized, double-blind, placebo-controlled, parallel trial receiving 35 mg of tocotrienols with 20 mg of alpha-tocopherol versus 20 control subjects who received only 20 mg of alpha-tocopherol. As would be expected, there were no significant changes in any lipid measurement. The dose of tocotrienol was too low in this study based on previous and subsequent human trials, and the dose of alpha-tocopherol was too high, which inhibited any effect of the tocotrienols on lipid levels as noted previously in other studies.

There may be differences among the tocotrienols in their ability to prevent the oxidation of LDL cholesterol (O'Byrne et al. 2000). Subjects were administered placebo or purified alpha-, gamma-, or delta-tocotrienyl acetates at 250 mg/day for 8 weeks, following a low fat diet for 4 weeks. Serum levels were measured and indicated adequate hydrolysis, absorption, and retention in the circulation for each of the tocotrienols. However, the serum concentration of alpha-tocotrienol was twice that of gamma-tocotrienol and 10 times greater than that of delta-tocotrienol despite equivalent doses. Alpha-tocotrienyl acetate increased *in vitro* LDL oxidative resistance by 22% ($p < 0.001$) and decreased its rate of oxidation ($p < 0.01$). The delta-tocotrienyl acetate resulted in significantly greater reductions in the rate of LDL oxidation and the amount of conjugated dienes formed (both $p < 0.05$). However, none of the preparations reduced serum lipids in the subjects.

Mustad et al. (2002) evaluated three commercially available tocotrienol supplements at a dose of 200 mg/day or a safflower oil placebo for 28 days in 67 hypercholesterolemic men and women in a double-blind, randomized, parallel-design study. No significant differences in mean lipid or glucose concentrations were observed among the four treatment groups. However, the composition analysis of the products indicated that all three had high concentrations of alpha-tocopherol, which reduced the tocotrienol effects, while the gamma or delta concentration of tocotrienols was low in two of the products. Therefore, this study was not an adequate evaluation of the effects of purified tocotrienols on serum lipids.

Quershi et al. (2002) demonstrated a dose–response of TRF-25 in 90 subjects given 25, 50, 100, and 200 mg/day of the TRF while on an AHA Step 1 diet. The TRF-25 was derived from stabilized and heated rice brans with alpha-, gamma-, delta-, and desmethyl and didesmethyl tocotrienols. The dose of 100 mg/day produced the maximum decrease of 20% in total cholesterol, 25% in LDL, 14% in apolipoprotein B, and 12% in triglycerides (all with $p < 0.05$).

Baliarsingh et al. (2005) evaluated tocotrienols as TRF 3 mg/kg body weight in 19 Type 2 diabetic subjects for 60 days and found significant reductions in total cholesterol of 30% and LDL of 42%. There were no changes in serum glucose or HDL. The TRF fraction was obtained from edible grade rice bran oil and contained 7.5% alpha-tocopherol, 14.6% alpha-tocotrienol, 2.2% beta-tocotrienol, 38.8% gamma-tocotrienol, 29.9% delta-tocotrienol, 4.5% delta-tocopherol, and 2.4% unidentified tocotrienols.

Wahlqvist (1992) evaluated 44 subjects over 20 weeks with hyperlipidemia treated with a palm-vitee oil containing 30% alpha-tocopherol as well as gamma- and delta-tocotrienols and found no changes in serum lipids. The high percent of alpha-tocopherol may have inhibited the effects of the tocotrienols on lipids.

Rice bran oil (Lichtenstein et al. 1994; Gerhardt and Gallo 1998; Cicero and Gaddi 2001; Nagao et al. 2001; Ausman et al. 2005; Kuriyan et al. 2005; Most et al. 2005; Wilson et al. 2007) has numerous components that improve the lipid profile. It contains unsaponifiables (up to 4.4%), including plant sterols (43%), four methyl sterols (10%), triterpene alcohols (29%), and less polar components such as squalene and tocotrienols (19%). Rice bran oil also contains 25% saturated fats, 40% polyunsaturated fatty acid (PUFA), and 40% monounsaturated fatty acid (MUFA). Oryzanol has a greater effect on lowering plasma non-HDL cholesterol and raising plasma HDL than ferulic acid, possibly through a greater capacity to increase fecal excretion of cholesterol and its metabolites (Nagao et al. 2001). However, ferulic acid may have greater antioxidant capacity by its ability to maintain serum vitamin E levels (Wilson et al. 2007). The average reduction in LDL is about 7%–14% (Gerhardt and Gallo 1998; Most et al. 2005).

19.5 SUMMARY AND CONCLUSIONS

Tocotrienols are natural derivatives of vitamin E that demonstrate significant reductions in total and LDL cholesterol in humans. The gamma and delta isomers as well as the desmethylated derivatives have the most potent lipid-lowering effects with reductions in LDL of 8%–27% and increase of Apo B degradation. Tocotrienols reduce formation and increase the degradation of HMG-CoA reductase, and increase LDL receptors. There is a dose-dependent effect that appears to be maximum at about 200 mg/day of gamma/delta-tocotrienols and 100 mg/day of the desmethylated derivatives. The lipid-lowering efficacy is reduced in the presence of a concentration of tocopherols exceeding 20%. Tocotrienols are most effective if taken in conjunction with an AHA lipid-lowering diet along with other healthy lifestyle changes. Tocotrienols should be taken in the evening with a meal at least 12 h after ingestion of any tocopherols, especially if the concentration of alpha-tocopherol is over 20% of the total vitamin E ingested in one day. In addition, the alpha- and delta-tocotrienols exhibit reduction in LDL oxidation and reduce carotid artery stenosis progression. There is suggestive evidence that gamma- and delta-tocotrienols may also reduce serum glucose (Junior et al. 2005; Russell et al. 2005). The annatto plant, which is a natural food color additive with high carotenoid content, has the highest natural amount of delta-tocotrienols (90%) and gamma-tocotrienols (10%) compared to rice bran oil and palm oil (Junior et al. 2005; Russell et al. 2005). Rice bran oil also contains oryzanol, which may reduce intestinal cholesterol absorption. A high-grade extraction process of rice bran oil with TRF-25 may have advantages due to the higher concentration of desmethylated tocotrienols that appear to reduce LDL even more than the gamma and delta isomers. There are no adverse effects noted in any of the clinical studies in humans. Several recent reviews have confirmed the efficacy and safety of tocotrienols in the treatment of dyslipidemia (Houston et al. 2009; Houston and Sparks 2010; Nigar et al. 2010).

19.6 CLINICAL RECOMMENDATIONS

Dyslipidemic patients should follow the AHA Step 1 lipid-lowering diet, portfolio or paleolithic diets, and consume 200 mg of gamma-/delta-tocotrienols in a purified form or 100 mg of TRF-25 at night with food. Tocopherols should be <20% of the total vitamin E consumed per day, and should be taken in the morning to avoid reduced efficacy of tocotrienols. The gamma and delta isomers are the most potent lipid lowering isomers. Both isomers enhance LDL-lowering effects of statins by an additional 15%. Gamma-tocotrienol may be most effective when used in conjunction with a statin, but more studies are needed to document this use (Song and DeBose-Boyd 2006). Other natural products enhance the effects of gamma- and delta-tocotrienols in the treatment of dyslipidemia, such as pantethine, phytosterols, red yeast rice, and fiber (Houston et al. 2009; Houston and Sparks 2010; Nigar et al. 2010). The addition of alpha-tocotrienol in small doses to reduce LDL oxidation may also be of benefit.

REFERENCES

Ausman, L. M., N. Rong et al. (2005). Hypocholesterolemic effect of physically refined rice bran oil: Studies of cholesterol metabolism and early atherosclerosis in hypercholesterolemic hamsters. *J Nutr Biochem* **16**(9): 521–529.

Baliarsingh, S., Z. H. Beg et al. (2005). The therapeutic impacts of tocotrienols in type 2 diabetic patients with hyperlipidemia. *Atherosclerosis* **182**(2): 367–374.

Cicero, A. F. and A. Gaddi (2001). Rice bran oil and gamma-oryzanol in the treatment of hyperlipoproteinaemias and other conditions. *Phytother Res* **15**(4): 277–289.

Correll, C. C., L. Ng et al. (1994). Identification of farnesol as the non-sterol derivative of mevalonic acid required for the accelerated degradation of 3-hydroxy-3-methylglutaryl-coenzyme A reductase. *J Biol Chem* **269**(26): 17390–17393.

Gerhardt, A. L. and N. B. Gallo (1998). Full-fat rice bran and oat bran similarly reduce hypercholesterolemia in humans. *J Nutr* **128**(5): 865–869.

Hosomi, A. and M. Arita (1997). Affinity for alpha-tocopherol transfer protein as a determinant of the biological activities of vitamin E analogs. *FEBS Lett* **405**: 105–108.

Houston, M. C., S. Fazio et al. (2009). Nonpharmacologic treatment of dyslipidemia. *Prog Cardiovasc Dis* **52**(2): 61–94.

Houston, M. C. and W. Sparks (2010). Effect of combination pantethine, plant sterols, green tea extract, delta-tocotrienol and phytolens on lipid profiles in patients with hyperlipidemia. *JANA* **13**(1): 15–20.

Iqbal, J., M. Minhajuddin et al. (2003). Suppression of 7,12-dimethylbenz[alpha]anthracene-induced carcinogenesis and hypercholesterolaemia in rats by tocotrienol-rich fraction isolated from rice bran oil. *Eur J Cancer Prev* **12**(6): 447–453.

Junior, A. C., L. M. Asad et al. (2005). Antigenotoxic and antimutagenic potential of an annatto pigment (norbixin) against oxidative stress. *Genet Mol Res* **4**(1): 94–99.

Khor, H. T., D. Y. Chirng et al. (1995). Tocotrienols inhibit HMG-CoA reductase activity in the guinea pig. *Nutr Res* (15): 537–544.

Kuriyan, R., N. Gopinath et al. (2005). Use of rice bran oil in patients with hyperlipidaemia. *Natl Med J India* **18**(6): 292–296.

Lichtenstein, A. H., L. M. Ausman et al. (1994). Rice bran oil consumption and plasma lipid levels in moderately hypercholesterolemic humans. *Arterioscler Thromb* **14**(4): 549–556.

Mensink, R. P., A. C. van Houwelingen et al. (1999). A vitamin E concentrate rich in tocotrienols had no effect on serum lipids, lipoproteins, or platelet function in men with mildly elevated serum lipid concentrations. *Am J Clin Nutr* **69**(2): 213–219.

Minhajuddin, M., Z. H. Beg et al. (2005). Hypolipidemic and antioxidant properties of tocotrienol rich fraction isolated from rice bran oil in experimentally induced hyperlipidemic rats. *Food Chem Toxicol* **43**(5): 747–753.

Most, M. M., R. Tulley et al. (2005). Rice bran oil, not fiber, lowers cholesterol in humans. *Am J Clin Nutr* **81**(1): 64–68.

Mustad, V. A., C. A. Smith et al. (2002). Supplementation with 3 compositionally different tocotrienol supplements does not improve cardiovascular disease risk factors in men and women with hypercholesterolemia. *Am J Clin Nutr* **76**(6): 1237–1243.

Nagao, K., M. Sato et al. (2001). Feeding unsaponifiable compounds from rice bran oil does not alter hepatic mRNA abundance for cholesterol metabolism-related proteins in hypercholesterolemic rats. *Biosci Biotechnol Biochem* **65**(2): 371–377.

Nigar, P., F. Burke et al. (2010). Role of dietary supplements in lowering low density lipoprotein cholesterol: A review. *J Clin Lipidol* **4**(4): 248–258.

O'Byrne, D., S. Grundy et al. (2000). Studies of LDL oxidation following alpha-, gamma-, or delta-tocotrienyl acetate supplementation of hypercholesterolemic humans. *Free Radic Biol Med* **29**(9): 834–845.

Parker, R. A., B. C. Pearce et al. (1993). Tocotrienols regulate cholesterol production in mammalian cells by post-transcriptional suppression of 3-hydroxy-3-methylglutaryl-coenzyme A reductase. *J Biol Chem* **268**(15): 11230–11238.

Pearce, B. C., R. A. Parker et al. (1992). Hypocholesterolemic activity of synthetic and natural tocotrienols. *J Med Chem* **35**(20): 3595–3606.

Pearce, B. C., R. A. Parker et al. (1994). Inhibitors of cholesterol biosynthesis. 2. Hypocholesterolemic and antioxidant activities of benzopyran and tetrahydronaphthalene analogues of the tocotrienols. *J Med Chem* **37**(4): 526–541.

Qureshi, A. A. (1996). Tocopherol attenuates the impact of gamma-tocotrienol on HMG-CoA reductase activity in chickens. *J Nutr* **126**: 389–394.

Qureshi, A. A., B. A. Bradlow et al. (1995). Response of hypercholesterolemic subjects to administration of tocotrienols. *Lipids* **30**(12): 1171–1177.

Qureshi, A. A., W. C. Burger et al. (1986). The structure of an inhibitor of cholesterol biosynthesis isolated from barley. *J Biol Chem* **261**(23): 10544–10550.

Qureshi, A. A., B. C. Pearce et al. (1996). Dietary alpha-tocopherol attenuates the impact of gamma-tocotrienol on hepatic 3-hydroxy-3-methylglutaryl coenzyme A reductase activity in chickens. *J Nutr* **126**(2): 389–394.

Qureshi, A. A., D. M. Peterson et al. (2001). Novel tocotrienols of rice bran suppress cholesterogenesis in hereditary hypercholesterolemic swine. *J Nutr* **131**(2): 223–230.

Qureshi, A. A., N. Qureshi et al. (1991a). Dietary tocotrienols reduce concentrations of plasma cholesterol, apolipoprotein B, thromboxane B2, and platelet factor 4 in pigs with inherited hyperlipidemias. *Am J Clin Nutr* **53**(4 Suppl): 1042S–1046S.

Qureshi, A. A., N. Qureshi et al. (1991b). Lowering of serum cholesterol in hypercholesterolemic humans by tocotrienols (palmvitee). *Am J Clin Nutr* **53**(4 Suppl): 1021S–1026S.

Qureshi, A. A., S. A. Sami et al. (2002). Dose-dependent suppression of serum cholesterol by tocotrienol-rich fraction (TRF25) of rice bran in hypercholesterolemic humans. *Atherosclerosis* **161**(1): 199–207.

Russell, K. R., E. Y. Morrison et al. (2005). The effect of annatto on insulin binding properties in the dog. *Phytother Res* **19**(5): 433–436.

Serbinova, E., V. Kagan et al. (1991). Free radical recycling and intramembrane mobility in the antioxidant properties of alpha-tocopherol and alpha-tocotrienol. *Free Radic Biol Med* **10**(5): 263–275.

Song, B. L. and R. A. DeBose-Boyd (2006). Insig-dependent ubiquitination and degradation of 3-hydroxy-3-methylglutaryl coenzyme a reductase stimulated by delta- and gamma-tocotrienols. *J Biol Chem* **281**(35): 25054–25061.

Teoh, M. K., J. M. Chong et al. (1994). Protection by tocotrienols against hypercholesterolaemia and atheroma. *Med J Malaysia* **49**(3): 255–262.

Tomeo, A. C., M. Geller et al. (1995). Antioxidant effects of tocotrienols in patients with hyperlipidemia and carotid stenosis. *Lipids* **30**(12): 1179–1183.

Wahlqvist, M. L., Z. Krivokuca-Bogetic et al. (1992). Differential serum responses to tocopherols and tocotrienols during vitamin E supplementation in hypercholesterolemic individuals without change in coronary risk factors. *Nutr Res* **12**: S181–S201.

Wilson, T. A., R. J. Nicolosi et al. (2007). Rice bran oil and oryzanol reduce plasma lipid and lipoprotein cholesterol concentrations and aortic cholesterol ester accumulation to a greater extent than ferulic acid in hypercholesterolemic hamsters. *J Nutr Biochem* **18**(2): 105–112.

Yap, S. P., K. H. Yuen et al. (2001). Pharmacokinetics and bioavailability of alpha-, gamma- and delta-tocotrienols under different food status. *J Pharm Pharmacol* **53**(1): 67–71.

Yu, S. G., A. M. Thomas et al. (2006). Dose-response impact of various tocotrienols on serum lipid parameters in 5-week-old female chickens. *Lipids* **41**(5): 453–461.

20 Tocotrienols and Vascular Effects

Aida Hanum Ghulam Rasool

CONTENTS

20.1 INTRODUCTION

The term "vitamin E" is used as the collective name for eight naturally occurring molecules (δ-, α-, β-, and γ-tocopherols and tocotrienols) which qualitatively showed the biological activity of tocopherol. Tocotrienols differ from tocopherols in their hydrocarbon tail; tocotrienols have an unsaturated isoprenoid tail while tocopherols have a saturated one. In this chapter, the term "tocotrienol-rich vitamin E (TRE)" indicates vitamin E preparations where the predominant vitamin E in the preparation is tocotrienols. This term is used, as almost all the available marketed tocotrienol preparations and natural tocotrienols exist together with tocopherols (Rasool and Wong 2007). For example, between 70% and 80% of vitamin E obtained from palm oil consists of a mixture of the different tocotrienol isomers while the rest are tocopherols.

Tocopherols and tocotrienols differ in terms of their pharmacodynamic effects. Tocotrienols are potent antioxidants (Serbinova et al. 1991), with reported health benefits which include cholesterol lowering (Qureshi et al. 1995, 1996, 1997, 2001, 2002; Raederstorff et al. 2002; Baliarsingh et al. 2005), cardiovascular protection (Tomeo et al. 1995; Black et al. 2000), antidiabetic, neuroprotective effects which include attenuation of diabetic neuropathy and alcohol-induced neuropathy (Khanna et al. 2006; Kuhad and Chopra 2009; Tiwari et al. 2009), and supporting bone formation (Mehat et al. 2010). In this chapter, we discuss the effects of tocotrienols on arterial compliance and vascular structure and function.

20.2 ANTIOXIDANTS AND CARDIOVASCULAR PROTECTIVE EFFECTS

Cardiovascular diseases, particularly coronary artery disease (CAD), are the most important cause of morbidity and mortality in developed countries. They are also a significant contributor of morbidity in developing countries. Stroke is another devastating cardiovascular illness and is one of the most common causes of severe disability in many developed and developing countries. Atherosclerotic plaque formation is believed to be the underlying basis for CAD, besides contributing to the occurrence of stroke. The plaque consists of a collection of variable amounts of cholesterol, smooth muscle cells, fibrous tissue, and inflammatory cells in the intima, separated by a fibrin cap from the flowing blood in the arterial lumen (Yusoff 2002). The plaque often grows with time, gradually narrowing the coronary lumen. This progressively decreases the blood supply to myocardial tissues supplied by the coronary artery. When a critical narrowing of the coronary lumen occurs, myocardial ischemia—clinically known as angina pectoris—follows. Initially, angina occurs on exertion because it is then that the blood supply, restricted by the narrowed lumen, is not able to provide for the increased demand in blood supply to nourish tissues requiring more energy during exertion. Later, myocardial infarction may occur as a result of plaque rupture and abrupt coronary occlusion, which is due to acute thrombus formation made worse by coronary stenosis.

Free radicals are widely reported to contribute to the development of atherosclerotic plaque and vascular diseases. Free radicals are molecules with one or more unpaired electrons, which are usually highly reactive toward biomolecules. Free radicals are involved in the formation of oxidized low-density lipoprotein (LDL-C), which contributes to the formation of atherosclerotic plaques. Oxidized LDL-C, not unoxidized LDL-C, is engulfed by intimal macrophages, transforming them into foam cells that develop into fatty streaks, the precursors of the atherosclerotic plaque. Foam cell formation also leads to endothelial injury and dysfunction. This further facilitates passage of LDL-C from the flowing blood into the intima, accelerating the process of vascular damage (Steinberg et al. 1989). Oxidized LDL-C accumulates in the vascular wall (Yla-Herttuala et al. 1989), where it is cytotoxic (Morel et al. 1983) and chemotactic for monocytes (Quinn et al. 1987), leading to the accumulation of vascular inflammatory cells and perhaps, the production of more free radicals that can inactivate endothelium-derived vasodilators. Because of the contribution of free radicals to plaque formation and vascular diseases, and the ability of antioxidants to neutralize these radicals, the relationship between antioxidants and cardiovascular incidence is intriguing to many. Antioxidant supplementation may be able to alleviate atherosclerotic damage caused by excessive production of reactive oxygen species (ROS). They may be especially useful in medical conditions associated with high oxidative stress such as diabetes. Thus, a number of studies had been conducted assessing the relationship between plasma antioxidant levels and cardiovascular diseases, and later, the effect of antioxidant supplementation on cardiovascular diseases.

The most abundant lipid soluble antioxidant in human plasma is vitamin E. It has received significant attention as a possible means of preventing and/or reducing cardiovascular complications. It is the principal lipid soluble chain breaking antioxidant in human tissues, membrane, and plasma, and a major chain-breaking antioxidant that prevents the propagation of free radical reactions in membranes and lipoproteins. Vitamin E is also the predominant antioxidant in LDL-C (Esterbauer et al. 1991). The oxidation of LDL-C *in vitro* is limited by vitamin E (Reaven et al. 1993; O'Byrne et al. 2000).

Animal studies supported the beneficial role of vitamin E in vascular health. Alpha-tocopherol is incorporated into vascular tissue (Keaney et al. 1996) and influences leukocyte adhesion to endothelial cells (Faruqi et al. 1994), monocyte transmigration, and oxidant-mediated cytotoxicity (Hennig et al. 1987). Vitamin E also inhibits protein kinase C activation in vascular smooth muscle cells. Stimulation of protein kinase C impairs endothelium-dependent arterial relaxation and receptor-mediated stimulation of endothelial nitric oxide production (Keaney et al. 1996).

In humans, supplementary vitamin E is effective in reducing the progression of atherosclerosis in subjects with previous coronary artery bypass graft surgery not treated with lipid-lowering drugs (Kritchevsky et al. 1995). Reduction in the progression of common carotid atherosclerosis was seen during 3 year treatment with combined supplementation of both vitamin E and vitamin C (Schroder et al. 2000). Large prospective cohort studies have demonstrated that intake of vitamin E from certain foods and supplements was associated with a reduced risk of major coronary events in postmenopausal women and subjects above the age of 40 (Rimm et al. 1993; Stampfer et al. 1993; Kushi et al. 1996). Results from randomized controlled clinical trials are inconsistent. The Cambridge Heart Antioxidant Study and Secondary Prevention with Antioxidants of Cardiovascular Disease in End Stage Renal Disease reported that antioxidant supplementation decreased the risk of cardiovascular diseases (Boaz et al. 2000; Stephens et al. 1996).

However, other interventional clinical trials had not shown benefits conferred by vitamin E supplementation (The Heart Outcomes Prevention Evaluation Study Investigators 2000; Collins et al. 2002). Variability in the type of antioxidants used, study population and their existing medical conditions, dosage regime, and study outcome parameters may influence these conflicting results. All these interventional clinical trials used the tocopherol vitamin E. Have we been studying the wrong vitamin E in its use for health maintenance, disease prevention, and therapeutic benefits for vascular diseases?

20.3   TOCOTRIENOLS AND VASCULOPROTECTIVE EFFECTS

Tocotrienols have several properties deemed beneficial in terms of cardiovascular diseases (Rasool and Wong 2007). Their potent antioxidant activity enables them to increase LDL-C oxidative resistance and decrease its rate of oxidation (O'Byrne et al. 2000). The role of oxidized LDL-C in the formation of foam cells and subsequent atherosclerosis has been already discussed.

Tocotrienols have lipid-lowering activity. They inhibit 3-hydroxy-3-methylglutaryl-coenzyme A reductase (HMG-CoA reductase) activity, the key enzyme involved in cholesterol synthesis *in vivo* (Pearce et al. 1992; Parker et al. 1993). This lipid-lowering property had been proved in animal studies (Raederstorff et al. 2002; Budin et al. 2009) and supported by many human studies (Qureshi et al. 1997, 2001, 2002; Baliarsingh et al. 2005; Ajuluchukwu et al. 2007)

Tocotrienols, especially δ-tocotrienols, have strong anti-inflammatory activity (Wu et al. 2008; Qureshi et al. 2011b). Inflammation is one of the factors contributing to atherosclerosis development. Serum tumor necrosis factor-alpha (TNF-α) levels were decreased by approximately 80% in avians fed with δ-tocotrienol-supplemented diet for 4 weeks. This was associated with reduction in serum total cholestrol (TC) and LDL-C (Qureshi et al. 2011b). Tocotrienols also have antithrombotic effects. Collagen- and adenosine diphosphate (ADP)-induced platelet aggregations were shown to be significantly inhibited not only by α-tocotrienols but also by TRE containing a mixture of α-, δ-, and γ-tocotrienols (Qureshi et al. 2011a). In the same study, tocotrienols were also shown to inhibit platelet-mediated thrombus formation as assessed using the cyclic flow reductions model. These suggest a potential therapeutic benefit in conditions such as stroke and myocardial infarction, which should be confirmed in clinical studies.

Animal studies suggested beneficial roles of TRE in the pathogenesis of atherosclerotic lesions (Black et al. 2000; Nafeeza et al. 2001; Budin et al. 2009). Nafeeza et al. (2001) investigated the effects of 10 weeks TRE ingestion on the microscopic development of atherosclerosis and lipid peroxidation in the aorta of cholesterol-fed rabbits. The aortic content of malondialdehyde (MDA) was lowest in rabbits that received the TRE compared to the groups that did not. The degree of intimal thickening was higher in the cholesterol-fed rabbits without TRE compared to the cholesterol-fed rabbits with TRE. The continuity of the internal elastic lamina was preserved in the cholesterol-fed rabbits with TRE, but appeared disrupted in the cholesterol-fed rabbits without TRE.

TRE has the potential to reduce oxidative damage and damage to the aortic wall in streptozotocin (STZ)-induced diabetic rats (Budin et al. 2009). Normally, STZ-induced diabetic rats have a damaged ultrastructural organization of the aorta. Examination of thoracic aorta wall via electron microscope showed that TRE supplementation resulted in improvement in the morphological changes of the aortic wall of diabetic rats as shown by reduced vascular smooth muscle proliferation and degeneration, more regular elastic lamina, smoother intima surface, and endothelial cells that still exhibited squamous characteristics. These observations were associated with the TRE-treated rats having lower serum glucose and glycated hemoglobin concentrations, lower levels of plasma TC, LDL-C and triglycerides (TG), and higher high-density lipoprotein cholesterol (HDL-C) compared to the untreated group. Oxidative stress markers were also improved with increased levels of superoxide dismutase activity, lowered plasma and aorta MDA (index of lipid peroxidation), and lower oxidative DNA damage.

Tocotrienols markedly inhibited the surface expression of vascular cell adhesion molecule-1 (VCAM-1 expression) in TNF-α activated human umbilical vein endothelial cells (HUVECs). In addition, the surface expression of intercellular adhesion molecule-1 and E-selectin were also reduced (Theriault et al. 2002). A marked decrease in monocytic cell adherence was also observed, and the decrease was higher compared to tocopherol. Similarly, Naito et al. (2005) showed that tocotrienols displayed a higher inhibitory effect on adhesion molecule expression and monocytic cell adherence to human aortic endothelial cells (HAECs) compared to tocopherol. By so doing, tocotrienols may inhibit the migration of circulating monocytes into the subendo-thelial space that occurs through these adhesion molecules. The authors proposed that the higher inhibitory effects of tocotrienols may be dependent on their intracellular accumulation; tocotri-enols accumulated in HAECs to levels approximately 25- to 95-fold greater than α-tocopherol (Naito et al. 2005).

Besides improving vascular structure, animal studies have also shown tocotrienols to be useful in improving vascular function. Endothelial dysfunction is the earliest vascular pathol-ogy that occurs before clinical vasculopathy occurs. It is defined as impairment in endothe-lium-mediated relaxation. Spontaneously hypertensive rats (SHRs) are known to have impaired endothelium-dependent relaxation. Segments of thoracic aorta from SHRs fed with palm based tocotrienol rich diet for 12 weeks had their endothelium-dependent vasodilatation restored (Abeywardena et al. 1997). This was supported by a study by Muhanis et al. showing tocotri-enols not only improved endothelium-dependent relaxation in SHR, but also in STZ-induced diabetic rats. As in humans, aortas of both the STZ-induced diabetic rats and SHRs exhibited impaired endothelium-dependent relaxation compared to the Wistar Kyoto Rat (WKY) aorta (Muharis et al. 2010).

In humans, a promising study on the vascular effects of TRE was conducted on 50 patients with hyperlipidemia and carotid atherosclerosis (Tomeo et al. 1995). Patients on 240 mg daily palm TRE over 18 months revealed, by bilateral duplex ultrasonography, carotid atherosclerotic regression in 28% and progression in 8% of the TRE-treated patients. None in the control group exhibited regression, while 40% of the control group showed progression. The improvement in progression of carotid atherosclerosis in the TRE-treated group was associated with improved oxidative stress as shown by reduced serum thiobarbituric acid reactive substances (TBARS).

In humans, impairment in endothelial function can be manifested by reduced arterial compliance/increased arterial stiffness. Arterial compliance is in large part dependent on endothe-lial function; thus, optimum arterial compliance relies on the presence of an intact endothelium. Therefore, measuring arterial compliance allows us a simple and non-invasive way to detect preclin-ical vasculopathy. Ability to detect subtle changes to the endothelial function and early detection of vascular pathology will allow early preventive measures and monitoring of the effects of treatment on the vascular function.

20.4   ARTERIAL COMPLIANCE AND ITS SIGNIFICANCE

Impairment in arterial compliance produces a condition of arterial stiffness. Arterial stiffness is an index of macrovascular health and is considered an early marker for vascular dysfunction before development of clinical vascular pathology. Increased arterial stiffness is a strong independent pre-dictor of cardiovascular outcome, not only in patients with diseases, but also in normal subjects (Laurent et al. 2001; Cruickshank et al. 2002; Willum-Hansen et al. 2006). The parameters widely used to assess arterial stiffness include aortic femoral pulse wave velocity (PWV) and central aug-mentation index (AI). Higher values of PWV and central AI indicate increased arterial stiffness and reduced compliance. PWV has been widely validated and provides additional risk prediction above and beyond classical risk factors; it is now included as a parameter for target organ damage evalua-tion in the 2007 Guidelines for Hypertension of the European Society of Hypertension (Mancia and ESH-ESC Task Force on the Management of Arterial Hypertension 2007). PWV is an independent predictor of coronary heart disease and stroke in healthy subjects (Mattace Raso et al. 2006), as well as of incident hypertension (Najjar et al. 2008). Stiff arteries (reduced arterial compliance) cause premature return of reflected waves in late systole, increased pressure load on ventricle, reducing ejection fraction, and increasing myocardial oxygen demand. Arterial stiffness also results in higher systolic blood pressure with a relative decrease in diastolic blood pressure (which could reduce coronary blood flow).

Arterial stiffening is modifiable and has been shown to be reversible in studies with several dietary interventions, including hormone replacement (Rajkumar et al. 1997), fish oil (McVeigh et al. 1994), flaxseed oil (Nestel et al. 1997a), and soy isoflavones (Nestel et al. 1997b). Arterial compliance as assessed by PWV and AI can be improved in those with conditions associated with increased arterial stiffness such as diabetes, and even in healthy volunteers by certain dietary antioxidants such as vitamin C and dark chocolate (Wilkinson et al. 1999; Mulan et al. 2002; Vlachopoulos et al. 2005a). More recently, a study by Shargorodsky et al. (2010) showed that 6 months supplementation with antioxidants consisting of vitamins C, E, coenzyme Q10, and selenium significantly increased arterial compliance in patients with multiple cardiovascular risk factors. The improvement in arterial compliance was associated with improvement in glucose and lipid metabolism and decrease in blood pressure.

20.5 TOCOTRIENOLS AND ARTERIAL COMPLIANCE

Vitamin E has the potential to improve arterial compliance due to its antioxidant property and effect on the vascular endothelium. The endothelium produces endothelium-derived relaxing factor (EDRF) that helps maintain vascular relaxation. Free radicals increase break down of EDRF (Rubanyi and Vanhoutte 1986). Antioxidants such as vitamin E help to quench/neutralize these free radicals, thus increasing the presence of EDRF and promoting vascular relaxation. The endothelium may also directly, or via substances it produces, cause changes in smooth muscle tone that affects arterial stiffness. Certainly, vitamin E, a strong antioxidant and the most abundant lipid soluble antioxidant in the biological membrane has been shown to prevent endothelial dysfunction in animal studies (Andersson et al. 1994; Stewart-Lee et al. 1994).

Rasool et al. conducted two studies to assess the effect of TRE on arterial compliance in humans. As these were preliminary studies, they were conducted in a generally healthy population. The first study involved giving a normal preparation of TRE predominantly containing α-tocotrienols for 2 months to determine their effects on arterial compliance. In this study, the group given 160 mg TRE daily showed significant improvement after treatment for the parameter central AI, a marker of systemic arterial compliance (Rasool et al. 2006). This was associated with a significant fall in central (aortic) systolic blood pressure. In the second study, the effects of oral supplementation with a self-emulsifying preparation of TRE on arterial compliance were studied. The self-emulsifying preparation of TRE was reported to produce higher blood levels of tocotrienols compared to the normal preparations (Yap and Yuen 2004). The self-emulsifying preparation predominantly contained γ-tocotrienol at 43% followed by α-tocotrienol at 24% and δ-tocotrienol. Three doses of the self-emulsifying preparations were used, that were 50, 100, and 200 mg daily, given for 2 months (Rasool et al. 2008). Significant improvement in systemic arterial compliance as assessed using the parameter central AI was seen in all the TRE-treated groups after treatment (Figure 20.1). At daily doses of 100 and 200 mg, significant improvement in aortic compliance, assessed using the parameter aortic femoral PWV was also observed (Figure 20.1). The self-emulsifying preparation of TRE has a smaller percentage of tocopherol at 23% of its tocol content compared to 26% in the normal preparation. A smaller percentage of tocopherol in the vitamin E content of TRE is believed to be more beneficial in the ability of the TRE to reduce plasma cholesterol (Qureshi et al. 1996, 1989). Thus, it appears that tocotrienols are able to improve arterial compliance and reduce arterial stiffness in humans. There were no other studies conducted on the effects of tocotrienol on arterial stiffness or vascular endothelial function in humans.

The exact mechanisms whereby tocotrienols improved arterial compliance have not been determined. Improvement in arterial stiffness can occur due to effects on the arterial function or structural alterations

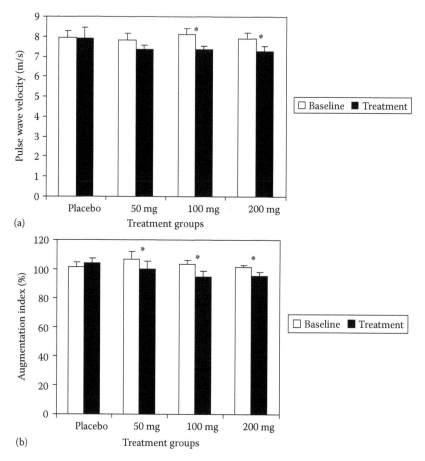

(a)

(b)

FIGURE 20.1   (a) PWV and (b) central AI values at baseline and after 2 months' treatment for groups receiving placebo, 50, 100, and 200 mg TRE daily. Lower PWV and AI values indicate better arterial compliance. * Indicates significant reduction in parameter after treatment compared to baseline. (From Rasool, A.H. et al., *Arch. Pharm. Res.*, 31(9), 1212, 2008. With permission.)

to the vascular wall. Improvements in arterial compliance in response to ingestion of antioxidants could occur within a few weeks. Thus, vascular functional improvement is probably involved, although structural alterations to the vascular wall affecting arterial compliance by antioxidants could also occur with longer supplementation period. Tocotrienol's potent antioxidant effect may be a contributor to the improved arterial compliance seen in humans; however, other mechanisms may also play a role.

Tocotrienol's antioxidant effect may play a role in improving endothelial function and increasing arterial compliance. TRE improves parameters of oxidative stress in humans (Tomeo et al. 1995; O'Byrne et al. 2000; Nafeeza et al. 2001; Ismail et al. 2002). The endothelium produces substances such as EDRF or nitric oxide (NO) to help vascular dilatation and maintain optimum vascular health. Recent evidence suggested that NO is important in regulating arterial stiffness (Wilkinson et al. 2002). NO is a potent vasodilator and has important antiatherogenic actions, which include inhibition of smooth muscle cell proliferation, monocyte adhesion, and platelet adhesion and aggregation. Free radicals, such as the superoxide anion, inactivate EDRF, reducing EDRF-mediated vasorelaxation and vasculoprotective effects (Rubanyi and Vanhoutte 1986). This can increase peripheral resistance, causing arterial stiffness. Tocotrienols have the ability to neutralize these free radicals, and thus may protect against arterial stiffness. A study by Naito et al. (2005) reported that tocotrienols showed good intracellular accumulation in HAECs: to levels approximately 25- to 95-fold greater than that of α-tocopherol (Naito et al. 2005). This may increase the effectiveness of its effect on the endothelium.

Elevated plasma oxidized LDL-C levels may be involved in the pathogenesis of increased arterial stiffness and vascular dysfunction, independent of cardiovascular disease (CVD) risk factors (Brinkley et al. 2009). In multivariate analyses of data from more than 2000 patients, oxidized LDL-C levels were associated with PWV after adjustment for demographics and traditional CVD risk factors; higher levels of oxidized LDL-C increased PWV values, indicating increased arterial stiffness. Individuals in the highest oxidized LDL-C tertile were 30%–55% more likely to have high arterial stiffness compared to those with lower oxidized LDL-C values. Administration of oral α-tocotrienols for 8 weeks in hypercholesterolemics has been shown to increase *in vitro* LDL-C oxidative resistance by 22% and decreased its rate of oxidation (O'Byrne et al. 2000). This may be another mechanism whereby the antioxidant effect of tocotrienols reduces arterial stiffness.

Reductions in blood pressure, especially systolic blood pressure, if present, may produce an improvement in arterial compliance. In the study by Rasool et al. improvement in arterial compliance in the group given TRE at 160 mg daily is associated with a significant reduction in aortic systolic blood pressure. Reduction in blood pressure due to tocotrienols may occur due to changes in endothelium-derived factors. This had been suggested by Ganafa et al. (2002), who showed that rats fed with palm oil containing tocotrienols had reduced age-dependent increase in mean arterial pressure (Ganafa et al. 2002). The reduction in blood pressure was associated with elevated levels of prostacyclin, NO, and aortic cyclic guanosine monophosphate (cGMP). Both prostacyclin and NO are endogenous vasodilators. Newaz et al. (2003) showed that TRE is beneficial in attenuating the effects of free radicals on blood pressure (Newaz and Nawal 1999). In their earlier study, the effects of γ-tocotrienol on lipid peroxidation and total antioxidant status of SHRs were determined. SHR lipid peroxide levels were significantly higher in plasma of SHR and blood vessels compared to that of normal rats. Superoxide dismutase (SOD) activity was lower in SHR compared to normal rats. After 3 months of treatment with γ-tocotrienol, all treated groups have reduced lipid peroxide levels in blood vessels. All treated groups also showed increased total antioxidant status and improved SOD activity. The same group later investigated the role of γ-tocotrienol on blood endothelial nitric oxide synthase (NOS) activity in SHR given 3 months of γ-tocotrienol supplementation (Newaz et al. 2003). NOS is the enzyme mediating formation of the vasodilator NO at the endothelium; compared to control rats, SHR has lower NOS activity in blood vessels. Upon treatment with γ-tocotrienol, increased NOS activity with concomitant reduction in blood pressure was observed. In their study, NOS activity in treatment groups showed a significant negative correlation with blood pressure.

Inflammation could increase arterial stiffness; one mechanism is via its effect on NO bioavailability (Vlachopoulos et al. 2005b). Acute inflammation impairs normal endothelial performance and reduces NO bioavailability (Hingorani et al. 2000; Clapp et al. 2004). Pro-inflammatory cytokines such as IL-6 have a direct adverse effect on NO-dependent vasorelaxation of experimental aortas (Orshal and Khalil 2004). Inflammation can also provoke structural and/or functional changes in the extracellular matrix of the aortic wall by increasing the levels of matrix metalloproteinase-9 (MMP-9). MMP-9 levels are associated with aortic stiffness in both healthy subjects and patients with isolated systolic hypertension (Yasmin et al. 2005). Tocotrienols have potent anti-inflammatory property (Wu et al. 2008; Qureshi et al. 2011b); reduction in the inflammatory marker TNF-α was seen in chickens fed with tocotrienol-rich diet. In human monocytic cells, tocotrienols significantly blocked lipopolysaccharide (LPS) induction of inducible NOS and cyclooxygenase-2 enzyme (COX-2) expression (without affecting the constitutive COX expression). Tocotrienols also caused a significant decrease in the transcription of pro-inflammatory cytokines.

Tocotrienol may improve arterial compliance through its effect on the vascular smooth muscle. TRE has been shown to reduce oxidative damage and damage to the aortic wall in STZ-induced rats (Budin et al. 2009). TRE supplementation resulted in improvement in the morphological changes of the aortic wall (observed via electron microscopy) of diabetic rats as shown by reduced vascular smooth muscle proliferation and degeneration, more regular elastic lamina, and smoother intima surface. The level of MDA, an oxidative stress marker was also improved in the aorta.

20.6 FUTURE DIRECTIONS

Assessment of vascular dysfunction by measuring arterial stiffness is a way to detect early pathological changes to the vascular system, and allows the monitoring of pharmacological and non-pharmacological interventions to the vascular health. Animal studies had proven the benefit of tocotrienols in improving vascular function in hypertensive and diabetic rat models. Studies in generally healthy humans support this by showing improved arterial compliance with oral TRE. It is likely that the vascular protective effects of vitamin E will also be observed, perhaps to a higher extent in those with medical conditions associated with increased arterial stiffness and those with high oxidative stress. This has been suggested, where 4 months of vitamin E significantly augmented endothelium-dependent relaxation only in hypercholesterolemic smokers (known to have high oxidative stress) but not in non-smoking subjects (Heitzer et al. 1999). Increased oxygen-derived free radicals leading to inactivation of EDRF were suggested as one major cause of endothelial dysfunction seen in smokers.

Diabetes mellitus is a major global public health problem affecting approximately 3% of the world population. This figure is higher in certain populations such as in Malaysia, a developing country where the prevalence was reported to be approximately 12.5% of the population. Diabetes is a medical condition associated with increased oxidative stress, where the hyperglycemic environment coupled with a compromised blood supply overloads the metabolic capacity of the mitochondria, producing oxidative stress (Brownlee 2001). Excess formation of ROS and reactive nitrogen eventually overloads the natural antioxidant capacity of the cell, resulting in injuries to lipids, proteins, and DNA, contributing to medical complications such as endothelial dysfunction that lead to small and large vascular diseases such as CADs, stroke, retinopathy, nephropathy, and peripheral neuropathy. Tocotrienol as a potent antioxidant could prevent this ROS-mediated cell damage and has the potential to ameliorate these cardiovascular complications in diabetes. Muharis et al. (2010) had shown that tocotrienols significantly improved endothelial function in both diabetic and SHR aorta in rats while another experimental study reported the benefit of TRE in ameliorating complications due to diabetes neuropathy (Kuhad 2009). Similar observations may be observed in diabetic humans also known to have high oxidative stress. Benefit may also be seen in hypertensive patients, since this population also has impaired endothelial function and increased arterial stiffness. These are areas that should be further explored.

REFERENCES

Abeywardena, M.Y., Head, R.J., and Gapor, A. 1997. Modulation of vascular endothelial function by palm oil antioxidants. *Asia Pacific J Clin Nutr* 6: 68–71.

Ajuluchukwu, J.N., Okubadejo, N.U., Mabayoje, M. et al. 2007. Comparative study of the effect of tocotrienols and tocopherol on fasting serum lipid profiles in patients with mild hypercholesterolemia: A preliminary report. *Niger Postgrad Med J* 14: 30–33.

Andersson, T.L., Matz, J., Ferns, A.A., and Anggard, E.E. 1994. Vitamin E reverse cholesterol induced endothelial dysfunction in the rabbit coronary circulation. *Atherosclerosis* 111: 39–45.

Baliarsingh, S., Beg, Z.H., and Ahmad, J. 2005. The therapeutic impacts of tocotrienols in type 2 diabetic patients with hyperlipidemia. *Atherosclerosis* 182: 367–374.

Black, T.M., Wang, P., Maeda, N., and Coleman, R.A. 2000. Palm tocotrienols protect ApoE+/− mice from diet-induced atheroma formation. *J Nutr* 130 (10): 2420–2426.

Boaz, M., Smetana, S., Weinstein, T. et al. 2000. Secondary prevention with antioxidants of cardiovascular disease in endstage renal disease (SPACE): Randomised, placebo controlled trial. *Lancet* 356: 1213–1218.

Brinkley, T.E., Nicklas, B.J., Kanaya, A.M., and the Health ABC study. 2009. Plasma oxidized low-density lipoprotein levels and arterial stiffness in older adults: The health ABC study. *Hypertension* 53: 846–852.

Brownlee, M. 2001. Biochemistry and molecular cell biology of diabetic complications. *Nature* 414: 813–820.

Budin, S.B., Othman, F., Louise, S.J., Abu Bakar, M., Das, S., and Mohamed, J. 2009. The effects of palm oil tocotrienol rich fraction supplementation on biochemical parameters, oxidative stress and the vascular wall of streptozotocin induced diabetic rats. *Clinics* 64: 235–244.

Clapp, B.R., Hingorani, A.D., Kharbanda, R.K. et al. 2004. Inflammation-induced endothelial dysfunction involves reduced nitric oxide bioavailability and increased oxidant stress. *Cardiovasc Res* 64: 172–178.

Collins, R., Peto, R., and Armitage, J. 2002. The MRC/BHF Heart Protection Study: Preliminary results. *Int J Clin Pract* 56: 53–56.

Cruickshank, K., Riste, L., Anderson, S.G., Wright, J., Dunn, G., and Gosling, R.G. 2002. Aortic pulse wave velocity and its relationship to mortality in diabetes and glucose intolerance; and integrated index of vascular function. *Circulation* 106: 2085–2090.

Esterbauer, H., Dieber-Rotheneder, M., Striegl, G., and Waeg, G. 1991. Role of vitamin E in preventing the oxidation of low density lipoprotein. *Am J Clin Nutr* 53: 314S–321S.

Faruqi, R., de la Motta, C., and DiCorleto, P. 1994. Alpha tocopherol inhibits agonist induced monocytic cell adhesion to cultured human endothelial cells. *J Clin Invest* 94: 592–600.

Ganafa, A.A., Socci, R.R., Eatman, D., Silvestrov, N., Abukhalaf, I.K., and Bayorh, M.A. 2002. Effect of palm oil on oxidative stress-induced hypertension in Sprague-Dawley rats. *Am J Hypertens* 15: 725–731.

Heitzer, T., Hertuala, S., Wild, E., Louma, J., and Drexler, H. 1999. Effect of vitamin E on endothelial vasodilator function in patients with hypercholesterolemia, chronic smoking or both. *J Am Coll Cardiol* 33: 499–505.

Hennig, B., Enoch, C., and Chow, C.K. 1987. Protection by vitamin E against endothelial cell injury by linoleic acid hydroperoxides. *Nutr Res* 7: 1253–1260.

Hingorani, A.D., Cross, J., Kharbanda, R.K. et al. 2000. Acute systemic inflammation impairs endothelium dependent dilatation in humans. *Circulation* 102: 994–999.

Ismail, N., Harun, A., Yusof, A.A., Zaiton, Z., and Marzuki, A. 2002. Role of vitamin E on oxidative stress in smokers. *Malays J Med Sci* 9: 34–42.

Keaney, J.F., Guo, Y., Cunningham, D., Shwaery, G.T., Xu, A., and Vita, J.A. 1996. Vascular incorporation of alpha tocopherol prevents endothelial dysfunction due to oxidised LDL by inhibiting protein kinase C stimulation. *J Clin Invest* 98: 386–394.

Khanna, S.R., Parinandi, N.L., Maurer, M., and Sen, C.K. 2006. Characterization of the potent neuroprotective properties of the natural vitamin E alpha-tocotrienol. *J Neurochem* 98 (5): 1474–1486.

Kritchevsky, S.B., Shimakawa, T., Tell, G.S. et al. 1995. Dietary antioxidants and carotid artery wall thickness. The ARIC study. *Circulation* 92: 2142–2150.

Kuhad, A. and Chopra, K. 2009. Attenuation of diabetic nephropathy by tocotrienol: involvement of NFkB signaling pathway. *Life Sci* 84 (9–10): 296–301.

Kuhad, A. and Chopra, K. 2009. Tocotrienol attenuates oxidative-nitrosative stress and inflammatory cascade in experimental model of diabetic neuropathy. *Neuropharmacology* 57 (4): 456–462.

Kushi, L.H., Folsorn, A.R., Princas, R.J., Mink, P.J., Wu, Y., and Bostick, R.M. 1996. Dietary antioxidant vitamins and death from coronary heart disease in postmenopausal women. *New Engl J Med* 334: 1156–1162.

Laurent, S., Boutouyrie, P., Asmar, R., Gautier, I., Laloux, B., Guize, L., Ducimetiere, P., and Benetos, A. 2001. Aortic stiffness is an independent predictor of all cause and cardiovasular mortality in hypertensive patients. *Hypertension* 37 (5): 1236–1241.

Mancia, G., and ESH-ESC Task Force on the Management of Arterial Hypertension. 2007. 2007 ESH-ESC Practice guidelines for the management of arterial hypertension. *J Hypertens* 25: 1751–1762.

Mattace Raso, F., van der Cammen, T.J., Hofman, A. et al. 2006. Arterial stiffness and risk of coronary heart disease and stroke—The Rotterdam Study. *Circulation* 113: 657–663.

McVeigh, G., Brennan, G.M., Cohn, J.N., Finkelstein, S.M., Hayes, R.J., and Johnston, G.D. 1994. Fish oil improves arterial compliance in non-insulin dependent diabetes mellitus. *Arterioscler Thromb* 14: 1425–1429.

Mehat, M.Z., Shuid, A.N., Mohamed, N., and Soelaiman, I.N. 2010. Beneficial effects of vitamin E isomer supplementation on static and dynamic bone histomorphometry parameters in normal male rats. *J Bone Miner Metab* 28: 503–509.

Morel, D.W., Hessler, G.M., and Chisolm, G.M. 1983. Low density lipoprotein cytotoxicity induced by free radical peroxidation of lipid. *J Lipid Res* 24: 1070–1076.

Muharis, S.P., Md Top, A.G., Murugan, D., and Mustafa, M.R. 2010. Palm oil tocotrienol fractions restore endothelium dependent relaxation in aortic rings of streptozotocin-induced diabetic and spontaneously hypertensive rats. *Nutr Res* 39: 209–216.

Mulan, B.A., Young, I.S., Fee, H., and McCance, D.R. 2002. Ascorbic acid reduces blood pressure and arterial stiffness in type 2 diabetes. *Hypertension* 40: 840–849.

Nafeeza, M.I., Norzana, A.G., Jalaluddin, H.L., and Gapor, M.T. 2001. The effects of a tocotrienol-rich fraction on experimentally induced atherosclerosis in the aorta of rabbits. *Malays J Pathol* 23: 17–25.

Naito, Y., Shimozawa, M., Kuroda, M. et al. 2005. Tocotrienols reduce 25-hydroxycholesterol-induced monocyte-endothelial cell interaction by inhibiting the surface expression of adhesion molecules. *Atherosclerosis* 180: 19–25.

Najjar, S.S., Scuteri, A., Shetty, V. et al. 2008. Pulse wave velocity is an independent predictor of the longitudinal increase in systolic blood pressure and of incident hypertension in the Baltimore longitudinal study of aging. *J Am Coll Cardiol* 51: 1377–1383.

Nestel, P.J., Pomeroy, S.E., Sasahara, T. et al. 1997a. Arterial compliance in obese subjects is improved with dietary plant n-3 fatty acid from flaxseed oil despite increased LDL oxidizability. *Arterioscler Thromb Vasc Biol* 17: 1163–1167.

Nestel, P.J., Yamashita, T., and Sasahara, T. 1997b. Soy isoflavones improve systemic arterial compliance but not plasma lipids in menopausal and perimenopausal women. *Arterioscler Thromb Vasc Biol* 17: 3392–3398.

Newaz, M.A. and Nawal, N.N. 1999. Effect of gamma tocotrienol on blood pressure, lipid peroxidation and total antioxidant status in spontaneously hypertensive rats (SHR). *Clin Exp Hypertens* 21: 1297–1313.

Newaz, M.A., Yousefipour, Z., Nawal, N., and Adeeb, N. 2003. Nitric oxide synthase activity in blood vessels of spontaneously hypertensive rats: Antioxidant protection by gamma-tocotrienol. *J Physiol Pharmacol* 54: 319–327.

O'Byrne, D., Grundy, S., Packer, L. et al. 2000. Studies of LDL oxidation following alpha, gamma or delta tocotrienol acetate supplementation of hypercholesterolemic humans. *Free Radic Biol Med* 29: 834–845.

Orshal, J.M. and Khalil, R.A. 2004. Interleukin-6 impairs endothelium-dependent NO-cGMP mediated relaxation and enhances contraction in systemic vessels of pregnant rats. *Am J Physiol Regular Integr Comp Physiol* 286: R1013–R1023.

Parker, R.A., Pearce, B.C., Clark, R.W., Gordon, D.A., and Wright, J.J. 1993. Tocotrienols regulate cholesterol production in mammalian cells by post transcriptional suppression of 3 hydroxy-3methylglutaryl-coenzyme A reductase. *J Biol Chem* 268: 11230–11238.

Pearce, B.C., Parker, R.A., Deason, M.E., Qureshi, A.A., and Wright, J.J. 1992. Hypocholesterolemic activity of synthetic and natural tocotrienols. *J Med Chem* 35: 3595–3606.

Quinn, M.T., Parthasarathy, S., Fong, L.G., and Steinberg, D. 1987. Oxidatively modified low density lipoproteins: A potential role in recruitment and retention of monocyte/macrophages during atherogenesis. *Proc Natl Acad Sci USA* 84: 2995–2998.

Qureshi, A.A., Bradlow, B.A., Brace, L., Manganello, J., Peterson, D.M., Pearce, B.C., Wright, J.J., Gapor, A., and Elson, C.E. 1995. Response of hypercholesterolemic subjects to administration of tocotrienols. *Lipids* 30: 1171–1177.

Qureshi, A.A., Bradlow, B.A., Salser, W.A., and Brace, L.D. 1997. Novel tocotrienols of rice bran modulate cardiovascular disease risk parameters of hypercholesterolemic humans. *J Nutr Biochem* 8: 290–298.

Qureshi, A.A., Karpen, C., Qureshi, N., Papasian, C.J., Morrison, D.C., and Folts, J.D. 2011a. Tocotrienols induced inhibition of platelet thrombus formation and platelet aggregation in stenosed canine coronary arteries. *Lipids Health Dis* 10: 1–13.

Qureshi, A.A., Pearce, B.C., Gapor, N.R.M., Peterson, D.M., and Elson, C.E. 1996. Dietary alpha tocopherol attenuates the impact of gamma tocotrienol on hepatic 3-hydroxy-3-methylglutaryl coenzyme A reductase activity in chickens. *J Nutr* 126: 389–394.

Qureshi, A.A., Peterson, D. Elson, C.E., Mangels, A,R,, and Din, Z.Z. 1989. Stimulation of avian cholesterol metabolism by alpha tocopherol. *Nutr Rep Int* 40: 993–1001.

Qureshi, A.A., Reis, J.C., Qureshi, N., Papasian, C.J., Morrison, D.C., and Schaefer, D.M. 2011b. Delta tocotrienol and quercetin reduce serum levels of nitric oxide and lipid parameters in female chickens. *Lipids Health Dis* 10: 1–22.

Qureshi, A.A., Sami, S.A., Salser, W.A., and Khan, F.A. 2001. Synergistic effect of tocotrienol-rich fraction (TRF(25)) of rice bran and lovastatin on lipid parameters in hypercholesterolemic humans. *J Nutr Biochem* 12: 318–329.

Qureshi, A.A., Sami, S.A., Salser, W.A., and Khan, F.A. 2002. Dose-dependent suppression of serum cholesterol by tocotrienol-rich fraction (TRF25) of rice bran in hypercholesterolemic humans. *Atherosclerosis* 161: 199–207.

Raederstorff, D., Elste, V., Aebischer, C., and Weber, P. 2002. Effect of either gamma-tocotrienol or a tocotrienol mixture on the plasma lipid profile in hamsters. *Ann Nutr Metab* 46: 17–23.

Rajkumar, C., Kingwell, B.A., Cameron, J.D. et al. 1997. Hormonal therapy increases arterial compliance in postmenopausal women. *J Am Coll Cardiol* 30: 350–356.

Rasool, A.H., Rahman, A.R., Yuen, K.H., and Wong, A.R. 2008. Arterial compliance and vitamin E blood levels with a self emulsifying preparation of tocotrienol rich vitamin E. *Arch Pharm Res* 31: 1212–1217.

Rasool, A.H., Yuen, K.H., Khalid, Y., Wong, A.R., and Rahman, A.R.A. 2006. Dose dependent elevation of plasma tocotrienol levels and its effect on arterial compliance, plasma total antioxidant status and lipid profile in healthy humans supplemented with tocotrienol rich vitamin E. *J Nutr Sci Vitaminol* 52: 473–478.

Rasool, A.H. and Wong, A.R. 2007. Tocotrienol rich vitamin E: A review of clinical studies. *International Medical Journal* 14: 139–143.

Reaven, P.D., Khouw, A., Beltz, W.F., Parthasarathy, S., and Witzturo, J.L. 1993. Effect of antioxidant combinations in humans. Protection of LDL by vitamin E but not by beta-carotene. *Arterioscler Thromb Vasc Biol* 13: 590–600.

Rimm, E.B., Stampfer, M.J., Ascherio, A., Giovannucci, E., Colditz, G.A., and Willett, W.C. 1993. Vitamin E consumption and the risk of coronary heart disease in men. *New Engl J Med* 320: 1450–1456.

Rubanyi, G.M. and Vanhoutte, P.M. 1986. Superoxide anion and hyperoxia inactivate endothelial derived relaxing factor. *Am J Physiol* 25: 822H–827H.

Schroder, H., Navarro, E., Tramullas, A., Mora, J., and Galiano, D. 2000. Nutritional antioxidant status and oxidative stress in professional basketball players: Effects of a three compound antioxidant supplement. *Int J Sports Med* 21: 146–150.

Serbinova, E., Kagan, V., Han, D., and Packer, L. 1991. Free radical recycling and intramembrane mobility in the antioxidant properties of alpha tocopherol and alpha-tocotrienol. *Free Radic Biol Med* 10: 263–275.

Shargorodsky, M., Debby, O., Matas, Z., and Zimlichman, R. 2010. Effect of long term treatment with antioxidants (vitamin C, vitamin E, coenzyme Q10 and selenium) on arterial compliance, humoral factors and inflammatory markers in patients with multiple cardiovascular risk factors. *Nutr Metab (Lond)* 7: 55.

Stampfer, M.J., Hennekens, C.H., Manson, J.E., Colditz, G.A., Rosner, B., and Willett, W.C. 1993. Vitamin E consumption and the risk of coronary disease in women. *New Engl J Med* 328: 1444–1449.

Stephens, N.G., Parsons, A., Schofield, P.M. et al. 1996. Randomised controlled trial of vitamin E in patients with coronary disease: Cambridge Heart Antioxidant Study (CHAOS). *Lancet* 347: 781–786.

Steinberg, D., Parthasarathy, S., Carew, T.E., Khoo, J.C., and Witztum, J.L. 1989. Beyond cholesterol. Modifications of low-density lipoprotein that increase its atherogenicity. *N Engl J Med* 320: 915–924.

Stewart-Lee, A.L., Forster, L.A., Nourooz-Zadeh, J., Ferns, G.S., and Angard, E.E. 1994. Vitamin E protects against impairment of endothelium mediated relaxations in cholesterol-fed rabbits. *Arterioscler Thromb* 14: 494–499.

The Heart Outcomes Prevention Evaluation Study Investigators. 2000. Vitamin E supplementation and cardiovascular events in high risk patients. *New Engl J Med* 342: 154–160.

Theriault, A., Chao, J.T., and Gapor, A. 2002. Tocotrienol is the most effective vitamin E for reducing endothelial expression of adhesion molecules and adhesion to monocytes. *Atherosclerosis* 160: 21–30.

Tiwari, V., Kuhad, A., and Chopra, K. 2009. Tocotrienol ameliorates behavioral and biochemical alterations in the rat model of alcoholic neuropathy. *Pain* 145 (1–2): 129–135.

Tomeo, A.C., Geller, M., Watkins, T.R., Gapor, A., and Bierenbaum, M.L. 1995. Antioxidant effects of tocotrienols in patients with hyperlipidemia and carotid stenosis. *Lipids* 30: 1179–1183.

Vlachopoulos, C., Aznaouridis, K., Alexopoulos, N., Economou, E., Andreadou, I., and Stefanadis, C. 2005a. Effect of dark chocolate on arterial function in healthy individuals. *Am J Hypertens* 18: 785–791.

Vlachopoulos, C., Dima, I., Aznaouridis, K. et al. 2005b. Acute systemic inflammation increases arterial stiffness and decreases wave reflections in healthy individuals. *Circulation* 112: 2193–2200.

Wilkinson, A.B., Megson, I.L., MacCallum, H., Sogo, N., Cockroft, J.R., and Webb, D.J. 1999. Oral vitamin C reduces arterial stiffness and platelet aggregation in humans. *J Cardiovasc Pharmacol* 34: 690–693.

Wilkinson, I.B., Qasem, A., McEniery, C.M., Webb, D.J., Avolio, A.P., and Cockroft, J.R. 2002. Nitric oxide regulates local arterial distensibility in vivo. *Circulation* 105: 213–217.

Willum-Hansen, T., Staessen, J.A., Torp-Pedersen, C., Rasmussen, S., Thijs, L., Ibsen, H., and Jeppesen, J. 2006. Prognostic value of aortic pulse wave velocity as index of arterial stiffness in the general population. *Circulation* 113 (5): 601–603.

Wu, S.J., Liu, P.L., and Ng, L.T. 2008. Tocotrienol-rich fraction of palm oil exhibits anti-inflammatory property by suppressing the expression of inflammatory mediators in human monocytic cells. *Mol Nutr Food Res.* 52: 921–929.

Yap, S.P. and Yuen, K.H. 2004. Influence of lipolysis and droplet size on tocotrienol absorption from self-emulsifying formulations. *Int J Pharm* 281: 67–78.

Yasmin, Wallace, S., McEniery, C.M. et al. 2005. Matrix Metalloproteinase-9 (MMP-9), MMP-2, and serum elastase activity are associated with systolic hypertension and arterial stiffness. *Arterioscler Thromb Vasc Biol* 25: 372–378.

Yla-Herttuala, S., Palinski, W., Rosenfeld, M.E. et al. 1989. Evidence for the presence of oxidatively modified low density lipoprotein in atherosclerotic lesions of rabbit and man. *J Clin Invest* 84: 1086–1095.

Yusoff, K. 2002. Vitamin E in cardiovascular disease: Has the die been cast? *Asia Pacific J Clin Nutr* 11: S443–S447.

21 Prolongevity Effects of Tocotrienols

Trials in Caenorhabditis elegans

Noriko Kashima, Yukiko Fujikura, Tomomi Komura,
Keiji Terao, Barrie Tan, and Yoshikazu Nishikawa

CONTENTS

21.1 INTRODUCTION

The legend of "The Fountain of Youth" shows that rejuvenation, as well as anti-senescence that slows down the processes of aging to extend the maximum and mean lifespan, has been a human desire probably since humans first appeared on this planet (Gruman, 2003). Several theories have been proposed to explain the mechanism of senescence such as the mutation accumulation theory (Medawar, 1952), the antagonistic pleiotropy theory (Williams, 1957), and the disposable soma theory (Kirkwood and Holliday, 1979). Among such theories, the free radical theory is considered a convincing theory (Harman, 2003). Free radicals, for example, singlet oxygen, hydrogen peroxide, and hydroxide radicals that are produced during oxygen metabolism react with the polyunsaturated fatty acid residues of plasma membranes. Such interaction with the membrane results in oxidative damage to subcellular organelles that is of particular significance for lysosomes, mitochondria, and the nuclear envelope (Goldstein et al., 1993).

Host defenses have evolved to prevent plasma membranes from the harmful effects of free radicals, including the production of hydrophilic and hydrophobic antioxidants such as ascorbic acid, uric acid, glutathione, cysteine, histidine peptides, creatine, carotenoids, bilirubin, catechol estrogens, ubiquinone, and of antioxidant enzymes, including selenium glutathione peroxidase, superoxide dismutase, and catalase (Goldstein et al., 1993). Based on the free radical theory of senescence, it is predicted that antioxidants would be useful to achieve longevity. However, it has recently been established that free radicals are also important both for causing hormesis that effects longevity (Ristow and Zarse, 2010; Van Raamsdonk and Hekimi, 2010) and for the modulation of specific signaling pathways that control intracellular levels of reactive oxygen species (Muller et al., 2007). Even though the relationship between free radicals and senescence has not yet been completely elucidated, it is likely that the biological processes that determine adult lifespan can be controlled (Mykytyn, 2010).

Vitamin E (VE) is an antioxidant that has been predicted to be important for defense against free radicals since it is found in cell membranes (Burton et al., 1983; Ingold et al., 1987). Although the role of VE in the longevity of humans is not well understood, epidemiological research on healthy centenarians reported that high levels of vitamin A and VE seem to be important in promoting their extreme longevity (Mecocci et al., 2000). A recent cohort study also suggested that VE could increase the life expectancy of initially healthy populations (Hemila and Kaprio, 2011).

A few experimental studies with rodents succeeded in showing that VE supplementation could ameliorate oxidative stress *in vivo* (Lass and Sohal, 2000) and extend lifespan (Navarro et al., 2005; Selman et al., 2008). However, this longevity might have been brought about by alleviation of the severity of autoimmune disease or by anti-cancer effects and may thus be independent of any antioxidant effect (Banks et al., 2010). In contrast, the group of Meydani et al. reported that diet supplementation with antioxidants that was initiated during middle age did not appear to affect lifespan (Lipman et al., 1998). However the beneficial effect of such supplementation should be demonstrated in connection with age-associated diseases in which oxidative stress is intimately involved (Meydani et al., 1998).

Since survival assays take time to carry out even if short-lived rodents are used, the effects of dietary antioxidant supplementation on oxidative stress and lifespan remain to be clarified. An efficient strategy for directly screening whether food factors or candidates for prolongevity therapy have any effect on lifespan is to determine whether supplementation can affect lifespan in short-lived invertebrate species that are used as alternative models for aging in humans (Kenyon, 2001).

Caenorhabditis elegans is a small free-living soil nematode that has been extensively used as an experimental system for biological studies because of its simplicity, transparency, ease of cultivation, and suitability for genetic analysis (Riddle et al., 1997). This worm has a particular advantage for aging studies since it has a short and reproducible lifespan (Finch and Ruvkun, 2001). We have previously shown that food and nutrients can influence senescence and host defenses of *C. elegans* (Ikeda et al., 2007; Komura et al., 2010; Shibamura et al., 2009). In this study, we first surveyed prior studies of the effects of VE on longevity, and subsequently evaluated whether tocotrienol(s) (T3) could prolong the lifespan of the worms and contribute to host defenses. Tocotrienols were administered to the worms as supplements, and their lifespan and resistance to *Salmonella* Enteritidis and *Legionella pneumophila* were compared with those of worms fed only *Escherichia coli* (OP50), an international standard food for *C. elegans*.

21.2   VITAMIN E FOR PROLONGEVITY OF INVERTEBRATES

VE is a mixture of several related tocopherols (Tp) and T3 isomers: T3 differ from Tp in that they have a short farnesyl tail containing double bonds instead of a longer phytyl side chain without double bonds (Tan and Brzuskiewicz, 1989). Most studies concerning VE have concentrated on alpha-Tp rather than on T3 because more than 90% of VE homologues in animal tissues are Tp.

Treatment of *C. elegans* with VE increased mean lifespan when the worms were cultured in axenic medium (Zuckerman and Geist, 1983) or in monoxenic nematode growth medium (NGM) (Harrington and Harley, 1988). However, although Tp was effective when it was administered during the larval period and resulted in a decrease in the total number of progeny and a delay in the time to peak reproduction, the observed longevity was produced by slowing growth and development (Ishii et al., 2004). These data did not support the theory that the lifespan extension was brought about due to free-radical scavenging by VE even though alpha-Tp can reportedly protect worms (Shashikumar and Rajini, 2011) and flies (Bahadorani et al., 2008) from oxidative stress. In a later study, Zou et al. (2007) reported that gamma-Tp, but not alpha-Tp, slightly extended the lifespan of nematodes, but that any benefits of gamma-Tp were suppressed by a detrimental effect of alpha-Tp supplementation.

Adachi and Ishii reported that administration of VE composed of 22% alpha-Tp, 24% alpha-T3, 37% gamma-T3, and 12% delta-T3 could extend mean lifespan and reduce the accumulation of protein carbonyl, which is an indicator of oxidative damage during aging. Conversely, alpha-Tp acetate did not affect these parameters (Adachi and Ishii, 2000). VE also protected against ultraviolet B-induced oxidative stress when it was administered before or after irradiation, and this protective effect was later reconfirmed using mice (Shibata et al., 2010).

21.3 BENEFICIAL EFFECTS OF TOCOTRIENOLS IN *C. elegans*

21.3.1 LONGEVITY INDUCED BY TOCOTRIENOLS

Based on the aforementioned reports, including our own (Shibamura et al., 2009), we were interested in determining whether antioxidants could extend the lifespan of *C. elegans*. However, despite the increased use of these nematodes in a variety of studies, there was no efficient method for the oral administration of the chemicals because, although *C. elegans* is a bacteriophagous nematode, it has been suggested that it cannot adapt to ingestion of solutions (Avery and Thomas, 1997). Dietary supplements of antioxidants were previously reported to have positive effects on longevity (Brown et al., 2006; Kampkötter et al., 2008; Melov et al., 2000; Wilson et al., 2006; Wu et al., 2002), while other studies reported controversial results (Bass et al., 2007; Goldstein et al., 1993; Keaney et al., 2004; Larsen and Clarke, 2002). These discrepancies are likely due to the lack of a proper method for the administration of these substances. To date, there are no conclusive data regarding the effect of VE on the prolongation of the lifespan of these nematodes.

We previously succeeded in orally administering substances to *C. elegans*, both hydrophilic substances using liposomes (Shibamura et al., 2009) as well as hydrophobic chemicals as inclusion compounds with gamma-cyclodextrin (CyD) (Kashima et al., 2012). In the latter study, the effect of T3 on the lifespan of nematodes was compared following T3 administration using both the CyD method and conventional method. Using the new CyD method, we showed obvious effects of T3 on the lifespan of *C. elegans* and inhibitory effects of Tp on the beneficial effects of T3.

For that study, worms of the *C. elegans* Bristol strain N2 were propagated on NGM using standard techniques (Stiernagle, 1999). The CyD inclusion compound (6.6 mg; wet weight) containing 86 µg of T3 was spread on the surface of a peptone-free NGM (mNGM) plate (10.0 mL of mNGM, 5 cm diameter plate) with OP50 (10 mg per plate), and nematodes were placed onto the plate. The CyD inclusion compound functioned as an efficient carrier of T3 for nematode uptake by mimicking bacterial particles.

The lifespan of the nematodes that ingested CyD inclusion compounds containing VE (Oryza Oil & Fat Chemical, Ichinomiya, Aichi, Japan) was longer than that of control worms maintained on mNGM containing CyD alone (Figure 21.1). This VE product was composed of alpha-T3 (4.9%), beta-T3 (0.5%), gamma-T3 (61.3%), delta-T3 (4.2%), alpha-Tp (1.2%), beta-Tp (0.6%), gamma-Tp (4.5%), and delta-Tp (0.7%). Thus, T3 accounted for more than 70% of the VE product whereas Tp accounted for 7%. The lifespan of the nematodes treated using the conventional administration method, in which the same amount of T3 was dissolved in ethanol and added into the mNGM, was indistinguishable from that of the control.

To date, most studies that use VE have been performed using alpha-Tp. However, in the last decade, T3, which is another component of VE, has been attracting increasing attention. T3s have been shown to exert powerful hypocholesterolemic, anti-cancer and neuroprotective properties that are often not exhibited by Tp (Nesaretnam, 2008; Sen et al., 2007). The earlier-described study showed a clear prolongevity effect of T3 that was consistent with that previously reported by Adachi and Ishii (2000). Since our method is very efficient at delivering hydrophobic antioxidants to nematodes, significant prolongevity effects were observed at a concentration of 0.2 µmol (86 µg) per mNGM plate, which is a 10-fold lower concentration than that used by Adachi and Ishii. This delivery mechanism should therefore facilitate clarification of the effects of hydrophobic compounds such as T3 on prolongevity in future studies.

The effects of T3 decreased when Tp was administered with T3 (Figure 21.2A), although an inclusion compound containing alpha-Tp alone showed no effects on lifespan (Figure 21.2B). When each isoform of T3, alpha-, gamma-, or delta-T3 was individually administered in an inclusion compound as a dietary supplement, the lifespan of worms supplemented with delta- and gamma-T3 was more prolonged compared to that of worms supplemented with alpha-T3 (Figure 21.3A and B).

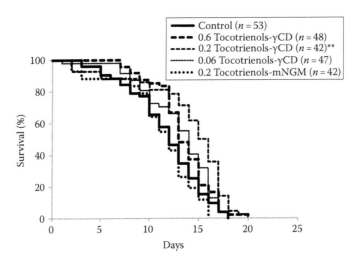

FIGURE 21.1 Survival curves of nematodes supplemented with tocotrienols. After hatching, nematodes were grown on *E. coli* OP50 for 3 days. The adult worms were then divided into groups and each group was placed on an mNGM plate onto which CyD inclusion compounds containing tocotrienols had been pre-spread at a concentration of 0.6, 0.2, or 0.06 μmol. The control plate was pre-spread with CyD alone. The plates were incubated at 25°C, and live and dead worms were determined every 24 h. A worm was considered dead if it failed to respond to gentle touch with a worm picker. Worms that died from sticking to the wall of the plate were not scored. Worms were transferred every day to fresh plates to avoid contamination from progeny. Each assay was carried out in duplicate and repeated two or three times to confirm reproducibility. For conventional administration, the worms were maintained on mNGM in which 0.2 μmol tocotrienol was dissolved. Nematode survival was calculated using the Kaplan–Meier method, and survival differences were tested for significance using the log rank test. **$p < 0.01$, compared to the control.

Zou et al. (2007) reported that gamma-Tp, but not alpha-Tp, extended the lifespan of nematodes and that the benefits of gamma-Tp were suppressed by alpha-Tp supplementation. In that study, the prolongevity effects of T3 were inhibited by simultaneous administration of alpha-Tp. Although the mechanism of this inhibition has not yet been elucidated, Qureshi et al. (1996) also reported that alpha-Tp could not exert the prolongevity and other beneficial effects of T3 and, in fact, inhibited the effects of T3. Nematodes reportedly absorb T3s better than Tp; however, uptake of T3 by cells is likely to be suppressed by alpha-Tp, and co-administration of T3 with Tp could reduce the availability of T3 to cells (Ikeda et al., 2003). Recently, Johnson and Kornfeld (2010) reported that the *C. elegans cgr-1* (*CRAL/TRIO and GOLD domain suppressor of activated ras*) gene is a functional ortholog of the mammalian alpha-Tp associated protein-1 (TAP-1) and that TAP-1 is involved in Ras signaling rather than in simple transport of Tp. Thus, the suppression of the T3-beneficial effects on longevity by alpha-Tp may not be explained simply by the competition for the transporter TAP-1.

The reason why desmethyl T3s (T3s with fewer methyl groups) were more effective than alpha-T3 is possibly explained by the number of methyl groups at the chromanol group of T3 (Tan and Mueller, 2008). Delta-T3 is monomethylated at the C8 position of the chromanol, making it the least substituted, and therefore the most potent, isomer of the four T3 compounds. Gamma-T3 is dimethylated at the C7 and C8 positions of the chromanol and may be the second most potent isomer.

The presence of lipofuscin, the so-called age pigment that accumulates with aging, was analyzed in nematodes at 5, 7, 10, and 15 days of age (Gerstbrein et al., 2005). Lipofuscin is thought to be generated by oxidative degeneration and autophagy of cellular components. Age-dependent accumulation of lipofuscin in the intestinal cells of worms has been demonstrated previously (Klass, 1977). However, CyD-mediated oral supplementation with T3 did not alter lipofuscin accumulation irrespective of the prolongevity effect. Antioxidants and lifespan extension are not always associated with a reduction in the age pigment (Braeckman et al., 2002; Kampkötter et al., 2007). Furthermore,

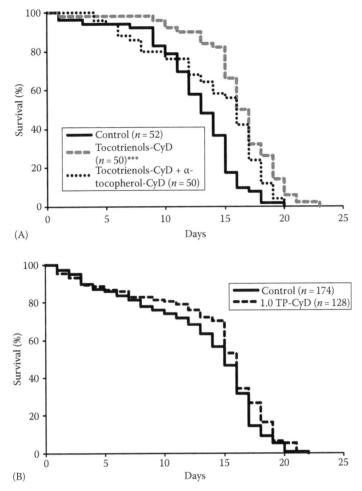

FIGURE 21.2   Inhibition of the prolongevity effect of tocotrienols by alpha-tocopherol. Survival curves of nematodes supplemented with tocotrienols. After hatching, nematodes were grown on *E. coli* OP50 for 3 days. (A) The adult worms were then divided into two groups and placed on mNGM plates that had been pre-spread with a CyD inclusion compound containing $0.2\,\mu mol$ tocotrienols with or without the same amount of alpha-tocopherol. The control plate was pre-spread with CyD alone. (B) Alpha-tocopherol ($1.0\,\mu mol$) was administered without tocotrienols. All experiments were then performed as described in the legend to Figure 21.1. ***$p < 0.001$, compared to the control.

it is possible that T3 extends longevity through an antioxidant-independent mechanism as well as through its neuroprotective effect (Sen et al., 2004), in spite of the fact that it is 40- to 60-fold more powerful as an antioxidant than Tp (Serbinova et al., 1991). Indeed, a variety of lipophilic antioxidants, with the exception of curcumin, that were ingested as inclusion compounds failed to extend the worms' lifespan at the dosages used in this study (Figure 21.4A through E). Studies are currently in progress to elucidate the mechanism by which T3 exerts its prolongevity effects.

21.3.2   IMMUNONUTRITION BY TOCOTRIENOLS

Age at infection is likely one of the most important determinants of disease morbidity and mortality (Miller and Gay, 1997). Because aging is accompanied by functional and metabolic alterations in cells and tissues, senescence of the immune system results in an age-related increase in infections, malignancy, and autoimmunity (Grubeck-Loebenstein, 1997; Moulias et al., 1985). Elderly humans have increased mortality due to many different types of infections (Bradley and Kauffman, 1990).

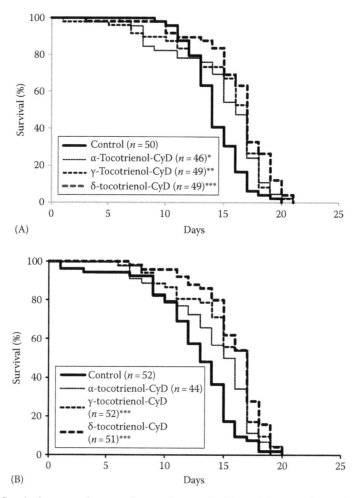

(A)

(B)

FIGURE 21.3 Survival curves of nematodes supplemented with each isomer of tocotrienol. After hatching, nematodes were grown on *E. coli* OP50 for 3 days. The adult worms were then divided into groups and placed on mNGM plates that had been pre-spread with a CyD inclusion compound containing 0.2 μmol of alpha-, gamma-, or delta-tocotrienol. The control plate was pre-spread with CyD alone. All experiments were then performed as described in the legend to Figure 21.1A and B; the results of two separate experiments are shown. $*p < 0.05$, $**p < 0.01$, $***p < 0.001$, compared to the control.

Whether nutritional control can retard senescence of immune function and decrease mortality from infectious diseases has not yet been established; the difficulty of establishing a study model has made this a challenging topic to investigate. Although some studies have shown that nutritional control successfully improves the expression of biomarkers relating to immunological functions (Bogden and Louria, 2004), few reports have shown a beneficial influence of nutrition on immunity and the resultant outcome of experimental infection (Effros et al., 1991; Hayek et al., 1997).

Since Tan et al. (1999) reported that *Pseudomonas aeruginosa* can cause a nematocidal infection, *C. elegans* has been recognized as an alternative to mammalian models of infection with bacterial pathogens (Kurz and Tan, 2004; Nicholas and Hodgkin, 2004; Tan et al., 1999). In recent years, *C. elegans* has become one of the most important experimental animals in the field of innate immune research, similar to the fruit fly *Drosophila* (Kurz and Tan, 2004; Nicholas and Hodgkin, 2004; Schulenburg et al., 2004).

To examine the effects of T3 on host defense, 7–8 day old worms were fed the *S.* Enteritidis strain SE1 or the *L. pneumophila* serogroup 1 strain JR32 instead of OP50. CyD-mediated oral supplementation with T3 failed to enhance the host defense to *Salmonella* (data not shown). However, when

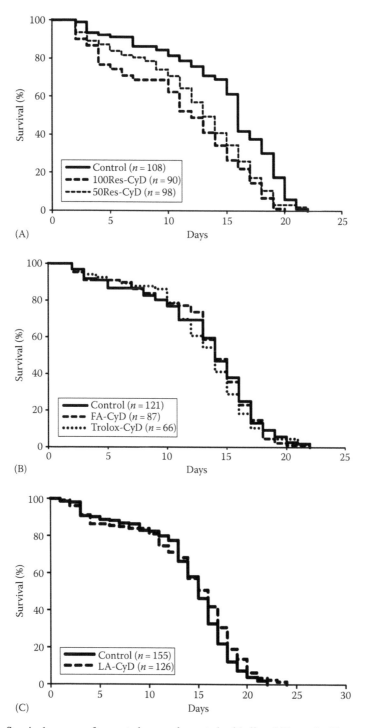

FIGURE 21.4 Survival curves of nematodes supplemented with lipophilic antioxidants. After hatching, nematodes were grown on *E. coli* OP50 for 3 days. The adult worms were then divided into groups and placed on mNGM plates that had been pre-spread with a CyD inclusion compound containing (A) resveratrol (Res), (B) ferulic acid (FA) or trolox, (C) alpha-lipoic acid (LA), (D) quercetin, or (E) curcumin. The control plate was pre-spread with CyD alone. All experiments were then performed as described in the legend to Figure 21.1. ***$p < 0.001$, compared to the control.

(*continued*)

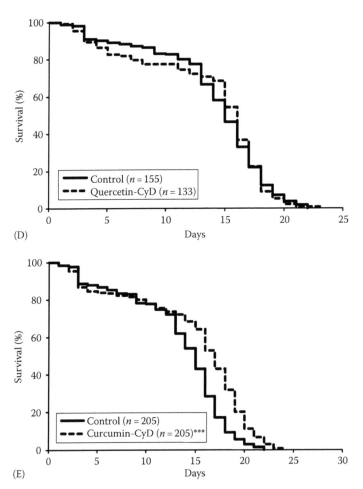

FIGURE 21.4 (continued)   Survival curves of nematodes supplemented with lipophilic antioxidants. After hatching, nematodes were grown on *E. coli* OP50 for 3 days. The adult worms were then divided into groups and placed on mNGM plates that had been pre-spread with a CyD inclusion compound containing (A) resveratrol (Res), (B) ferulic acid (FA) or trolox, (C) alpha-lipoic acid (LA), (D) quercetin, or (E) curcumin. The control plate was pre-spread with CyD alone. All experiments were then performed as described in the legend to Figure 21.1. ***$p < 0.001$, compared to the control.

nematodes were exposed to *L. pneumophila* that functions as an opportunistic pathogen in aged nematodes (Komura et al., 2010), T3s were protective against the infection (Kashima et al., 2012).

Protein damage occurs specifically at the site of the host–pathogen interaction; reactive oxygen species produced by the host are a source of protein damage during infection (Mohri-Shiomi and Garsin, 2008). It is possible that T3 could reverse the reactive oxygen species-mediated protein damage that occurred due to the opportunistic pathogen *Legionella*, although it did not work against the highly virulent *Salmonella* infection. Alternatively, the protective effect of T3 might be explained by an antioxidant-independent action since T3 reportedly inhibits inflammatory signaling pathways such as nuclear factor-kappa B (Ahn et al., 2007; Shibata et al., 2010).

21.4   CONCLUSION

Gamma-CyD is an excellent vehicle for oral delivery of hydrophobic substances to *C. elegans*. Using this method, oral supplementation with T3 efficiently prolonged the lifespan of worms, while a conventional method of T3 administration failed to affect longevity at the same dosage. Delta- and gamma-T3 were more effective at increasing longevity than alpha-T3. In contrast, Tp inhibited the beneficial effects of T3. T3 could prevent opportunistic infection of *L. pneumophila* in older worms, possibly through anti-senescence effects. Delta- and gamma-T3 are candidate "Fountain-of-Youth" substances.

ACKNOWLEDGMENTS

This study was supported in part by a Grant from the Osaka City University Graduate School of Human Life Science from 2009 to 2011. The nematodes used in this study were kindly provided by the Caenorhabditis Genetics Center, which is funded by the NIH National Center for Research Resources (NCRR).

REFERENCES

Adachi, H., N. Ishii. 2000. Effects of tocotrienols on life span and protein carbonylation in *Caenorhabditis elegans*. *J Gerontol A Biol Sci Med Sci* 55: B280–B285.

Ahn, K. S., G. Sethi, K. Krishnan, B. B. Aggarwal. 2007. gamma-tocotrienol inhibits nuclear factor-kappa B signaling pathway through inhibition of receptor-interacting protein and TAK1 leading to suppression of antiapoptotic gene products and potentiation of apoptosis. *J Biol Chem* 282: 809–820.

Avery, L., J. H. Thomas. 1997. Feeding and defecation. In *C. elegans II*, 2nd edn., D. L. Riddle, T. Blumenthal, B. J. Meyer, J. R. Priess (eds.), pp. 679–716. Cold Spring Harbor, NY: Cold Spring Harbor Laboratory Press.

Bahadorani, S., P. Bahadorani, J. P. Phillips, A. J. Hilliker. 2008. The effects of vitamin supplementation on *Drosophila* life span under normoxia and under oxidative stress. *J Gerontol A Biol Med Sci* 63: 35–42.

Banks, R., J. R. Speakman, C. Selman. 2010. Vitamin E supplementation and mammalian lifespan. *Mol Nutr Food Res* 54: 719–725.

Bass, T. M., D. Weinkove, K. Houthoofd, D. Gems, L. Partridge. 2007. Effects of resveratrol on lifespan in *Drosophila melanogaster* and *Caenorhabditis elegans*. *Mech Ageing Dev* 128: 546–552.

Bogden, J. D., D. B. Louria. 2004. Nutrition and immunity in the elderly. In *Diet and Human Immune Function*, D. A. Hughes, J. Gail Darlington, A. Bendich (eds.), pp. 79–101. Totowa, NJ: Humana Press.

Bradley, S. F., C. A. Kauffman. 1990. Aging and the response to salmonella infection. *Exp Gerontol* 25: 75–80.

Braeckman, B. P., K. Houthoofd, K. Brys et al. 2002. No reduction of energy metabolism in Clk mutants. *Mech Ageing Dev* 123: 1447–1456.

Brown, M. K., J. L. Evans, Y. Luo. 2006. Beneficial effects of natural antioxidants EGCG and alpha lipoic acid on life span and age-dependent behavioral declines in *Caenorhabditis elegans*. *Pharmacol Biochem Behav* 85: 620–628.

Burton, G. W., A. Joyce, K. U. Ingold. 1983. Is vitamin-E the only lipid-soluble, chain-breaking antioxidant in human blood plasma and erythrocyte membranes. *Arch Biochem Biophys* 221: 281–290.

Effros, R. B., R. L. Walford, R. Weindruch, C. Mitcheltree. 1991. Influences of dietary restriction on immunity to influenza in aged mice. *J Gerontol* 46: B142–B147.

Finch, C. E., G. Ruvkun. 2001. The genetics of aging. *Annu Rev Genomics Hum Genet* 2: 435–462.

Gerstbrein, B., G. Stamatas, N. Kollias, M. Driscoll. 2005. In vivo spectrofluorimetry reveals endogenous bio-markers that report healthspan and dietary restriction in *Caenorhabditis elegans*. *Aging Cell* 4: 127–137.

Goldstein, P., E. McCann-Hargrove, L. Magnano. 1993. Hypervitaminosis E and gametogenesis in *Caenorhabditis elegans*. *Cytobios* 73: 121–133.

Grubeck-Loebenstein, B. 1997. Changes in the aging immune system. *Biologicals* 25: 205–208.

Gruman, G. J. 2003. *A History of Ideas about the Prolongation of Life*. New York: Springer Pub. Co.

Harman, D. 2003. The free radical theory of aging. *Antioxid Redox Signal* 5: 557–561.

Harrington, L. A., C. B. Harley. 1988. Effect of vitamin E on lifespan and reproduction in *Caenorhabditis elegans*. *Mech Ageing Dev* 43: 71–78.

Hayek, M. G., S. F. Taylor, B. S. Bender et al. 1997. Vitamin E supplementation decreases lung virus titers in mice infected with influenza. *J Infect Dis* 176: 273–276.

Hemila, H., J. Kaprio. 2011. Vitamin E may affect the life expectancy of men, depending on dietary vitamin C intake and smoking. *Age Ageing* 40: 215–220.

Ikeda, S., T. Tohyama, H. Yoshimura, K. Hamamura, K. Abe, K. Yamashita. 2003. Dietary alpha-tocopherol decreases alpha-tocotrienol but not gamma-tocotrienol concentration in rats. *J Nutr* 133: 428–434.

Ikeda, T., C. Yasui, K. Hoshino, K. Arikawa, Y. Nishikawa. 2007. Influence of lactic acid bacteria on longevity of *Caenorhabditis elegans* and host defense against *Salmonella enterica* serovar Enteritidis. *Appl Environ Microbiol* 73: 6404–6409.

Ingold, K. U., A. C. Webb, D. Witter, G. W. Burton, T. A. Metcalfe, D. P. R. Muller. 1987. Vitamin-E remains the major lipid-soluble, chain-breaking antioxidant in human plasma even in individuals suffering severe vitamin-E deficiency. *Arch Biochem Biophys* 259: 224–225.

Ishii, N., N. Senoo-Matsuda, K. Miyake et al. 2004. Coenzyme Q10 can prolong *C. elegans* lifespan by lowering oxidative stress. *Mech Ageing Dev* 125: 41–46.

Johnson, K. G., K. Kornfeld. 2010. The CRAL/TRIO and GOLD domain protein TAP-1 regulates RAF-1 activation. *Dev Biol* 341: 464–471.

Kampkötter, A., C. Gombitang Nkwonkam, R. F. Zurawski et al. 2007. Effects of the flavonoids kaempferol and fisetin on thermotolerance, oxidative stress and FoxO transcription factor DAF-16 in the model organism *Caenorhabditis elegans*. *Arch Toxicol* 81: 849–858.

Kampkötter, A., C. Timpel, R. F. Zurawski et al. 2008. Increase of stress resistance and lifespan of *Caenorhabditis elegans* by quercetin. *Comp Biochem Physiol B Biochem Mol Biol* 149: 314–323.

Kashima, N., Y. Fujikura, T. Komura et al. 2012. Development of a method for oral administration of hydrophobic substances to *Caenorhabditis elegans*: Pro-longevity effects of oral supplementation with lipid-soluble antioxidants. *Biogerontology* 13: 337–344.

Keaney, M., F. Matthijssens, M. Sharpe, J. Vanfleteren, D. Gems. 2004. Superoxide dismutase mimetics elevate superoxide dismutase activity in vivo but do not retard aging in the nematode *Caenorhabditis elegans*. *Free Radic Biol Med* 37: 239–250.

Kenyon, C. 2001. A conserved regulatory system for aging. *Cell* 105: 165–168.

Kirkwood, T. B. L., R. Holliday. 1979. Evolution of aging and longevity. *Proc R Soc Lond B Biol Sci* 205: 531–546.

Klass, M. R. 1977. Aging in the nematode *Caenorhabditis elegans*: Major biological and environmental factors influencing life span. *Mech Ageing Dev* 6: 413–429.

Komura, T., C. Yasui, H. Miyamoto, Y. Nishikawa. 2010. *Caenorhabditis elegans* as an alternative model host for *Legionella pneumophila* and the protective effects of *Bifidobacterium infantis*. *Appl Environ Microbiol* 76: 4105–4108.

Kurz, C. L., M. W. Tan. 2004. Regulation of aging and innate immunity in *C. elegans*. *Aging Cell* 3: 185–193.

Larsen, P. L., C. F. Clarke. 2002. Extension of life-span in *Caenorhabditis elegans* by a diet lacking coenzyme Q. *Science* 295: 120–123.

Lass, A., R. S. Sohal. 2000. Effect of coenzyme Q(10) and alpha-tocopherol content of mitochondria on the production of superoxide anion radicals. *FASEB J* 14: 87–94.

Lipman, R. D., R. T. Bronson, D. Wu et al. 1998. Disease incidence and longevity are unaltered by dietary antioxidant supplementation initiated during middle age in C57BL/6 mice. *Mech Ageing Dev* 103: 269–284.

Mecocci, P., M. C. Polidori, L. Troiano et al. 2000. Plasma antioxidants and longevity: A study on healthy centenarians. *Free Radical Biol Med* 28: 1243–1248.

Medawar, P. B. 1952. *An Unsolved Problem of Biology*. London, U.K.: H. K. Lewis.

Melov, S., J. Ravenscroft, S. Malik et al. 2000. Extension of life-span with superoxide dismutase/catalase mimetics. *Science* 289: 1567–1569.

Meydani, M., R. D. Lipman, S. N. Han et al. 1998. The effect of long-term dietary supplementation with antioxidants. In *Towards Prolongation of the Healthy Life Span: Practical Approaches to Intervention*, D. Harman, R. Holliday, M. Meydani (eds.), pp. 352–360. New York: New York Academy of Sciences.

Miller, E., N. Gay. 1997. Effect of age on outcome and epidemiology of infectious diseases. *Biologicals* 25: 137–142.

Mohri-Shiomi, A., D. A. Garsin. 2008. Insulin signaling and the heat shock response modulate protein homeostasis in the *Caenorhabditis elegans* intestine during infection. *J Biol Chem* 283: 194–201.

Moulias, R., A. Devillechabrolle, B. Lesourd et al. 1985. Respective roles of immune and nutritional factors in the priming of the immune response in the elderly. *Mech Ageing Dev* 31: 123–137.

Muller, F. L., M. S. Lustgarten, Y. Jang, A. Richardson, H. Van Remmen. 2007. Trends in oxidative aging theories. *Free Radical Biol Med* 43: 477–503.

Mykytyn, C. E. 2010. A history of the future: the emergence of contemporary anti-ageing medicine. *Sociol Health Illn* 32: 181–196.

Navarro, A., C. Gomez, M. J. Sanchez-Pino et al. 2005. Vitamin E at high doses improves survival, neurological performance, and brain mitochondrial function in aging male mice. *Am J Physiol Regul Integr Comp Physiol* 289: R1392–R1399.

Nesaretnam, K. 2008. Multitargeted therapy of cancer by tocotrienols. *Cancer Lett* 269: 388–395.

Nicholas, H. R., J. Hodgkin. 2004. Responses to infection and possible recognition strategies in the innate immune system of *Caenorhabditis elegans*. *Mol Immunol* 41: 479–493.

Qureshi, A. A., B. C. Pearce, R. M. Nor, A. Gapor, D. M. Peterson, C. E. Elson. 1996. Dietary alpha-tocopherol attenuates the impact of gamma-tocotrienol on hepatic 3-hydroxy-3-methylglutaryl coenzyme A reductase activity in chickens. *J Nutr* 126: 389–394.

Riddle, D. L., T. Blumenthal, B. J., Meyer, J. R. Priess. 1997. Introduction to C. *elegans*. In *C. elegans II*, 2nd edn., D. L. Riddle, T. Blumenthal, B. J. Meyer, J. R. Priess (eds.), pp. 1–22. Cold Spring, NY: Cold Spring Harbor Laboratory Press.

Ristow, M., K. Zarse. 2010. How increased oxidative stress promotes longevity and metabolic health: The concept of mitochondrial hormesis (mitohormesis). *Exp Gerontol* 45: 410–418.

Schulenburg, H., C. L. Kurz, J. J. Ewbank. 2004. Evolution of the innate immune system: The worm perspective. *Immunol Rev* 198: 36–58.

Selman, C., J. S. McLaren, C. Mayer et al. 2008. Lifelong alpha-tocopherol supplementation increases the median life span of C57BL/6 mice in the cold but has only minor effects on oxidative damage. *Rejuvenation Res* 11: 83–95.

Sen, C. K., S. Khanna, S. Roy. 2004. Tocotrienol: The natural vitamin E to defend the nervous system? *Ann NY Acad Sci* 1031: 127–142.

Sen, C. K., S. Khanna, S. Roy. 2007. Tocotrienols in health and disease: The other half of the natural vitamin E family. *Mol Aspects Med* 28: 692–728.

Serbinova, E., V. Kagan, D. Han, L. Packer. 1991. Free-radical recycling and intramembrane mobility in the antioxidant properties of alpha-tocopherol and alpha-tocotrienol. *Free Radical Biol Med* 10: 263–275.

Shashikumar, S., P. S. Rajini. 2011. Alpha-tocopherol ameliorates cypermethrin-induced toxicity and oxidative stress in the nematode *Caenorhabditis elegans*. *Indian J Biochem Biophys* 48: 191–196.

Shibamura, A., T. Ikeda, Y. Nishikawa. 2009. A method for oral administration of hydrophilic substances to *Caenorhabditis elegans*: Effects of oral supplementation with antioxidants on the nematode lifespan. *Mech Ageing Dev* 130: 652–655.

Shibata, A., K. Nakagawa, Y. Kawakami, T. Tsuzuki, T. Miyazawa. 2010. Suppression of gamma-tocotrienol on UVB induced inflammation in HaCaT keratinocytes and HR-1 hairless mice via inflammatory mediators multiple signaling. *J Agric Food Chem* 58: 7013–7020.

Stiernagle, T. 1999. Maintenance of C. *elegans*. In *C elegans: A Practical Approach*, I. A. Hope (ed.), pp. 51–67. New York: Oxford University Press.

Tan, B., L. Brzuskiewicz. 1989. Separation of tocopherol and tocotrienol isomers using normal-phase and reverse-phase liquid chromatography. *Anal Biochem* 180: 368–373.

Tan, B., A. M. Mueller. 2008. Tocotrienols in cardiometabolic diseases. In *Tocotrienols: Vitamin E beyond Tocopherols*, R. R. Watson, V. R. Preedy (eds.), pp. 257–273. New York: CRC Press.

Tan, M. W., S. Mahajan-Miklos, F. M. Ausubel. 1999. Killing of *Caenorhabditis elegans* by *Pseudomonas aeruginosa* used to model mammalian bacterial pathogenesis. *Proc Natl Acad Sci USA* 96: 715–720.

Van Raamsdonk, J. M., S. Hekimi. 2010. Reactive oxygen species and aging in *Caenorhabditis elegans*: Causal or casual relationship? *Antioxid Redox Signal* 13: 1911–1953.

Williams, G. C. 1957. Pleiotropy, natural-selection, and the evolution of senescence. *Evolution* 11: 398–411.

Wilson, M. A., B. Shukitt-Hale, W. Kalt, D. K. Ingram, J. A. Joseph, C. A. Wolkow. 2006. Blueberry polyphenols increase lifespan and thermotolerance in *Caenorhabditis elegans*. *Aging Cell* 5: 59–68.

Wu, Z., J. V. Smith, V. Paramasivam et al. 2002. *Ginkgo biloba* extract EGb 761 increases stress resistance and extends life span of *Caenorhabditis elegans*. *Cell Mol Biol* 48: 725–731.

Zou, S. G., J. Sinclair, M. A. Wilson et al. 2007. Comparative approaches to facilitate the discovery of prolongevity interventions: Effects of tocopherols on lifespan of three invertebrate species. *Mech Ageing Dev* 128: 222–226.

Zuckerman, B. M., M. A. Geist. 1983. Effects of vitamin E on the nematode *Caenorhabditis elegans*. *Age* 6: 1–4.

22 Anti-Tyrosinase Activity of Tocotrienol in Skin Blemishes

Daniel Yee Leng Yap

CONTENTS

22.1   INTRODUCTION TO MELANOGENESIS

Melanin pigments are responsible for skin and hair colors. They play an important role in the defense against harmful ultraviolet radiation (Fitzpatrick et al. 1949; Tomita et al. 1984). In the body, the formation of pigment melanin occurs within the melanosome of skin melanocytes (Mason 1949; Fitzpatrick et al. 1950). This process is regulated by melanogenic enzymes such as tyrosinase and tyrosinase-related protein 1/2 (TRP1/2) (Chen and Chavin 1966). Specifically, these proteins catalyze the rate-limiting, two-part reaction in melanin biosynthesis: the hydroxylation of L-tyrosine to 3,4-dihydroxyphenylalanine (DOPA) and its subsequent oxidation to dopaquinone (Korner and Pawelek 1982). Modulation of tyrosinase activities therefore represents a key process for the regulation of cutaneous melanogenesis (Korner and Pawelek 1982). In addition, because increased levels of epidermal pigmentation (melanogenesis process) is a hallmark of cosmetic problems (e.g., skin blemishes, melasma) and malignant skin diseases (e.g., melanoma), the control of tyrosinase activity may provide a basis for treating patients with this type of malignancies.

The regulatory mechanisms governing melanogenesis are complex (Fitzpatrick et al. 1950; Chen and Chavin 1966). A number of biochemical agents (Khan et al. 2006) are known to either stimulate or inhibit melanogenesis in cultured melanocyte cell lines. Melanocyte stimulating hormones (MSH) (Wong and Pawelek 1973), microphthalmia-associated transcription factors (MITF) (Hodgkinson et al. 1993; Hemesath et al. 1994; Steingrimsson et al. 1994), cyclic adenosine monophosphate (AMP) derivatives (Johnson and Pastan 1972), cholera toxins (Pawelek 1976), and UVB rays (Choi et al. 2002) stimulate tyrosinase promoter activities and thus lead to higher melanogenesis. Conversely, the exogenous tyrosinase inhibitors such as kojic acid derivatives (Cabanes et al. 1994), sodium lactate (Usuki et al. 2003), retinoic acid (Talwar et al. 1993), aloesin (Jin et al. 1999), phenylthiourea (Hall and Orlow 2005), hormone-derived inhibitory oligopeptides (Abu Ubeid et al. 2009), hydroxytetronic acid (Perricone 2002), benzoyl compounds (Khan et al. 2006), hydroquinone (Smith et al. 1988), alcohol-extracted diol and triol analogs (Khan et al. 2006), and ascomycete-derived enzymes (Ragnelli et al. 1992) inhibit melanogenesis. More recently, the utilization of endogeneous gene-silencing short ribonucleic acid (RNA), such as microRNA (miRNA) and small hairpin RNA (shRNA), provides a powerful new strategy vis-à-vis modulation of melanogenesis *in vivo*, particularly for hyperpigmentation treatment via inhibition of tyrosinase (Wu et al. 2008; Lee et al. 2010; Zhu et al. 2010). Although most of these tyrosinase inhibitors work well *in vitro*, only a few of them are able to induce decent hypopigmenting effects in clinical trials without side effects (Gupta et al. 2006). An increasing number of studies on the ways by which these agents regulate melanin-generating cells may increase our understanding of the mechanisms that govern the melanogenesis process, potentially allowing for improvements in skin-whitening cosmetics and better modalities for melanoma therapy.

22.2 TOCOTRIENOLS: THE SUPER VITAMIN E

Tocotrienols (T3) are important plant vitamin E constituents. Together with tocopherols (TP), they provide a significant source of antioxidant activity to all living cells (Ahmad et al. 2005; Mazlan et al. 2006). This common antioxidant attribute reflects the similarity in chemical structures between T3 and TP, which differ only in their structural isoprenoid side chains (a farnesyl group for T3 versus a saturated phytyl side chain for TP). The common volatile hydrogen atom from the hydroxyl group on their chromanol ring acts to scavenge the chain-propagating peroxyl free radicals. Depending on the locations of the methyl groups on their chromanol ring, T3 and TP can each be categorized into the following four isomeric forms: alpha (α), beta (β), gamma (γ), and delta (δ).

Concerning their functional role in oilseeds, the eight forms of vitamin E are vital in preventing lipid peroxidation, thus ensuring seedling longevity and healthy germination (Cahoon et al. 2003; Sattler et al. 2004). Apart from these common functions, T3 and TP accumulation kinetics exhibit significant differences that depend on the physical geography of oilseed plants. For example, the T3 family is found in a limited number of tropical oilseeds like *Elaeis guineensis* (palm) and *Bixa orellana* (annatto). In contrast, TP is found ubiquitously in various tissues of temperate oilseeds like *Glycine max* (soybean), *Zea mays* (maize), and *Olea europaea* (olive). The relationship between T3 accumulations in tropical oilseeds can be explained by its inherently stronger ability to counteract the higher oxidative burdens (UV radiation, temperature stress, and disease insult) faced by the tropical oilseeds (Jenkins et al. 1997; Smirnoff 1998).

Apart from the antioxidant and anti-cancer properties of T3 covered by other chapters in this volume (Yap et al. 2008; Chang et al. 2009; Yap et al. 2010a,b), it was recently shown that the strong antioxidant property of δ-T3 decreased melanin levels in murine B16 melanocyte cells by inhibiting the oxidative reactions of tyrosinase (Michihara et al. 2009). However, it was unclear from the report whether or not other T3 isomers also inhibited tyrosinase activity, in addition to the synergistic interaction of T3 with other tyrosinase inhibitors. The palm α-T3-rich fraction was also shown to suppress tyrosinase activity in primary human skin melanocyte cells (Makpol et al. 2009). Although it was concluded that α-T3 is the most active agent suppressing tyrosinase activity, there was no α-TP control sample included in the study to eliminate the possible interference from TP. Of note, the experimental data may also have been misinterpreted because the palm T3-rich fraction (TRF) is known to consist of 75% T3 rather than α-T3, as claimed by the authors.

22.3 DISSECTING THE ANTI-TYROSINASE EFFECT OF T3 ISOMERS

Using the treatment dosage that did not affect the cell proliferation rate, B16 melanocyte cells were treated with α-TP, γ-, and δ-T3 isomers and various tyrosinase inhibitors (kojic acid and sodium lactate). The reverse transcription polymerase chain reaction (RT-PCR) results showed that the mRNA transcript of the tyrosinase gene was not affected by T3 treatments (Yap et al. 2010). However, Western blotting results indicated that $20\,\mu M$ γ- and δ-T3 treatments resulted in remarkable suppression of tyrosinase protein expression in B16 melanocyte cells. The suppression of tyrosinase protein expression without concomitant reduction in mRNA levels suggested a post-transcription regulation mediated by intronic RNAs (Wu et al. 2008).

In contrast to T3's potent anti-tyrosinase activity, $20\,\mu M$ treatments with kojic acid and sodium lactate did not result in observable downregulation of the tyrosinase protein level. The use of a higher dose of kojic acid and sodium lactate (0.05% or $\geq 3\,mM$), however, led to significant inhibition of tyrosinase protein expression. Similar inhibition of tyrosinase protein expression was also demonstrated for other types of skin-whitening agents (Q10, vitamin C, tranexamic acid, arbutin, glycyrrhetinic acid) above the $20\,\mu M$ treatment dosage (Figure 22.1).

For the dose response of tyrosinase suppression by all components of palm TRF to be studied, B16 melanocyte cells were treated with an increasing dosage of all palm TRF isomers, including α-TP. As shown in Figure 22.1, only γ- and δ-T3 induced significant suppression of tyrosinase in a dose-dependent manner. In addition, treatment of B16 melanocyte cells with $20\,\mu M$ of the palm TRF mixture and its acetate also resulted in consistent suppression of tyrosinase protein expression. The level of suppression by palm TRF was comparable to that using γ- and δ-T3 isomers alone.

For the time response of tyrosinase suppression by γ- and δ-T3, α-TP, and tyrosinase inhibitors to be investigated, B16 melanocyte cells were treated with a single dose of γ- and δ-T3 isomers, α-TP, sodium lactate, and kojic acid for up to 48 h. Suppression of tyrosinase protein expression by γ- and δ-T3 isomers was shown to be enhanced by increasing the treatment period from 24 to 48 h (Yap et al. 2010). However, the opposite observation was determined when the treatment period for sodium lactate and kojic acid increased from 24 to 48 h, suggesting that the inhibition by the two agents may be short lived. As expected, α-TP did not result in tyrosinase suppression within 48 h.

22.4 γ- AND δ-T3 REDUCE TYROSINASE ACTIVITY AND MELANIN CONTENT

The melanin synthesis rates and total melanin content per cell were determined in both control and treated mediums. After tyrosinase activity was normalized for differences in cell growth by dividing the total activity by the cell number, it was found that B16 melanocyte cells treated with γ- and δ-T3 and palm TRF had <40% of the tyrosinase activity that was present in the controls. The inhibition of tyrosinase activity continued for up to 9 days after treatment. On day 9, it was found that B16 melanocyte cells treated with γ-T3 had <15% of the tyrosinase activity that was present in the controls. Figure 22.2 shows that the tyrosinase activity on day 9 following γ-T3 treatment was comparable to that treated with 0.05% kojic acid. With the low γ-T3 treatment concentration taken into consideration, the inhibition of tyrosinase activity by γ- and δ-T3 was at least 150-fold more potent than kojic acid and sodium lactate. On day 9, the melanin content of B16 melanocyte cell cultures treated with γ- and δ-T3 was 55% and 30% lower than that of the controls, respectively. The melanin content of B16 melanocyte cells following γ-T3 treatment was marginally lower than that in the treatment samples using 4.5 mM sodium lactate and 3.5 mM kojic acid.

22.5 γ- AND δ-T3 AS HYPOPIGMENTATION AGENT: *IN VITRO* AND *IN VIVO* EVIDENCE

For the ability of γ- and δ-T3, palm TRF, and tyrosine inhibitors to inhibit the induction of melanogenesis in B16 melanocyte cells to be tested, studies were conducted to examine the pigmentation level of cell pellets and xenografted solid tumors in immunocompromised mice. In Figure 22.3a, the amount of pigment is demonstrated directly by photographs of cell pellets treated with 5 days of blank, δ-T3, γ-T3, α-TP, palm TRF, $20\,\mu M$ sodium lactate, $20\,\mu M$ kojic acid, 0.05% sodium lactate,

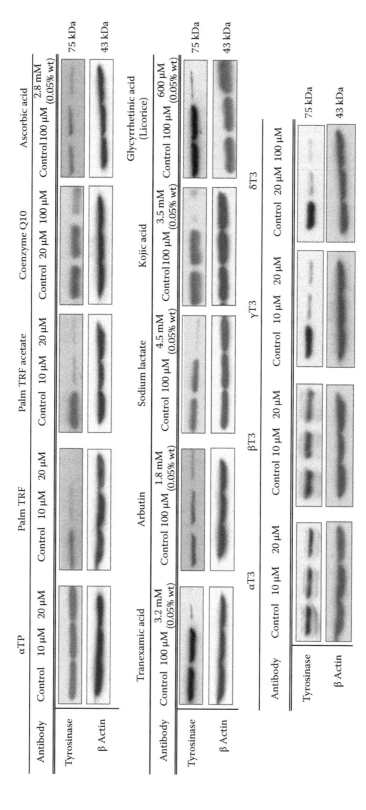

FIGURE 22.1 Treatment of B16 melanocyte cells with 20 mM of γ- and δ-T3 and a high concentration (0.05% wt) of other skin whitening agents for 24 h suppresses tyrosinase protein expression. Of note, αTP has no impact on the suppression of tyrosinase protein expression.

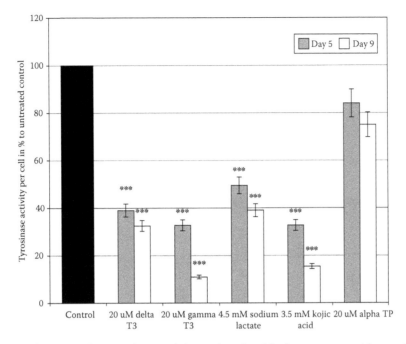

FIGURE 22.2 Time-dependent tyrosinase activity on days 5 and 9 after treatment with γ- and δ-T3, αTP, kojic acid, and sodium lactate. Bar chart, average for three assay measurements; bars, standard deviation. Note that γ-T3 significantly suppressed the activity of tyrosinase on day 9. Of note, α-TP has no impact on the suppression of tyrosinase enzymatic activity.

and 0.05% kojic acid (left to right panels). Lighter pigmentation was observed in samples treated with γ-T3, δ-T3, palm TRF, 0.05% sodium lactate, and 0.05% kojic acid. In Figure 22.3b, not only was the pigmentation of solid tumors lighter in color after 14 days of T3 supplementation compared with that of the controls but the tumor size was also significantly smaller for the γ-T3 and δ-T3 groups. Immunoblot of tyrosinase in solid tumors indicates that the γ-T3-treated B16 solid tumors have lower tyrosinase protein expression (Yap et al. 2010).

22.6   γ- AND δ-T3 REDUCE HYPERPIGMENTATION IN HUMAN SUBJECTS

Human clinical trial provides credible scientific evidence to support qualified health claims. To this end, several clinical studies are currently being conducted to investigate whether T3 is able to induce decent hypopigmenting effects in human subjects. Figure 22.3c shows a typical photograph of age spots on the face of one trial subject, before and after 1 month treatment using Kose Prime cream containing 2% γ- and δ-T3. The age spots in treated subjects showed observable skin lightening compared with the control subjects, who did not show improvement (n = 13).

22.7   γ- AND δ-T3 SYNERGIZE WITH OTHER ANTI-TYROSINASE AGENTS

Many of the natural products, such as quinone derivatives (Devkota et al. 2007) and phenolic licorice extracts (Nerya et al. 2003; Fu et al. 2005; Tengamnuay et al. 2006), which are extracted from plants, have been shown to have anti-melanogenesis effects. Previous studies have shown that many of these natural products inhibit tyrosinase activity in a synergistic manner via different mechanisms of action (Schved and Kahn 1992; Jin et al. 1999). To test whether T3 acts synergistically with tyrosinase inhibitors, studies were conducted to compare the effects of palm TRF alone or in

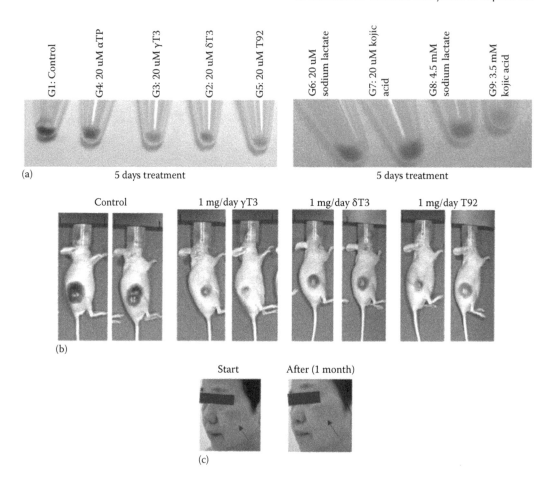

(a) 5 days treatment   5 days treatment

(b)

(c)

FIGURE 22.3 (a) B16 melanocyte cells were sub-cultured, treated for γ- and δ-T3, α-TP, palm TRF, kojic acid, and sodium lactate, then harvested. Photographs of the cell pellets were taken. Note that treatments of B16 melanocyte cells with 20 µM of γ- and δ-T3, palm TRF, and 0.05% kojic acid led to lighter cell pigmentation. Conversely, 20 µM of α-TP, kojic acid, and sodium lactate produced cell pellets with comparable pigmentation level to controls. (b) B16 melanocyte cells pre-treated with 20 µM of γ- and δ-T3, or palm TRF for 1 week were xenografted onto the flank of nude mice. This was followed by a 2 week supplementation of γ- and δ-T3, or palm TRF at the dose of 1 mg/day. Photographs of the solid tumors were taken at the end of a 2 week treatment. (c) Photographs of aged spots on the face of one subject, before and after 1 month treatment using Kose Prime cream containing 2% palm γ- and δ-T3. The control subjects did not show improvement in age spot (*n* = 13).

combination with other anti-tyrosinase agents. As shown in Figure 22.4a, the tyrosinase activities per cell following palm TRF co-treatment with kojic acid or sodium lactate are significantly lower than those treated with palm TRF, kojic acid or sodium lactate alone. Using Western blotting, γ-T3 co-treatment with kojic acid enhanced the suppression of tyrosinase protein expression when compared to treatments of γ-T3 or kojic acid alone. A similar synergistic interaction was also observed when γ-T3 was combined with alpha arbutin, hydroquinone, and L-glutathione (Figure 22.4b).

In the past, kojic acid, a by-product of the fermentation process of malting rice, was considered a mild inhibitor of the formation of pigment in animal tissues (Cabanes et al. 1994). The synthetic derivatives of kojic acid were recently improved to show a 100-fold increase in tyrosinase inhibitory activity compared to native kojic acid. Since long-term usage of kojic acid has indicated dermal toxicity (Kim et al. 2004), its combination with γ- and δ-T3 may provide a dose-sparing strategy that can improve anti-melanogenesis efficacy while reducing long-term side effects.

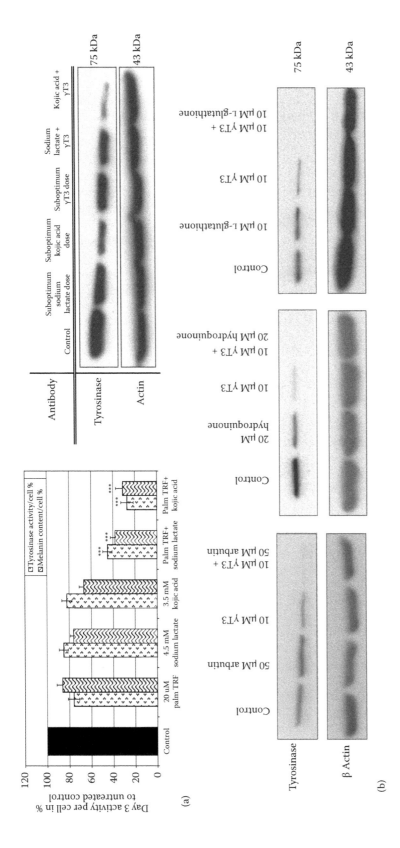

FIGURE 22.4 (a) B16 melanocyte cells were treated with 20 μM of palm TRF and 0.05% of either sodium lactate or kojic acid for 72 h. The suppression of tyrosinase activity and melanin content following co-treatment were significantly greater than the cells treated with either agent alone. Using Western blotting, 5 μM of γ-T3 co-treatment with 0.01% of kojic acid for 24 h resulted in enhanced suppression of tyrosinase protein. (b) B16 melanocyte cells were treated with γ-T3 and other anti-tyrosinase agents for 24 h. The suppression of tyrosinase protein expression following co-treatment was significantly greater than the cells treated with either agent alone.

In contrast, sodium lactate has been reported to be effective in treating pigmentary lesions, such as melasma and post-inflammatory hyperpigmentation, by directly targeting tyrosinase catalytic activity (Usuki et al. 2003). Thus, the synergistic interaction with γ- and δ-T3 cannot be easily determined by using Western blotting, but through its tyrosinase activity and melanin content (Yap et al. 2010).

22.8 γ- AND δ-T3 BLOCK UV-INDUCED MELANOGENESIS, NOT ITS ACETATE FORM

Because ultraviolet light (UVB) was previously reported to stimulate skin melanin synthesis (Fitzpatrick et al. 1949; Sharma et al. 1979) via a different mechanism from the constitutive tyrosinase action in melanin-generating cells, investigations were also conducted to evaluate the ability of T3 to block UVB-induced melanogenesis in B16 melanocyte cells. For an appropriate UVB irradiation dose to be derived, MTT cell proliferation rates were compared following different doses of UVB exposure. B16 melanocyte cells exposed to ≥12 h have a reduced cell proliferation rate, as evidenced by the activation of critical apoptotic molecules (cleaved caspase 3 and PARP) (Yap et al. 2010). Therefore, the UVB exposure of cells was limited to <12 h to avoid interference from apoptotic responses. Figure 22.5 showed the time-dependent suppression of UVB-induced tyrosinase protein over-expression. Although δ-T3 was more potent than γ-T3 in suppressing short-term (<1 min) UVB-induced tyrosinase activation, its long-term inhibitory effect was comparable. Surprisingly, palm TRF acetate and α-TP were not able to block UVB-induced activation of tyrosinase. This observation suggested that the mechanism for UVB-induced tyrosinase activation differs from that of its constitutive expression and that the native form of palm TRF, in particular γ- and δ-T3, may be a more robust tyrosinase inhibitor that exerts its inhibitory effects via multiple signaling pathways (Nylander et al. 2000; Galibert et al. 2001).

22.9 γ- AND δ-T3, AND PALM TRF, BUT NOT α-TP, SUPPRESS CONSTITUTIVE MELANIN SYNTHESIS

Two recent reports (Makpol et al. 2009; Michihara et al. 2009) suggested the possible regulation of melanin synthesis by T3. Michihara et al. examined the effect of δ-T3 on melanin content using mouse B16 melanocyte cells and concluded that the melanin content was significantly reduced as a result of a concomitant decrease of the protein level of tyrosinase. Although the study reported strong inhibition of tyrosinase protein and mRNA by using Western blotting and RT-PCR, the experimental results had a major drawback. A case in point is that the authors have not investigated the apoptotic response of B16 melanocyte cells following 24 h treatments with 50 and 100 μM of δ-T3. Based on our study, treatment of B16 melanocyte cells at 50–100 μM of δ-T3 has led to a significant decrease in cell proliferation rates (42% and 90%, respectively) and apoptosis. The activation of apoptosis at these treatment doses was also confirmed by using Western blotting for cleaved caspase 3 and poly ADP ribosome polymerase (PARP; Yap et al. 2010). Given the possible interference from apoptotic responses, the authors may not have sufficient evidence to conclude that tyrosinase suppression at mRNA and protein levels were caused by δ-T3 treatment. Alternatively, they may have investigated the tyrosinase protein expression using a lower treatment dose of δ-T3.

In the second study (Makpol et al. 2009), the authors concluded that treatment of primary skin melanocytes with α-T3-rich TRF reduced tyrosinase activity and melanin content compared to that of the controls. Although the results suggest that at least two members of palm TRF are potent against melanogenesis, we were unable to reproduce the results despite repeated trials. In contrast, treatment of B16 melanoma cells with purified α-TP and α-T3 both did not result in observable suppression of tyrosinase at the mRNA and protein levels (Yap et al. 2010). Further evaluation of the research protocol suggested that the researchers may have used the full spectrum palm TRF containing γ- and δ-T3, which are active against tyrosinase, rather than palm TRF,

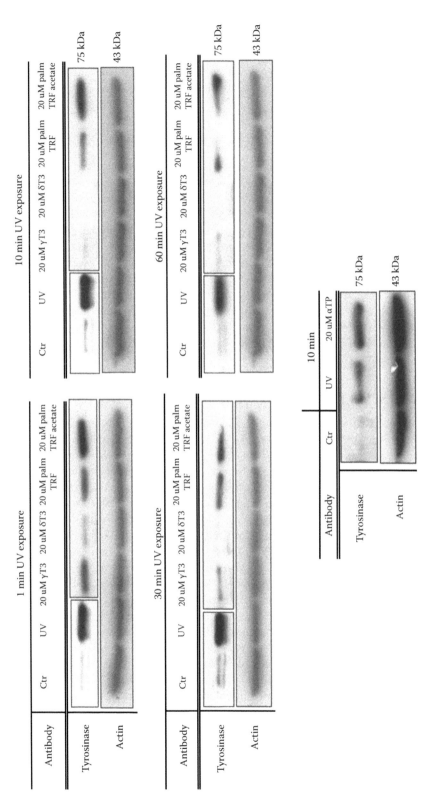

FIGURE 22.5 Using Western blotting, the activation of tyrosinase by UVB is completely blocked by γ- and δ-T3 after 60 min of incubation time. The same experiment shows that palm TRF only partially blocked UVB-induced tyrosinase activation. In contrast, palm TRF acetate had no activity against UVB-induced tyrosinase activation. Of note, treating B16 melanocyte cells with 20 μM of α-TP does not reverse UVB-induced tyrosinase activation.

which contains only 75% α-T3 and 25% TP, as claimed. Of note, typical palm TRF contains ~75% T3 instead of αT3. Basing our findings on our results using individual palm isomers, we speculate that it was the γ- and δ-T3 within the palm TRF that suppressed tyrosinase activity of primary skin melanocytes. Such a study using palm TRF is difficult to interpret because TRF contains a mixture of α-TP and α-, β-, γ-, and δ-T3, plant phytosterols, carotenoids, and squalene, in addition to a determination of the most potent active ingredients and the respective mechanisms of action.

22.10 γ- AND δ-T3: HYPOPIGMENTATION AGENTS BEYOND ANTIOXIDATION

One surprising finding was that palm TRF acetate suppresses tyrosinase protein expression at comparable strengths to γ- and δ-T3 (Yap et al. 2010). Two possible reasons exist to explain the observation. First, the anti-melanogenesis effect may be unrelated to the antioxidant properties of γ- and δ-T3, but associated with the unsaturated isoprenoid side chain. This explanation is nonclassic since it is thought that the antioxidant properties of T3 decrease melanin levels by inhibiting the oxidative enzymatic reactions, including tyrosinase or other enzymes in melanosomes (Raper 1927; Mason 1948). Second, it remains possible that palm TRF acetate is absorbed and hydrolyzed by B16 melanoma cells to the native palm TRF (Brisson et al. 2008), thus conferring the inhibitory effect on the tyrosinase gene. Nonetheless, the aforementioned conjectures do not have strong scientific evidence and require more experimental investigations to dissect the role played by isoprenoid side chains as well as various ester forms of vitamin E and its intermediate metabolites. In addition, it is also vital to include members from the TP and T3 family since the bulk of vitamin E knowledge generated in PubMed has been directed at tocopherols.

22.11 FUTURE RESEARCH TO DELINEATE T3 MODE OF ACTION

Recent studies indicated that a low concentration of γ- and δ-T3 reduces tyrosinase protein and melanin production. Given that γ- and δ-T3 are lipid-soluble agents that have high bioavailability in skin layers (Ikeda et al. 2000, 2001), the utilization of γ- and δ-T3 alone, or in combination with other anti-tyrosinase agents, provides a potentially innovative strategy for human skin care and therapeutic applications. Although the inhibitory effect of T3 on tyrosinase is well documented, its upstream regulatory mechanism has not been adequately studied. More recent data using human melanocyte cells suggested that γ-T3 modulates tyrosinase protein expression through a series of miRNAs (Yap and Xu 2011). To date, >50 native miRNAs capable of silencing human tyrosinase have been identified (Griffiths-Jones et al. 2006, 2008). Thus, one of the future research efforts should emphasize on dissecting the upstream regulatory mechanism that possibly involves miRNA roles (Figure 22.6). By utilizing T3-mediated miRNA strategy, many cosmetic and therapeutic applications can be developed, offering more long-term effectiveness, better target specificity (Elbashir et al. 2001a,b; Sledz et al. 2003), and higher safety in skin gene manipulation.

In addition, a high-throughput metabolomics technique (Zeisel 2007; Oresic 2009) should also be employed to better profile alterations in the metabolic end-products of cellular processes that result in reduced skin pigmentation. The main advantage of this technique, compared to other "omics" platforms, is its capability to analyze small biomolecules found in biofluids like sweat, and provide an instantaneous snapshot of the physiology of skin cells in response to T3. For example, comparison of metabolite profiles of sweat from different individuals can be used to identify specific metabolic changes leading to the understanding of biochemical pathways, complex biomarker combinations, and disease regression. Such type of approach is also meaningful to identify individuals who will most likely benefit from T3 treatment, and may be developed into future means for consumers to adapt their T3 requirements based on their health and nutritional status (Kussmann et al. 2006, 2008). Last but not the least, research emphasis should also be on the impact of the indigenous gut microbial consortia on T3 metabolism and absorption before

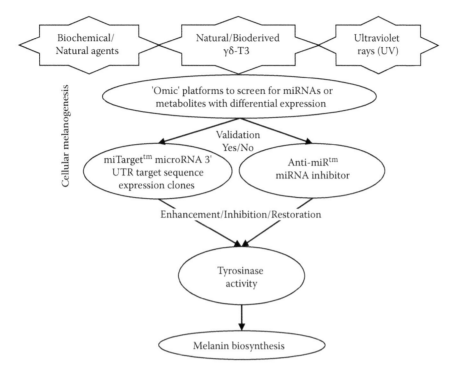

FIGURE 22.6 Future research on T3 mechanism of action should emphasize on pursuing the upstream miRNA regulatory mechanism which leads to tyrosinase suppression.

interaction with human cells at the molecular level. To this end, increasing investigations showed that humans are colonized by a complex and dynamic community of microorganisms (Savage 1977) that collectively acts as a metabolically active vehicle affecting T3 metabolism and absorption (Hooper et al. 2002; Backhed et al. 2005). The microbiota may preferentially degrade dietary T3 that is otherwise available to elucidate its various health benefits in the human body, or vice versa: One such example is the key role played by gut microbial in the conversion of dietary genistin to genistein (Coldham et al. 2002).

22.12 LAST HURDLE: CLINICAL EVIDENCE TO SUPPORT QUALIFIED HEALTH CLAIMS

Compared to TP, there is a shortage of published human clinical trials directed to prove unequivocally T3 efficacy in human populations. A consideration for major T3 companies is that an acceptable level of return of investment (ROI) may not be made on the huge clinical development cost needed to bring T3 through placebo-controlled clinical trials to market. Sales of a new anti-tyrosinase agent like T3 may also be limited due to the existence of many substitutes (Smith et al. 1989) and cheaper agents (Arung et al. 2005) already in the market. Concerns have also been raised that today's regulatory procedures make approval difficult for new anti-tyrosinase agents as they are compared head-to-head against established agents in diseased states, while therapeutic side effects are not adequately weighted. As a suggestion, T3 companies may enter their T3 products into credible clinical trials to support their claims of safety and efficacy. Emphasis should also be on the use of effective γδT3-based formulation to avoid reliance on feeble claims. Although well conceived clinical trials are expensive and take months to complete, their value in promoting product marketability, and preventing liability and adverse regulatory enforcement far outweighs the cost and struggle to bring T3 from bench to bedside (Wolfram et al. 2006).

ACKNOWLEDGMENTS

The experimental work was performed at the Dermatology Lab of Davos Life Science Pte Ltd. and supported by a research grant from Kuala Lumpur Kepong (KLK) Berhad (2006–2011). The results were published in *Pigment Cell & Melanoma Research* 2010.

REFERENCES

Abu Ubeid, A., L. Zhao, Y. Wang, and B. M. Hantash. 2009. Short-sequence oligopeptides with inhibitory activity against mushroom and human tyrosinase. *J Invest Dermatol* 129 (9):2242–2249.

Ahmad, N. S., B. A. Khalid, D. A. Luke, and S. Ima Nirwana. 2005. Tocotrienol offers better protection than tocopherol from free radical-induced damage of rat bone. *Clin Exp Pharmacol Physiol* 32 (9):761–770.

Arung, E.T., I.W. Kusuma, Y. M. Iskandar, S. Yusatake, K. Shimizu, and R. Kondo. 2005. Screening of Indonesian plants for tyrosinase inhibitory activity. *J Wood Sci* 51 (5):520–525.

Backhed, F., R. E. Ley, J. L. Sonnenburg, D. A. Peterson, and J. I. Gordon. 2005. Host–bacterial mutualism in the human intestine. *Science* 307 (5717):1915–1920.

Brisson, L., S. Castan, H. Fontbonne, C. Nicoletti, A. Puigserver, and H. Ajandouz el. 2008. Alpha-tocopheryl acetate is absorbed and hydrolyzed by Caco-2 cells comparative studies with alpha-tocopherol. *Chem Phys Lipids* 154 (1):33–37.

Cabanes, J., S. Chazarra, and F. Garcia-Carmona. 1994. Kojic acid, a cosmetic skin whitening agent, is a slow-binding inhibitor of catecholase activity of tyrosinase. *J Pharm Pharmacol* 46 (12):982–985.

Cahoon, E. B., S. E. Hall, K. G. Ripp, T. S. Ganzke, W. D. Hitz, and S. J. Coughlan. 2003. Metabolic redesign of vitamin E biosynthesis in plants for tocotrienol production and increased antioxidant content. *Nat Biotechnol* 21 (9):1082–1087.

Chang, P. N., W. N. Yap, D. T. Lee, M. T. Ling, Y. C. Wong, and Y. L. Yap. 2009. Evidence of gamma-tocotrienol as an apoptosis-inducing, invasion-suppressing, and chemotherapy drug-sensitizing agent in human melanoma cells. *Nutr Cancer* 61 (3):357–366.

Chen, Y. M. and W. Chavin. 1966. Incorporation of carboxyl groups into melanin by skin tyrosinase. *Nature* 210 (5031):35–37.

Choi, S., S. K. Lee, J. E. Kim, M. H. Chung, and Y. I. Park. 2002. Aloesin inhibits hyperpigmentation induced by UV radiation. *Clin Exp Dermatol* 27 (6):513–515.

Coldham, N. G., C. Darby, L. Hows, L. J. King, A. Q. Zhang, and M. J. Sauer. 2002. Comparative metabolism of genistin by human and rat gut microflora: Detection and identification of the end-products of metabolism. *Xenobiotica* 32 (1):45–62.

Devkota, K. P., M. T. Khan, R. Ranjit, A. M. Lannang, Samreen, and M. I. Choudhary. 2007. Tyrosinase inhibitory and antileishmanial constituents from the rhizomes of *Paris polyphylla*. *Nat Prod Res* 21 (4):321–327.

Elbashir, S. M., J. Harborth, W. Lendeckel, A. Yalcin, K. Weber, and T. Tuschl. 2001a. Duplexes of 21-nucleotide RNAs mediate RNA interference in cultured mammalian cells. *Nature* 411 (6836):494–498.

Elbashir, S. M., W. Lendeckel, and T. Tuschl. 2001b. RNA interference is mediated by 21- and 22-nucleotide RNAs. *Genes Dev* 15 (2):188–200.

Fitzpatrick, T. B., S. W. Becker, Jr., A. B. Lerner, and H. Montgomery. 1950. Tyrosinase in human skin: Demonstration of its presence and of its role in human melanin formation. *Science* 112 (2904):223–225.

Fitzpatrick, T. B., A. B. Lerner et al. 1949. Mammalian tyrosinase; melanin formation by ultraviolet irradiation. *Arch Derm Syphilol* 59 (6):620–625.

Fu, B., H. Li, X. Wang, F. S. Lee, and S. Cui. 2005. Isolation and identification of flavonoids in licorice and a study of their inhibitory effects on tyrosinase. *J Agric Food Chem* 53 (19):7408–7414.

Galibert, M. D., S. Carreira, and C. R. Goding. 2001. The Usf-1 transcription factor is a novel target for the stress-responsive p38 kinase and mediates UV-induced tyrosinase expression. *EMBO J* 20 (17):5022–5031.

Griffiths-Jones, S., R. J. Grocock, S. van Dongen, A. Bateman, and A. J. Enright. 2006. miRBase: microRNA sequences, targets and gene nomenclature. *Nucleic Acids Res* 34 (Database issue):D140–D144.

Griffiths-Jones, S., H. K. Saini, S. van Dongen, and A. J. Enright. 2008. miRBase: Tools for microRNA genomics. *Nucleic Acids Res* 36 (Database issue):D154–D158.

Gupta, A. K., M. D. Gover, K. Nouri, and S. Taylor. 2006. The treatment of melasma: A review of clinical trials. *J Am Acad Dermatol* 55 (6):1048–1065.

Hall, A. M., and S. J. Orlow. 2005. Degradation of tyrosinase induced by phenylthiourea occurs following Golgi maturation. *Pigment Cell Res* 18 (2):122–129.

Hemesath, T. J., E. Steingrimsson, G. McGill, M. J. Hansen, J. Vaught, C. A. Hodgkinson, H. Arnheiter, N. G. Copeland, N. A. Jenkins, and D. E. Fisher. 1994. Microphthalmia, a critical factor in melanocyte development, defines a discrete transcription factor family. *Genes Dev* 8 (22):2770–2780.

Hodgkinson, C. A., K. J. Moore, A. Nakayama, E. Steingrimsson, N. G. Copeland, N. A. Jenkins, and H. Arnheiter. 1993. Mutations at the mouse microphthalmia locus are associated with defects in a gene encoding a novel basic-helix-loop-helix-zipper protein. *Cell* 74 (2):395–404.

Hooper, L. V., T. Midtvedt, and J. I. Gordon. 2002. How host–microbial interactions shape the nutrient environment of the mammalian intestine. *Annu Rev Nutr* 22:283–307.

Ikeda, S., T. Niwa, and K. Yamashita. 2000. Selective uptake of dietary tocotrienols into rat skin. *J Nutr Sci Vitaminol (Tokyo)* 46 (3):141–143.

Ikeda, S., K. Toyoshima, and K. Yamashita. 2001. Dietary sesame seeds elevate alpha- and gamma-tocotrienol concentrations in skin and adipose tissue of rats fed the tocotrienol-rich fraction extracted from palm oil. *J Nutr* 131 (11):2892–2897.

Jenkins, M. E., T. C. Suzuki, and D. W. Mount. 1997. Evidence that heat and ultraviolet radiation activate a common stress-response program in plants that is altered in the uvh6 mutant of *Arabidopsis thaliana*. *Plant Physiol* 115 (4):1351–1358.

Jin, Y. H., S. J. Lee, M. H. Chung, J. H. Park, Y. I. Park, T. H. Cho, and S. K. Lee. 1999. Aloesin and arbutin inhibit tyrosinase activity in a synergistic manner via a different action mechanism. *Arch Pharm Res* 22 (3):232–236.

Johnson, G. S. and I. Pastan. 1972. N 6,O 2′-dibutyryl adenosine 3′,5′-monophosphate induces pigment production in melanoma cells. *Nat New Biol* 237 (78):267–268.

Khan, S. B., M. T. Hassan Khan, E. S. Jang, K. Akhtar, J. Seo, and H. Han. 2010. Tyrosinase inhibitory effect of benzoic acid derivatives and their structure-activity relationships. *J Enzyme Inhib Med Chem* 25 (6):812–817.

Khan, M. T., S. B. Khan, and A. Ather. 2006. Tyrosinase inhibitory cycloartane type triterpenoids from the methanol extract of the whole plant of *Amberboa ramosa* Jafri and their structure-activity relationship. *Bioorg Med Chem* 14 (4):938–943.

Kim, H., J. Choi, J. K. Cho, S. Y. Kim, and Y. S. Lee. 2004. Solid-phase synthesis of kojic acid-tripeptides and their tyrosinase inhibitory activity, storage stability, and toxicity. *Bioorg Med Chem Lett* 14 (11):2843–2846.

Korner, A. and J. Pawelek. 1982. Mammalian tyrosinase catalyzes three reactions in the biosynthesis of melanin. *Science* 217 (4565):1163–1165.

Kussmann, M., F. Raymond, and M. Affolter. 2006. OMICS-driven biomarker discovery in nutrition and health. *J Biotechnol* 124 (4):758–787.

Kussmann, M., S. Rezzi, and H. Daniel. 2008. Profiling techniques in nutrition and health research. *Curr Opin Biotechnol* 19 (2):83–99.

Lee, Y. S., D. W. Kim, S. Kim, H. I. Choi, Y. Lee, C. D. Kim, J. H. Lee, S. D. Lee, and Y. H. Lee. 2010. Downregulation of NFAT2 promotes melanogenesis in B16 melanoma cells. *Anat Cell Biol* 43 (4):303–309.

Makpol, S., N. N. M. Arifin, Z. Ismail, K. H. Chua, Y. Anum, M. Yusof, and W. Z. W. Ngah. 2009. Modulation of melanin synthesis and its gene expression in skin melanocytes by palm tocotrienol rich fraction. *Afr J Biochem Res* 3 (12):385–392.

Mason, H. S. 1948. The chemistry of melanin; mechanism of the oxidation of dihydroxyphenylalanine by tyrosinase. *J Biol Chem* 172 (1):83–99.

Mason, H. S. 1949. The chemistry of melanin; mechanism of the oxidation of catechol by tyrosinase. *J Biol Chem* 181 (2):803–812.

Mazlan, M., T. Sue Mian, G. Mat Top, and W. Zurinah Wan Ngah. 2006. Comparative effects of alpha-tocopherol and gamma-tocotrienol against hydrogen peroxide induced apoptosis on primary-cultured astrocytes. *J Neurol Sci* 243 (1–2):5–12.

Michihara, A., S. Morita, Y. Hirokawa, S. Ago, K. Akasaki, and H. Tsuji. 2009. Delta tocotrienol causes decrease of melanin content in mouse melanoma cells. *J Health Sci* 55 (2):314–318.

Nerya, O., J. Vaya, R. Musa, S. Izrael, R. Ben-Arie, and S. Tamir. 2003. Glabrene and isoliquiritigenin as tyrosinase inhibitors from licorice roots. *J Agric Food Chem* 51 (5):1201–1207.

Nylander, K., J. C. Bourdon, S. E. Bray, N. K. Gibbs, R. Kay, I. Hart, and P. A. Hall. 2000. Transcriptional activation of tyrosinase and TRP-1 by p53 links UV irradiation to the protective tanning response. *J Pathol* 190 (1):39–46.

Oresic, M. 2009. Metabolomics, a novel tool for studies of nutrition, metabolism and lipid dysfunction. *Nutr Metab Cardiovasc Dis* 19 (11):816–824.

Pawelek, J. M. 1976. Factors regulating growth and pigmentation of melanoma cells. *J Invest Dermatol* 66 (4):201–209.

Ragnelli, A. M., G. Pacioni, P. Aimola, B. Lanza, and M. Miranda. 1992. Truffle melanogenesis: Correlation with reproductive differentiation and ascocarp ripening. *Pigment Cell Res* 5 (5 Pt 1):205–212.

Raper, H. S. 1927. The tyrosinase-tyrosine reaction: Production from tyrosine of 5: 6-Dihydroxyindole and 5: 6-Dihydroxyindole-2-carboxylic acid—The precursors of melanin. *Biochem J* 21 (1):89–96.

Sattler, S. E., L. U. Gilliland, M. Magallanes-Lundback, M. Pollard, and D. DellaPenna. 2004. Vitamin E is essential for seed longevity and for preventing lipid peroxidation during germination. *Plant Cell* 16 (6):1419–1432.

Savage, D. C. 1977. Microbial ecology of the gastrointestinal tract. *Annu Rev Microbiol* 31:107–133.

Schved, F. and V. Kahn. 1992. Synergism exerted by 4-methyl catechol, catechol, and their respective quinones on the rate of DL-DOPA oxidation by mushroom tyrosinase. *Pigment Cell Res* 5 (1):41–48.

Sharma, R. C., R. Ali, and O. Yamamoto. 1979. Effect of UV light on biological activity of tyrosinase in buffer solution. *J Radiat Res (Tokyo)* 20 (2):186–195.

Sledz, C. A., M. Holko, M. J. de Veer, R. H. Silverman, and B. R. Williams. 2003. Activation of the interferon system by short-interfering RNAs. *Nat Cell Biol* 5 (9):834–839.

Smirnoff, N. 1998. Plant resistance to environmental stress. *Curr Opin Biotechnol* 9 (2):214–219.

Smith, C. J., K. B. O'Hare, and J. C. Allen. 1988. Selective cytotoxicity of hydroquinone for melanocyte-derived cells is mediated by tyrosinase activity but independent of melanin content. *Pigment Cell Res* 1 (6):386–389.

Smith, T. J., J. T. Warren, Jr., and E. L. Kline. 1989. Retinoic acid blockade of imidazole-induced tyrosinase expression in B16 melanoma cultures: Similar effects of the active retinoid and triiodothyronine. *Biochem Biophys Res Commun* 162 (1):288–293.

Steingrimsson, E., K. J. Moore et al. 1994. Molecular basis of mouse microphthalmia (mi) mutations helps explain their developmental and phenotypic consequences. *Nat Genet* 8 (3):256–263.

Talwar, H. S., C. E. Griffiths, G. J. Fisher, A. Russman, K. Krach, S. Benrazavi, and J. J. Voorhees. 1993. Differential regulation of tyrosinase activity in skin of white and black individuals *in vivo* by topical retinoic acid. *J Invest Dermatol* 100 (6):800–805.

Tengamnuay, P., K. Pengrungruangwong, I. Pheansri, and K. Likhitwitayawuid. 2006. *Artocarpus lakoocha* heartwood extract as a novel cosmetic ingredient: Evaluation of the *in vitro* anti-tyrosinase and *in vivo* skin whitening activities. *Int J Cosmet Sci* 28 (4):269–276.

Tomita, Y., A. Hariu, C. Kato, and M. Seiji. 1984. Radical production during tyrosinase reaction, dopa-melanin formation, and photoirradiation of dopa-melanin. *J Invest Dermatol* 82 (6):573–576.

Usuki, A., A. Ohashi, H. Sato, Y. Ochiai, M. Ichihashi, and Y. Funasaka. 2003. The inhibitory effect of glycolic acid and lactic acid on melanin synthesis in melanoma cells. *Exp Dermatol* 12 (Suppl 2):43–50.

Wolfram, S., Y. Wang, and F. Thielecke. 2006. Anti-obesity effects of green tea: From bedside to bench. *Mol Nutr Food Res* 50 (2):176–187.

Wong, G. and J. Pawelek. 1973. Control of phenotypic expression of cultured melanoma cells by melanocyte stimulating hormones. *Nat New Biol* 241 (111):213–215.

Wu, D. T. S., J. S. Chen, D. C. Chang, and S. L. Lin. 2008. Mir-434-5p mediates skin whitening and lightening. *Clin Cosmet Investig Dermatol* 1:19–35.

Yap, W. N., P. N. Chang, H. Y. Han, D. T. Lee, M. T. Ling, Y. C. Wong, and Y. L. Yap. 2008. Gamma-tocotrienol suppresses prostate cancer cell proliferation and invasion through multiple-signalling pathways. *Br J Cancer* 99 (11):1832–1841.

Yap, W. N., N. Zaiden, S. Y. Luk, D. T. Lee, M. T. Ling, Y. C. Wong, and Y. L. Yap. 2010a. In vivo evidence of gamma-tocotrienol as a chemosensitizer in the treatment of hormone-refractory prostate cancer. *Pharmacology* 85 (4):248–258.

Yap, W. N., N. Zaiden, Y. L. Tan, C. P. Ngoh, X. W. Zhang, Y. C. Wong, M. T. Ling, and Y. L. Yap. 2010b. Id1, inhibitor of differentiation, is a key protein mediating anti-tumor responses of gamma-tocotrienol in breast cancer cells. *Cancer Lett* 291 (2):187–199.

Yap, W. N., N. Zaiden, C. H. Xu, A. Chen, S. Ong, V. Teo, and Y. L. Yap. 2010c. Gamma- and delta-tocotrienols inhibit skin melanin synthesis by suppressing constitutive and UV-induced tyrosinase activation. *Pigment Cell Mel Res* 23 (5):688–692.

Yap, Y. L. and C. H. Xu. 2011. Synergistic interaction of at least one vitamin e component and tyrosinase inhibitors for dermatological applications. WIPO patent WO2011129765, October 20, 2011.

Zeisel, S. H. 2007. Nutrigenomics and metabolomics will change clinical nutrition and public health practice: Insights from studies on dietary requirements for choline. *Am J Clin Nutr* 86 (3):542–548.

Zhu, Z., J. He et al. 2010. MicroRNA-25 functions in regulation of pigmentation by targeting the transcription factor MITF in Alpaca (*Lama pacos*) skin melanocytes. *Domest Anim Endocrinol* 38 (3):200–209.

23 Tocotrienols and Bone Health

Ima Nirwana Soelaiman, Norazlina Mohamed,
Ahmad Nazrun Shuid, and Norliza Muhammad

CONTENTS

23.1 INTRODUCTION

The pathogenesis of osteoporosis is multifactorial. Oxygen-derived free radicals are involved in the formation and activation of osteoclasts (Garrett et al., 1990), leading to an increase in bone resorption and bone loss. Bone histomorphometric studies have shown that ferric nitrilotriacetate (Fe-NTA), an oxidizing agent, increased osteoclast numbers (Ebina et al., 1991) and impaired mineralization (Takeuchi et al., 1997). Osteoporotic women had significantly higher plasma superoxide dismutase (SOD) enzyme activity and higher malondialdehyde (MDA) levels while glutathione peroxidase (GSH-Px) enzyme activity and nitric oxide (NO) levels were similar when compared to non-osteoporotic controls (Ozgocmen et al., 2007). A negative correlation was found between SOD and lumbar bone mineral density (BMD) levels (r = −0.328; p = 0.021). The same trend was observed between NO and lumbar BMD (r = −0.473; p = 0.001) and femoral neck BMD values (r = −0.540; p = 0.000) (Yalin et al., 2005). Low bone mineral density was associated with increased 8-iso-prostaglandin $F_{2\alpha}$, an oxidative stress biomarker (Basu et al., 2001). Based on the close association between free radicals and osteoporosis, there is reason to believe that antioxidants, notably the tocotrienols, may be effective in the prevention and treatment of osteoporosis. The most easily available source of tocotrienols in Malaysia is from palm oil. Palm cooking oil contains 178.33 ppm α-tocopherol, 188.50 ppm α-tocotrienol, 260.83 ppm γ-tocotrienol, and 69.83 ppm δ-tocotrienol (Siti Khadijah, 2011). Our studies mainly used tocotrienols extracted from palm oil in the form of tocotrienol mixtures as well as the pure γ-isomer. We used the rat as our animal model since previous studies have shown that their bone anatomy, bone remodeling, and response to treatment are similar to humans (Abe et al., 1993, Mosekilde, 1995).

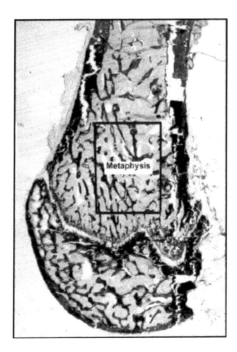

FIGURE 23.1 Longitudinal section of the distal femur showing the margin for sampling in the metaphyseal region. The metaphyseal region was located 3–7 mm from the lowest point of the growth plate and 1 mm from the lateral cortex, excluding the endocortical region. (From Hermizi, H. et al., *Calcif. Tissue Int.*, 84, 67, 2009.)

23.2 TOCOTRIENOLS, OXIDATIVE STRESS, AND BONE

Our early studies found that ferric-nitrilotriacetate (Fe-NTA), a strong oxidizing agent, decreased calcium content of bone, and this was prevented by supplementation with tocotrienol mixture (Yee and Ima-Nirwana 1998). Bone histomorphometry was done to better quantify the effects of tocotrienols on bone. The histomorphometry was done on the distal end of the femur (Figure 23.1) and the nomenclature adopted was according to Parfitt et al. (1987). Measurement was done using an image analyzer (Quantimet 520; Cambridge Instruments, Woburn, MA, USA) with the VideoTest-Master software (Video-Test, St. Petersburg, Russia).

The bone histomorphometric studies found that tocotrienols 60 mg/kg/day for 8 weeks prevented the loss in bone structure by increasing osteoblast number and reducing osteoclast number (Figures 23.2 and 23.3) (Nazrun et al., 2005).

Photomicrograph of the bone using Von Kossa stain showed less bony trabeculae in the group treated with Fe-NTA (F), with apparent recovery seen in the Fe-NTA group with supplemented tocotrienols (F + P) (Figure 23.4).

23.3 TOCOTRIENOLS AND ESTROGEN-DEFICIENT OSTEOPOROSIS

Lack of estrogen enhanced osteoclastic activity, which leads to increased erosion depth and trabecular perforation (Parfitt, 2000). Estrogen deficiency lowered antioxidant defences in osteoclasts resulting in increased osteoclastic resorption (Lean et al., 2003). The levels of lipid peroxidation and hydrogen peroxide were increased and enzymatic antioxidants like SOD, GPx, and GST were decreased in ovariectomized rats (Muthusami et al., 2005). We found that tocotrienols prevented the structural bone loss due to ovariectomy by preventing the increase in osteoclasts, while maintaining an increase in osteoblasts (Figures 23.5 and 23.6, Table 23.1) (Norliza, 2007).

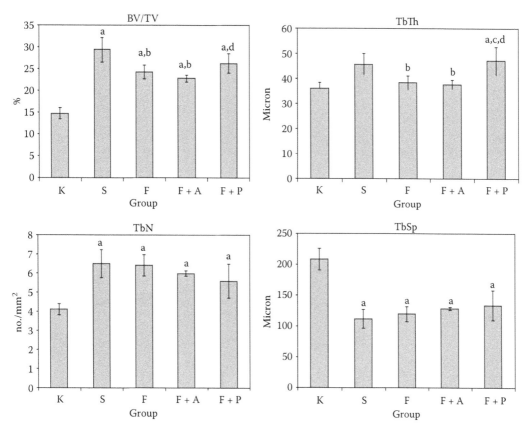

FIGURE 23.2 Structural bone histomorphometric parameters. BV/TV, bone volume/total volume; TbTh, trabecular thickness; TbN, trabecular number; TbSp, trabecular separation; a, significant from baseline control group (K); b, significant from normal control group (S); c, significant from Fe-NTA-treated group (F); d, significant from α-tocopherol supplemented group (F + A); F + P, tocotrienol supplemented group. Significance taken at $p < 0.05$. (From Nazrun et al., *Curr. Top. Pharmacol.*, 9(2), 107, 2005.)

23.4 TOCOTRIENOLS AND NICOTINE-INDUCED OSTEOPOROSIS

Nicotine appeared to stimulate osteoclast resorption in a porcine marrow cell model (Henemyre et al., 2003), increased serum interleukin-1 levels (Norazlina et al., 2004), and reduced left femoral calcium content in male rats (Ima-Nirwana et al., 2005). Animal studies have shown that nicotine exposure leads to oxidative stress (Wetscher et al., 1995, Kalpana and Menon, 2004). Smoking is implicated as a risk factor for osteoporosis and therefore increased the susceptibility for fractures in both men and women (Kapoor and Jones, 2005, Chapurlat, 2008). Our own studies found that treatment of rats with intraperitoneal nicotine 7 mg/kg/day for 2 months reduced bone volume and osteoblast number, increased osteoclast number, and impaired bone formation and mineralization; and stopping the nicotine for 2 months did not improve or reverse the impairment (Table 23.2, Figure 23.7) (Hapidin et al., 2011).

Following that, we treated male rats for 2 months with nicotine, stopped the nicotine, and supplemented with three types of vitamin E: tocotrienol-enhanced fraction (TEF), γ-tocotrienol (GTT), and α-tocopherol (ATF). All three types of vitamin E were given by oral gavage, 60 mg/kg/day for an additional 2 months (Table 23.3).

The structural histomorphometric parameters showed that all the three vitamin E types were able to improve bone volume (BV/TV), trabecular thickness (TbTh), and trabecular number (TbN). The osteoclast number (OsN) and eroded surface (ES/BS) was also reduced in the three vitamin E groups.

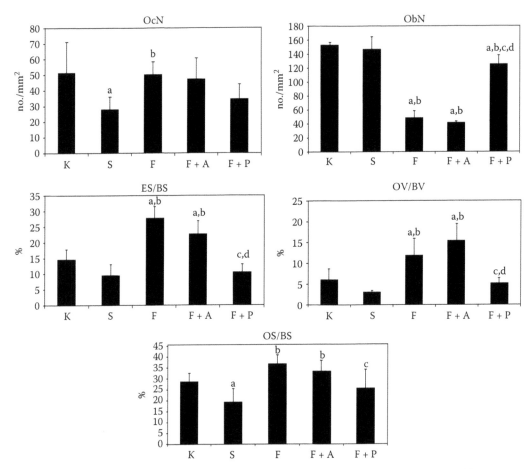

FIGURE 23.3 Cellular (static) bone histomorphometric parameters. OcN, osteoclast number; ObN, osteoblast number; ES/BS, eroded surface/bone surface; OV/BV, osteoid volume/bone volume; OS/BS, osteoid surface/bone surface. Same letters indicate significant difference at $p < 0.05$. (From Nazrun et al., *Curr. Top. Pharmacol.*, 9(2), 107, 2005.)

The improvement showed by the three vitamin E groups were even better than the baseline and age-matched control groups, with the γ-tocotrienol isomer showing the highest efficacy (Table 23.4, Figure 23.8) (Hermizi et al., 2009).

In order to measure the dynamic histomorphometric parameters, the rats were injected with calcein, a fluorochrome that is taken up by calcium and is incorporated into growing bone. The intraperitoneal injection was done 9 and 2 days before sacrifice. When the undecalcified, unstained bone was viewed under a fluorescent microscope, two greenish fluorescent lines (double-labeled surface, dLs) seen distinctly indicate significant bone growth, whereas a single line (single-labeled surface, sLs) indicates failure of bone growth within the 7 days in between the injections (Figure 23.9). The mineral apposition rate (MAR) and bone formation rate (BFR) were calculated by the software from the sLs and dLs data (Table 23.3).

Our results showed that the vitamin E-treated groups, especially the γ-tocotrienol (GTT) group had less sLs, and this was confirmed quantitatively (Table 23.4, Figure 23.10). Consequently the mineral apposition rate and bone formation rate were higher in the vitamin E groups. Again the improvements were even better than the control groups, with the GTT group showing the highest efficacy among the three types of vitamin E (Table 23.4) (Hermizi et al., 2009).

We have thus shown that tocotrienol was able to prevent as well as reverse bone loss seen in oxidative stress, estrogen deficiency, and nicotine exposure. In fact, it was clearly seen in the

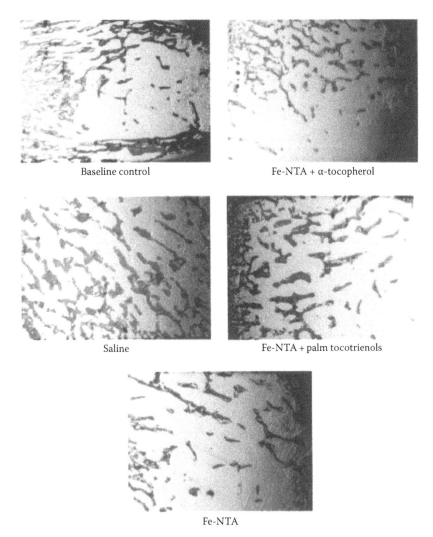

Baseline control

Fe-NTA + α-tocopherol

Saline

Fe-NTA + palm tocotrienols

Fe-NTA

FIGURE 23.4 The bony trabeculae stained black by Von Kossa. The effects of Fe-NTA and tocotrienol supplementation can be seen (×5 magnification). (From Nazrun, A.S. et al., *Curr. Top. Pharmacol.*, 9(2), 107, 2005.)

nicotine-induced osteoporosis study that the tocotrienols significantly improved the histomorphometric parameters compared to the baseline control and age-matched control groups. This led us to hypothesize that besides its antiresorptive action, tocotrienols may also have bone anabolic properties. This will further increase its anti-osteoporotic effects, and may even increase peak bone mass in normal subjects.

23.5 EFFECTS OF TOCOTRIENOLS ON LIPID PEROXIDATION AND ANTIOXIDANTS IN BONE

Lipids accumulated in the bone undergo oxidation, and oxidized lipids exert adverse effects on bone by targeting osteoclastic and osteoblastic cells (Parhami et al., 1997). Oxidized lipids promote bone resorption (Garrett et al., 1990) by recruitment and differentiation of osteoclast precursor cells and also by inhibiting osteoblast differentiation (Parhami et al., 2000). Our earlier studies have proven that treating rats with an oxidizing agent (Fe-NTA) caused bone loss and can lead to osteoporosis,

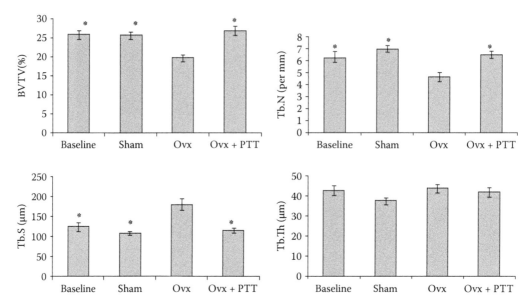

FIGURE 23.5 Structural bone histomorphometric parameters. BV/TV, bone volume/total volume; TbTh, trabecular thickness; TbN, trabecular number; TbSp, trabecular separation; Baseline, baseline control group; sham, sham-operated group; Ovx, ovariectomized group; Ovx + PTT, ovx + tocotrienols group; *indicates significant difference from Ovx at $p < 0.05$. (From Norliza, M., Thesis, Universiti Kebangsaan Malaysia, Selangor, Malaysia, 2007.)

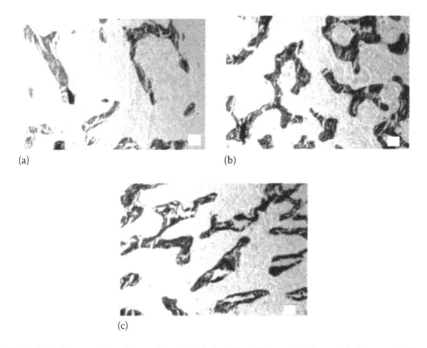

FIGURE 23.6 The bony trabeculae stained black by Von Kossa. (a) Ovx; (b) Sham; (c) Ovx + PTT. Supplementing tocotrienols to ovariectomized rats clearly prevented the bone loss seen in the ovariectomized group (×5 magnification). (From Norliza, M., Thesis, Universiti Kebangsaan Malaysia, Selangor, Malaysia, 2007.)

TABLE 23.1
Cellular (Static) Bone Histomorphometric Parameters

	Baseline	Sham	Ovx	Ovx + PTT
Oc.S (%)	2.7 ± 0.35*	3.08 ± 0.26*	7 ± 0.88	2.95 ± 0.25*
Ob.S (%)	9.9 ± 0.66*,a	9.49 ± 0.38*,a	21.54 ± 1.47	19.7 ± 1.12[b]
OS/BS (%)	7.52 ± 1.2*	6.27 ± 0.97*	21.18 ± 0.85	10.27 ± 1.37*
OV/BV (%)	3.59 ± 0.55*	3.08 ± 0.58*	11.15 ± 0.72	5.46 ± 0.32*

Source: Norliza M., 2007, Thesis, Universiti Kebangsaan Malaysia, Selangor, Malaysia.
OcN, osteoclast number; ObN, osteoblast number; ES/BS, eroded surface/bone surface; OV/BV, osteoid volume/bone volume; OS/BS, osteoid surface/bone surface.
[a,b] Different letters indicate significant difference at p < 0.05.
* Indicates significant difference from Ovx at p < 0.05.

TABLE 23.2
Bone Histomorphometric Parameters in Male Sprague-Dawley Rats

	C	N2	N4	NC
BV/TV (%)	31.26 ± 0.98	25.01 ± 1.55*	24.53 ± 1.13*	25.34 ± 1.12*
Tb.Th (μm)	52.17 ± 1.40	46.23 ± 2.14	43.99 ± 1.45*	45.44 ± 1.66*
Tb.N (mm⁻¹)	6.04 ± 0.23	5.52 ± 0.28	5.55 ± 0.18	5.63 ± 0.33
Tb.Sp (μm)	116.95 ± 5.82	146.65 ± 9.32	141.97 ± 5.72	143.73 ± 11.14
Ob.S/BS (%)	57.69 ± 0.65	46.94 ± 3.77*	43.50 ± 0.97*	44.67 ± 2.60*
Oc.S/BS (%)	18.50 ± 1.78	24.44 ± 1.81*,**	24.20 ± 0.97*,**	23.56 ± 0.55
sLS/BS (%)	41.47 ± 2.22	55.87 ± 2.03*	57.90 ± 1.27*	55.07 ± 1.46*
dLS/BS (%)	48.00 ± 1.80	28.36 ± 1.24*	27.86 ± 1.20*	30.83 ± 2.00*
MAR (μm/day)	0.89 ± 0.02	0.40 ± 0.01*	0.44 ± 0.01*,**	0.51 ± 0.01*,**,***
BFR/BS (μm³/μm² daily)	60.91 ± 1.73	22.03 ± 0.47*	24.88 ± 0.64*,**	29.63 ± 0.65*,**,***

Source: Hermizi, H. et al., *Calcif. Tissue Int.*, 88, 41, 2011.
C, control (no treatment, 4 months); N2, nicotine (7 mg/kg nicotine, 2 months); N4, nicotine (7 mg/kg nicotine, 4 months); NC, nicotine cessation (7 mg/kg nicotine, 2 months + no treatment, 2 months); n = 7.
Values expressed as mean ± SEM. p < 0.05 is considered significant. *p < 0.05 compared with C group, ** p < 0.05 compared with N2 group, ***p < 0.05 compared with N4 group.

and supplementation with an antioxidant, tocotrienol, was able to prevent the bone loss (Nazrun et al., 2005). In order to determine the lipid peroxidation activity in the bone itself, we measured that level of thiobarbituric acid reactive substances, TBARS and the activity of the antioxidant enzyme, glutathione peroxidase in grounded femoral rat bones.

In this study 3 month old male Sprague-Dawley rats, weighing 200–250 g, were divided into seven groups and administered either tocopherol acetate or palm tocotrienol mixture using oral gavage needles in different doses as follows: (1) vehicle olive oil (age-matched control); (2) ATF30 group, receiving 30 mg/kg α-tocopherol acetate; (3) ATF60 group, receiving 60 mg/kg α-tocopherol acetate; (4) ATF100 group, receiving 100 mg/kg α-tocopherol acetate; (5) TT30 group, receiving 30 mg/kg palm tocotrienol mixture; (6) TT60 group, receiving 60 mg/kg palm tocotrienol mixture; and (7) TT100 group, receiving 100 mg/kg palm tocotrienol mixture (Sandra et al., 2008). The rats were not subjected to any osteoporotic stress. The vitamin E treatment was given for 4 months.

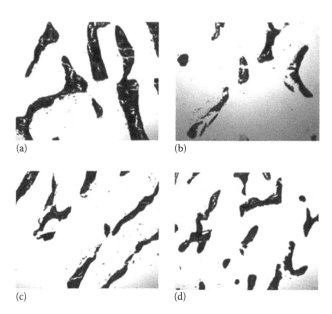

FIGURE 23.7 Photomicrographs of trabecular bone. Undecalcified section (×100 magnification) shows trabecular bone (black) with white background stain using von Kossa method in five groups. Note that all test groups (N2, N4, and NC) showed lower trabecular bone volume (BV/TV) relative to the C group. (a) C, control (no treatment, 4 months); (b) N2, nicotine (7 mg/kg nicotine, 2 months); (c) N4, nicotine (7 mg/kg nicotine, 4 months); (d) NC, nicotine cessation (7 mg/kg nicotine, 2 months; no treatment, 2 months). (Hermizi, H. et al., *Calcif. Tissue Int.* 88, 41, 2011.)

TABLE 23.3
Animal Groupings and Treatment

Groups	Treatment Phases	
	First 2 Months	**Following 2 Months**
Baseline (B, n = 7)	Killed at the commencement of the study	
Control (C, n = 7)	Normal saline (+olive oil)	Normal saline (+olive oil)
Nicotine (N, n = 7)	Nicotine 7 mg/kg (+olive oil)	Killed
Nicotine cessation (NC, n = 7)	Nicotine 7 mg/kg (+olive oil)	Normal saline (+olive oil)
Tocotrienol-enhanced fraction (TEF, n = 7)	Nicotine 7 mg/kg (+olive oil)	TEF 60 mg/kg (+normal saline)
γ-Tocotrienol (GTT, n = 7)	Nicotine 7 mg/kg (+olive oil)	GTT 60 mg/kg (+normal saline)
α-Tocopherol group (ATF, n = 7)	Nicotine 7 mg/kg (+olive oil)	ATF 60 mg/kg (+normal saline)

Source: Hermizi, H. et al., *Calif. Tissue Int.*, 84, 67, 2009.
Nicotine was given intraperitoneally, 7 mg/kg/day; vitamin E was given by oral gavage, 60 mg/kg/day.

The results showed that the group given the highest dose of tocotrienols (TT100) had significantly lower lipid peroxidation level, which was reflected in the lowest thiobarbituric acid reactive substances, TBARS (malondialdehyde) values compared to all the other groups, including the age-matched control group (Figure 23.11). Both ATF and TT increased the activity of the antioxidant enzyme, glutathione peroxidase, in a dose-dependent manner. However, only TT100 was able to raise the activity to above that of the control group (Figure 23.12). These results showed that the tocotrienols are better antioxidants in the bone compared to α-tocopherol (Maniam et al., 2008).

TABLE 23.4
Results of Bone Histomorphometric Parameters

Group	BV/TV (%)	Tb.Th (μm)	Tb.N (mm^{-1})	Oc.S/BS (%)	ES/BS (%)	sLS/BS (%)	MAR (μm/day)	BFR/BS (μm^3/μm^2/day)
B	30.8 ± 2.00	47.0 ± 2.31	6.7 ± 0.80	15.9 ± 0.80	23.0 ± 1.61	42.5 ± 1.41	0.9 ± 0.01	57.7 ± 1.65
C	31.3 ± 0.98	52.2 ± 1.40	6.0 ± 0.23	18.5 ± 1.78	20.7 ± 0.27	41.5 ± 2.22	0.9 ± 0.02	60.9 ± 1.73
N	25.0 ± 1.55[a,b]	46.2 ± 2.14	5.5 ± 0.28	24.4 ± 1.81[a,b]	31.3 ± 0.47[a,b]	55.9 ± 2.03[a,b]	0.4 ± 0.01[a,b]	22.0 ± 0.65[a,b]
NC	25.3 ± 1.12[b]	45.4 ± 1.66	5.6 ± 0.33	23.6 ± 0.55[a,b]	30.0 ± 0.47[a,b]	55.1 ± 1.46[a,b]	0.5 ± 0.01[a,b]	29.6 ± 0.65[a,b]
TEF	40.8 ± 0.52[a,b,c,d]	61.2 ± 1.49[a,b,c,d]	6.8 ± 0.20	9.0 ± 0.47[a,b,c,d]	12.6 ± 0.79[a,b,c,d]	22.3 ± 1.64[a,b,c,d]	1.2 ± 0.03[a,b,c,d]	93.6 ± 2.13[a,b,c,d]
GTT	44.9 ± 0.89[a,b,c,d]	65.3 ± 2.15[a,b,c,d]	7.0 ± 0.24[c]	8.7 ± 0.20[a,b,c,d]	11.6 ± 0.31[a,b,c,d]	23.3 ± 1.62[a,b,c,d]	1.4 ± 0.04[a,b,c,d,e]	111.2 ± 5.61[a,b,c,d,e]
ATF	41.8 ± 1.53[a,b,c,d]	59.6 ± 2.05[a,c,d]	7.1 ± 0.41[c,d]	13.1 ± 1.21[b,c,d]	17.0 ± 0.55[b,c,d,e,f]	27.9 ± 1.93[a,b,c,d]	1.3 ± 0.05[a,b,c,d,f]	95.2 ± 5.45[a,b,c,d,f]

Source: Hermizi, H. et al., *Calif. Tissue Int.*, 84, 67, 2009.
Values expressed as mean ± SEM. $p < 0.05$ is considered significant.

[a] Significantly different from B group.
[b] Significantly different from C group.
[c] Significantly different from N group.
[d] Significantly different from NC group.
[e] Significantly different from TEF group.
[f] Significantly different from GTT group.

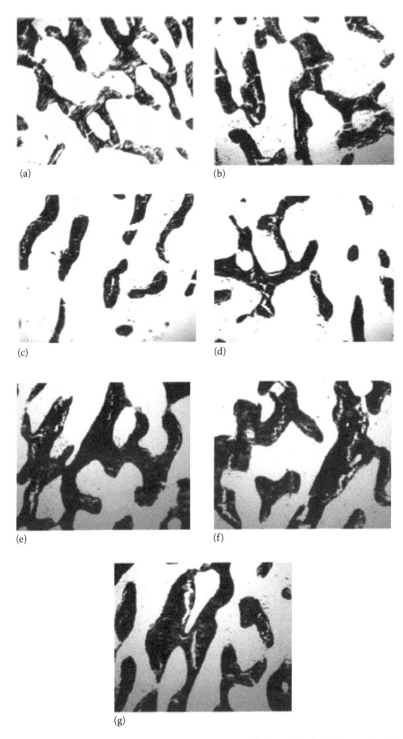

FIGURE 23.8 Photomicrographs of trabecular bone. Undecalcified section (×100 magnification) shows trabecular bone (black) with white background stained using the von Kossa method in seven groups: (a) B, baseline control; (b) C, control; (c) N, nicotine; (d) NC, nicotine cessation; (e) TEF, tocotrienol-enhanced fraction; (f) GTT, γ-tocotrienol; and (g) ATF, α-tocopherol groups. Note that the vitamin E-treated groups (TEF, GTT, ATF) showed thicker and more abundant trabeculae relative to the other groups. (From Hermizi, H. et al., *Calcif. Tissue Int.*, 84, 67, 2009.)

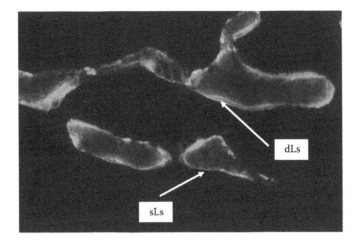

FIGURE 23.9 Photomicrograph showing single-labeled surface (sLs) and double-labeled surface (dLs).

23.6 TOCOTRIENOLS AND BONE STRENGTH

The current antiosteoporotic drugs are mainly bone resorption inhibitors that act by suppressing bone resorption in order to stabilize the bone mass (Canalis et al., 2007). Anabolic agents are required to restore the density of osteoporotic bone. An anabolic agent for bone is defined as an agent that increases bone strength by increasing bone mass substantially as a result of an overall increase in bone remodeling in favor of the formation phase rather than the resorption phase (Riggs and Parfitt 2005). Our recent study had shown that vitamin E did not stop at treating nicotine-induced osteoporosis but continued to improve the structural and cellular properties of trabecular bone until they were significantly above the control values (Hermizi et al., 2009).

To study whether tocotrienols have bone anabolic properties, we determined the bone structural histomorphometry and bone biomechanical strength in normal male rats not subjected to any osteoporotic stress. The bone histomorphometry showed that γ-tocotrienol improved bone structure better than the control group, while α-tocopherol did not have much effect (Figures 23.13 and 23.14; Shuid et al., 2010).

Strength and biomechanical properties of the femoral bones were assessed using an Instron Universal Testing Machine (model 5560; Instron, Canton, MA) equipped with the Bluehill 2 software. The femur was placed in the three-point bending configuration, whereby it was placed on two lower supports that were 5 mm apart. The force was applied at the mid-diaphysis on the anterior surface such that the anterior surface was in compression and the posterior surface in tension until the bone fractures (Figure 23.15). The main parameters of the biomechanical test can be divided into extrinsic and intrinsic: the extrinsic parameters (load, displacement, and stiffness) measure the properties of whole bones whereas the intrinsic parameters (stress, strain, and Young's modulus of elasticity) measure the material of the bone (Figure 23.16; Shuid et al., 2010).

Gamma-tocotrienol was found to improve every biomechanical parameter as compared to the control group, while α-tocopherol did not show much effect (Figures 23.17 and 23.18; Shuid et al., 2010).

The results from this study showed that γ-tocotrienol was highly effective in improving the structure and strength of normal bones. This indicates that γ-tocotrienol may have bone anabolic properties besides its antiresorptive properties. Thus, it has the potential to improve the peak bone mass when supplemented to normal adults.

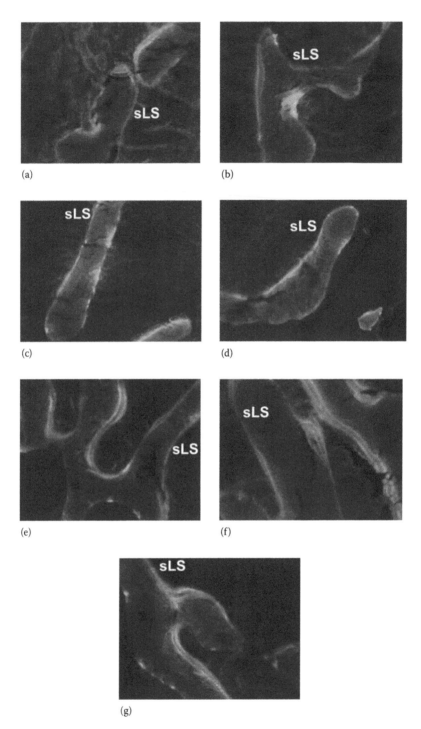

(a)   (b)

(c)   (d)

(e)   (f)

(g)

FIGURE 23.10 Photomicrograph shows calcein labels along trabecular bone, demonstrated using fluorescence microscopy in an undecalcified section without staining (magnification ×200): (a) B, baseline control; (b) C, control; (c) N, nicotine; (d) NC, nicotine cessation, (e) TEF, tocotrienol-enhanced fraction; (f) GTT, γ-tocotrienol; and (g) ATF (α-tocopherol) groups. Note that N and NC groups showed thin interlabeled distance compared to the other groups, indicating more sLs. The vitamin E-treated groups (TEF, GTT, ATF) had less sLS and more dLs relative to the other control groups. (From Hermizi, H. et al., *Calcif. Tissue Int.*, 84, 67, 2009.)

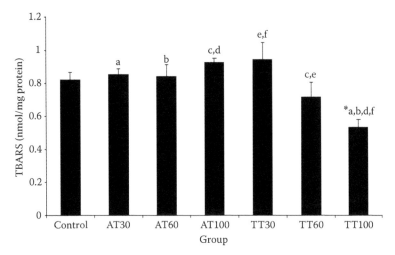

FIGURE 23.11 Effect of α-tocopherol (ATF) and palm tocotrienol (TT) supplementation on lipid peroxidation in the femur of adult male rats. Values marked by the same letters indicate significant difference between groups at $p < 0.05$; *indicates significant difference from the control group at $p < 0.05$. TBARS, thiobarbituric acid-reactive substances. (From Sandra, M. et al., *Basic Clin. Pharmacol. Toxicol.*, 103, 55, 2008.)

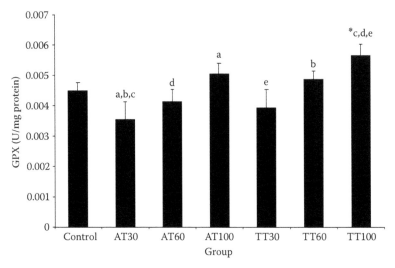

FIGURE 23.12 Effect of α-tocopherol (ATF) and palm tocotrienol (TT) on the specific activity of glutathione peroxidase (GPX) in the femur of adult male rats. Values marked by the same letters indicate significant difference between groups at $p < 0.05$; *$p < 0.05$, significantly different from control group. (From Sandra, M. et al., *Basic Clin. Pharmacol. Toxicol.*, 103, 55, 2008.)

23.7 CONCLUSION

Osteoporosis is a common disease especially affecting the elderly population. The complications of osteoporosis, such as pain, deformities, reduced mobility, and fractures cause significant morbidity and even mortality. The current drugs used to treat osteoporosis vary in safety and efficacy. In general, the more highly efficacious drugs have more side effects. Toxicity studies of tocotrienols

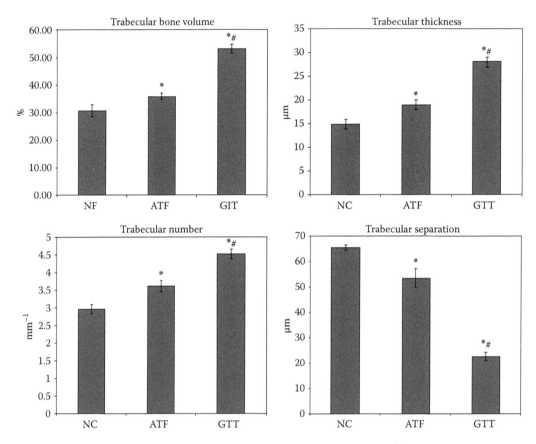

FIGURE 23.13 Structural bone histomorphometry. NC normal control group, ATF a-tocopherol group, and GTT c-tocotrienol group. *Indicates significant difference compared to NC group; # indicates significant difference compared to ATF group (p < 0.05). Data are expressed as mean ± SEM. (Nazrun, A.S. et al., *J. Bone Miner. Metab.,* 28(2), 149, 2010.)

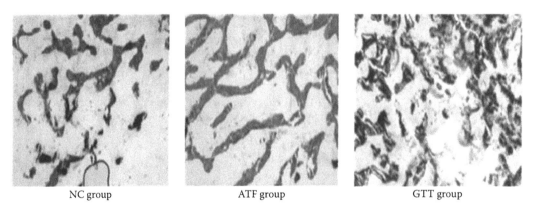

FIGURE 23.14 Photomicrographs of undecalcified rat femur stained with Von Kossa (950). The trabeculae are stained black. Grossly, GTT and ATF groups appear to have more trabeculae than the NC group; the GTT group has more trabeculae than the ATF group. NC vehicle, ATF 60 mg/kg α-tocopherol, and GTT 60 mg/kg γ-tocotrienols. (Nazrun, A.S. et al., *J. Bone Miner. Metab.,* 28(2), 149, 2010.)

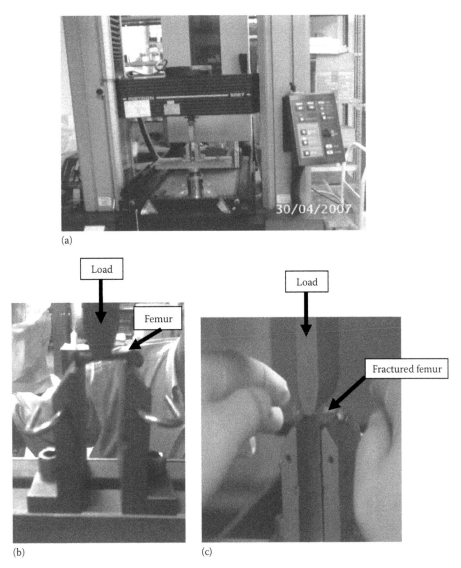

FIGURE 23.15   (a) Instron Universal Testing Machine; (b) Three-point bending configuration; (c) The rat femur fractures.

have found that it has a wide safety margin and is safe at the effective doses used (Nakamura et al., 2001, Ima-Nirwana et al., 2011). From the results of the studies shown earlier, it is clear that tocotrienols improve bone structure and strength in our animal models. It has demonstrated antiresorptive as well as anabolic effects on bone. As shown by the studies of Nazrun et al. (2005) and Sandra et al. (2008), the protective effects of the tocotrienols on bone are most probably due to its antioxidant properties. In view of all these findings, we conclude that tocotrienol has the potential to be developed as an antiosteoporotic agent. In addition to its efficacy and safety profile, its convenient oral administration and easy availability make it an attractive agent to be used in the long term to increase peak bone mass as well as to prevent and treat osteoporosis. However, further studies need to be conducted to elucidate its molecular mechanisms of action. Clinical studies are also needed to determine the efficacy and safety in humans.

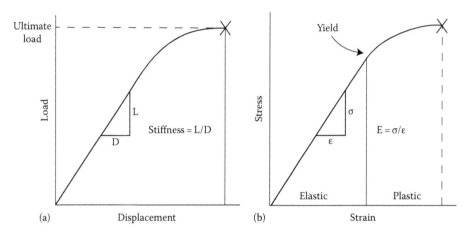

FIGURE 23.16   (a) Load-displacement curve measures extrinsic properties of bone (load, displacement, and stiffness). (b) Stress-strain curve measures intrinsic properties of bone (viscoelasticity, stress, and strain). (From Helfrich, M.H. and Ralston, S.H. (eds.), Bone research protocols, In: *Methods in Molecular Medicine*, Humana Press, Totowa, NJ, Vol. 80, p. 450, 2003.)

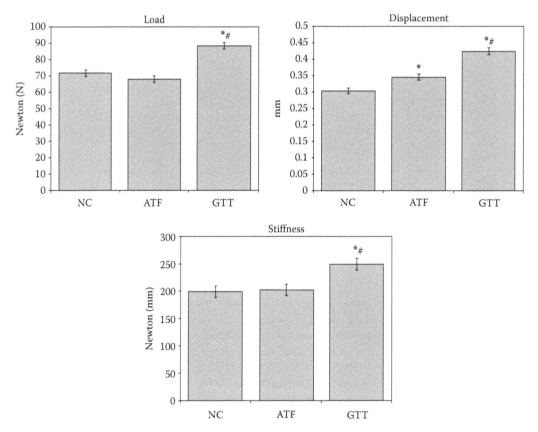

FIGURE 23.17   Extrinsic parameters of bone strength. *Indicates significant differences compared to NC group; # indicates significant differences compared to ATF group at ($p < 0.05$). Data are expressed as mean ± SEM. NC normal control group, ATF α-tocopherol group, and GTT γ-tocotrienol group. (Nazrun, A.S. et al., *J. Bone Miner. Metab.*, 28(2), 149, 2010.)

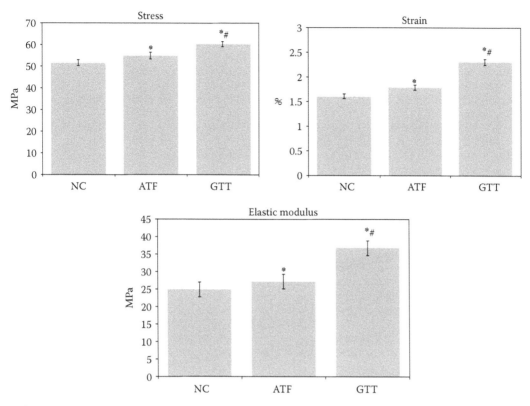

FIGURE 23.18 Intrinsic properties of bone. *Indicates significant differences compared to NC group; # indicates significant differences compared to ATF group at (p < 0.05). Data are expressed as mean ± SEM. NC normal control group, ATF α-tocopherol group, and GTT γ-tocotrienol group. (Nazrun, A.S. et al., *J. Bone Miner. Metab.,* 28(2), 149, 2010.)

REFERENCES

Abe T, Chow JW, Lean JM, Chambers TJ. 1993. Estrogen does not restore bone lost after ovariectomy in the rat. *J Bone Miner Res* 8(7):831–838.

Basu S, Whiteman M, Mattey DL, Halliwell B. 2001. Raised levels of F2-isoprostanes and prostaglandin F2á in different rheumatic diseases. *Ann Rheum Dis* 60:627–631.

Canalis E, Giustina A, Bilezikian JP. 2007. Mechanisms of anabolic therapies for osteoporosis. *N Engl J Med* 357:905–916.

Chapurlat R. 2008. Epidemiology of osteoporosis. *J Soc Biol* 202: 251–255.

Ebina Y, Okada S, Hamazaki S, Toda Y, Midorikawa O. 1991. Impairment of bone formation with aluminum and ferric nitrilotriacetate complexes. *Calcif Tissue Int* 48(1):28–36.

Garret IR, Boyce BF, Oretto ROC, Bonewald L, Poser J, Mundy GR. 1990. Oxygen-derived free radicals stimulate osteoclastic bone resorption in rodent bone in vitro and in vivo. *J Clin Invest* 85:632–639.

Hapidin H, Othman F, Soelaiman IN, Shuid IN, Mohamed N. 2011. Effects of nicotine administration and nicotine cessation on bone histomorphometry and bone biomarkers in Sprague–Dawley male rats. *Calcif Tissue Int* 88:41–47.

Helfrich, MH, Ralston, SH. (eds.). 2003. Bone research protocols. In: *Methods in Molecular Medicine*, Vol. 80, Totowa, NJ: Humana Press, p. 450.

Henemyre CL, Scales DK, Hokett SD, Cuenin MF, Peacock ME, Parker MH, Brewer PD, Chuang AH. 2003. Nicotine stimulates osteoclast resorption in a porcine marrow cell model. *J Periondontol* 74:1440–1446.

Hermizi H, Faizah O, Ima-Nirwana S, Ahmad Nazrun S, Norazlina M. 2009. Beneficial effects of tocotrienol on bone histomorphometric parameters in Sprague-Dawley male rats after nicotine cessation. *Calcif Tissue Int* 84:67–74.

Ima-Nirwana S, Cheng CT, Norazlina M. 2005. Effects of nicotine on bone mineral density and calcium homeostasis in male Sprague-Dawley rats. *Curr Top Pharmacol* 9(2):125–129.

Ima-Nirwana S, Nursyazwani Y, Nazrun AS, Norliza M, Norazlina M. 2011. Subacute and subchronic toxicity of palm vitamin E in mice. *J Pharmacol Toxicol* 6(2):166–173.

Kalpana C, Menon VP. 2004. Protective effect of curcumin on circulatory lipid peroxidation and antioxidant status during nicotine-induced toxicity. *Toxicol Mech Methods* 14:339–343.

Kapoor D, Jones TH. 2005. Smoking and hormones in health and endocrine disorders. *Eur J Endocrinol* 152:491–499.

Lean JM, Davies JT, Fuller K. 2003. A crucial role for thiol antioxidants in estrogen-deficiency bone loss. *J Clin Invest* 112(6):915–923.

Maniam S, Mohamed N, Shuid AN, Soelaiman IN. 2008. Palm tocotrienol exerted better antioxidant activities in bone than α-tocopherol. Basic *Clin Pharmacol Toxicol* 103:55–60.

Mosekilde L, 1995. Assessing bone quality—Animal models in preclinical osteoporosis research. *Bone* 7(4):343S–352S.

Muthusami S, Ramachandran I, Muthusamy B, Vasudevan G, Prabhu V, Subramaniam V, Jagadeesan A, Narasimhan S. 2005. Ovariectomy induces oxidative stress and impairs bone antioxidant system in adult rats. *Clin Chim Acta* 360(1–2):81–86.

Nakamura H, Furukawa F, Nishikawa A, Miyauchi M, Son HY, Imazawa T, Hirose M. 2001. Oral toxicity of a toctrienol preparation in rats. *Food Chem Toxicol* 39(8):799–805.

Nazrun AS, Luke DA, Khalid BAK, Ima-Nirwana S. 2005. Vitamin E protects from free-radical damage on femur of rats treated with ferric nitrilotriacetate. *Curr Top Pharmacol* 9(2):107–115.

Norazlina M, Nik Farideh YMK, Arizi A, Faisal A, Ima-Nirwana S, 2004. Effects of nicotine on bone resorbing cytokines in male rats. *Int Med J* 3(2):1–9. www.e-imj.com/Vol3-No2/Vol-3-No2-B10htm

Norliza M. 2007. The effects of vitamin E supplementation on bone metabolism in ovariectomised rats based on histomorphometric and biochemical parameters. Thesis. Universiti Kebangsaan Malaysia, Selangor, Malaysia.

Ozgocmen S, Kaya H, Fadillioglu E, Aydogan R, Yilmaz Z. 2007. Role of antioxidant systems, lipid peroxidation and nitric oxide in postmenopausal osteoporosis. *Mol Cell Biochem* 295(1–2):45–52.

Parfitt AM. 2000. Skeletal heterogeneity and the purposes of bone remodeling: Implications for the understanding of osteoporosis. In: *Osteoporosis*. 2nd edn. Marcus R, Feldman D, Kelsey J (eds.), San Diego, CA: Academic Press, pp. 433–447.

Parfitt AM, Drezner MK, Glorieux FH, Kanis JA, Malluche H, Meunier PJ, Ott SM, Recker RR. 1987. Bone histomorphometry: Standardization of nomenclature, symbols and units. *J Bone Miner Res* 2(6):595–610.

Parhami F, Garfinkel A, Demer LL. 2000. Role of lipids in osteoporosis. *Aterioscler Thromb Vasc Biol* 20:2346–2348.

Parhami F, Marrow AD, Balucan J, Leitinger N, Watson AD, Tintut Y. et al. 1997. Lipid oxidation products have opposite effects on calcifying vascular cell and bone cell differentiation, a possible explanation for the paradox of arterial calcification in osteoporotic patients. *Aterioscler Thromb Vasc Biol* 17:680–687.

Riggs BL, Parfitt AM. 2005. Drugs used to treat osteoporosis: The critical need for a uniform nomenclature based on their action on bone remodeling. *J Bone Miner Res* 20:177–184.

Shuid AN, Mehat Z, Mohamed N, Muhammad N, Soelaiman IN. 2010. Vitamin E exhibits bone anabolic actions in normal male rats. *J Bone Miner Metab* 28(2):149–156.

Siti Khadijah A. 2011. Effects of heated palm oil and soy oil on factors related to atherosclerosis in ovariectomised rats. Thesis. Universiti Kebangsaan Malaysia, Selangor, Malaysia.

Takeuchi K, Okada S, Yukihiro S, Inoue H. 1997. The inhibitory effects of aluminium and iron on bone formation, in vivo and in vitro study. *Pathophysiology* 4:97–104.

Wetscher GJ, Bagchi M, Bagchi D, Perdikis G, Hinder PR, Glaser K, Hinder RA. 1995. Free radical production in nicotine treated pancreatic tissue. *Free Radic Biol Med* 18(5):877–882.

Yalin S, Bagis S, Polat G, Dogruer N, Cenk Aksit S, Hatungil R, Erdogan C. 2005. Is there a role of free oxygen radicals in primary male osteoporosis? *Clin Exp Rheumatol* 23(5):689–692.

Yee JK, Ima-Nirwana S. 1998. Palm vitamin E protects bone against ferric-nitrilotriacetate-induced impairment of bone calcification. *Asia Pac J Pharmacol* 13:1–7.

24 Tocotrienol and Physiology of Reproduction

M.H. Rajikin, N. Mokhtar, A. Chatterjee, and Y.S. Kamsani

CONTENTS

24.1 INTRODUCTION

The majority of earlier studies on vitamin E have focused on its total forms without considering single isoform. Compared to tocopherols, tocotrienols have been poorly studied (Sen et al., 2006, 2007b; Miyamoto et al., 2009). The research trend has, however, been shifted to isoforms of vitamin E other than alpha-tocopherol, namely, the tocotrienols (TCT) (Rahmat et al., 1993). TCT is now found to possess neuroprotective, anticancer, antioxidant, and cholesterol-lowering properties that are different from tocopherol (TCP) isomers (Sen et al., 2004). Deficiency of Vitamin E also causes degenerative diseases such as gamma ataxia and Duchenne muscular dystrophy-like muscle degeneration (Aggarwal et al., 2010). It has been documented that many of the beneficial effects of α-tocotrienol are not shared by α-tocopherol (Sen et al., 2006). Since α-TCT shows better mobility through the cell membrane (Suzuki et al., 1993), tocotrienols are believed to have much more potent antioxidant properties than α-tocopherol (Serbinova et al., 1991). In cardiovascular diseases, efficacy of δ- and γ-TCT, the most potent isomers in supporting cardiac health such as coronary heart disease, ischemia-induced arrhythmia, and reduced heart rate accompanied by improved myocardial efficiency are well evident (Rasool et al., 2008). In addition, the beneficial effect of TCT in preventing osteoporosis by increasing bone formation and suppressing bone resorption has been documented (Maniam et al., 2008).

Geva et al. (1996) have proposed a promising potential effect of tocotrienol to improve fertility status. A woman is considered fertile when she has the ability to conceive, maintain the pregnancy, and deliver a healthy baby. Defect at any stage of these processes, even at the stage of folliculogenesis, may lead to infertility. The importance of vitamin E was first observed in the 1930s where rats fed with a vitamin E-deficient diet developed uterine discoloration (Barrie, 1938). A significant decrease in vitamin E along with other antioxidant vitamins has been reported in a population of women with habitual abortion (Simsek et al., 1998). Moreover, in an abnormal pregnancy, vitamin E concentrations are found to be lowered compared to normal pregnancy (Perkins, 2006). The activity of superoxide dismutase (SOD), the endogenous oxygen ion scavenger is also found to be significantly reduced in women whose pregnancy ended in miscarriage compared to healthy pregnant women (Jenkins et al., 2000). Reproduction encompasses very complex physiological processes. Each process of reproduction such as oogenesis, fertilization, embryo cleavage and development, decidual cell reaction, implantation, pregnancy outcome, and parturition is influenced by systemic as well as local factors. In oogenesis itself, other complex processes also take part such as cumulus and corona cell expansion and loosening, cytoplasmic and nuclear maturation.

Knowledge regarding the possible role of TCT, if any in all these processes, is indeed lacking. Tocopherol was found in a small concentration in the follicular fluid of women who underwent *in vitro* fertilization (IVF) compared to the plasma. However, further studies are needed to explore the underlying mechanism of its role in aiding reproductive success (Schweigert et al., 2003).

Scientists have also found the involvement of vitamin E in male reproduction. Male rats treated with α-tocopherol at a dose of 100 mg/kg for 120 days postpartum showed significant reduction in lipid peroxidation, a decrease in cellular apoptosis and an increase in the maturation of seminiferous epithelium (Vigueras-Villasenor et al., 2011). Similar beneficial effects of vitamin E have also been documented in rats treated at a dose of 60 mg/kg body weight for 60 days (Mat Nor et al., 2006). The test animals showed a consistent increase in the quality of sperm and testicular cells (Mat Nor et al., 2006). The antioxidant action of vitamin E has been tested on 13 healthy smokers who received a substantial amount of α-tocopherol supplementation for 2 weeks. Results showed a significant reduction of lipid peroxidation in the subjects involved (Hoshino et al., 1990). While examining the antioxidant as well as free radical scavenging effects, tocotrienols appear to be superior to tocopherols (Suzuki et al., 1993). It has been shown that α-tocopherol transfer protein (TTP)-deficient female mice are infertile (Terasawa et al., 2000). However, restoration of fertility of TTP knockout mice following oral supplementation of α-tocotrienol suggests that distribution of α-tocotrienol to vital organs is relatively TTP-independent (Khanna et al., 2005)

We have recently reported that TCT-rich vitamin E is able to reverse the nicotine-induced retarded embryogenesis and pregnancy loss in rats (Mokhtar et al., 2008). We have also found that TCT-rich vitamin E supplementation in the nicotine-treated rats have lower plasma malondialdehyde (MDA), a biomarker for oxidative stress, as compared to its nicotine-treated counterpart (Mokhtar et al., 2008). In addition, supplementation of 60 mg/kg γ-TCT significantly reduces fetal loss in the nicotine-treated mice (Kamsani et al., 2011). These findings clearly indicate that γ-TCT, a potent antioxidant, has a huge potential in the regulation of reproductive processes. However, the molecular mechanism of TCT in reproduction is still open for further investigations.

24.2 PHYSIOLOGY OF REPRODUCTION

During folliculogenesis, the preovulatory oocyte undergoes meiotic maturation that results in the cytoplasmic and chromosomal changes. This is followed by ovulation, where the oocyte is then transported into the fallopian tube for fertilization. During transport, spermatozoa undergo capacitation and acrosome reaction in order to enable them to penetrate the oocyte. Following fertilization, the oocyte becomes an embryo, which while being transported along the fallopian tube undergoes cleavage to 2, 4, 8, and 16 cells, morula, and blastocyst (Figure 24.1A through H).

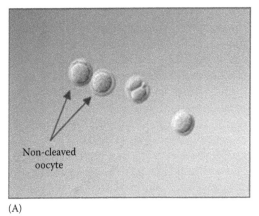

(A)

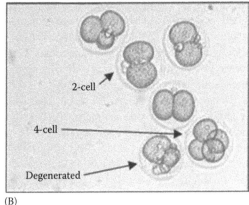

(B)

FIGURE 24.1 Development of preimplantation mice embryos incubated in 5% CO_2 at 37°C using the Whitten medium (M16). (A) shows a single non-cleaved oocyte, (B) shows a two- to four-cell embryos,

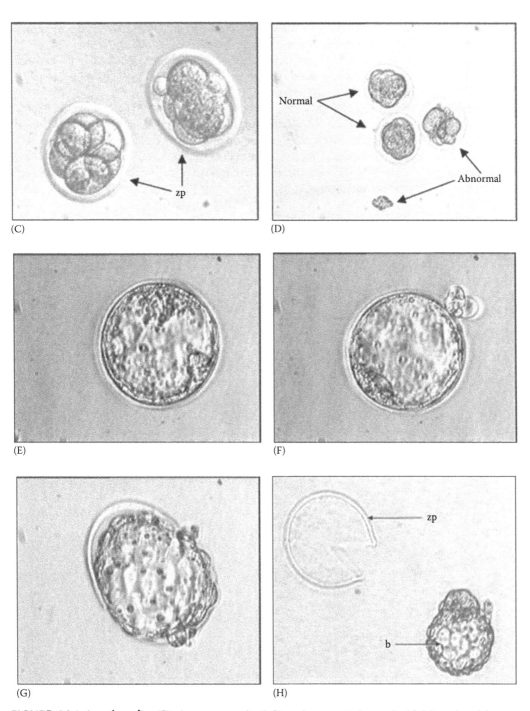

FIGURE 24.1 (continued) (C) shows a morula (left) and compacted morula (right) enclosed in zona pellucida (zp), (D) shows a compacted morula (normal and abnormal), (E) shows an expanded blastocyst, (F) shows an early stage of a hatching blastocyst, (G) shows a late stage of a hatching blastocyst, and (H) shows a fully hatched blastocyst.

The developing conceptus (blastocyst) will be implanted in the uterus. Understanding the mechanism of fertilization in mammals through the *in vivo* process is difficult. Thus, imitating such natural processes within a defined environmental condition will enable researchers to study not only the mechanism of fertilization, but also the micromanipulating technique to collect embryos. Therefore, assisted reproductive technologies (ART) have become an important tool in the study of reproduction, where the manipulation of various determining factors such as medium, pH, concentration of chemical agents, osmolarity, and temperature can be achieved.

Previous reports have shown that the presence of tocopherol in the ovarian fluid may play an important role in oogenesis, preimplantation embryo development, and embryo hatching (Dalvit et al., 2005; Sen et al., 2007a; Jeong et al., 2009). An accumulation of α- and γ-TCT in the egg yolk of zebra finches (Royale et al., 2003) suggests that the deposition of these antioxidants occurs from the dietary intake of the mother to the egg. The scanning (Figure 24.2A through C) and the transmission electron microscopic (Figure 24.3A through I) studies showed that TCT partially reduced the hazardous effects of nicotine by

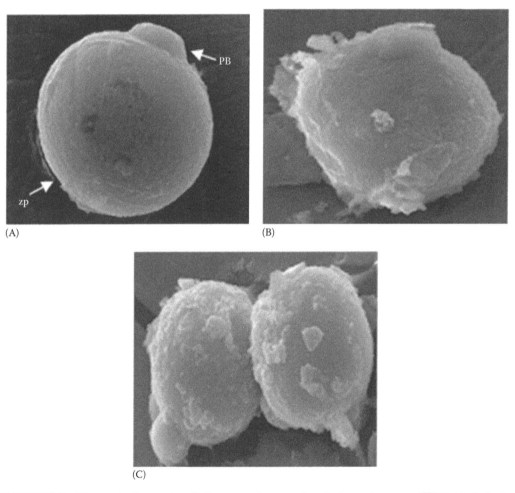

(A)

(B)

(C)

FIGURE 24.2 Changes in the oocytes of all groups using scanning electron microscopy (SEM). (A) A single oocyte with spherical shape obtained from the control group. The surface looks smooth and the zona pellucida intact. The polar body is clearly seen and labeled as PB. (B) The shape and outline of an oocyte from the nicotine-treated mice are not clearly visible. The zona pellucida is also torn and becomes irregular. The polar body was also present. (C) The outline of an oocyte from mice given nicotine with γ-tocotrienol is clearly visible and looks spherical in shape, similar to that of the control mice. The zona pellucida is still intact, although the outer surface is still rough and irregular. (From Rajikin, M.H. et al., *Med. Sci. Monit.*, 15, 378, 2009.)

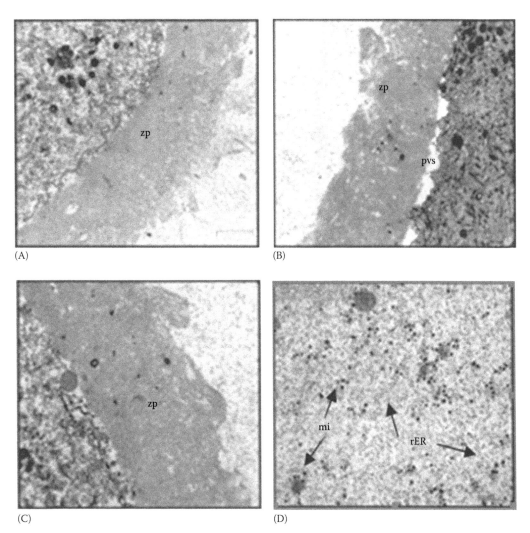

FIGURE 24.3 Transmission electron microscope photographs (TEM) showing the layers of the oocyte from the control (A), nicotine-treated (B), and nicotine plus γ-tocotrienol (C) groups. (A) The zona pellucida (zp) is intact and smooth. The previtelline space (pvs) is tight between the zp and the ooplasm. (B) The zp is torn and loose in the oocyte obtained from nicotine-treated mice. The previtelline space is brightly stained between the zp and the inner side of the oocyte and is greater in size. (C) Supplementation of γ-tocotrienol resulted in an intact and smooth zp. The pvs is also tight, that is, similar to the control mice. Photographs showing the cytoskeletal structures of the oocytes under transmission electron microscope of the control (D), nicotine-treated (E), and nicotine with γ-tocotrienol (F) groups. (D) Less dense rough endoplasmic reticulum (rER) and no detectable vesicles. (E), Dense rER with numerous vesicles in the ooplasm. The mitochondria (mi) in both the groups were evenly distributed. (F) Supplementation of γ-tocotrienol showed less rER and no visible vesicles, as found in the control group. Photographs showing the cytoskeletal structures of the oocytes obtained from the control (G), nicotine-treated (H), and nicotine with γ-tocotrienol (I) groups. (G) A denser matrix with the presence of cristae and fewer remnants of dead cells (rdc). (H) A low number of mitochondria with less dense matrix and no cristae. A large number of vesicles (v) or multivesicular bodies (mv) with multiple areas of rdc or fibrogranular substances. (I) A greater number of mitochondria and dense matrix. The vesicles were also fewer and not prominent. The number of rdc was also less. (From Rajikin, M.H. et al., *Med. Sci. Monit.*, 15, 378, 2009.)

(*continued*)

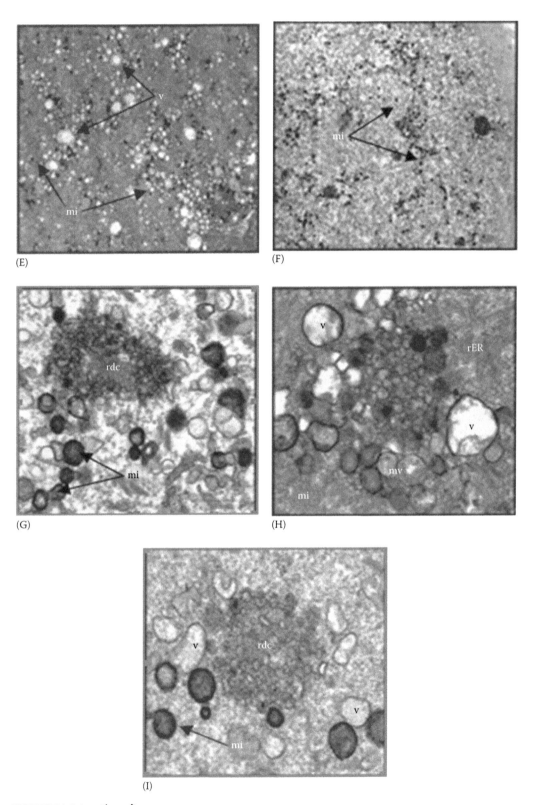

FIGURE 24.3 (continued)

retaining the smooth boundary of the zona pellucida with the tight perivitelline space, less rough endoplasmic reticulum with no visible vesicles and a lower amount of dense mitochondrial matrix (Rajikin et al., 2009). It has, moreover, been shown that supplementation of γ-TCT reduced the plasma MDA concentration compared to that of nicotine-treated controls, which agrees with the findings that TCT reduces the oxidative stress by scavenging free radicals such as hydroxyl (OH^-) and peroxyl (ROO^-) (Brigelius-Floher and Traber, 1999; Mokhtar et al., 2008). Preovulatory maturation of oocytes is known to depend on the stimulation of follicle-stimulating hormone (FSH) followed by luteinizing hormone (LH) surge prior to ovulation. Other sex steroids such as estrogen, progesterone, and testosterone are also involved not only in the process of oocyte maturation, but also in reproduction in general. Following oocyte maturation, the process of fertilization and embryonic development depend on the specific level of estrogen, progesterone, and testosterone. Therefore, the normal function of the hypothalamic-pituitary-ovarian axis in the reproductive processes is crucial.

However, there are two issues to be looked into: whether the pro-oxidant has any effects on the pituitary-ovarian profile, which subsequently determines the maternal endometrial decidualization and fetal outcome, and whether TCT exerts any beneficial effects to maintain endometrial decidualization and fetal outcome while there is generation of excess free radicals.

A study on mice has shown that 10 mg/kg/day corticosterone, a stress hormone induces retarded embryo development which could be reversed by the supplementation of 60 mg/kg/day TCT (Azme et al., 2010a). Supplementation of 120 mg/kg/day TCT also reverses embryonic loss in corticosterone-treated mice (Azme et al., 2010b).

24.3 MOLECULAR MECHANISM OF TOCOTRIENOL

Tocotrienol has great potential to be involved in the formation of new blood vessels in the reproductive system. Angiogenesis in reproduction can easily be observed following the regeneration of endometrial lining during the follicular phase of menstruation. In pregnancy, angiogenesis can also be seen starting from the trophoblast that grows into the endometrium to form a cord until the placenta is formed. Placenta formation is essential to supply nutrients to the embryo *in utero*. In pathological conditions such as cancer, angiogenesis is a process that is related with the cells' survival (Skobe et al., 1997). A recent study on γ-TCT showed that it can inhibit angiogenesis based on the *in vivo* evidence on the number of blood vessels formed on the chick chorioallantoic membrane assay (Li et al., 2011). The *in vivo* evidence of TCT was observed, in which the ICR mice implanted with DLD-1-induced angiogenesis and treated with TCT at 10 mg/day for 5 days showed a significant reduction in the angiogenesis index (Miyazawa et al., 2008). Supporting evidence was also seen in human umbilical vein endothelial cells (HUVEC) treated with TCT at a dose between 5 and 20 μmol/L, which showed a reduction in the migration of cells and the length of tube formation assay (Miyazawa et al., 2008). The mRNA expression of pro-angiogenic cytokines, IL 8 and IL 6, as well as the vascular endothelial growth factor (VEGF) were reduced in HUVEC and mouse mammary cancer cells treated with TCT (Selvaduray et al., 2011). To date, there are no data that describe the role of TCT in promoting or inhibiting angiogenesis in the reproductive system.

All forms of tocotrienols are better than tocopherol in inhibiting normal mammary cell growth (Sylvester et al., 2001). The action was thought to be mediated through the epidermal growth factor (EGF). In addition, γ-TCT has the ability to reduce the cell progression from the G1 to S phase of the cell cycle as seen in the *in vitro* study of mammary tumor cells (Samant et al., 2010). This has provided a basis to study the role of TCT in the cell proliferation during the follicular phase of the menstrual cycle or even in the development of the placenta.

24.4 SUMMARY

Vitamin E as a fertility factor was discovered in 1938. Since then, relatively little has been studied about the role of tocotrienol, the unsaturated analogues of vitamin E in reproduction and fertility. Female reproduction is a complex system that consists of the hypothalamic GnRH-adenohypophyseal gonadotrophs axis, ovary, fallopian tube, uterus, and the placenta. The complexity of the reproductive process is further comprehended by the fact that this process involves not only female but also male factors. Since tocotrienol is more efficiently delivered to several vital organs compared to tocopherol (Suzuki et al., 1993), its beneficial effects have been briefed in this chapter. However, the role of TCT in relation to reproduction in general warrants further investigation.

REFERENCES

Aggarwal BB, Sundaram C, Prasad S, and Kannappan R. 2010. Tocotrienols, the vitamin E of the 21st century: Its potential against cancer and other chronic diseases. *Biochem Pharmacol*; 80: 1613–1631.

Azme N, Rajikin MH, Nor-Ashikin MNH, and Satar N. 2010a. Cessation of embryonic development in mice treated with corticosterone. *Proceedings of the 19th Scientific Conference on Endocrine Society, Malaysia*, Langkawi, Malaysia, December 14–16.

Azme N, Rajikin MH, Nor-Ashikin MNH, and Satar N. 2010b. Fetal resorption in corticosterone-induced oxidative stress in mice. *J Endocr Metab;* Suppl Issue 1(2): 81.

Barrie, MM. 1938. Vitamin E deficiency in the rat: Fertility in the female. *Biochem J*; 32(12): 2134–2137.

Brigelius-Flohe R and Traber MG. 1999. Vitamin E: Function and metabolism. *FASEB J*; 13(10): 1145–1155.

Dalvit G, Llanes S, Descalzo A, Insani M, Beconi M, and Cetica P. 2005. Effect of alpha-tocopherol and ascorbic acid on bovine oocyte *in vitro* maturation. *Reprod Domest Anim*; 40: 93–97.

Geva E, Bartoov B, Zabludovsky N, Lessing, JB, Lerner-Geva L, and Amit A. 1996. The effect of antioxidant treatment on human spermatozoa and fertilization rate in an in vitro fertilization program. *Fertil Steril*; 66(3): 430–434.

Hoshino E, Shariff R, Van Gossum A, Allard JP, Pichard C, Kurian R, and Jeejeebhoy KN. 1990. Vitamin E suppresses increased lipid peroxidation in cigarette smokers. *JPEN J Parenter Enteral Nutr*; 14(3): 300–305.

Jenkins C, Wilson R, Roberts J, Miller H, McKillop J, and Walker J. 2000.Antioxidents: Their role in pregnancy and miscarriage. *Antioxid Redox Signal*; 2: 623–627.

Jeong NH, Song ES, Lee JM, Lee KB, Kim MK, Cheon JE, Lee JK, Son SK, Lee JP, Kim JH, Hur SY, and Kwon YI. 2009. Plasma carotenoids, retinol and tocopherol levels and the risk of ovarian cancer. *Acta Obstet Gynecol*; 88: 457–462.

Kamsani YS, Rajikin MH, Chatterjee A, Nor-Ashikin MNK, and Satar N. 2011. Effects of gamma tocotrienol on the rate of blastocyst implantation and fetal outcome in mice induced with nicotine (personal communication).

Khanna S, Patel V, Rink C, Roy S, and Sen CK. 2005. Delivery of orally supplemented alpha-tocotrienol to vital organs of rats and tocopherol-transport protein deficient mice. *Free Radic Biol Med*; 39: 1310–1319.

Li Y, Sun WG, Liu HK, Qi GY, Wang Q, Sun XR, Chen BQ, and Liu JR. 2011. Gamma-Tocotrienol inhibits angiogenesis of human umbilical vein endothelia cell induced by cancer cell. *J Nutr Biochem* 22(12): 1127–1136.

Maniam S, Mohamed N, Shuid AN, and Soelaiman IN. 2008. Palm tocotrienol exerted better antioxidant activities in bone than α-tocopherol. *Bas Clin Pharm Toxicol*; 103: 55–60.

Mat Nor M, Nor-Asmaniza AB, Phang HT, and Muhammad HR. 2006. Effects of nicotine and co administration of nicotine and Vitamin E on testis and sperm quality of adult rats. *Malays Appl Biol*; 35(2): 47–52.

Miyamoto K, Shiozaki M, Shibata M, Koike M, Uchiyama Y, and Gotow T. 2009. Very-high-dose alpha-tocopherol supplementation increases blood pressure and causes possible adverse central nervous system effects in stroke-prone spontaneously hypertensive rats. *J Neurosci Res*; 87: 556–566.

Miyazawa T, Shibata A, Nakagawa K, and Tsuzuki T. 2008. Anti-angiogenic function of tocotrienol. *Asia Pac J Clin Nutr*; 17 Suppl 1: 253–256.

Mokhtar N, Rajikin MH, and Zakaria Z. 2008. Role of tocotrienol-rich palm vitamin E on pregnancy and pre-implantation embryos in nicotine-treated rats. *Biomed Res*;19: 181–184.

Perkins A. 2006. Endogenous anti-oxidant in pregnancy and preeclampsia. *Aust NZ J Obstet Gynecol*; 46: 77–83.

Rahmat A, Ngah WZ, Shamaan NA, Gapor A, and Abdul Kadir K. 1993. Long-term administration of tocotrienols and tumor-marker enzyme activities during hepatocarcinogenesis in rats. *Nutrition*; 9(3): 229–232.

Rajikin MH, Latif ES, Megat Radzi MAR, Mat Top AG, and Mokhtar N. 2009. Deleterious effects of nicotine on the ultrastructure of oocytes: Role of γ-tocotrienol. *Med Sci Monit*;15: 378–383.

Rasool AHG, Rahman AR, Yuen KH, and Wong AR. 2008. Arterial compliance and vitamin E blood levels with a self emulsifying preparation of tocotrienol rich vitamin E. *Arch Pharm Res*; 31(9): 1212–1217.

Royale NJ, Surai PF, and Hartley IR. 2003. The effect of variation in dietary intake on maternal deposition of antioxidants in zebra finch eggs. *Funct Ecol*; 17: 472–481.

Samant GV, Wali VB, and Sylvester PW. 2010. Anti-proliferative effects of gamma-tocotrienol on mammary tumour cells are associated with suppression of cell cycle progression. *Cell Prolif*; 43(1): 77–83.

Schweigert FJ, Steinhagen B, Raila J, Siemann A, Peet D, and Buscher U. 2003. Concentrations of carotenoids, retinol and alpha-tocopherol in plasma and follicular fluid of women undergoing IVF. *Hum Reprod*; 18 (6): 1259–1264.

Selvaduray KR, Radhakrishnan AK, Kutty MK, and Nesaretnam K. In Press, 2012. Palm tocotrienols decrease levels of pro-angiogenic markers in human umbilical vein endothelial cells (HUVEC) and murine mammary cancer cells. *Genes Nutr*; 7(1): 53–61.

Sen, C.K, Khanna S, and Roy S. 2004. Tocotrienol: The natural vitamin E to defend the nervous system? *Ann NY Acad Sci*; 1031: 127–142.

Sen CK, Khanna S, and Roy S. 2006. Tocotrienols: Vitamin E beyond tocopherols. *Life Sci*; 78: 2088–2098.

Sen CK, Khanna S, and Roy S. 2007a. Tocotrienols in health and disease: The other half of the natural vitamin E family. *Mol Aspects Med*; 28: 692–728.

Sen CK, Khanna S, Rink C, and Roy S. 2007b. Tocotrienols: The emerging face of natural vitamin E. *Vitam Horm*; 76: 203–261.

Serbinova E, Kagan V, Han D, and Packer L. 1991. Free radical recycling and intramembrane mobility in the antioxidant properties of alpha-tocopherol and alpha-tocotrienol. *Free Radic Biol Med*; 10: 263–275.

Simsek M, Naziroglu M, Simsek H, Cay M, Aksakal M, and Kumru S. 1998. Blood plasma levels of lipoperoxide, glutathione peroxide, beta carotene, vitamin A and E in women with habitual abortion. *Cell Biochem Funct*; 16: 227–231.

Skobe M, Rockwell P, Goldstein N, Vosseler S, and Fusenig N.E. 1997. Halting angiogenesis suppresses carcinoma cell invasion. *Nat Med*; 3(11): 1222–1227.

Suzuki YJ, Tsuchiya M, Wassall SR, Choo YM, Govil G, Kagan V.E, and Packer L. 1993. Structural and dynamic membrane properties of alpha-tocopherol and alpha-tocotrienol: Implication to the molecular mechanism of their antioxidant potency. *Biochemistry*; 32: 10692–10699.

Sylvester PW, McIntyre BS, Gapor A, and Briski KP. 2001. Vitamin E inhibition of normal mammary epithelial cell growth is associated with a reduction in protein kinase Ca activation. *Cell Prolif*; 34: 347–357.

Terasawa Y, Ladha Z, Leonard SW, Morrow JD, Newland D, Sanan D, Packer L, Traber MG, and Farese Jr. RV. 2000. Increased atherosclerosis in hyperlipidemic mice deficient in alpha-tocopherol transfer protein and vitamin E. *Proc Natl Acad Sci USA*; 97: 13830–13834.

Vigueras-Villasenor R.M, Ojeda I, Gutierrez-Perez O, Chavez-Saldana M, Cuevas O, Maria D.S, and Rojas-Castaneda J.C. 2011. Protective effect of alpha-tocopherol on damage to rat testes by experimental cryptorchidism. *Int J Exp Pathol*; 92(2): 131–139.

25 Tocotrienol and Tocopherol in Stress-Induced Gastric Mucosal Injury

Nafeeza Mohd Ismail and Ibrahim Abdel Aziz Ibrahim

CONTENTS

25.1 INTRODUCTION

Stress-induced pathological changes can affect the psychological and physiological balances (Selye 1956). In studies related to stress, rats have been widely used. There is an established model for producing gastric lesions, which we refer to as stress-induced gastric mucosal injury (SIGMI). SIGMI can be produced by various methods such as restraint stress (Brodie et al. 1962; Galvine 1985; Hayase and Takeuchi 1986), water immersion restraint stress (WIRS) (Kitagawa et al. 1979; Arai et al. 1987), and cold restraint stress (Galvine et al. 1986; Al-Moutairy and Tariq 1996).

The pathological basis for the development of gastric lesion is multifactorial. It includes factors that disrupt the gastric mucosal integrity such as changes in gastric acid, mucus, and bicarbonate secretions, inhibition of gastric mucosal prostaglandin (PG) synthesis, reduction of gastric mucosal blood flow (Kwiecień et al. 2004; Brzozowski et al. 2006, 2008a), as well as changes in stress hormone levels (Ainsah et al. 1999; Filaretova et al. 1999; Dronjak et al. 2004) and gastric motility (Allen and Leonarn 1988; Aase 1989; Güzel et al. 1998; Ephgrave et al. 2000; DuBay et al. 2003). Stress-induced gastric wall contractions and the compression of the intramural vessels are also probably responsible for the degeneration of the mucosal cell leading to the impairment of gastric microcirculation, which precipitates SIGMI (Dai and Ogle 1975). It is also proposed that an increase in catecholamine level during stress causes vasoconstriction (Nur Azlina and Nafeeza 2008). These changes can ultimately result in SIGMI (Ephgrave et al. 1998). A recent study has also shown the involvement of oxidative stress in the pathogenesis of stress-induced gastric ulcer (Jia et al. 2007). In this chapter, we discuss the non-antioxidative functions of palm vitamin E (PVE), which is a combination of 74% tocotrienol (TT) and 25% tocopherol (TF) against SIGMI.

25.2 EFFECTS OF PALM VITAMIN E AND α-TOCOPHEROL ON STRESS HORMONES

25.2.1 EFFECT ON PLASMA ADRENOCORTICOTROPIN AND CORTICOSTERONE

Ibrahim et al. (2011) reported that the exposure to WIRS caused a remarkable increase in plasma adrenocorticotropin (ACTH) and corticosterone levels (Figures 25.1 and 25.2). These findings are in agreement with the other studies. Klenerová et al. (2003) and Lou et al. (2008) found that plasma ACTH and corticosterone levels were elevated in rats exposed to WIRS. Other studies using different models of stress, such as restraint or cold restraint stress, also demonstrated a similar finding, that is, a rise in these stress hormones (Ainsah et al. 1999; Filaretova et al. 1999; Dronjak et al. 2004; Nur Azlina and Nafeeza 2008).

It has been demonstrated that stress induces activation of the hypothalamus–pituitary–adrenal (HPA) axis (Stark et al. 2006). When exposed to stress, the first system to respond is the autonomic nervous system, which sends a message to the hypothalamus. The hypothalamus, in turn, releases corticotropin-releasing factor (CRF), which is picked up by the nearby pituitary. This neuropeptide stimulates the pituitary to release ACTH into the bloodstream. ACTH stimulates the production and release of glucocorticoids (corticosterone in rats, cortisol in humans) from the adrenal glands. Corticosterone stimulates the release of glucose from body stores, which provides energy to the body to fight off the danger or to run away from it. Once the threat is over, the mediators return to baseline levels due to negative feedback on the HPA axis (McEwen 2002; Carrasco and Van de Kar 2003).

Corticosteroids are known to be a sensitive marker of the degree of stress experienced by the animal (Kheir-Eldin et al. 2001). The elevation of plasma corticosterone in stressed rats noted by Ibrahim et al. (2012) is in agreement with the results of Al-Shabanah et al. (1996), Ainsah et al. (1999), Klenerová et al. (2003), Lou et al. (2008), and Nur Azlina and Nafeeza (2008). This elevation could be explained on the basis that stress induces the activation of the HPA axis causing increased

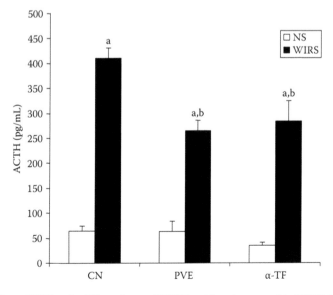

FIGURE 25.1 Effect of PVE and α-TF on plasma ACTH level in rats exposed to WIRS. Each bar represents mean ± SEM ($n = 10$). a vs non-stressed group ($p < 0.01$). b vs stressed control (CN + WIRS) ($p < 0.01$).

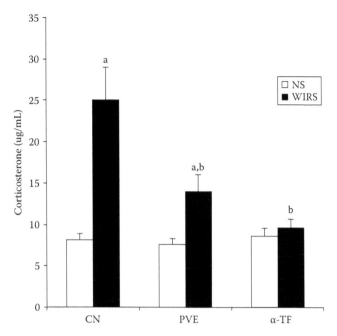

FIGURE 25.2 Effect of PVE and α-TF on plasma corticosterone level in rats exposed to WIRS. Each bar represents mean ± SEM ($n = 10$). a vs non-stressed group (CN + NS) ($p < 0.01$). b vs stressed control (CN + WIRS) ($p < 0.01$).

secretion of pituitary endorphins, ACTH, and adrenal corticosteroids such as corticosterone. The plasma corticosterone level is the most striking hormonal change found in stress and is used as a sensitive index of stress (Ainsah et al. 1999). On the other hand, the increase in corticosterone level is a well-known physiological response to stress (Lim and Funder 1983).

Hellhammer et al. (1983) reported that the corticosterone levels were greatly increased in the blood of both the lesion and the non-lesion groups compared to the controls. In addition, Weiss (1971) found that the severity of stress ulceration correlated positively with the levels of plasma corticosterone, and proposed that steroids, in quantities that the animal is capable of secreting, may contribute to the production of ulcers. Further support for this idea came from the observation that animals with hippocampal lesions exhibit increased plasma corticosterone levels and develop more gastric erosions during stress (Murphy et al. 1979). Nur Azlina and Nafeeza (2008) also showed that the increase in the corticosterone level was correlated to the increased incidence of SIGMI as seen in the stressed control rats. Thus, the corticosterone rise during stress can be considered as an ulcerogenic factor. However, Murison et al. (1989) observed that metyrapone treatment, slightly reduced corticosterone levels under stress, had no effect on lesion development. Bakker and Murison (1989) studied the administration of CRF to rats aged 100–220 days and then exposed to WIRS. The age of the animals itself was not a significant factor for both basal levels of plasma corticosterone and for the extent of restraint-induced SIGMI. However, after CRF administration, only the young animals had a significant increase in plasma corticosterone levels, and postrestraint gastric ulcerations were more severe in older rats. The increased corticosterone secretion during stress is related to the increased occurrence of SIGMI but it is not the sole causative agent for the pathogenesis of SIGMI (Bakker and Murison 1989). However, this suggests a new role of corticosterone produced during stress in gastric ulceration. Filaretova (2006) demonstrated that an acute rise of corticosterone during stress increased the resistance of the stomach to stress injury. However, it is difficult to relate the increased corticosteroid secretion to stress induced lesions formation because adrenalectomy had been reported to either increase (Brodie and Hanson 1960) or inhibit (Sethbhadki et al. 1970) the production of stress-induced lesions.

The data by Ibrahim et al. (2011) showed that vitamin E supplementations (PVE or α-tocopherol [α-TF]) at the dose of 60 mg/kg body weight for 28 days were able to decrease stress by reducing the plasma ACTH and corticosterone levels. Shaheen et al. (1993) showed that intraperitoneal injection of 5 mg/kg body weight of vitamin E for 6 days in rats prior to a single swimming test diminished the stress-induced elevation of corticosterone. Ainsah et al. (1999) reported the rats treated with 90 or 150 mg vitamin E/kg rat chow for 8 weeks had a significant reduction in plasma corticosterone compared to the controls. Therefore, the supplementation of vitamin E reduced the release or effects of endorphins, thus decreasing the effects of stress on rats' locomotor activity and plasma corticosterone levels. Furthermore, Taniguchi et al. (2001) indicated that vitamin E suppresses the elevation of the plasma corticosterone concentration in animals, possibly by inhibiting the conversion of cholesterol ester to free cholesterol in the adrenal gland (Taniguchi et al. 2001). In addition, vitamin E reduced the stress-induced changes in brain metabolism including sodium, potassium, and adenosine triphosphatase activities, thus showing that inhibition of lipid peroxidation altered the response marker to stress (Shaheen et al. 1993).

Nur Azlina and Nafeeza (2008) reported that TT and TF were capable of reducing the plasma corticosterone level in restraint stress condition. Rats fed with TT and TF showed no increase in corticosterone level even after being stressed, which indicates that TT and TF are capable of maintaining the corticosterone level in the stress-induced rats. Nevertheless, in the study by Ibrahim et al. (2011), the exposure to WIRS for 3.5 h increased the plasma corticosterone level significantly in the PVE stressed group but not in the α-TF stressed group in comparison to the PVE non-stressed and α-TF non-stressed groups, respectively (Ibrahim et al. 2011). This indicates that α-TF has the ability to maintain the corticosterone level in stress conditions but not TT. However, the exposure to WIRS for 3.5 h increased the plasma ACTH level significantly in both PVE and α-TF stressed groups compared to the non-stressed groups, respectively. The reason for this discrepancy is unclear. It is possible that PVE which in combination of 21% α-TF, 17% α-tocotrienol, 4% γ-tocopherol, 33% γ-tocotrienol, and 24% δ-tocotrienol is not as potent as 100% α-TF, which was able to maintain the corticosterone level in stress. The other reason could be related to the duration of stress and the different models of stress used in the study by Nur Azlina and Nafeeza (2008). It is well known that restraint stress alone is a milder stress model which was shown by an increase in corticosterone level of only 18.6% (Nur Azlina and Nafeeza 2008), compared to the effect of WIRS which induced a critical increase in corticosterone by 32% and this demonstrates the difference between two stress models (Ibrahim et al. 2011).

The ability to reduce the stress-induced increase in corticosterone level by PVE in acute and more extensive stress may be lower. Thus, it is a possibility that a higher dose of PVE is needed to achieve the effect similar to treatment with α-TF alone. In the study by Nur Azlina and Nafeeza (2008), there was no significant difference in pre- and poststressed plasma corticosterone levels between TT- and α-TF-treated groups. Thus, treatment with both TT and α-TF can block the increase in corticosterone levels due to stress. In their study, however, a pure mixture of TT was used.

25.2.2 Effect on Plasma Catecholamines (Noradrenaline and Adrenaline)

Ibrahim (2010) study demonstrated that the exposure to WIRS after 3.5 h increased the noradrenaline and adrenaline levels significantly (Figures 25.3 and 25.4). These findings are in agreement with results previously described by Perveen et al. (2003), Bodnar et al. (2004), and Watanabe et al. (2008). These observations support the hypothesis that the adrenal catecholamines play a physiological role in response to stressful situations. Catecholamines are significantly involved in the regulation of homeostasis of an organism at rest and especially during stressful situations. Stress induces the increase in both plasma adrenaline and noradrenaline levels. A study by Hamada et al. (1993) found that rats exposed to stress develop SIGMI associated with a reduction in brain noradrenaline content and an increase in plasma catecholamines and corticosterone levels. Similarly, in the study by Nur Azlina and Nafeeza (2008), rats exposed to restraint stress had a higher level of plasma noradrenaline compared to the non-stressed rats.

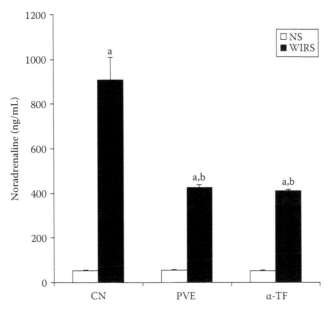

FIGURE 25.3 Effect of PVE and α-TF on plasma noradrenaline level in rats exposed to WIRS. Each bar represents mean ± SEM (n = 10). a vs non-stressed group (CN + NS) (p < 0.05). b vs stressed control (CN + WIRS) (p < 0.05).

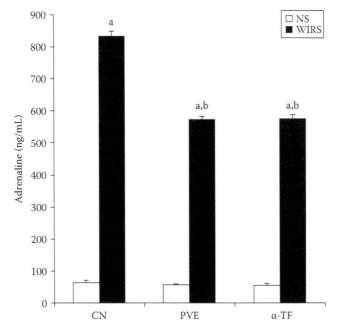

FIGURE 25.4 Effect of PVE and α-TF on plasma adrenaline level in rats exposed to WIRS. Each bar represents mean ± SEM (n = 10). a vs non-stressed group (CN + NS) (p < 0.05). b vs stressed control (CN + WIRS) (p < 0.05).

During stress, the underlying mechanisms involved are the activation of the HPA and sympathetic–adrenal medullary (SAM) systems, causing the release of corticosterone along with noradrenaline and adrenaline. Furthermore, the elevations of catecholamines may generate free radicals (Cariello 2000), which may be cytotoxic and mediate tissue damage by injuring cellular membranes and releasing intracellular components. It is widely accepted that the pathogenesis of gastric mucosal lesions involves oxygen-derived free radicals, while the role of lipid peroxidation, induced by stress, remains uncertain. Among various stressors used in animals, the most reproducible results in forming SIGMI were obtained by restraint stress (Hirota et al. 1990; Salim 1990; Brzozowski et al. 2000b; Nur Azlina and Nafeeza 2007).

In the study by Ibrahim (2010), the noradrenaline and adrenaline levels of stressed PVE and α-TF groups were reduced significantly in comparison to the stressed control. Nur Azlina and Nafeeza (2008) reported that the increase in the noradrenaline level was blocked in rats given TT supplementation but not in rats receiving α-TF. This finding suggests that TT but not α-TF is more potent in blocking the effects of stress. In terms of an increase in catecholamine levels, TT was able to inhibit stress-induced increase in noradrenaline, which correlates with its ability to block the formation of lesions in rats exposed to stress. However, with α-TF supplementation the finding suggests that the inability of α-TF to totally block the incidence of SIGMI could partly be due to its inability to block the effect of stress at the higher concentrations. From what has been discussed earlier, vitamin E was shown to play an important role in reducing the elevated catecholamines level induced by stress. In addition, the finding of their studies demonstrated that the PVE and α-TF were able to improve the stress-induced lesions by reducing noradrenaline and adrenaline levels. However, no significant difference between the PVE and α-TF groups was observed. Both treatments were able to improve the effects of stress by reducing the levels of noradrenaline and adrenaline (Ibrahim 2010).

Ibrahim (2010) showed that PVE and α-TF supplementation reduced the plasma noradrenaline and adrenaline levels significantly compared to stressed control rats. Moreover, the noradrenaline and adrenaline levels in the PVE and α-TF stressed groups were not different from their non-stressed groups, respectively. PVE and α-TF were unable to totally block the formation of SIGMI in rats exposed to stress; vitamin E could only reduce lesion formation, most probably by reducing the noradrenaline and adrenaline levels.

In the study by Nur Azlina and Nafeeza (2008), rats were restrained for 2 h daily for four consecutive days. It is possible that the rats became adapted to the stressor. However, in the study by Ibrahim (2010), rats were exposed to a single WIRS for 3.5 h, and this led to the increased levels of noradrenaline by 92% and adrenaline by 89%. This indicates that the WIRS model is a more significant stressor, which induced a higher increase in noradrenaline and adrenaline levels in the blood when compared to restraint alone.

Campese and Shaohua (2007) reported that rats fed with a vitamin-E-fortified diet manifested a significant reduction in noradrenaline secretion from the posterior hypothalamus. A vitamin-E-fortified diet mitigated the formation of reactive oxygen species (ROS) in the brain, and this was associated with reduction in sympathetic nervous system activity and blood pressure in rats with phenol-induced renal injury.

Kirshenbaum et al. (1990) reported that administration of vitamin E (50 mg/kg intraperitoneally), given 24 and 1 h before adrenaline infusion, significantly increased the amount of adrenaline required to produce pathological arrhythmias. Vitamin E pretreatment did not have any detrimental effect on the pressure readings nor did it have any influence on adrenaline-induced pressure changes. The data suggest that a combination therapy with vitamin E may allow therapeutic use of higher concentrations of adrenaline required to improve function in failing hearts with a reduced risk of arrhythmias.

25.3 EFFECT OF PALM VITAMIN E AND α-TOCOPHEROL ON GASTRIC MOTILITY

25.3.1 Effect on Plasma Acetylcholine Products

Ibrahim et al. (2012) reported that the exposure to WIRS for 3.5 h increased the plasma acetylcholine (Ach) products level significantly in rats (Figure 25.5). Previous studies had reported the effect of stress on the hippocampus, which is a part of the forebrain that is located in the medial temporal lobe. It belongs to the limbic system and plays major roles in short-term memory and spatial navigation,

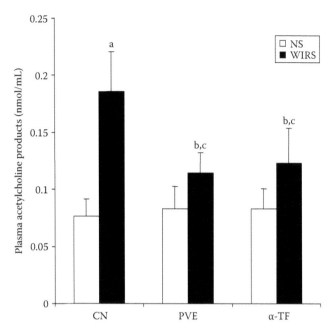

FIGURE 25.5 Effect of PVE and α-TF on plasma Ach products in rats exposed to WIRS. Each bar represents mean ± SEM ($n = 10$). a vs non-stressed control (CN + NS) ($p < 0.05$). b vs stressed control (CN + WIRS) ($p < 0.05$). c vs non-stressed group ($p < 0.05$).

especially in the hippocampal cholinergic system. The hippocampal cholinergic system seems to be activated after WIRS (Finkelstein et al. 1985; Gonzalez and Pazos 1992). The septo-hippocampal cholinergic system is activated by several kinds of stressful stimuli, for instance, acute or chronic restraint stress (Imperato et al. 1991; Mark et al. 1996; Tajima et al. 1996; Mizuno and Kimura, 1997; Mitsushima et al. 2003), repeated foot shocks (Dazzi et al. 1995), or cold (Fatranska et al. 1989).

Whereas some studies demonstrated a significant correlation between increased plasma corticosterone and hippocampal Ach levels (Mitsushima et al. 2003), another study did not find this correlation (Imperato et al. 1991). This suggests that the increase in hippocampal Ach levels may not always reflect an emotional response to stress. In addition, it is possible that the hippocampal cholinergic system will only be involved in certain stressful situations. Therefore, it is important to use a model that has been shown to involve the hippocampus when attempting to determine the importance of the hippocampal cholinergic system in the modulation of stress.

Mark et al. (1996) reported that in response to the stressful event, Ach release was significantly increased in the prefrontal cortex (186%; $p < 0.01$) and hippocampus (168%; $p < 0.01$) but not in the amygdala or nucleus accumbens. The sole effect observed in the amygdala and nucleus accumbens occurred upon release from the restrainer, at which point Ach levels were significantly elevated in both areas (amygdala: 150%; $p < 0.05$; nucleus accumbens: 13%; $p < 0.05$). An enhanced Ach release was also evident during this sample period in the hippocampus and prefrontal cortex. These data demonstrate an enhancement of cholinergic activity in response to stress in two Ach projection systems (hippocampus and prefrontal cortex) but not in the intrinsic Ach system of the nucleus accumbens or the extrinsic innervation of the amygdala. In addition, Tajima et al. (1996) investigated the role of the hippocampal cholinergic neurons during WIRS in rats, in which Ach release was increased by the immobilization state of WIRS.

Ach is synthesized in certain neurons by the enzyme choline acetyltransferase from the compounds choline and acetyl-CoA. The enzyme acetylcholinesterase converts Ach into the inactive metabolites choline and acetate. This enzyme is abundant in the synaptic cleft, and its role in rapidly clearing free Ach from the synapse is essential for proper muscle function.

The major limitation in the study by Ibrahim et al. (2012) appears to be the lack of information on the ACh levels in the gastric tissue. Under the study protocol, the gastric tissue was too scanty to measure the ACh, and reference was made to its level in the blood. Despite its short half-life in plasma, such measurements of ACh in plasma have been reported in a number of previous works (Kawashima et al. 1987; Watanabe et al. 1987; Fujii et al. 1995, 1997).

To the best of our knowledge, there are few studies conducted on the effects of vitamin E on Ach levels. Lee et al. (2001) reported the effects of vitamin E on the levels of neurotransmitters and acetylcholinesterase activity in the brains of rats treated with scopolamine, an inducer of dementia. Brain acetylcholinesterase activity was markedly reduced by scopolamine injection. However, the supplementation of vitamin E in the diet significantly increased the reduced brain acetylcholinesterase activity up to the level of the scopolamine-untreated group. This shows that supplementation with vitamin E might be useful in maintaining brain acetylcholinesterase activity at the normal level. Thus, there is a possible role of vitamin E in reducing Ach levels.

Similarly, Ibrahim et al. (2012) demonstrated that the supplementation of 60 mg/kg of PVE and α-TF for 28 days reduced the plasma Ach products significantly in rats exposed to WIRS. These findings indicate the possibilities of vitamin E to protect against the increase in Ach during stress, which leads to a reduction in the vagal simulated gastric motility as discussed in the next section. Although the mechanism of Ach reduction is unclear, it is possible that vitamin E acts by increasing the acetylcolinesterase activity as previously shown by Lee et al. (2001).

25.3.2 Effect on Gastric Motility

Ibrahim et al. (2012) reported that WIRS for 3.5 h caused a marked increase in gastric motility by increasing the frequency and amplitude of gastric contractions (Figures 25.6 through 25.8). The increase in motility had been previously reported by many studies including Yano et al. (1978), Garrick et al. (1986a), Koo et al. (1986), Ito et al. (1993), Ephgrave et al. (1997, 2000), and DuBay et al. (2003). The increase in gastric motility had been implicated as one of the important factors

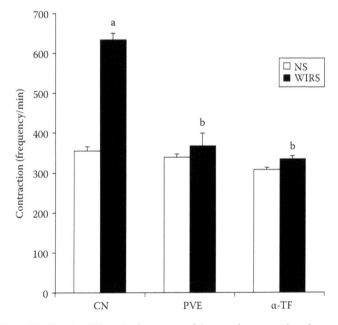

FIGURE 25.6 Effect of PVE and α-TF on the frequency of the gastric contractions in rats exposed to WIRS. Each bar represents mean ± SEM ($n = 10$). a vs non-stressed control (CN + NS) ($p < 0.05$). b vs stressed control (CN + WIRS) ($p < 0.05$).

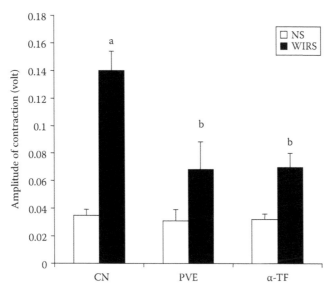

FIGURE 25.7   Effect of PVE and α-TF on the amplitude of the gastric contractions in rats exposed to WIRS. Each bar represents mean ± SEM ($n = 10$). a vs non-stressed control group (CN + NS) ($p < 0.05$). b vs stressed control (CN + WIRS) ($p < 0.05$).

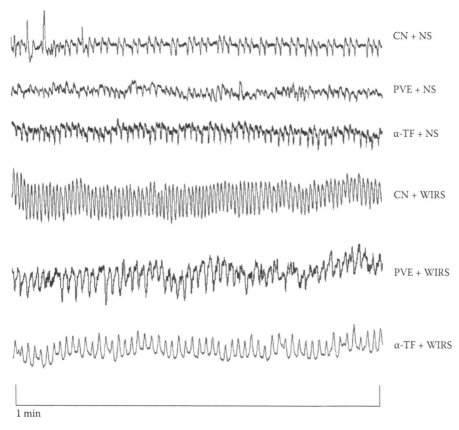

FIGURE 25.8   Representative electrogastrogram (EGG) tracings of the gastric motility for non-stressed (NS) and WIRS rats in PVE- and α-TF-treated and control (CN) groups.

leading to the formation of SIGMI. Regular frequencies and amplitudes were recorded in the control group. In rats with gastric motility disorder induced by WIRS, the contractions were disordered and irregular. There was an obvious difference in frequency and high amplitudes of the contractions between the stressed and non-stressed control groups. Shen et al. (2006) reported that in the cold-restrained stressed rats, frequency and amplitude of contractions were disordered and irregular. The frequency and amplitude of gastric motility were significantly higher than those in the control group. The decrease in gastric mucosal blood flow and increased gastric motility play an important role in inducing gastric mucosal lesions under stress conditions (Wang and Zhu 1995).

Gastric motility is regulated by a complex hierarchy of neurons and hormones and by intrinsic properties of the gastric smooth muscle. It is certain that Ach is the most dominant agonist to stimulate gastrointestinal contractions (Kaneko et al. 2001). The gastric motility is related to stress, which activates the release of Ach from postganglionic terminals of the vagus nerve and neurons of the intramural (metasympathetic) nervous system (Ibrahim et al. 2012). This elevation of the Ach will then induce the contractions in the rat stomach (Petroianu and Weinberg 1986; Buharalioglu and Akar 2002). On the other hand, the development of the lesions depends on the gastric motility. A high amplitude and prolonged duration of gastric contractions will augment the development of lesions (Garrick et al. 1986a,b, 1987). High-amplitude contractions may diminish mucosal blood flow (Livingston et al. 1988; Tarnasky et al. 1990).

During cold water immersion restraint stress (CWIR), a characteristic pattern of phasic high-amplitude, prolonged contractions was present (Garrick et al. 1986a,b, 1987). Autoradiographic assessment of gastric mucosal blood flow during a contraction induced by CWIR showed alternating regions of low flow and hyperemia in the gastric corpus (Livingston et al. 1988). These findings suggest that strong phasic gastric contractions might result in foci of relative ischemia, followed by hyperemia upon cessation of contraction.

During stress, the gastric smooth muscles contract intensively, resulting in disturbance of the blood circulation, decrease in gastric mucosal blood flow, and increased permeability of the vascular wall. As a result, gastric ulcer occurs (Mersereau and Hinchey 1988; Ueki et al. 1988). Ito et al. (1993) reported that gastric motility appears to play an important role in the pathogenesis of ulceration by causing ischemic change along the folds. Garrick et al. (1986a) suggested that the longer duration of cold-restraint stress increased the amplitude and frequency of gastric contractions along with the formation of gastric erosions. In addition, mucosal erosions following the stimulation of gastric contractions induced by vagal or direct electrical stimulation. Livingston et al. (1991) demonstrated that strong gastric contractions cause mucosal ischemia. Considering the presence of heterogeneity of mucosal lesions, the assessment of blood flow in the specific topographical area is necessary even in the same mucosa, which implies that evaluation of blood flow and/or tissue oxygen pressure should be applied for the flat and fold formation area.

Nakade et al. (2006) demonstrated that restraint stress significantly increased gastric contractions of the antrum and pylorus in response to solid food ingestion. It was also shown that the increased gastric motility was restored to basal levels immediately after termination of the restraint stress loading. Because atropine, hexamethonium, and vagotomy blocked restraint stress-induced augmentation of gastric motility, the vagal cholinergic pathway might be involved in this event. This indicates that the central nervous system (CNS) produces several neuropeptides in response to restraint stress. Another possibility could be that cold-restraint stress increases thyrotropin-releasing hormone (TRH) in the brain stem, which stimulates gastric motility and liquid emptying (Tache et al. 2001).

Tani et al. (1990) suggested the significance of hemodynamic redistribution of mucosal blood flow by hypermotility induced by 2-deoxy-D-glucose vagal stimulation, based on their observations on frozen and transparent specimens. Their study suggested that gastric hypermotility results in congestive change at the crest and ischemic change at the base of the folds. During WIRS, the significant decrease in gastric blood flow is considered to be common. In other words, the distortion of the form of gastric contractions might result in the temporary restriction of blood flow to the mucosa to produce anoxic damage. The reduction of blood flow may be purely mechanical—the tightly contracted muscles in the stomach wall would simply block the small blood vessels traversing through it. The restriction of blood flow might also involve vascular contraction or the shunting of blood away from the mucosa, thereby accentuating anoxic damage (Garrick et al. 1986a).

Ibrahim et al. (2012) demonstrated that PVE and α-TF were able to decrease gastric motility in stressed rats. They found that stress increased the level of Ach that might stimulate stomach contractions. Rats pretreated with vitamin E and then subjected to stress had a reduced Ach level. The study also observed that the plasma Ach level was lower in rats treated with PVE and α-TF. Thus, reduction in the stomach motility may therefore be associated with the vitamin E effect on the release or metabolism of the Ach (Ibrahim et al. 2012).

To the best of our knowledge, there is no study conducted regarding the effect of vitamin E on gastric motility. However, there was a study done to investigate the effects of antioxidant on gastric motility after stress in rats. Wang et al. (2006) reported that the antioxidant puerarin significantly attenuated gastric mucosal damage induced by WIRS by inhibiting the gastric motility. It decreased the percentage of gastric contraction time and number of violent contractions, which contributed to gastric motility inhibition. PVE and α-TF might have the same effects as puerarin, where we also observed a significantly lower gastric contraction and frequency in rats treated with PVE and α-TF. The absence of difference in the effects by PVE and α-TF on gastric motility after stress suggests an equal effectiveness of these two types of vitamin E on gastric motility.

25.4 EFFECTS OF PALM VITAMIN E AND α-TOCOPHEROL ON GASTRIC PROSTAGLANDIN E_2 CONTENT

PGs are known to play an important role in maintaining the mucosal integrity. It is one of the major groups of chemical mediators in the mammalian body, involved in numerous physiological reactions, such as inflammation and cellular differentiation (Srinivasan and Kulkarni 1989). PGs, especially PGE_2, also have cytoprotective effects on gastric mucosa by increasing epithelial mucus and bicarbonate secretions (Kauffman et al. 1980; Keogh et al. 1997), amelioration of mucosal blood flow (Morris et al. 1998), and inhibition of free radical and enzyme release from neutrophils (Gryglewski et al. 1987).

PG synthesis depends upon the activity of cyclooxygenase (COX), a rate-limiting enzyme in the synthesis of eicosanoids (Eberhart and Dubois 1995). Two isoforms of COX have been identified in many cells: a constitutive enzyme designated COX-1 and an inducible isoform known as COX-2 (Masferrer et al. 1996). COX-1 appears to be responsible for the production of PGs that are physiologically important for homeostatic functions, such as maintenance of the mucosal integrity and mucosal blood flow (Vane and Botting 1995). Under physiological conditions, prostanoid synthesis depends upon the availability of arachidonic acid and COX-1 activity. The latter is a major target of non-steroidal anti-inflammatory agents causing mucosal damage in the stomach (Kargman et al. 1996). In contrast, COX-2 is not constitutively expressed in most tissues but is dramatically upregulated during inflammation. The overexpression of the gene for COX-2 was demonstrated *in vitro* after the stimulation of COX-2 mRNA by proinflammatory cytokines such as interleukin-1b or tumor necrosis factor (Brzozowski et al. 1999).

Ibrahim et al. (2008) reported that the gastric PGE_2 content after 3.5 h WIRS to be significantly suppressed as compared to that in the control group (Figure 25.9). This finding is consistent with previous reports by Konturek et al. (1995) and Kato et al. (2002). Brzozowski et al. (1999) suggested that the expression of COX-2 mRNA after WIRS might be due to deficient PGE_2 generation in the gastric mucosa. Thus, this expression might reflect the suppression of PGE_2 generation, because COX-2 plays a crucial role in the healing of gastric ulcers (Kato et al. 2002).

Brzozowski et al. (1999) showed that the exposure to ischemia reperfusion produced a significant decrease in PGE_2 generation in the gastric mucosa but it was gradually restored during mucosal recovery from SIGMI, suggesting that endogenous PG may be involved in the spontaneous healing

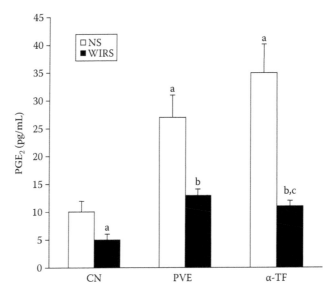

FIGURE 25.9 Effect of PVE and α-TF on gastric PGE_2PGE_2 content in rats exposed to WIRS. Each bar represents mean $\pm$ SEM ($n = 10$). a vs non-stressed control (CN + NS) ($p < 0.05$). b vs stressed control (CN + WIRS) ($p < 0.05$). c vs α-TF non-stressed (α-TF + NS) ($p < 0.05$).

of these lesions. This is supported by the fact that PGE_2 generation reached higher values during the course of healing of ulcerated gastric mucosa than it did in non-ulcerated mucosa (Lesch et al. 1998). This higher amount of PGE_2 was also detected at the site of ulceration rather than in non-ulcerated mucosa (Brzozowski et al. 1999). In addition, the recovery period of PGE_2 generation, starts increasing significantly after 3 h until 10 days in ulcerated gastric mucosa in comparison to non-ulcerated gastric mucosa after ischemia reperfusion (Brzozowski et al. 1999).

Takeuchi et al. (1999) found that 16,16-dimethyl PGE_2 administrated to rats that were exposed to hypothermic-stress led to a reduction in the formation of SIGMI. A study by Auguste et al. (1990) found that hypothermic-restraint stress produced gastric ulcer formation and significantly reduced PGE_2 in rats. It was reported that verapamil stimulates PGE_2 synthesis and its protective effect against stress-induced mucosal damage seems to be mediated by PGE_2. In addition, Gitlin et al. (1988) found hypothermic-restraint stress reduced gastric PGE_2 content compared to the non-stressed group.

Ibrahim et al. (2008) reported that the gastric PGE_2 content of non-stressed PVE and α-TF groups were increased significantly compared to the non-stressed control group, and the gastric PGE_2 content of stressed PVE and α-TF groups was significantly higher compared to the stressed control. Vitamin E improves the gastric PGE_2 content, by stimulating PG synthesis via the activation of the calcium-dependent phospholipase enzyme A_2 and inhibition of the lipooxygenase enzyme (Hirata 1981). Thus, pretreatment of vitamin E may prevent gastric mucosal damage caused by stress via increasing PGE_2 level. This result suggests that vitamin E was able to heal the SIGMI immediately after exposure to WIRS by increasing the gastric PGE_2 contents, and it acts to protect the gastric mucosa from ulcers.

Nur Azlina et al. (2005b) found that the mean gastric PGE_2 contents in all groups were not significantly different, despite the reduction in PGE_2 content after exposure to stress repeatedly for 2 h throughout four continuous days. However, it was increased in groups supplemented with tocotrienol or tocopherol. Furthermore, Nafeeza and Kang (2005) reported that the combination of two antioxidant agents (tocopherol–tocotrienol, tocopherol–ubiquinone, or tocotrienol–ubiquinone) had a higher level of gastric PGE_2 content compared to the control.

25.5 EFFECTS OF PALM VITAMIN E AND α-TOCOPHEROL ON GASTRIC ACIDITY

25.5.1 EFFECT ON GASTRIC ACIDITY

Gastric acidity is the primary aggressive factor in the gastric mucosa that is believed to take part in the formation of SIGMI by exposure to stress. It was reported that WIRS might lead to changes of gastric acid secretion (Li et al. 2006). Some studies indicate that WIRS increases acid secretion (Kitagawa et al. 1979; Al Moutaery 2003; Brzozowski et al. 2004a), while other studies showed gastric acid secretion decreases during WIRS (Hayase and Takeuchi 1986; Gutierrez-Cabano 1999).

In the study by Ibrahim et al. (2008), WIRS for 3.5 h reduced the gastric acidity (about 45%) significantly (Figure 25.10). Hayase and Takeuchi (1986) found that in pylorus-ligated rats, acid secretion decreased in response to restraint alone or restraint plus water immersion stress for 3.5 h. There was also a significant difference in the gastric juice volume and acid output between the control and restraint plus water immersion groups. In their study, rats that were exposed to longer duration stress for 7 h exhibited a significant increase in acid secretory activity in terms of the juice volume and the acid output, as compared to those of the controls. These disparities in the results may be due to a longer exposure to WIRS that led to increased gastric acidity in rats.

The discrepancy in outcomes of gastric acidity related to stress have been associated with different models of stress generation, duration of stress exposure, and methods of gastric acidity measurement. In a previous study, rats in which pylorus was tied demonstrated a reduction in gastric acid secretion when they were exposed to restraint stress or WIRS, whereas an increase in gastric acidity was observed when the lumen in rats exposed to WIRS was perfused, but not in rats exposed to restraint stress alone (Hayase and Takeuchi 1986).

A study by Nur Azlina et al. (2003) with a different model of stress (restraint stress alone) showed that gastric acid concentration reduced 30%, compared to that of rats exposed to restraint stress for 2 h every day for 4 days. Hayase and Takeuchi (1986) found that gastric acid secretion of rats exposed to restraint stress had slightly decreased and reached 60% from the normal secretion after 2 h of restraint stress. Similar findings were reported in previous studies, which confirmed that

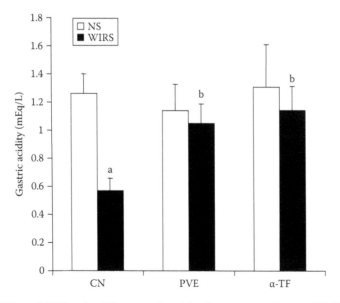

FIGURE 25.10 Effect of PVE and α-TF on gastric acidity in rats exposed to WIRS. Each bar represents mean ± SEM ($n = 10$). a vs non-stressed control (CN + NS) ($p < 0.05$). b vs stressed control (CN + WIRS) ($p < 0.05$).

restraint stress in rats reduced the secretion and gastric acid concentration (Dai and Ogle 1974; Ogle et al. 1985; Hayase and Takeuchi 1986; Koo et al. 1986; Arai et al. 1987).

It is possible that the reduction in the gastric acidity in stress is a result of the dysfunction of gastric acid secreting cells. The dysfunction could be due to ischemia of the parietal cells as a result of the compromised gastric microcirculation under stress conditions (Hayase and Takeuchi 1986). The relationship between the gastric acidity and the gastric blood flow had been shown previously by various researchers (Hayase and Takeuchi 1986; Wong et al. 2002).

The alteration of blood flow in stress has been studied deeply; one of the reasons suggested was a reduction in blood flow (Schoenberg et al. 1984). This happens because when the body responds to the stress, the blood flow rises in the vital organs to prepare the body for "fight or flight" response. This response leads to a decrease in blood flow to organs that function in digesting, reproduction, and immunity. The increasing of corticosterone during stress in the rats also leads to the increase of noradrenaline and adrenaline levels, which ultimately cause vasoconstriction and reduction of gastric blood flow (Hayase and Takeuchi 1986).

The reduction in gastric blood flow during stress could be due to hypergastric motility. This increase in gastric motility was related with the increase in the vagal activity during stress, where vagotomy and atropine were found to have the ability to reduce the formation of SIGMI (Mersereau and Hinchey 1981). Alteration in gastric contraction reduces the gastric blood flow and leads to the damage by anoxia of the tissue. The reduction in the gastric microcirculation leads to ischemia of gastric mucosa. During this period of ischemia, the parietal cells are damaged which leads to an overall hypofunction of the acid secretory system and may cause a reduction of gastric acidity.

Esplugues et al. (1996) also suggested that the inhibition of gastric acid secretion could be a defense mechanism during stress, and it is mediated by a nervous reflex involving a neuronal pathway that includes nitric oxide (NO) synthesis in the brain, specifically in the dorsal motor nucleus of the vagus. This suggests that the reduction in gastric acidity induced by stress is not caused by one factor only, but may involve several physiological factors that occur during stress.

The reduction in the gastric acidity during stress directly suggests that the gastric acidity is not an important factor in the formation of SIGMI. Although gastric acidity has been accepted widely as an aggressive factor in the gastric mucosa and may be responsible as a mediator for different kinds of SIGMI, many studies believed that in no stress period, gastric mucosa is resistant to a high concentration of acid. However, in stress, the defense mechanism of gastric mucosa is impaired by the increased gastric contraction and reduction in gastro-protective function as result of ischemia, which causes damaging effects on the gastric mucosa even though there is reduced gastric acid concentration.

Ibrahim et al. (2008) found that the gastric acidity of PVE and α-TF groups was significantly increased after exposure to WIRS compared to the control. This finding indicates the ability of PVE and α-TF to improve the gastric acidity by minimizing damage to the gastric acid secreting cells, probably by scavenging free radicals that are produced during the stress.

Nur Azlina et al. (2003) compared different preparations of vitamin E in an effort to determine if any of these preparations could improve acid reduction in stress. It was found that the diet deficient in vitamin E caused a reduction in gastric acidity in stressed rats. Adding tocopherol to the vitamin E deficient diet caused a reduction in gastric acid concentration induced by stress. However, the gastric acid concentrations in the tocotrienol and tocomin groups were comparable, with or without stress exposure. Tocomin contains many antioxidants other than tocopherol and tocotrienol such as phytosterol and ubiquinone. This reflects that tocotrienol can inhibit the suppression of gastric acid in restraint stressed rats. As there was no difference, they postulated that the tocotrienol component in the tocomin group was responsible for the effects. This outcome led to the suggestion that tocotrienol and tocomin conferred protection on the changes in the gastric acidity induced by stress. This is a possibility of preservation of a normal gastric mucosal blood flow during stress, and can then prevent ischemia thus protecting from hypofunction of the parietal cells.

Al-Moutairy and Tariq (1996) on the other hand found that giving vitamin E (α-TF) at a high dose (300 mg/kg body weight) reduced the secretion of gastric acid in non-stressed rats. Therefore, one of the protective functions of vitamin E suggested was its antisecretory activity. It was found that rats given vitamin E, but not exposed to stress, had a similar acid concentration compared to the non-stressed control. The difference between their study and this study is in the dose of tocopherol used. Al-Moutairy and Tariq (1996) used 300 mg/kg α-TF compared to 60 mg/kg in this study. Hence, there is a possibility that at a higher dose, α-TF could produce an antisecretory effect.

The mechanism of how vitamin E can decrease gastric acid secretion is not clear. There is proof that shows gastric acid secretion to be a calcium-dependent process (Coruzzi et al. 1986). Calcium administration by intravenous or intragastric routes increased the gastric acid secretions significantly (Harty et al. 1984), whereas verapamil, which is a calcium antagonist, was shown to reduce gastric acid secretion stimulated by calcium (Al Bekairi et al. 1994).

Vitamin E can also reduce calcium influx in cell membranes (Hall et al. 1991). Therefore, the antisecretory effect of PVE and α-TF in the study could be due to reduced calcium influx in cell membranes, or they might also function in the maintenance of normal gastric blood flow as discussed earlier.

25.5.2 Effect on Plasma Gastrin Level

Ibrahim et al. (2008) reported that the exposure to WIRS for 3.5 h leads to a reduced gastrin level (Figure 25.11). This finding is in agreement with Aricioğlu et al. (1996), Nur Azlina et al. (2005b), Papovich et al. (1992), and Zhang et al. (2008) who used different models of stress. Papovich et al. (1992) reported that serum gastrin level in stressed rats, which developed gastric ulcers, was lower than that of the normal rats. Aricioğlu et al. (1996) study showed a decrease in gastrin levels in cold-restraint stressed rats, and Nur Azlina et al. (2005b) proved that stress reduced serum gastrin levels in rats exposed to 2 h of repeated restraint stress. The reduction in the gastrin level may not only cause lower acid secretion, but also a decrease in the protective effects of gastrin on the gastric mucosa, which can eventually lead to formation of lesions in an impaired mucosa (Nur Azlina et al. 2005b).

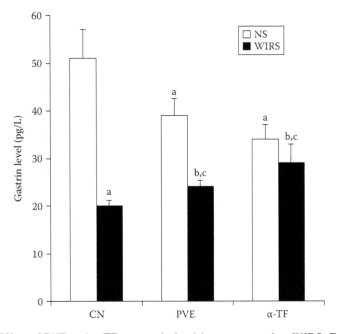

FIGURE 25.11 Effect of PVE and α-TF on gastrin level in rats exposed to WIRS. Each bar represents mean ± SEM ($n = 10$). a vs non-stressed control (CN + NS) ($p < 0.05$). b vs stressed control (CN + WIRS) ($p < 0.05$). c vs non-stressed group ($p < 0.05$).

Previous studies showed that the mechanism of gastric protection that prevents the damage of the gastric mucosa is developed by the same factor that causes the rising of gastric acid secretion (Takeuchi et al.1987; Tanaka et al. 1997). For instance, gastrin, which is known to increase gastric acid secretion, is also an important defense mechanism in the stomach, where it acts by improving blood flow and thickening the mucus gel on the gastric mucosa (Tanaka et al. 1998). The whole effect is to create a balance of both factors: destructive and gastroprotective, thus preventing the injury on the gastric mucosa in conditions of hypergastric acidity.

The healing by a gastrin analog was reported to protect the gastric mucosa from injury induced by ethanol (Komuro et al. 1992; Konturek et al. 1995; Stroff et al. 1995) and stress (Takeuchi and Johnson 1979; Sakamoto et al. 1985). Takeuchi and Johnson (1979) found that giving liquid diet to rats that reduced gastrin secretion improved the lesion in the stomach induced by stress, while giving pentagastrin to rats exposed to stress was found to protect the gastric mucosa from gastric lesion formation. They also showed that SIGMI formation had a high correlation with the reduction in DNA and ribonucleic acid (RNA) synthesis in the gastric mucosa, which caused the inability for the epithelial cell renewal and repair led to gastric erosion during stress. Gastrin tropic effects are known to stimulate DNA and RNA synthesis, thus conferring their protective function.

Takeuchi and Johnson (1979) suggested that rats with low endogenous gastrin are more susceptible to produce gastric ulcers induced by stress compared to rats that have normal levels of gastrin. This shows that reducing gastrin level during stress may be one of the important factors in the formation of gastric lesions. Johnson and Guthrie (1980) compared pentagastrin and epidermal growth factor (EGF) in gastric mucosa and found that both EGF and pentagastrin significantly increased DNA synthesis of the oxyntic gland mucosa. This may be apart from gastrin protective function. Another study by Lenz and Druge (1990) found that in rats exposed to physical restraint, gastric acid stimulation was blocked by 50% with administration of pentagastrin. Treatment with gastrin had been shown to significantly increase the rate of repair of ulcers and blood flow to the ulcer margins, which led to upregulation of COX-2 mRNA and COX-2 proteins in the mucosa (Sakamoto et al. 1985).

Administration of gastrin analog had also been reported to protect rats against ethanol-induced gastric injuries (Konturek et al. 1995; Stroff et al.1995). Thus, it could be important to preserve gastrin levels in conditions susceptible to gastric mucosal damage. Ibrahim et al. (2008) showed that the gastrin level in the stressed PVE group and α-TF group were significantly increased compared to the stressed control. In addition, the current study shows that the effect of stress on gastrin can be blocked by supplementation of PVE and α-TF, where the gastrin level was found to be comparable in both stressed and non-stressed rats.

Nur Azlina et al. (2005b) showed that the effect of stress on gastrin level could be blocked by supplementation of tocotrienol, where it was found that the serum gastrin level was comparable in both stressed and non-stressed rats. However, the serum gastrin level cannot be blocked by tocopherol supplementation. Their finding also supports the possibility that the protective effect of tocotrienol against gastric lesion formation caused by stress can be in part due to preservation of the endogenous gastrin. In the study by Ibrahim et al. (2008), the plasma gastrin levels of both stressed PVE and α-TF groups were reduced significantly when compared with the non-stressed groups. These protective effects of gastrin may be preserved during stress conditions by supplementation with PVE and α-TF.

25.6 EFFECTS OF PALM VITAMIN E AND α-TOCOPHEROL AGAINST STRESS-INDUCED GASTRIC MUCOSAL INJURY

Previous studies have demonstrated that SIGMI can develop in experimental animals following psychological or physical stress (Das and Banerjee 1993; Nur Azlina et al. 2005a). Gastric lesions caused by stress, alcohol, *Helicobacter pylori* infection, and non-steroidal anti-inflammatory drugs have been shown to be mediated largely through the generation of ROS that seem to play an important role in producing lipid peroxides (Nur Azlina et al. 2005a; Brzozowski et al. 2008a; Park et al. 2008; Mita et al. 2008).

In stress studies, rats have been widely used. There are some established models for producing SIGMI from various methods of stress. Nur Azlina et al. (2005a) had shown that rats exposed to restraint stress for 2 h every day for 4 days developed lesions in their gastric glandular mucosa. Singh et al. (2008) also reported that the cold-restraint stress caused a considerable ulceration in the form of hemorrhagic mucosal lesions in stomach. However, exposure to WIRS for 3.5 h resulted in an immediate appearance of multiple gastric lesions in the gastric mucosa (Konturek et al. 2001). Ulcerations in rats exposed to WIRS were typically spherical or oblong and superficially covered with blood (Landeira-Fernandez 2004). In the study by Ibrahim et al. (2008), WIRS model was used because it could induce acute gastric injury with a reliable reproducibility of SIGMI (Figures 25.12 and 25.13).

Previous studies had used macroscopic investigation whereby the gastric lesion was measured and given a score to assess the level of injury of gastric-mucosa-induced stress. In the study by Nur Azlina et al. (2005a), the gastric lesion score was given based on the total area of the gastric mucosal lesion. However, the severity of the lesion was low in their study. In the study by Ibrahim et al. (2008), the assessment of gastric lesions was determined by measuring each lesion in millimeter along its greatest diameter. The total length in each group of rats was averaged and expressed as the lesion index following the method previously described by Wong et al. (2002).

A study by Ibrahim et al. (2008) showed that animals exposed to WIRS for 3.5 h developed gastric mucosa lesions, thus confirming the reproducibility of this model for the study. The pathological basis for the development of these lesions is multifactorial and includes factors which disrupt gastric mucosal integrity, such as gastric acid secretion, inhibition of gastric mucosal PG synthesis, reduction of gastric mucosal blood flow, and inhibition of gastric mucus and bicarbonate secretion (Güzel et al. 1998; Önen et al. 2000). The formation of the SIGMI might be due to the increased

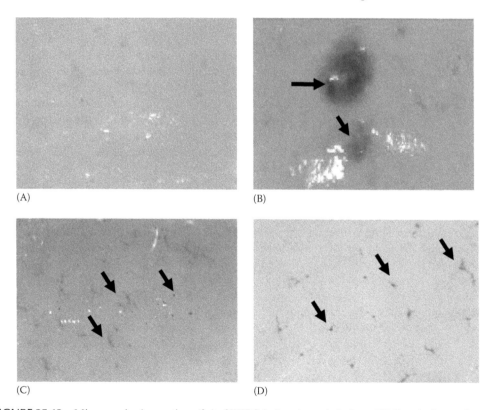

(A) (B) (C) (D)

FIGURE 25.12 Microscopic observations (3×) of WIRS-induced gastric lesions. (A) Gastric tissue of normal rat (no lesions). (B) Gastric tissue of a rat exposed to 3.5 h of WIRS (developed gastric ulcer as shown by the arrow). (C) Gastric tissue of a rat exposed to 3.5 h of WIRS and PVE (developed petechial hemorrhage as shown by the arrows). (D) Gastric tissue of a rat exposed to 3.5 h of WIRS and α-TF.

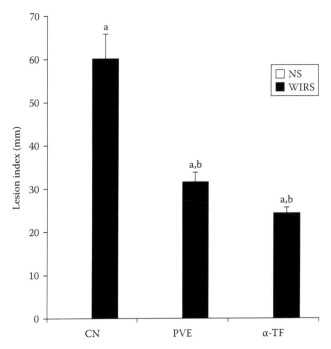

FIGURE 25.13 Effect of PVE and α-TF pretreatments for 28 days on gastric lesions in rats exposed to WIRS. Each bar represents mean ± SEM ($n = 10$). a vs non-stressed group (NS) ($p < 0.05$). b vs stressed control (CN + WIRS) ($p < 0.05$).

gastric contractions, which resulted in temporary restriction of blood flow to the mucosa. This restriction of the blood flow might also involve vascular contraction or the shunting of blood away from the mucosa, thereby accentuating anoxic damage (Garrick et al. 1986a; Ephgrave et al. 1998). The stress-induced strong vasocontractions of the gastric wall and compression of the intramural vessels are probably responsible for some degenerative changes in the mucosal cells leading to the impairment of gastric microcirculation and finally SIGMI (Konturek et al. 1998).

Ibrahim et al. (2008, 2011) and (Ibrahim 2010) reported that the supplementations of PVE and α-TF at 60 mg/kg for 28 days prior to exposure to stress reduced the gastric mucosal injury (Figure 25.12). This finding is similar to other studies (Kamsiah et al. 2002; Nafeeza et al. 2002; Nur Azlina et al. 2005a). In the study by Nur Azlina et al. (2005a), it was reported that supplementation with tocotrienol and tocopherol was able to reduce the formation of lesions in the gastric mucosa after restraint stress insult. However, no difference between these two agents was observed, showing equal effectiveness in preventing stress-induced gastric injury. Tocotrienol and tocopherol intake prevents the occurrence of SIGMI by strengthening the gastric mucosal barrier against stress-induced elevation of lipid peroxidation.

The study by Kamsiah et al. (2002) examined the effects of various doses of PVE and tocopherol on the prevention of aspirin-induced gastric lesions. The gastric lesions index was found to be significantly lower in all the vitamin E groups compared to the control, but there was no significant difference in ulcer indices between PVE- and tocopherol-treated groups. However, PVE administration at a dose of 100 mg/kg body weight and 150 mg/kg body weight was more effective in preventing aspirin-induced gastric lesions than TF at a dose of 30 mg/kg body weight, as the gastric mucosal thickness in these PVE groups were significantly higher compared to the other groups (Kamsiah et al. 2005). Another study by Nafeeza et al. (2000) also mentioned that the supplementation with PVE reduced the formation of ethanol induced gastric lesions.

Similarly, exposure to WIRS has been shown to increase the incidence of gastric mucosal lesions, and this increase was lowered by the administration of various antioxidants (Ohta et al. 2005; Brzozowski et al. 2005). A study by Ohta et al. (2005) had demonstrated that WIRS for 6 h reduced gastric α-TF concentration, but pre-administration of ascorbic acid partially reversed this reduction. Hence, in the present study, the prevention of the harmful effects of the stress may be mediated by the antioxidant activity possessed by the PVE and α-TF, by either directly or indirectly reducing the formation of free radicals, which causes SIGMI (Nur Azlina et al. 2005a). Furthermore, Brzozowski et al. (2005) confirmed that the pretreatment with grapefruit seed extract, which had antioxidative activity, applied topically in doses ranging from 8 to 64 mg/kg caused a significant reduction in SIGMI.

A study by Al Moutairy and Tariq (1996) also found that a single dose of α-TF (300 mg/kg) before stress could reduce the formation of gastric lesions in rats that were exposed to a cold-restraint stress for 2 h. Their study found that vitamin E could decrease the formation of gastric lesions in terms of size and number, but failed to stop the formation of gastric lesions comprehensively. However, Ozdil et al. (2004) had reported that the ascorbic acid (vitamin C), DL-α-TF acetate (vitamin E), and sodium selenite (selenium) improved gastric mucosal injury in rats induced by ethanol.

All the earlier findings indicated that antioxidants improved the integrity of gastric mucosal epithelium and reduced the degree of damage in the mucosal architecture (Nordmann 1994). Microscopic evaluation of gastric mucosa of the antioxidant-treated groups revealed a significant reduction in injury formation (Ozdil et al. 2004). It could correlate these findings with the free radical trapping activity of the antioxidants.

The vitamin E protective mechanism and its role on human health are still not well understood. The characteristic of the vitamin E antioxidant, especially its effect on polyunsaturated fatty acids (PUFAs), may improve cell membrane integrity. It may cause gastric tissue to become more resistant toward gastric aggressive factors like acid and pepsin. The outcome of the study by Ibrahim et al. (2008) and other previous studies suggested that vitamin E has a significant protective effect against stress-induced gastric lesions (Ozdil et al. 2004; Nur Azlina et al. 2005a). Based on this, there is a possibility that it can be used as treatment in stress-induced gastric lesion.

25.7 CONCLUSION

In light of the data reviewed earlier, we conclude that the exposure to WIRS for 3.5 h causes SIGMI formation. Supplementation with PVE and α-TF was able to reduce the SIGMI formation significantly compared to the stressed control group. The exposure to WIRS for 3.5 h elevated stress hormones, which include ACTH, corticosterone, noradrenalin, and adrenalin, and these increases were reduced by PVE and α-TF. WIRS reduced gastric PGE$_2$ content, plasma gastrin level, and gastric acidity, but the vitamin E pretreatments were able to significantly increase these parameters. The findings also show that WIRS causes the increase of gastric motility through the increase of plasma Ach product, which induced contraction in the rat stomach. Consequently, PVE and α-TF were able to reduce the gastric motility probably through blocking the changes by Ach via increasing the acetylcholinesterase concentration. The gastroprotective effects of PVE are comparable to α-TF in rats exposed to WIRS.

REFERENCES

Aase, S. 1989. Disturbances in the balance between aggressive and protective factors in the gastric and duodenal mucosa. *Scand J Gastroenterol* **24**: 17–23.

Ainsah, O., Nabishah, B.M., Osman, C.B., and Khalid, B.A.K. 1999. Naloxone and vitamin E block stress-induced reduction of locomotors activity and elevation of plasma corticosterone. *Exp Clin Endocrin Diabetes* **107**(7): 462–467.

Al Bekairi, A.M., Al Rajhi, A.M., and Tariq, M. 1994. Effect of verapamil and hydralazine on stress and chemically induced gastric ulcers in rats. *Pharm Res* **29**: 225–236.

Al Moutaery, A.R. 2003. Effect of centrophenoxine on water-immersion restraint stress-and chemically-induced gastric ulcers in rats. *Res Commun Mol Path Pharm* **113–114**: 39–56.

Allen, A. and Leonarn, J.A. 1988. The mucus barrier: Its role in gastroduodenal mucosal protection. *J Clin Gastroenterol* **10** (1): 593–598.

Al-Moutairy, A. and Tariq, M. 1996. Effect of vitamin E and selenium on hyphothermic restraint stress and chemically induced ulcers. *Dig Dis Sci* **41**(6): 1165–1171.

Al-Shabanah, O.A., Mostafa, Y.H., Hassan, M.T., Khairaldin, A.A., and Al Sawaf, H.A. 1996. Vitamin E protects against bacterial endotoxin-induced increase of plasma corticosterone and brain glutamate in the rat. *Res Commun Mol Pathol Pharmacol* **92**(1): 95–105.

Arai I., Hirose H., Muramatsu, M., and Aihara H. 1987. Effects of restraint and water-immersion stress and insulin on gastric acid secretion in rats. *Physiol Behav* **40**(3): 357–361.

Aricioğlu, A., Öz, E., Erbaş, D., and Gökçora, N. 1996. Effects of EGF and allopurinol on prostaglandin and lipid peroxide levels in mucosa of stomach in restraint cold stress. *Prostaglandins Leukot Essent Fatty Acids* **54**(4): 285–288.

Auguste, L.J., Sterman, H.R., Stein, T.A., Bailey, B., and Wise, L. 1990. Effect of verapamil on the gastric mucosal level of PGE$_2$ during stress. *J Surg Res* **49**(1): 34–36.

Bakker, H.K. and Murison, R. 1989. Plasma corticosterone and restraint induced gastric pathology: Age-related differences after administration of corticotropin releasing factor. *Life Sci* **45**: 907–916.

Bodnar, I., Mravec, B., Kubovcakava, L., Fekete, M., Nagy, G.M., and Kvetnansky, R. 2004. Immobilization stress-induced increase in plasma catecholamine levels is inhibited by a prolactoliberin (salsolinol) administration. *Ann NY Acad Sci* **1018**: 124–130.

Brodie, D.A. and Hanson, H.M. 1960. A study of the factors involved in the production of gastric ulcers by the restraint technique. *Gastroenterology* **38**: 353–360.

Brodie, D.A., Richard, W.M., Moreno, O.M. 1962. Effect of restraint on gastric acidity in the rat. *Am J Physiol* **202**(4): 812–814.

Brzozowski, T., Konturek, P.C., Chlopicki, S., Sliwowski, Z., Pawlik, M., Ptak-Belowska, A., Kwiecien, S. et al. 2008a. Therapeutic potential of 1-methylnicotinamide against acute gastric lesions induced by stress: Role of endogenous prostacyclin and sensory nerves. *J Pharmacol Exp Ther* **326**(1): 105–116.

Brzozowski, T., Konturek, P.C., Drozdowicz, D., Konturek, S.J., Zayachivska, O., Pajdo, R., Kwiecien, S., Pawlik, W.W., and Hahn, E.G. 2005. Grapefruit-seed extract attenuates ethanol-and stress-induced gastric lesions via activation of prostaglandin, nitric oxide and sensory nerve pathways. *World J Gastroenterol* **11**(41): 6450–6458.

Brzozowski, T., Konturek, P.C., Konturek, S.J., Drozdowicz, D., Kwiecień, S., Pajdo, R., Bielanski, W., and Hahn, E.G. 2000a. Role of gastric acid secretion in progression of acute gastric erosions induced by ischemia–reperfusion into gastric ulcers. *Eur J Pharmacol* **398**(1): 147–158.

Brzozowski, T., Konturek, P.C., Konturek, S.J. Drozdowicz, D., Pajdo, R., Pawlik, M., Brzozowska, I., and Hahn, E.G. 2000b. Expression of cyclooxygenase (COX)-1 and COX-2 in adaptive cytoprotetion induced by mild stress. *J Physiol* **94**: 83–91.

Brzozowski, T., Konturek, P.C., Konturek, S.J., Kwiecien, S., Drozdowicz, D., Bielanski, W., Pajdo, R. et al. 2004a. Exogenous and endogenous ghrelin in gastroprotection against stress-induced gastric damage. *Regul Pept* **120**(1–3): 39–51.

Brzozowski, T., Konturek, P.C., Konturek, S.J., Pajdo, R., Kwiecien, S., Pawlik, M., Drozdowicz, D., Sliwowski, Z., and Pawlik, W.W. 2004b. Ischemic preconditioning of remote organs attenuates gastric ischemia–reperfusion injury through involvement of prostaglandins and sensory nerves. *Eur J Pharmacol* **499**(1–2): 201–213.

Brzozowski, T., Konturek, P.C., Konturek, S.J., Sliwowski, Z., Drozdowicz, D., Stachura, J., Pajdo, R. and Hahn, E.G. 1999. Role of prostaglandins generated by cyclooxygenase-1 and cyclooxygenase-2 in healing of ischemia–reperfusion-induced gastric lesions. *Eur J Pharmacol* **385**(1): 47–61.

Brzozowski, T., Konturek, P.C., Sliwowski, Z., Pajdo, R., Drozdowicz, D., Kwiecien, S., Burnat, G., Konturek, S.J., and Pawlik, W.W. 2006. Prostaglandin/cyclooxygenase pathway in ghrelin induced gastroprotection against ischemia-reperfusion injury. *J Pharmacol Exp Ther* **319**: 477–487.

Buharalioğlu, C.K. and Akar, F. 2002. The reactivity of serotonin, acetylcholine and kcl-induced contractions to relaxant agents in the rat gastric fundus. *Pharm Res* **45**(4): 325–331.

Campese, V.M. and Shaohua, Y. 2007. A vitamin-E-fortified diet reduces oxidative stress, sympathetic nerve activity, and hypertension in the phenol-renal injury model in rats. *J Am Soc Hypertens* **1**(4): 242–250.

Cariello, A. 2000. Oxidative stress and glycemic regulation. *Metabolism* **49**(2): 27–29.

Carrasco, G.A. and Van de Kar, L.D. 2003. Neuroendocrine pharmacology of stress. *Eur J Pharmacol* **463**: 235–272.

Coruzzi, G., Adami, M., and Bertaccini, G. 1986. Effect of Ca^{2+} ions in gastric acid secretion by the rat isolated stomach. *Agents Actions* **18**: 201–204.

Das, D. and Banerjee, R.K. 1993. Effect of stress on the antioxidant enzymes and gastric ulceration. *Mol Cell Biochem* **125**(2): 115–125.

Dai, S. and Ogle, C.W. 1974. Gastric ulcers induced by acid accumulation and by stress in pylorus-occluded rats. *Eur J Pharmacol* **26**: 15–21.

Dai, S. and Ogle, C.W. 1975. Effects of stress and of autonomic blockers on gastric mucosal microcirculation in rats. *Eur J Pharmacol* **30**(1): 86–92.

Dazzi, L., Motzo, C., Imperato, A., Serra, M., Gessa, G.L., and Biggio, G. 1995. Modulation of basal and stress-induced release of acetylcholine and dopamine in rat brain by abecarnil and imidazenil, two anxioselective gamma- aminobutyric acid A receptor modulators. *J Pharmacol Exp Ther* **273**: 241–247.

Dronjak, S., Gavrilović, L., Filipović, D., and Radojčić, M.B. 2004. Immobilization and cold stress affect sympatho–adrenomedullary system and pituitary–adrenocortical axis of rats exposed to long-term isolation and crowding. *Physiol Behav* **81**: 409–415.

DuBay, D., Ephgrave, K.S., Cullen, J.J., and Broadhurst, K.A. 2003. Intracerebroventricular calcitonin prevents stress-induced gastric dysfunction. *J Sur Res* **110**: 188–192.

Eberhart, C.E. and Dubois, R.N. 1995. Eicosanoids and the gastrointestinal tract. *Gastroenterology* **109**: 285–301.

Ephgrave, K., Brasel, K., Cullen, J., and Broadhurst, K. 1998. Gastric mucosal protection from enteral nutrients: Role of motility. *J Amer Coll Surg* **186(4)**: 434–440.

Ephgrave, K.S., Cullen, J.J., Broadhurst, K., Kleiman-Wexler, R., Shirazi, S.S., and Schulze-Delrieu, K. 1997. Gastric contractions, secretions and injury in cold restraint. *Neurogastroenterol Motil* **9(3)**: 187–192.

Ephgrave, K.S., Scott, D.L., Ong, A., Cullen, J.J., and Broadhurst, K.A. 2000. Are gastric, jejunal, or both forms of enteral feeding gastroprotective during stress? *J Surg Res* **88(1)**: 1–7.

Esplugues, J.V., Barrachina, M.D., Beltran, B., Calaatayud S., Whittle, B.J., and Moncada, S. 1996. Inhibition of gastric acid secretion by stress: A protective reflex mediated by cerebral nitric oxide. *Proc Natl Acad Sci USA* **93(25)**: 14839–14844.

Fatranska, M., Budai, D., Gulya, K., and Kvetnansky, R. 1989. Changes in acetylcholine content, release and muscarinic receptors in rat hippocampus under cold stress. *Life Sci* **45**: 143–149.

Filaretova, L., Maltcev, N., Bogdanov, A., and Levkovich, Y. 1999. Role of gastric microcirculation in the gastroprotection by glucocorticoids released during water-restraint stress in rats. *Chin J Physiol* **42**: 145–152.

Filaretova, L. 2006. The hypothalamic–pituitary–adrenocortical system: Hormonal brain–gut interaction and gastroprotection. *Auton Neurosci: Basi Clin* **125**: 86–93.

Finkelstein, Y., Koffler, B., Rabey, J.M., and Gilad, G.M. 1985. Dynamics of cholinergic synaptic mechanisms in rat hippocampus after stress. *Brain Res* **343**: 314–319.

Fujii, T., Mori, Y., Tominaga, T., Hayasaka, I., and Kawashima, K. 1997. Maintenance of constant blood acetylcholine content before and after feeding in young chimpanzees. *Neurosci Lett* **227(1)**: 21–24.

Fujii, T., Yamada, S., Yamaguchi, N., Fujimoto, K., Suzuki, T., and Kawashima, K. 1995. Species differences in the concentration of acetylcholine, a neurotransmitter, in whole blood and plasma. *Neurosci Lett* **201(3)**: 207–210.

Galvine, G.B. 1985. Effects of morphine and naloxone on restraint-stress ulcers in rats. *Pharmacology* **31(1)**: 57–60.

Galvine, G.B., Kiernan, K., Hnatowich, M.R., and Labella, F.S. 1986. Effects of morphine and naloxone on stress ulcers formation and gastric acid secretion. *Eur J Pharmacol* **124**: 121–127.

Garrick, T., Buack, S., and Bass, P. 1986a. Gastric motility is a major factor in cold restraint-induced lesion formation in rats. *Am J Physiol* **250**: G191–G199.

Garrick, T., Leung, F.W., Buack, S., Hirabyashi, K., and Guth, P. 1986b. Gastric motility is stimulated but overall blood flow is unaffected during cold restraint in the rat. *Gastroenterology* **91**: 141–148.

Garrick, T., Yoshiaki, G., Buack, S., and Guth, P. 1987. Cimetidine and ranitidine protect against cold restraint-induced ulceration in the rat by suppressing gastric acid secretion. *Dig Dis Sci* **32**: 1261–1267.

Gitlin, N., Ginn, P., Kobayashi, K., and Arakawa, T. 1988. The relationship between plasma cortisol and gastric mucosa prostaglandin levels in rats with severe ulcers. *Aliment Pharm Ther* **2(3)**: 213–220.

Gonzalez, A.M., and Pazos, A. 1992. Modification of muscarinic acetylcholine receptors in the rat brain following chronic immobilization stress: An autoradiographic study. *Eur J Pharmacol* **223**: 25–31.

Gryglewski, R.J., Szczeklik, A., and Wandzilak, M. 1987. The effect of six prostaglandins, prostacyclin and iloprost on generation of superoxide anions by human polymorphonuclear leukocytes stimulated by zymosan or formyl- methionyl-leucyl-phenylalanine. *Biochem Pharmacol* **36**: 4209–4213.

Gutierrez-Cabano, C.A. 1999. Luminal acid in water-immersion stress and the antiulcer effect of axetazolamide in the rat gastric mucosa. *Acta Gastroenterol Latinoam* **29**: 25–31.

Güzel, C., Kurt, D., Sermet, A., Kanay, Z., Denli, O., and Canoruc, F. 1998. The effects of vitamin E on gastric ulcers and gastric mucosal barrier in stress induced rats. *Tr J Med Sci* **28**: 19–21.

Hall, E.D., Pazara, K.E., and Braughler, J.M. 1991. Effects of thialazid mesylate on postischemic brain lipid peroxidation and recovery of extracellular calcium in gerbils. *Stroke* **22**: 361–366.

Hamada, T., Kamisaki, Y., and Itoh, T. 1993. Inhibitory effect of bifemelane on stress-induced astric mucosal lesions. *Yonago Acta Medica* **36**: 35–46.

Harty, R.F., Maico, D.G., Brown, G.M., and McGuigan, J.E. 1984. Effect of calcium on cholinergic-stimulated gastrin release in the rat. *Mol Cell Endocrinol* **37**: 133–138.

Hayase, M. and Takeuchi, K. 1986. Gastric acid secretion and lesion formation in rats under-immersion stress. *Dig Dis Sci* **31**(2): 166–171.

Hellhammer, D.H., Hingtgen, J.N., Wade, S.E., Shea, P.A., and Aprison, M.H. 1983. Serotonergic changes in specific areas of rat brain associated with activity stress gastric lesions. *Psychosom Med* **45**(2): 115–122.

Hirata, F. 1981. The regulation of lipomodulin a phospholipaze inhibitor protein in rabbit neutrophils by phosporylation. *J Biol Chem* **256**: 7730–7733.

Hirota, M., Inoue, M., Ando, Y. 1990. Inhibition of stress-induced gastric mucosal injury by a long acting superoxide dismutase that circulates bound to albumin. *Arch Biochem Biophys* **280**: 269–273.

Ibrahim I.A. 2010. Effects of palm vitamin E and α-tocopherol on hormones and gastric parameters in rats exposed to water-immersion restraint stress. PhD thesis in Pharmacology, Faculty of Medicine, Universiti Kebangsaan Malaysia (UKM), Malaysia.

Ibrahim, A.I., Kamisah, Y., Nafeeza, M.I., and Nur Azlina, M.F. 2011. Modulation of gastric motility and gastric lesion formation in stressed rats given enteral supplementation of palm vitamin-E and α-tocopherol. *Int Med J* **18**: 47–52.

Ibrahim A.I., Kamisah Y., Nafeeza M.I., and Nur Azlina, M.F. 2012. The effects of palm vitamin E on stress hormone levels and gastric lesions in stress-induced rats. *Arch Med Sci* **8**(1): 22–29.

Ibrahim, I.A., Yusof, K., Ismail N.M., and Mohd-Fahami, N.A. 2008. Protective effect of palm vitamin E and α-tocopherol against gastric lesions induced by water immersion restraint stress in Sprague-Dawley rats. *Indian J Pharma* **40**: 73–77.

Imperato, A., Puglisi-Allegra, S., Casolini, P., and Angelucci, L. 1991. Changes in brain dopamine and acetylcholine release during and following stress are independent of the pituitary-adrenocortical axis. *Brain Res* **538**: 111–117.

Ito, M., Shichijo, K., and Sekine, I. 1993. Gastric motility and ischemic changes in occurrence of linear ulcer formation induced by restraint-water immersion stress in rat. *J Gastroenterol* **28**(3): 367–373.

Jia, Y.T., Ma, B., Wei, W., Xu, Y., Wang, Y., Tang, H.T., and Xia, Z.F. 2007. Sustained activation of nuclear factor-kappa B by reactive oxygen species is involved in the pathogenesis of stress-induced gastric damage in rats. *Crit Care Med* **35**(6): 1582–1591.

Johnson, L.R. and Guthrie, P.D. 1980. Stimulation of rat oxyntic gland mucosal growth by epidermal growth factor. *Am J Physiol* **238**: G45–G49.

Kamsiah, J., Gapor, M.T., Nafeeza, M.I., and Fauzee, A.M. 2002. Effect of various doses of palm vitamin E and tocopherol on aspirin-induced gastric lesions in rats. *Int J Exp Pathol* **83**(6): 295–302.

Kamsiah, J., Muhaizan, W., Gapor, M.T., and Roslin, O. 2005. Mucosal protective effects of vitamin E on aspirin-induced gastric lesions in rats. *Int J Pharmacol* **1**(1): 93–97.

Kaneko, H., Tomomasa, T., Watanabe, T., Takahashi, A., Tabata, M., Hussein, S., and Morikawa, A. 2001. Effect of vincristine on gastric motility in conscious rats. *Dig Dis Sci* **46**(5): 952–959.

Kargman, S., Charifson, S., Cartwiright, M., Frank, J., Riendean, D., Mancini, J., Evans, J. & O'Neill, G. 1996. Characterization of prostaglandin G/H synthase 1 and 2 in rat, dog, monkey and human gastrointestinal tract. *Gastroenterol* **111**: 445–454.

Kato, K., Murai, I., Asai, S., Takahashi, Y., Nagata, T., Komuro, S., Mizuno, S., Iwasaki, A., Ishikawa, K., and Arakawa, Y. 2002. Circadian rhythm of melatonin and prostaglandin in modulation of stress-induced gastric mucosal lesions in rats. *Aliment Pharm Ther* **2**: 29–34.

Kauffman, G.L., Jr., Reeve, J.J., Jr., and Grossman, M.I. 1980. Gastric bicarbonate secretion: effect of topical and intravenous 16, 16-dimethyl prostaglandin E_2. *Am J Physiol* **239**: G44–G48.

Kawashima, K., Oohata, H., Fujimoto, K., and Suzuki, T. 1987. Plasma concentration of acetylcholine in young women. *Neurosci Lett* **80**(3): 339–342.

Keogh, J.P., Allen, A., and Garner, A. 1997. Relationship between gastric mucus synthesis, secretion and surface gel erosion measured in amphibian stomach *in vitro*. *Clin Exp Pharm Physiol* **24**: 844–849.

Kheir-Eldin, A.A., Motawi, T.K., Gad, M.Z., and Abd-ElGawad, H.M. 2001. Protective effect of vitamin E, β-carotene and N-acetylcysteine from the brain oxidative stress induced in rats by lipopolysaccharide. *Int J Biochem Cell Biol* **33**(5): 475–482.

Kirshenbaum, L.A., Gupta, M., Thomas, T.P., and Singal, P.K. 1990. Antioxidant protection against adrenaline-induced arrhythmias in rats with chronic heart hypertrophy. *Can J Cardiol* **6**(2): 71–74.

Kitagawa, H., Fujiwara, M., and Osumi, Y. 1979. Effect of water-immersion stress on gastric secretion and mucosal blood flow in rats. *Gastroenterology* **77**: 298–302.

Klenerová V., Jurcovicova J., Kaminsky, O., Sida, P., Krejci, I., Hlinak, Z., and Hynie, S. 2003. Combined restraint and cold stress in rats: Effects on memory processing in passive avoidance task and on plasma levels of ACTH and corticosterone. *Behav Brain Res* **142**: 143–149.

Komuro, Y., Ishihara, K., and Ohara, S. 1992. Effects of tetragastrin on mucus glycoprotein in rat gastric mucosal protection. *Gastroenterol Jpn* **27**: 597–603.

Konturek, S.J. Brzozowski, T., and Bielamski, W. 1995. Role of endogenous gastrin in gastroprotection. *Eur J Pharmacol* **278**: 203–212.

Konturek, P.C., Brzozowski, T., Dudab, A., Kwiecienb, S., Löbera, S., Dembinskib, A., Hahna, E.G., and Konturek S.J. 2001. Epidermal growth factor and prostaglandin E$_2$ accelerate mucosal recovery from stress-induced gastric lesions via inhibition of apoptosis. *J Physiol—Paris* **95**: 361–367.

Konturek, P.C., Brzozowski, T., Konturek, S.J., and Dembinski, A. 1992. Role of epidermal growth factor, prostaglandin and sulfhydryls in stress-induced gastric lesions. *Gastroenterology* **99**: 1607–1615.

Konturek, P.C., Brzozowski, T., Konturek, S.J., Taut, A., Sliwowski, Z., Stachura, J., and Hahn, E.G. 1998. Activation of genes for growth factors and cyclooxygenase in rat gastric mucosa during recovery from stress damage. *Eur J Pharmacol* **342**: 55–65.

Koo, M.W.L., Cho, C.H., and Ogle, C.W. 1986. Luminal acid in stress ulceration and the antiulcer action of verapamil in rat stomachs. *J Pharm Pharmacol* **38**: 845–848.

Kwiecień, S., Brzozowski, T., Konturek, P.C., Pawlik, M.W., Pawlik, W.W., Kwiecień, N., and Konturek, S.J. 2004. Gastroprotection by pentoxyfilline against stress-induced gastric damage. Role of lipid peroxidation, antioxidizing enzymes and proinflammatory cytokines. *J Physiol Pharmacol* **55(2)**: 337–355.

Landeira-Fernandez, J. 2004. Analysis of the cold-water restraint procedure in gastric ulceration and body temperature. *Physiol Behav* **82(5)**: 827–833.

Lee, L., Kang, S.A., and Lee, H.O. 2001. Effect of supplementation of vitamin E and vitamin C on brain acetylcholinesterase activity and neurotransmitter levels in rats treated with scopolamine, an inducer of dementia. *J Nutr Sci Vitaminol* **47**: 323–328.

Lenz, H.J. and Druge, G. 1990. Neurohormonal pathways mediating stress-induced inhibition of gastric acid secretion in rats. *Gastroenterology* **98(6)**: 1490–1492.

Lesch, C.A., Gilbertsen, R.B., Song, Y., Dyer, R.D., Sehrier, D., Kraus, E.R., Sanchez, B., and Guglietta, A. 1998. Effect of novel anti-inflammatory compounds on healing of acetic acid-induced gastric ulcer in rats. *J Pharmacol Exp Ther* **287**: 301–306.

Li, Y.M., Lu, G.M., Zou, X.P., Li, Z.S., Peng, G.Y., and Fang, D.C. 2006. Dynamic functional and ultrastructural changes of gastric parietal cells induced by water immersion-restraint stress in rats. *World J Gastroenterol* **12(21)**: 3368–3372.

Lim, A.T.W. and Funder, J.W. 1983. Stress-induced changes in plasma, pituitary and hypothalamic immunoreactive β-endorphin: Effects of diurnal variation, adrenalectomy, corticosteroids, and opiate agonists and antagonists. *Neuroendocrinology* **36(3)**: 225–234.

Livingston, E.H., Howard, T.J., Garrick, T.R., Passaro, E.P., Jr., and Guth, P.H. 1991. Strong gastric contractions cause mucosal ischemia. *Am J Physiol Gastrointest Liver Physiol* **260**: 524–530.

Livingston, E.H., Scremin, O.U., Yasue, N., Garrick, T.R., and Guth, P.H. 1988. Cold restraint produces foci of marked ischemia in the rat gastric corpus. *Gastroenterology* **94**: A266.

Lou, L.X., Geng, B., Du, J.B., and Tang, C.S. 2008. Hydrogen sulphide-induced hypothermia attenuates stress-related ulceration in rats. *Clin Exp Pharmacol Physiol* **35(2)**: 223–228.

Lou, L.X., Geng, B., Yu, F., Zhang, J., Pan, C.S., Chen, L., Qi, Y.F., Ke, Y., Wang, X., and Tang, C.S. 2006. Endoplasmic reticulum stress response is involved in the pathogenesis of stress induced gastric lesions in rats. *Life Sci* **7(19)**:1856–1864.

Mark, G.P., Rada, P.V., and Shors, T.J. 1996. Inescapable stress enhances extracellular acetylcholine in the rat hippocampus and prefrontal cortex but not the nucleus accumbens or amygdala. *Neuroscience* **74**: 767–774.

Masferrer, J.L., Isakson, P.C., and Seibert, K. 1996. Cyclooxygenase-2 inhibitors. *Gastroenterol Clin North Am* **252**: 363–372.

McEwen, B.S. 2002. Mood disorders and allostatic load. *Biol Psychiatry* **54**: 200–207.

Mersereau, W.A. and Hinchey, E.J. 1981. Effect of gastric acidity on gastric ulceration induced by hemorrhage in the rat, utilizing a gastric chamber technique. *Gastroenterology* **64**: 1130–1135.

Mersereau, W.A. and Hinchey, E.J. 1988. Relationship between the gastric myoelectric and mechanical activity in the genesis of ulcers in indomethacin-insulin-treated rats. *Dig Dis Sci* **33(2)**: 200–208.

Mita, M., Satoh, M., Shimada, A., Okajima, M., Azuma, S., Suzuki, J.S., Sakabe, K., Hara, S., and Himeno, S. 2008. Metallothionein is a crucial protective factor against *Helicobacter pylori*-induced gastric erosive lesions in a mouse model. *Am J Physiol Gastrointest Liver Physiol* **294(4)**: G877–G884.

Mitsushima, D., Funabashi, T., Shinohara, K., and Kimura, F. 2003. Housing in a small cage attenuates stress response of the hippocampal acetylcholine release but not of the adrenocortical corticosterone release in male rats. *Psychoneuroendocrinology* **28**: 574–583.

Mizuno, T. and Kimura, F. 1997. Attenuated stress response of hippocampal acetylcholine release and adreno-cortical secretion in aged rats. *Neurosci Lett* **222**: 49–52.

Morris, G.P., Fallone, C.A., Pringle, G.C., and MacNaughton, W.K. 1998. Gastric cytoprotection is secondary to increased mucosal fluid secretion: A study of six cytoprotective agents in the rat. *J Clin Gastroenterol* **1**: S53–S63.

Murison, R., Overmier, J.B., Hellhammer, D.H., and Carmona, M. 1989. Hypothalamo- pituitary-adrenal manipulations and stress ulcerations in rats. *Psychoneuroendocrinology* **14**: 331–338.

Murphy, H.M., Wideman, C.H., and Brown, T.S. 1979. Plasma corticosterone levels and ulcer formation in rats with hippocampal lesions. *Neuroendocrinology* **28**:123–130.

Nafeeza, M.I. and Kang, T.T. 2005. Synergistic effects of tocopherol, tocotrienol, and ubiquinone in indometh-acin-induced experimental gastric lesions. *Int J Vitam Nutr Res* **75(2)**: 149–155.

Nafeeza, M.I., Fauzee, A.M., Kamsiah, J., and Gapor M.T. 2002. Comparative effects of a tocotrienol-rich fraction and tocopherol in aspirin-induced gastric lesions in rats. *Asia Pac J Clin Nutr* **11(4)**: 309–313.

Nafeeza, M.I., Syamsinaz, S.N., Renuvathani, M., Gapor, M.T., and Kamsiah, J. 2000. Protection by palm vitamin E against ethanol gastric injury is independent of gastric mucus quantity. *Mal J Biochem Mol Biol* **5**: 18–22.

Nakade, Y., Tsuchida, D., Fukuda, H., Iwa, M., Pappas, T.N., and Takahashi, T. 2006. Restraint stress augments postprandial gastric contractions but impairs antropyloric coordination in conscious rats. *Am J Physiol Regul Integr Comp Physiol* **290**: R616–R624.

Nordmann, R. 1994. Alcohol and antioxidant systems. *Alcohol and Alcohol* **29**: 513–522.

Nur Azlina, M.F., Khalid, B.A.K., and Nafeeza, M.I. 2003. Modulation of gastric acidity in rats given enteral supplementation of vitamin E and exposed to restraint stress. *Mal J Biochem Mol Biol* **8**: 26–29.

Nur Azlina, M.F. and Nafeeza, M.I. 2007. Phytonutrient: Effects on lipid peroxidation in experimental gastritis induced by restraint stress. *Int J Pharmacol* **3(3)**: 254–259.

Nur Azlina, M.F. and Nafeeza, M.I. 2008. Tocotrienol and α-tocopherol reduces corticosterone and noradrena-lin levels in rats exposed to restraint stress. *Pharmazie* **63(12)**: 890–892.

Nur Azlina, M.F., Nafeeza, M.I., and Khalid, B.A.K. 2005a. Effect of tocotrienol on lipid peroxidation in experimental gastritis induced by restraint stress. *Pak J Nutr* **4(2)**: 69–72.

Nur Azlina, M.F., Nafeeza, M.I., and Khalid, B.A.K. 2005b. A comparison between tocopherol and tocotrienol effects on gastric parameters in rats exposed to stress. *Asia Pac J Clin Nutr* **14(4)**: 358–365.

Ogle, C.W., Cho, C.H., Tong, M.C., and Koo, M.W.L. 1985. The influence of verapamil on the gastric effects of stress in rats. *Eur J Pharmacol* **112**: 399–404.

Ohta, Y., Kamiya, Y., Imai, Y., Arisawa, T., and Nakano, H. 2005. Role of gastric mucosal ascorbic acid in gas-tric mucosal lesion development in rats with water immersion restraint stress. *Inflammopharmacology* **13(1–3)**: 249–259.

Önen, A., Kanay, Z., Güzel, C., Kurt, D., and Ceylan, K. 2000. The effects of allopurinol on stomach mucosal barrier of rats subjected to ischemia-reperfusion. *Turk J Med Sci* **30(5)**: 449–452.

Ozdil, S., Bolkent, Ş., Yanardag, R., and Arda-Pirincci, P. 2004. Protective effects of ascorbic acid, DL-α-tocopherol acetate, and sodium selenate on ethanol- induced liver damage of rats. *Biol Trace Element Res* **97(2)**: 149–161.

Papovich, I.L., Butusova, I.A., Ivasivka, S.V., and Laramenko, M.S. 1992. Features of gastric reaction in rats with different susceptibilities to gastric mucosa lesions in immobilization-cold stress. *Bull Eksp Biol Med* **113(2)**: 126–127.

Park, S.W., Oh, T.Y., Kim, Y.S., Sim, H., Park, S.J., Jang, E.J., Park, J.S., Baik, H.W., and Hahm. K.B. 2008. *Artemisia asiatica* extracts protect against ethanol- induced injury in gastric mucosa of rats. *J Gastroenterol Hepatol* **23(6)**: 976–984.

Perveen, T., Zehra, S.F., Haider, S., Akhtar, N., and Haleem, D.J. 2003. Effects of 2 hrs. restraint stress on brain serotonin metabolism and memory in rats. *Pak J Pharm Sci* **16(1)**: 27–33.

Petroianu, A. and Weinberg, J. 1986. Motility of isolated mammalian gastric fundus. *Comp Biochem Physiol* **85C**: 57–59.

Sakamoto, T., Swierczek, J.S., and Ogden, X.C.D. 1985. Cytoprotective effect of pentagastrin and epidermal growth factor on stress ulcer formation. *Ann Surg* **201**: 290–295.

Salim, A.S. 1990. Role of oxygen-derived free radicals in the mechanism of acute and chronic duodenal ulcer-ation in the rat. *Dig Dis Sci* **35**: 73–79.

Schoenberg, M., Muhl, E., Sellin, D., Younes, M., Schildberg, F., and Hagluno, V. 1984. Posthypotensive gen-eration of superoxide free radicals-possible role in the pathogenesis of intestinal mucosa damage. *Acta Chir Scand* **150**: 301–309.

Selye, H. *The Stress of Life*. New York: McGraw-Hill, 1956.

Sethbhadki, S., Roth, J.L.A., and Pfeiffer, C.H. 1970. Gastric mucosal ulceration after epinephrine. A study of the etiologic mechanisms. *Dig Dis Sci* **15**: 1055–1065.

Shaheen, A.A., Hamdy, M.A., Kheir-Eldin, A.A., Lindstrom, P., and Abd El-Fattah, A.A. 1993. Effect of pretreatment with vitamin E or diazepam on brain metabolism of stressed rats. *Bioch Pharm* **46**(1): 194–197.

Shen, G.M., Zhou, M.Q., Xu, G.S., Xu, Y., and Yin, G. 2006. Role of vasoactive intestinal peptide and nitric oxide in the modulation of electroacupuncture on gastric motility in stressed rats. *World J Gastroenterol* **12**(38): 6156–6160.

Singh, S., Khajuria, A., Taneja, S.C., Khajuria, R.K., Singh, J., Johri, R.K., and Qazi, G.N. 2008. The gastric ulcer protective effect of boswellic acids, a leukotriene inhibitor from *Boswellia serrata*, in rats. *Phytomedicine* **15**(6–7): 408–415.

Srinivasan, B.D. and Kulkarni, P.S. 1989. Inhibitors of the arachidonic acid cascade in the management of ocular inflammation. *Prog Clin Biol Res* **312**: 229–249.

Stark, R., Wolf, O.T., Tabbert, K., Kagerer, S., Zimmermann, M., Kirsch, P., Schienle, A., and Vaitla, D. 2006. Influence of the stress hormone cortisol on fear conditioning in humans: Evidence for sex differences in the response of the prefrontal cortex. *NeuroImage* **32**(3): 1290–1298.

Stroff, T., Plate, S., and Respondek, M. 1995. Protection by gastrin in the rat stomach involves afferent neiro, calcitonin gene-related peptide, and nitric oxide. *Gastroenterology* **109**: 89–97.

Tache, Y., Martinez, V., Million, M., and Wang, L. 2001. Stress and the gastrointestinal tract. III. Stress-related alterations of gut motor function: Role of brain corticotropin-releasing factor receptors. *Am J Physiol Gastrointest Liver Physiol* **280**: 173–177.

Tajima, T., Endo, H., Suzuki, Y., Ikari, H., Gotoh, M., and Iguchi, A. 1996. Immobilization stress-induced increase of hippocampal acetylcholine and of plasma epinephrine, norepinephrine and glucose in rats. *Brain Res* **720**: 155–158.

Takeuchi, K. and Johnson, L.R. 1979. Pentagastrin protects against stress ulceration in rats. *Gastroenterology* **78**(2): 327–334.

Takeuchi, K., Nishiwaki, H., and Furukawa, O. 1987. Cytoprotection action of histamine against 0.6N HCl-induced gastric mucosal injury in rats; comparative study with adaptive cytoprotection induced by exogenous acid. *Jpn J Pharmacol* **22**: 335–344.

Takeuchi, K., Suzuki, K., Araki, H., Mizoguchi, H., Sugamoto, S., and Umdeda, M. 1999. Roles of endogenous prostaglandins and nitric oxide in gastroduodenal ulcerogenic responses induced in rats by hypothermic stress. *J Physiol Paris* **93**(5): 423–431.

Tanaka, S., Akiba, Y., and Kaunitz, J.D. 1998. Pentagastrin gastroprotection against acid is related to H2 receptor activation but not acid secretion. *Gut* **43**(3): 334–337.

Tanaka, S., Tache, Y., and Kaneko, H. 1997. Central vagal activation increases mucus gel thickness and surface cell intracellular pH in rat stomach. *Gastroenterology* **112**: 409–417.

Tani, K., Yamaguchi, T., and Binada, T. 1990. Gastric mucosal red blood cell distribution in gastric hypermotility. *Exp Ulcer* **17**: 200–201.

Taniguchi, N., Ohtsuka, A., and Hayashi, K. 2001. A high dose of vitamin E inhibits adrenal corticosterone synthesis in chickens treated with ACTH. *J Nutr Sci Vitam* **47**(1): 40–46.

Tarnasky, P.R., Livingston, E.H., Jacobs, K.M., Zimmerman, B.J., Guth, P.H., and Garrick, T.R. 1990. Role of oxyradicals in cold water immersion restraint-induced gastric mucosal injury in the rat. *Dig Dis Sci* **35**(2): 173–177.

Ueki, S., Takeuchi, K., and Okabe, S. 1988. Gastric motility is an important factor in the pathogenesis of indomethacin-induced gastric mucosal lesions in rats. *Dig Dis Sci* **33**(2): 209–216.

Vane, J.R. and Botting, R.M. 1995. New insights into the mode of action of anti- inflammatory drugs. *Inflamm Res* **44**: 1–10.

Wang, F.W., Li, J., Hu, Z.L., and Xie, Y.Y. 2006. Protective effect of puerarin on stress-induced gastric mucosal injury in rats. *Zhongguo Zhong Yao Za Zhi* **31**(6): 504–506.

Wang, Z.J. and Zhu, W.Y. 1995. *Cytoprotection*. Beijing, China: Beijing Medical University–China Union Medical University Joint Publishing Company, pp. 195–196.

Watanabe, M., Kimura, A., Akasaka, K., and Hayashi, S. 1987. Determination of acetylcholine in human blood. *Biochem Med Metab Biol* **36**(3): 355–362.

Watanabe, M., Tomiyama-Miyaji, C., Kainuma, E., Inoue, M., Kuwano, Y., Ren, H., Shen, J., and Abo, T. 2008. Role of alpha-adrenergic stimulus in stress-induced modulation of body temperature, blood glucose and innate immunity. *Immunol Lett* **115**(1): 43–49.

Weiss, J.M. 1971. Effects of coping behavior in different warning signal conditions on stress pathology in rats. *J Comp Physiol Psychol* **77**: 1–13.

Wong, D., Koo, M.W., Shin, V.Y., Liu, E.S., and Cho, C.H. 2002. Pathogenesis of nicotine treatment and its withdrawal on stress-induced gastric ulceration in rats. *Eur J Phramacol* **434**: 81–86.

Yano, S., Akahane, M., and Harada, M. 1978. Role of gastric motility in development of stress-induced gastric lesions of rats. *Jpn J Pharmacol* **28**: 607–615.

Zhang, H., Han, T., Sun, L.N., Huang, B.K., Chen, Y.F., Zheng, H.C., and Qin, L.P. 2008. Regulative effects of essential oil from *Atractylodes lancea* on delayed gastric emptying in stress-induced rats. *Phytomedicine* **15**: 602–611.

26 Structural Modification of Tocotrienols to Improve Bioavailability

Awantika Singh, Philip J. Breen, Sanchita Ghosh,
K. Sree Kumar, Kottayil I. Varughese, Peter A. Crooks,
Martin Hauer-Jensen, and Cesar M. Compadre

CONTENTS

26.1 INTRODUCTION

Tocotrienols have gained more attention in recent years because of their beneficial effects in many health-related problems not observed with the other component of the vitamin E family, the tocopherols (Agarwal et al., 2010; Berbee et al., 2009; Ghosh et al., 2009; Kulkarni et al., 2010; Sylvester et al., 2010; Tan, 2005). Structurally, tocopherols and tocotrienols, collectively known as tocols, are closely related in having a chromanol head and a lipophilic tail, but differing in the nature of the chromanol side chain. They show widely varying degrees of biological effectiveness. The biological activity of vitamin E constituents is governed not only by their chemical structure but also by their ability to be absorbed and delivered to the plasma and target tissues, and by their ability to be retained at the site of action in sufficient quantity to afford the desired pharmacological response.

Bioavailability is defined as the fraction of an ingested compound or nutrient that reaches the systemic circulation. Bioavailability of vitamin E is dependent on several factors, including its absorption, plasma transport, and delivery to the target tissue, as well as hepatic metabolism and oxidative stress (Traber, 2007). Orally administered tocotrienols have very limited bioavailability due to poor absorption and transport mechanisms within the body, which is, in turn, related to the high selectivity of the α-tocopherol transfer protein (ATTP) for α-tocopherol, the more common form of vitamin E in supplements.

Intestinal absorption of the tocols depends greatly on bile secretion and micelle formation. Vitamin E in the diet passes through the gastrointestinal tract, and is absorbed from the small intestine in a similar manner to other lipids and fatty acids. After ingestion, the vitamin E components

TABLE 26.1
Apparent Elimination Half-Life of Tocols

Tocols	$t_{1/2}$ (H)	References
RRR-α-tocopherol	44	Traber et al. (1994)
SRR-α-tocopherol	17	Traber et al. (1994)
γ-Tocopherol	13	Leonard et al. (2005)
α-Tocotrienol	4.4	Yap et al. (2001)
γ-Tocotrienol	4.3	Yap et al. (2001)
δ-Tocotrienol	2.3	Yap et al. (2001)

are, in turn, emulsified by bile, transported to the enterocytes in micelles, released at the enterocyte surface, and then transported into the enterocyte, predominantly in a carrier-mediated process. Abuasal et al. (2010) demonstrated that the intestinal absorption of γ-tocotrienols is a carrier-mediated process which undergoes saturation as the intestinal concentration of γ-tocotrienols increases.

After vitamin E, along with lipids and fatty acids, is absorbed into enterocytes, it is assembled into chylomicrons. Chylomicrons are then taken up by the lacteals and secreted into the lymphatic system via exocytosis. The tocol-containing chylomicrons then exit the thoracic duct and enter the circulation at the left brachiocephalic vein. Lipoprotein lipase hydrolyses chylomicrons (Cooper, 1997) by removing triglycerides, leading to the formation of chylomicron remnants. Various tissues of the body can take up the released lipids. The liver takes up chylomicron remnants and repacks them as very low-density lipoproteins (VLDLs). Vitamin E in VLDLs is then secreted from the liver into the blood by the action of ATTP.

The mean apparent elimination half-life of tocotrienols and tocopherols varies between 2.3 and 44 h, with tocotrienols exhibiting the lowest half-life values (Table 26.1).

This review focuses on structural modifications of tocotrienols that result in increased bioavailability. Delivery systems and formulation approaches that may improve absorption have been discussed elsewhere (Kumar et al., 2009; Yuen et al., 2009).

26.2   STRUCTURAL FACTORS AFFECTING TOCOTRIENOL BIOAVAILABILITY

As described by Neuzil et al. (2002) vitamin E analogues have three structural domains, comprising a phenolic OH group, crucial for redox and apoptotic activity, the chromane ring with variable methylation patterns, and a lipophilic side chain whose function is classically considered to promote incorporation of the molecule into the lipid bilayer of biological membranes. However, the farnesyl-like nature of the tail is also important for receptor recognition (Behery et al., 2010). Nevertheless, a review of the literature shows that the influence of the structural domains of the tocols on their bioavailability has been explored to only a limited extent. Tocopherol and tocotrienol general structures are illustrated in Figure 26.1.

Pharmacokinetic studies in humans have demonstrated that all tocotrienols are not equally bioavailable. Differences in the methylation pattern on the chromanol ring may account for the differences in bioavailability. In addition, bioavailability is dependent on fed and fasted conditions, and also on the route of administration (Yap et al., 2001, 2003; Yuen et al., 2009).

A study in humans using deuterated *RRR*- and *SRR*-α-tocopherol stereoisomers demonstrated a selective preference for the *RRR*-stereoisomer during VLDL secretion by the liver (Traber et al., 1990). Equal amounts of both stereoisomers of these deuterated tocopherols were absorbed in chylomicron fractions and also during a few hours after chylomicron secretion and catabolism, demonstrating no discrimination during absorption and chylomicron secretion by the intestine. However, the *RRR* isomer was preferentially secreted in the VLDL. This preferential incorporation into VLDL resulted in *RRR*-α-tocopherol

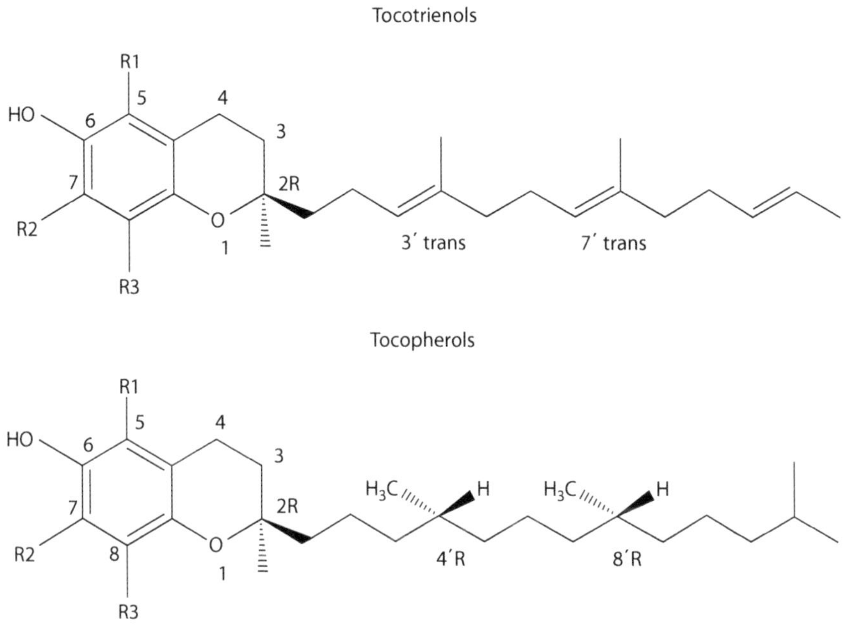

Tocotrienols

Tocopherols

	R1	R2	R3
Alpha (α)	CH_3	CH_3	CH_3
Beta (β)	CH_3	H	CH_3
Gamma (γ)	H	CH_3	CH_3
Delta (δ)	H	H	CH_3

FIGURE 26.1 Chemical structures of tocotrienols and tocopherols.

plasma curves which were larger and which declined more slowly than the *SRR*-α-tocopherol plasma curves (Traber et al., 1994). Hoppe and Krennrich (2000) reported a compilation of studies comparing various measures of bioequivalency of *RRR*-α-tocopherol to all rac-α-tocopherol. Values ranged from 0.98 to 2.62, with the most common value being 1.36. The authors cautioned that the value of the bio-availability ratio would not necessarily predict the biopotency ratio of the two stereoisomers in humans.

Natural tocotrienols represent a single isomeric structure (2*R*, 3'-*trans*, 7'-*trans*) (Kamal-Eldin and Appelqvist, 1996), whereas commercially available synthetic tocotrienols exist in the racemic 2*R/S* stereoisomeric forms. In addition to *R/S* form, the presence of double bonds at the 3' and 7' positions results in four *cis/trans* isomers for individual tocotrienols. Therefore, a total of eight isomers may exist for each tocotrienol (Table 26.2).

TABLE 26.2
Possible *cis/trans* Isomers of Tocotrienols

2	3'	7'
R	cis	cis
R	cis	trans
R	trans	cis
R	trans	trans
S	cis	cis
S	cis	trans
S	trans	cis
S	trans	trans

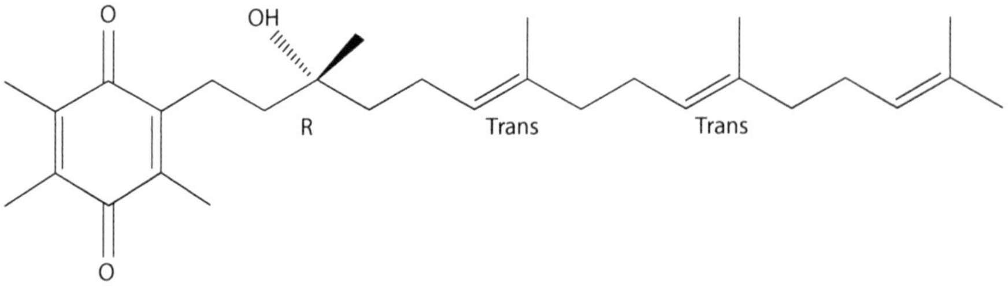

FIGURE 26.2   Structure of α-tocotrienol quinone (ATQ3).

Drotleff and Ternes (1999) studied the effect of *cis/trans* geometry on the bioavailability of α-tocotrienol in eggs from tocotrienol-fed laying hens. Tocotrienol side-chain isomers extracted from the eggs of synthetic α-tocotrienol-fed hens were compared with eggs of a control group of hens where no α-tocotrienol supplement was added to the diet. *Cis/trans* isomers of α-tocotrienol were not detected in eggs from the control group (non-supplemented diet). All four isomers were determined in the egg yolk of hens supplemented with a synthetic α-tocotrienol diet, demonstrating bioavailability of all four isomers. However, preference was observed for natural 2*R*, 3′-*trans*, 7′-*trans* form over the other isomers.

Although the integrity of the chromanol ring is important for biological activity, it is not an absolute requirement for bioavailability of the tocols. Pharmacokinetic studies have been performed to explore the bioavailability of α-tocotrienol quinone (ATQ3) (Figure 26.2), a metabolite of α-tocotrienol (Shrader et al., 2011). Bioavailability studies carried out in rats and dogs have shown that ATQ3 is orally bioavailable and that the presence of food increases the oral absorption and absolute bioavailability of ATQ3 (Shrader et al., 2011). These studies also reported that ATQ3 is readily distributed into brain and heart after intraperitoneal administration in mice and into retina after oral administration in dogs.

26.3   STRUCTURAL MODIFICATIONS TO IMPROVE BIOAVAILABILITY

Novel tocol prodrugs have been developed in an effort to overcome limitations in the oral absorption of the tocols. The properties of an ideal prodrug include sufficient water solubility and rapid conversion to the parent drug *in vivo*. An effective way to improve the aqueous solubility of poorly water-soluble drugs that contain a hydroxyl group is the formation of water-soluble ester prodrugs. Esterification can also prevent rapid metabolic inactivation. The phenolic hydroxyl group in the tocols can be easily esterified, and some of the resulting ester derivatives, such as aminoalkylcarboxylic acid esters, have enhanced aqueous solubility as well as improved stability to oxidation.

26.3.1   Succinates

Vitamin E succinate (VES) has been shown to possess antitumor activity (Malafa et al., 2006; Yin et al., 2007); however, this compound exhibits low efficacy due to limited bioavailability when given orally. In order to overcome the problem of poor oral bioavailability of VES, an ether analogue, *RRR*-α-tocopheryloxybutyl sulfonic acid (VEBSA) was developed (Ni et al., 2009) (Figure 26.3).

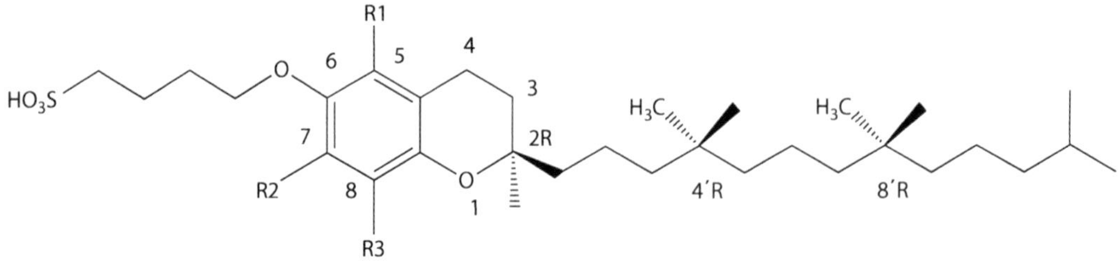

FIGURE 26.3   Structure of *RRR*-α-tocopheryloxybutyl sulfonic acid (VEBSA).

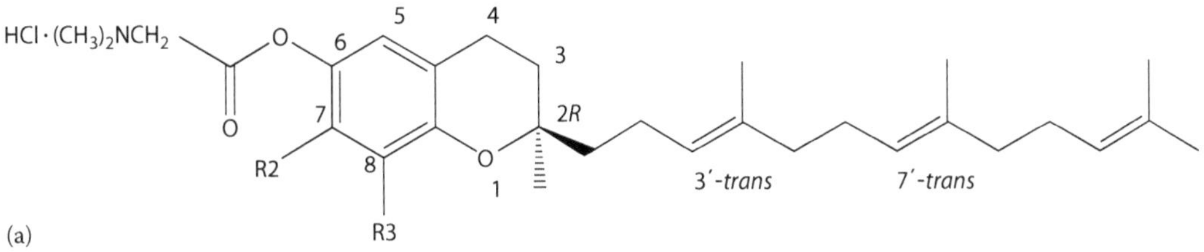

FIGURE 26.4 Structures of (a) 2R-γ-tocotrienyl *N,N*-dimethylaminoacetate hydrochloride and (b) γ-tocopheryl *N,N*-dimethylglycinate hydrochloride.

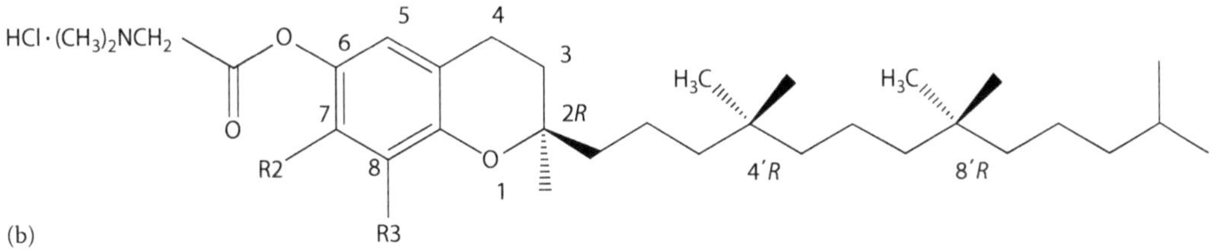

As compared VEBSA was given orally there was a significant increase in serum levels of VEBSA when compared to oral administration of VES. Results from this study indicate that VEBSA had a better bioavailability and antitumor effect when compared with VES *in vivo*.

26.3.2 HYDROCHLORIDES

Even though γ-tocopherol is associated with superior ability to scavenge reactive nitrogen species as compared to α-tocopherol, its high reactivity toward atmospheric oxygen and its poor water solubility limit its clinical usefulness. Takata et al. (2002) synthesized γ-tocopheryl *N, N*-dimethylglycinate hydrochloride (γ-TDMG) (Figure 26.4b) as a water-soluble ester prodrug to improve the physicochemical properties of γ-tocopherol. γ-TDMG showed a significant increase in water solubility, and γ-tocopherol was released upon enzymatic cleavage in the liver. There was also a significant increase in the plasma and liver concentration of γ-tocopherol after intravenous administration of γ-TDMG.

Water-soluble prodrugs may be an efficient way to deliver γ-tocotrienol orally. In this context a recent publication describes the synthesis of three different esters of γ-tocotrienol (Akaho et al., 2007). One of these ester derivatives, 2R-γ-tocotrienyl *N,N*-dimethylaminoacetate hydrochloride (Figure 26.4a) showed high water solubility and was rapidly converted to γ-tocotrienol by esterases in both rat and human liver. An intravenous injection of this compound increased the levels of γ-tocotrienol in plasma, liver, heart, and kidney.

26.3.3 MALEATES

A semisynthetic highly polar ester, α-tocotrienol maleate (Figure 26.5), has nearly 1000-fold greater water solubility compared to α-tocotrienol. This compound has enhanced chemical stability and

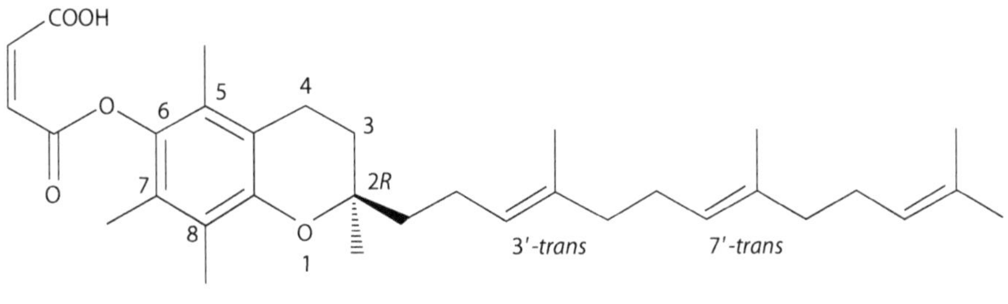

FIGURE 26.5 Structure of α-tocotrienol maleate.

bioactivity, and a slower decomposition rate in rat plasma. At nanomolar doses, this compound effectively inhibited the proliferation of malignant +SA mouse mammary epithelial cells (Behery et al., 2010).

26.4   TRANSPORT-TARGETED APPROACHES TO IMPROVE TOCOTRIENOL BIOAVAILABILITY

Tocotrienols have considerably shorter elimination half-lives than α-tocopherol (Table 26.1). This is likely due to the continual cycle of secretion of α-tocopherol by the liver via ATTP, followed by reuptake. Tocotrienols, which have less affinity for ATTP, have a longer residence time in the liver, putting them at higher risk for metabolism and biliary excretion. A shorter elimination half-life has a striking effect on the exposure time of a drug in the blood, as measured by area-under-the-plasma drug concentration vs. time curve (AUC).

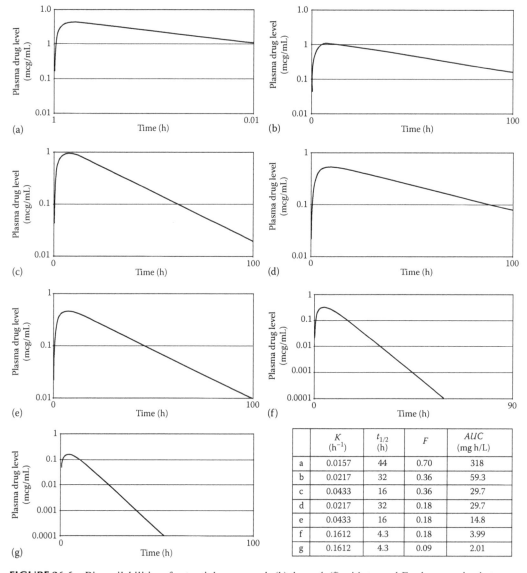

	K (h^{-1})	$t_{1/2}$ (h)	F	AUC (mg h/L)
a	0.0157	44	0.70	318
b	0.0217	32	0.36	59.3
c	0.0433	16	0.36	29.7
d	0.0217	32	0.18	29.7
e	0.0433	16	0.18	14.8
f	0.1612	4.3	0.18	3.99
g	0.1612	4.3	0.09	2.01

FIGURE 26.6   Bioavailabilities of potential compounds (b) through (f) with $t_{1/2}$ and F values ranging between those of α-tocopherol (a) and γ-tocotrienol (g).

Besides elimination half-life, another factor that contributes to a large AUC is the bioavailability factor *F*. In view of the earlier description of the sequence of events occurring during the absorption of fats and fat-soluble vitamins such as the tocols, it becomes apparent that a fraction of tocol molecules carried to the blood by the lymphatic system appears in the blood before reaching the liver, with a subsequent cycle of secretion and reuptake. It is this fraction of the dose of tocol molecules that constitutes the *F* value. This parameter, reflected in the size of the peak plasma tocol level, is a factor, along with elimination half-life, that determines the size of the *AUC*. Specifically, $AUC = FX_0/KV = Ft_{1/2}X_0/V$, where $t_{1/2}$ is elimination half-life, X_0 is administered dose, and *V* is volume of distribution. Differences among tocols in their transport across the enterocyte membrane constitute the most likely reason for differences in *F*, with carrier-mediated transport of trienols being rate-limiting; whereas, differences in the affinity of the tocols for ATTP would produce differences in the half-life.

Figure 26.6 simulates combinations of theoretical compounds with elimination half-lives longer than, and *F* parameters greater than, those of γ-tocotrienol. From this figure, it is clear that the development of a tocotrienol derivative with affinity for ATTP approaching that of the tocopherols would afford a compound having a plasma level vs. time profile likely to resemble one of the graphs in Figure 26.6, any one of which has superior bioavailability properties compared to γ-tocotrienol.

The key role of ATTP in regulating the pharmacokinetics of tocols has been elegantly demonstrated by the work of Traber et al. (1994), as illustrated in Figure 26.7. From these studies, it is clear that a tocol that does not bind efficiently to ATTP would have lower bioavailability than a tocol that binds efficiently to this transporter. The reason for this is that when a tocol that does not bind well to ATTP reaches the liver, it is cleared from the body by biliary excretion (Min et al., 2003). On the other hand, when α-tocopherol reaches the liver, it is re-secreted into the circulation by ATTP. For example, a synthetic isomer such as *SRR*-α-tocopherol, which does not bind efficiently to ATTP, shows a much more pronounced rate of disappearance from blood (Traber, 2007).

The x-ray crystal structure of ATTP has been solved independently by two groups (Meier et al., 2003; Min et al., 2003) (Figure 26.8). The ligand-binding pocket of ATTP closes once it

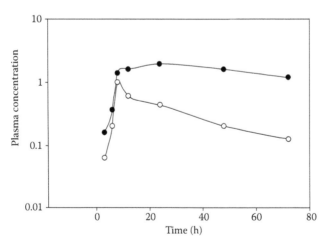

FIGURE 26.7 Concentration of α-tocopherol in the plasma in normal human subjects after administration of an oral dose containing 50 mg each of (●) *RRR*- and (○) *SRR*-α-tocopherol. Blood samples were obtained at the indicated time intervals. Naturally occurring *RRR*-α-tocopherol can bind efficiently to ATTP and thus can be re-secreted into circulation. A synthetic isomer *SRR*-α-tocopherol, which does not bind efficiently to ATTP, shows a much more pronounced rate of clearance from the blood. (Adapted from Traber, M.G., Vitamin E bioavailability, In: *The Encyclopedia of Vitamin E*, Preedy, V.R. and Watson R.R. (eds.), CABI Publishers, Oxford, U.K., 2007.).

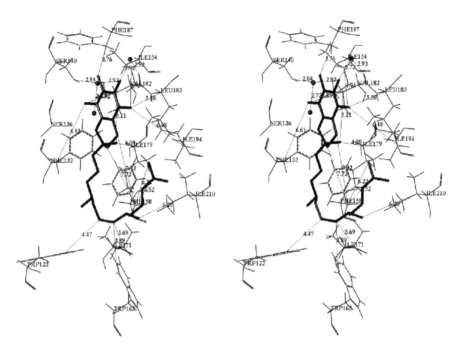

FIGURE 26.8 Stereo view of the ligand-binding pocket of ATTP in a complex with RRR-α-tocopherol. α-Tocopherol is represented as a capped-stick model (darker). (Adapted from Min, K.C. et al., *Proc. Natl. Acad. Sci. USA*, 100, 14713, 2003.) The dark circles represent water molecules in the binding cavity. The van der Waals interactions, between methyl groups of α-tocopherol and the ligand binding pocket, important for higher binding preference of these compounds over the other vitamin E components, are represented by faint lines.

accommodates α-tocopherol, causing this compound to fold in a unique way as it fits into the binding pocket of the transporter protein. ATTP transfers α-tocopherol from the hepatic cells into plasma (Arita et al., 1995); this protein is more specific for α-tocopherol, and no equivalent protein is known for the transfer of other tocopherols and tocotrienols. These other vitamers are metabolized and/or excreted due to their low affinity for ATTP. Thus, differential affinities of the various forms of vitamin E for the transport protein and their subsequent transfer into systemic circulation determine their bioavailability. The structural features influencing substrate binding to ATTP have been identified (Traber and Arai, 1999). The position and the number of the methyl groups on the chromane ring (especially the presence of a 5-methyl group, the presence of the phenolic hydroxyl group, the side chain structure, and the orientation of the binding pocket are critical structural elements that determine binding affinity for ATTP. The fully methylated *RRR* isomer of tocopherol has the highest binding affinity for ATTP compared to other vitamers. Other analogues of vitamin E such as α-tocotrienol, γ-tocopherol, and *SRR*-α-tocopherol have lower affinity for this protein.

Hosomi et al. (1997) have reported relative affinities of vitamin E analogs with ATTP. Experimental values were in the order: α-tocopherol (100%), β-tocopherol (38%), γ-tocopherol (9%), δ-tocopherol (1.6%), α-tocotrienol (12%), α-tocopherol acetate (1.7%), and α-tocopherol quinone (1.5%).

Based on the van der Waals interactions and hydrogen-bonding pattern between ATTP and α-tocopherol, the differential binding affinity of other vitamin E analogues can be explained. The 5′-methyl group of α-tocopherol has interactions with the residues I154, L183, and I194, and the 7′-methyl group interacts with the residues S140 and F187. These interactions explain the lower binding affinity of γ- and δ-tocopherol, which lacks a 5′-methyl group, and β- and δ-tocopherol, in which the 7′-methyl group is absent. The lower binding affinity of *SRR*-α-tocopherol for ATTP can be explained by the difference in the orientation of the binding pocket near residues I179 and

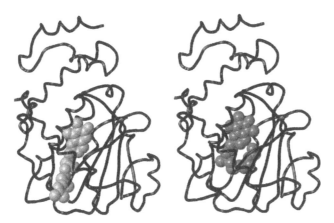

FIGURE 26.9 When α-tocopherol (right) binds to ATTP the protein encloses the molecule; on the other hand γ-tocotrienol (left) cannot adopt a conformation that allows efficient binding. Based on the x-ray crystal structure of AT bound to ATTP. (From Min, K.C. et al., *Proc. Natl. Acad. Sci. USA*, 100, 14713, 2003.)

V182 (Figure 26.8). Furthermore, modification of the phenolic OH group, as in α-tocopherol acetate and α-tocopherol quinone, also lowers the affinity for ATTP by disrupting H-bonding of the phenol hydroxyl group with a water molecule in the ligand pocket. The presence of unsaturation in the side chain of the tocotrienols accounts for their lower affinity for ATTP, which makes it impossible for such compounds to undergo the unique folding of the molecule inside the ligand-binding pocket of ATTP.

The very specific binding requirements of ATTP make α-tocopherol bind more efficiently than, for example, γ-tocotrienol. A prominent reason for this selectivity is that the tail of the tocopherol molecules is much more flexible than the tail of the tocotrienol molecules, allowing the tocopherol molecules to bend and adopt a conformation that can be enclosed into the binding pocket of the protein; whereas the conformationally restricted tocotrienol tail, because of the double bonds in the chain, cannot bend to adopt the appropriate conformation for binding to transporter protein (Figure 26.9).

Thus, from the earlier observations it is clear that ATTP could be used as a target for the development of novel tocol analogues with enhanced bioavailability, in what can be classified a transport-targeted approach. A compound that possesses ATTP affinity similar to that of α-tocopherol should have a comparable residence time in the blood, with a corresponding increase in bodily exposure to the compound.

To test this approach, we designed a series of novel compounds with enhanced conformational flexibility, which we have termed the "tocoflexols" (Compadre et al., 2011). In the tocoflexols, a mono- or dienyl chain is substituted for the trienyl chain of the farnesyl tail of the corresponding tocotrienol. Depending on the position and the number of the double bonds in the tail, there are 10 possible groups of tocoflexols. Taking into consideration the number of possible variations in the head group, there are potentially thousands of different combinations of compounds. Thus, to optimize resources and increase the chance of success, we subjected all the possible candidates to a rigorous computer-based virtual screening to determine those compounds with the highest potential for high affinity binding with ATTP (Figure 26.10).

The tocoflexols should also exhibit enhanced transport from the liver and improved distribution via the systemic circulation throughout the body to the various sites of action. By overcoming the rate-limiting step of transport from the liver, tocoflexols should have superior bioavailability with respect to the existing tocotrienols.

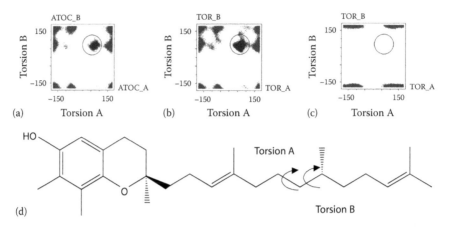

(a)   Torsion A   (b)   Torsion A   (c)   Torsion A

(d)

FIGURE 26.10 Example of the molecular dynamic-based screening of the potential of tocol deriva-tives for enhanced binding to ATTP. This figure shows the comparative molecular dynamics simulations analysis of the potential of the following molecules to bind to ATTP: (a) γ-tocoflexol (b) α-tocopherol, (c) γ-tocotrienol. The analysis shows that only γ-tocoflexol and α-tocopherol have the capability to adopt conformations that are capable of binding with high affinity to ATTP. In the molecules with favor-able conformations for binding, both torsion angles A and B must be around 60° (d). As shown in (c), γ-tocotrienol did not show any conformations in the favorable region. The circle shows the areas in which there should be conformations suitable for binding to ATTP. Molecular dynamics simulations were performed using SYBYL 8.1 (Tripos, Saint Louis, MO), *in vacuo* with a dielectric constant of 4 using an NVT ensemble. For the analysis 20 ns production simulation was conducted. A total of 100,000 conformations for each molecule were saved and the structural, dynamic, and energetic properties were derived from the analyses of these snapshots. The analysis presented in this figure was derived from these conformational populations.

26.5   CONCLUSIONS

Although the components of vitamin E are often considered as a family, the reality is that these compounds are substantially different in chemical, pharmacological, and pharmacokinetic properties, and individual components have different propensities with respect to these roles. Tocotrienols have been shown to have a remarkable profile of biological activities; however, in many cases their poor bioavailability limits their usefulness. In this context it was concluded that well-planned structural modification of tocotrienols might render molecules not only potent but also bioavailable. Although both the tocotrienols and the tocopherols are absorbed in the GI tract, they have very substantial differences in their bioavailability, due to differences in their elimina-tion half-lives. To this date only a limited number of efforts have been made to improve the bio-availability of tocotrienols by structural modification. In this review we advance the notion that the use of a transport-targeted approach would likely produce tocol analogues with an extended half-life. A set of such compounds, the tocoflexols, have been developed utilizing a state-of-the-art computer-aided molecular dynamics approach that permits the *in silico* selection of compounds with improved binding to ATTP. Thus, it is hoped that this novel approach may provide oppor-tunities for the development of structurally modified tocotrienols with improved bioavailability.

ACKNOWLEDGMENTS

Financial support: Defense Threat Reduction Agency grants number H.10027_07_AR_R to KSK and HDTRA1-07-0028 to Martin Hauer-Jensen, the National Center for Research Resources, award 1UL1RR029884, and the University of Arkansas for Medical Sciences College of Pharmacy Research Fund. The University of Arkansas holds patents on the tocoflexols. A potential royalty stream to AS, PJB, KSK, MH-J, and CMC may occur consistent with the University of Arkansas Policy.

REFERENCES

Abuasal, B., Sylvester, P. W., and Kaddoumi, A. 2010. Intestinal absorption of γ-tocotrienol is mediated by Niemann-Pick C1-like 1: In situ rat intestinal perfusion studies. *Drug Metabolism and Disposition* 38, 939–945.

Agarwal, B. B., Sundaram, C., Prasad, S., and Kannappan, R. 2010. Tocotrienols, the vitamin E of the 21st century: Its potential against cancer and other chronic diseases. *Biochemical Pharmacology* 80(11), 1613–1631.

Akaho, N., Takata, J., Fukushima, T., Matsunaga, K., Hattori, A., Hidaka, R., Fukui, K. et al. 2007. Preparation and in vivo evaluation of a water-soluble prodrug for 2R-gamma-tocotrienol and as a two step prodrug for 2,7,8-trimethyl-2S-(beta-carboxyethyl)-6-hydroxychroman (S-gamma-CEHC) in rat. *Drug Metabolism and Disposition* 35, 1502–1510.

Arita, M., Sato, Y., Miyata, A., Tanabe, T., Takahashi, E., Kayden, H. J., Arai, H., and Inoue, K. 1995. Human alpha-tocopherol transfer protein: cDNA cloning, expression and chromosomal localization. *Biochemical Journal* 306, 437–443.

Behery, F. A., Elnagar, A. Y., Akl, M. R., Wali, V. B., Abuasal, B., Kaddoumi, A., Sylvester, P. W., and El Sayed, K. A. 2010. Redox-silent tocotrienol esters as breast cancer proliferation and migration inhibitors. *Bioorganic and Medicinal Chemistry* 18(22), 8066–8075.

Berbee, M., Fu, Q., Boerma, M., Wang, J., Kumar, K. S., and Hauer-Jensen, M. 2009. Gamma-tocotrienol ameliorates intestinal radiation injury and reduces vascular oxidative stress after total body irradiation by an HMG-CoA reductase-dependent mechanism. *Radiation Research* 171(5), 596–605.

Compadre, C. M., Breen P. J., Hauer-Jensen, M., Breen, P. J., Varughese, K. I., and Kumar, S. 2011. Tocopherol derivatives and methods of use. wo 2011/153353A1, (accessed on 8 December, 2011).

Cooper, A. D. 1997. Hepatic uptake of chylomicron remnants. *Journal of Lipid Research* 38, 2173–2192.

Drotleff, A. M. and Ternes, W. 1999. Cis/trans isomers of tocotrienols occurrence and bioavailability. *European Food Research and Technology* 210, 1–8.

Ghosh, S. P., Kulkarni, S., Hieber, K., Toles, R., Romanyukha, L., Kao, T-C., Hauer-Jensen, M., and Kumar, K. S. 2009. Gamma-tocotrienol, a tocol antioxidant as a potent radioprotector. *International Journal of Radiation Biology* 85, 598–606.

Hoppe, P.P. and Krennrich, G. 2000. Bioavailability and potency of natural-source and *all-racemic* α-tocopherol in the human. *European Journal of Nutrition* 39, 183–193.

Hosomi, A., Arita, M., Sato, Y., Kiyose, C., Ueda, T., Igarashi, O., Arai, H., and Inoue, K. 1997. Affinity for alpha-tocopherol transfer protein as a determinant of the biological activities of vitamin E analogs. *FEBS Letters* 409,105–108.

Kamal-Eldin, A. and Appelqvist, L. A. 1996. The chemistry and antioxidant properties of tocopherols and tocotrienols. *Lipids* 31(7), 671–701.

Kulkarni, S., Ghosh, S. P., Satyamitra, M., Mog, S., Hieber, K., Romanyukha, L., Gambles, K. et al. 2010. Gamma-tocotrienol protects hematopoietic stem and progenitor cells in mice after total-body irradiation. *Radiation Research* 173, 738–747.

Kumar, K. S., Ghosh, S., and Hauer-Jensen, M. 2009. Gamma-tocotrienol: Potential as a countermeasure against radiological threat, In: *Tocotrienols: Vitamin E Beyond Tocopherols,* Watson R. R. and Preedy V. R. (eds.), CRC Press, Boca Raton, FL, pp. 379–398.

Leonard, S. W., Paterson, E., Atkinson, J. K., Ramakrishnan, R., Cross, C. E., and Traber, M. G. 2005. Studies in humans using deuterium-labeled α- and γ-tocopherol demonstrate faster plasma γ-tocopherol disappearance and greater γ-metabolite production. *Free Radical Biology and Medicine,* 38, 857–866.

Malafa, M. P., Fokum, F. D., and Andoh, J. 2006. Vitamin E succinate suppresses prostate tumor growth by inducing apoptosis. *International Journal of Cancer* 118, 2441–2447.

Meier, R., Tomizaki, T., Schulze-Briese, C., Baumann, U., and Stocker, A. 2003. The molecular basis of vitamin E retention: Structure of human a-tocopherol transfer protein. *Journal of Molecular Biology* 331, 725–734.

Min, K. C., Kovall, R. A., and Hendrickson, W. A. 2003. Crystal structure of human alpha-tocopherol transfer protein bound to its ligand: Implications for ataxia with vitamin E deficiency. *Proceedings of National Academic Science* 100, 14713–14718.

Neuzil, J., Kågedal, K., Andera, L., Weber, C., and Brunk, U. T. 2002. Vitamin E analogs: A new class of multiple action agents with anti-neoplastic and anti-atherogenic activity. *Apoptosis* 7(2), 179–187.

Ni, J., Mai, T., Pang, S-T., Haque, I., Huang, K., DiMagio, M. A., Xie, S. et al. 2009. In vitro and in vivo anticancer effects of the novel vitamin E ether analogue *RRR*-alpha-tocopheryloxybutyl sulfonic acid in prostate cancer. *Clinical Cancer Research* 15(3), 898–906.

Shrader, W. D., Amagata, A., Barnes, A., Enns, G. E., Hinman, A., Jankowski, O., Kheifets, V. et al. 2011. α-tocotrienol quinone modulates oxidative stress response and the biochemistry of aging. *Bioorganic and Medicinal Chemistry Letters* 21(12), 3693–3698.

Sylvester, P. W., Kaddoumi, A., Nazzal, S., and El Sayed, K. A. 2010. The value of tocotrienols in the prevention and treatment of cancer. *Journal of the American College of Nutrition* 29(3), 324S–333S.

Takata, J., Hidaka, R., Yamasaki, A., Hattori, A., Fukushima, T., Tanabe, M., Matsunaga, K., Karube, Y., and Imai, K. 2002. Novel d-gamma-tocopherol derivative as a prodrug for d-gamma-tocopherol and a two-step prodrug for S-gamma-CEHC. *Journal of Lipid Research* 43(12), 2196–2204.

Tan, B. 2005. Appropriate spectrum vitamin E and new perspectives on desmethyl tocopherols and tocotrienols. *Journal of the American Nutraceutical Association* 8(1), 35–42.

Traber, M. G. 2007. Vitamin E bioavailability In: *The Encyclopedia of Vitamin E*, Preedy, V. R. and Watson R. R. (eds.), CABI Publishers, Oxford, U.K., pp. 221–230.

Traber, M. G. and Arai, H. 1999. Molecular mechanisms of vitamin E transport. *Annual Review of Nutrition* 19, 343–355.

Traber, M. G., Burton, G. W., Ingold, K. U., and Kayden, H. J. 1990. RRR- and *SRR*-α-tocopherols are secreted without discrimination in human chylomicrons, but *RRR*- α-tocopherol is preferentially secreted in very low density lipoproteins. *Journal of Lipid Research* 31, 675–685.

Traber, M. G., Ramakrishnan, R., and Kayden, H. J. 1994. Human plasma vitamin E kinetics demonstrate rapid recycling of plasma RRR-α-tocopherol. *Proceedings of the National Academic Science USA* 91, 10005–10008.

Yap, S. P., Yuen, K. H., and Lim, A. B. 2003. Influence of route of administration on the absorption and disposition of alpha-, gamma- and delta-tocotrienols in rats. *Journal of Pharmacy and Pharmacology* 55(1), 53–58.

Yap, S. P., Yuen, K. H., and Wong, J. W. 2001. Pharmacokinetics and bioavailability of α-, γ-, and δ-tocotrienols under different food status. *Journal of Pharmacy and Pharmacology* 53(1), 67–71.

Yin, Y., Ni, J., Chen, M., DiMaggio, M. A., Guo, Y., and Yeh, S. 2007. The therapeutic and preventive effect of *RRR*-alpha-vitamin E succinate on prostate cancer via induction of insulin-like growth factor binding protein-3. *Clinical Cancer Research* 13(7), 2271–2280.

Yuen, K. H., Ng, B. H., and Wong, J. W. 2009. Absorption and disposition of tocotrienols. In: *Tocotrienols: Vitamin E Beyond Tocopherols*, Watson R. R. and Preedy V. R. (eds.), CRC Press, Boca Raton, FL, pp. 297–308.

Index

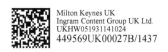

Milton Keynes UK
Ingram Content Group UK Ltd.
UKHW051931141024
449569UK00027B/1437

9 781138 199729